The Back Pain Revolution

To Sandra, with love
who shared it all
and made it all worthwhile.

About the author

Professor Gordon Waddell is a Scot born and bred. He has spent
most of his professional life in orthopedic surgery but as several
have commented 'I have never met an orthopedic surgeon like him!'
For 17 years he ran a Problem Back Clinic where he struggled with
many of the difficult clinical issues of back pain management. His
research has ranged through clinical assessment and health care
delivery, medico-legal issues and social policy. He received the first
Volvo Award on back pain research for his description of the 'Waddell
signs' in back pain and was the first person to receive a second
Volvo award for his biopsychosocial model of low back disability.
Although always a full time clinician, in 1992 he was appointed an
Honorary Professor in Orthopedic Surgery at the University of
Glasgow in recognition of his academic achievements. He is also
Visiting Professor at the Department of Medicine (Rheumatology),
University of Manchester and Associate Professor of Clinical
Research at the British School of Osteopathy.

For Churchill Livingstone

Editorial Director: Mary Law
Design Direction: Judith Wright

The Back Pain Revolution

Gordon Waddell DSc MD FRCS
Orthopedic Surgeon, Glasgow

Forewords by

Alf L. Nachemson MD PhD HonFRCSEng&Ed Hon MAA OS
Hon FBOA MHonSFCOT
Professor emeritus, Göteborg University, Sweden
Research Professor, Georgetown University, Washington DC, USA

Reed B. Phillips DC PhD
President, Los Angeles College of Chiropractic, USA

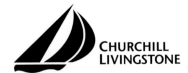
CHURCHILL
LIVINGSTONE

EDINBURGH LONDON NEW YORK PHILADELPHIA SYDNEY TORONTO 1998

CHURCHILL LIVINGSTONE
An imprint of Harcourt Publishers Limited

© Churchill Livingstone, an imprint of Harcourt Brace and
Company Limited 1998
© Harcourt Publishers Limited 1999

except:
Appendices 17A, D, E, 18A and B which are in the public
domain, and Appendix 17B which is under Crown copyright
and is reproduced with kind permission of the Controller,
HMSO.

⬡ is a registered trademark of Harcourt Publishers Limited

First published 1998
Reprinted 1999

ISBN 0 443 060398

British Library Cataloguing in Publication Data
A catalogue record for this book is available from the
British Library.

Library of Congress Cataloging in Publication Data
A catalog record for this book is available from the Library
of Congress.

Note
Medical knowledge is constantly changing. As new
information becomes available, changes in treatment,
procedures, equipment and the use of drugs become
necessary. The author and the publishers have, as far as
it is possible, taken care to ensure that the information
given in this text is accurate and up-to-date. However,
readers are strongly advised to confirm that the information,
especially with regard to drug usage, complies with latest
legislation and standards of practice.

The
publisher's
policy is to use
**paper manufactured
from sustainable forests**

Printed in the United Kingdom

Contents

Additional contributors

Chris J Main PhD FBPsS
Clinical Psychologist
Salford

David B Allan MB ChB FRCS
Orthopedic Surgeon
Glasgow

Clinical Guidelines and patient information material by:

The Agency for Health Care Policy and Research, US

The Clinical Standards Advisory Group, UK

The Royal College of General Practitioners, UK

The National Advisory Committee on Health and Disability and The Accident Rehabilitation and Compensation Insurance Corporation, New Zealand, including the *Guide to Assessing Psychosocial Yellow Flags*, by:

Nick Kendall, clinical psychologist, Christchurch, New Zealand
Steven Linton, clinical psychologist, Orebro, Sweden
Chris Main, clinical psychologist, Salford, England

The Back Book by:
Martin Roland, general practitioner, Manchester
Gordon Waddell, orthopedic surgeon, Glasgow
Jennifer Klaber Moffett, physiotherapist, York
Kim Burton, osteopath, Huddersfield
Chris Main, clinical psychologist, Salford
Ted Cantrell, rehabilitation physician, Southampton

Foreword

We are seeing a revolution growing out of the old orthopedic concept of the 'dynasty of the disc' into a more integrated biopsychosocial model of back pain. Gordon Waddell has been in the forefront of this revolutionary thinking during the last 20 years and this book now crowns his many years of scientific endeavours into this novel way of looking at the problem.

Chronic axial pain has become a major socio-economic burden. It is now a major problem which affects the availability of health care resources in all industrialized nations, as well as being a very difficult problem for the patients and for the health care providers.

The Back Pain Revolution with its comprehensive view on back pain is mainly aimed at the care providers, but in my view should also be mandatory reading for the policy makers in many countries. Psychologic and social factors can have significant effects on the onset of some symptoms, influence their ultimate course and definitely affect treatment results.

Throughout the 90s several new monographs on spinal disorders have been published each year – far more than are justified by the relatively scarce new scientific findings produced in the field. Most of these books, containing authoritative but single-minded 'how to' chapters by individual authors, have steered modern medicine related to back pain management in the entirely wrong direction. Although most of these authors (well known and skilful surgeons, chiropractors, ergonomists, physical therapists and others) pay lip service to the broader

approach including psychosociology, for most of the time they unfortunately fanfare as the solution their own 'Holy Grail' or special treatment. New evidence from the Cochrane reviews and other similar sources based on strict research have clearly shown how deficient the knowledge of these 'experts' really is. In the meantime evidence has been forthcoming that 'strengthening' patients by addressing their psychosocial needs can be effective in managing their symptoms. By helping patients to manage not just their disease but also to increase their coping skills and self control our treatment outcomes can be significantly improved in a cost effective manner. Our improved under-standing of these now proven facts about back pain management can be largely credited to Gordon Waddell.

The Back Pain Revolution is based on the ultimate new science of evidence-based medicine. It will influence how we treat painful but currently non-specific pain syndromes, including the common back pain, which have no apparent anatomic or pathologic cause. It will encourage and enable us to treat those suffering from these conditions with empathy and encouragement, not with needles and knives.

It is to be hoped that in the next millennium there will be another revolution in the treatment of back pain. New insights, already discernible, into psycho-neuro-endocrino-immunology, pain physiology and genetics of the ageing human frame may finally discover the real cause of back pain. Even then, clinicians will always have to treat patients, and should heed the wisdom of Gordon Waddell. If we don't, there will be serious consequences for our patients and for our industrialized societies. Progress in managing the back pain problem will be hampered by shifting scarce resources into inappropriate areas and money will be wasted on disability payments instead of being used to fund ground-breaking but expensive research to elucidate the many different causes of back pain.

1998   Alf L. Nachemson

A book is a continuous arrangement of words, tables and figures ordered in a fashion to enhance understanding, communicate knowledge, arouse emotion and change behavior. This can be an evolutionary achievement *à la* Michener or revolutionary *à la* Waddell.

A back is a continuous arrangement of vertebrae, muscles, tendons, ligaments, vessels of various sorts and nerves all encased by a smooth-textured outer covering of skin. The back is designed to support the human frame, protect the nervous system, provide attachments for muscles, give rise to movement and contribute to the expression of the individual. These functions of the back have been ascribed to evolution *à la* Darwin or creation as in the Bible.

An evolutionist might suggest that the back, a marvel in its own right, is incomplete in the evolutionary transition from a quadrupedal form of transportation to a bipedal form. Thus the explanation of back pain. The back has not yet adapted to the upright posture with its incumbent inequities of weight distribution, the irregularities of force translation resulting from free-form movement and the debilitating effects of passing through the process of ageing.

A creationist might suggest that the back has been created in the image of a perfect model. The back pain problem is the result of our failure to follow the traditional wisdom of a life-style that promotes health and well-being. We live in a world whose tide ebbs and flows largely on the rocky shores of physical experience while the emotional, social and spiritual are relegated to quiet, untraveled inlets and lagoons often thought too shallow to be of significance. But back pain is more than a physical experience. The apparent smooth surface of the emotional, social and spiritual lagoons may indeed be directly related to the cause of back pain and in a true chiastic fashion the emotional, social and spiritual calmness can be equally disturbed by genuine physical back pain.

But why a revolution? The author speaks not of guns or warfare. The revolution is truly a Kuhnian paradigm shift. Whether our backs are evolving to a higher order of structure and function or our emotional, social and spiritual well-being is degenerating to a lower order of civilisation matters not. The revolution is not in what our backs are doing to us but in what we are doing to the back!

Humans have lived with their backs for eons of time. It has been in roughly the last 100 years that we have taken it upon ourselves to take more notice of our backs. We have stretched our backs. We have twisted and curled our backs. We have adjusted our backs. We have placed great weights upon our backs and walked long distances. We have cooked our backs. We have refrigerated our backs. We have stimulated our backs with electric currents of various sorts, and with ultrasound waves, infrared waves, magnetic waves and X-rays. We have rubbed our backs with liniments, spirits, gels, perfumes and poultices. When all else fails, nay often before anything else is even tried, we stick our backs with needles, electrodes, catheters and scalpels, and quickly justify the need to cut it open, cut it out, fuse it, screw it, and wire it all in the name of improving function and reducing pain. It is little wonder that our backs are revolting–wouldn't yours? And why not pour a little salt into the wound by admitting that we never knew why the back hurt to begin with.

The application of our wisdom to the care of the back is only over-shadowed by the wisdom of our economic policies. The prize has gone to the highest bidder. If back pain could be treated for \$10 or \$10 000 and the patient had to pay, he or she would obviously opt for the lesser cost. Spurning the obvious wisdom of the patient, the medicalized, third-party reimbursement system selects the greater cost, the most invasive alternative.

You may ask 'But which is the more effective?'. Well, that depends on what is wrong with your back. But since we often do not know what causes back pain, we are inclined to trust only in the most highly trained to make the decision for us. It is of little consequence that the most highly trained is also the most expensive care-giver. If the only tool in your possession is a hammer, you will treat every challenge as if it is a nail. Does the same hold true if you replace the hammer with a scalpel?

If not knowing what is causing the back to hurt (implying that we really do not know what to do to stop the pain) is not enough to make John Doe Patient rebel against his costly care, try this one on for comfort. What will John say when he learns that there is not only an absence of consensus on what to do for his hurting back, but there is geographical variation in treatment in excess of seven-fold and professional variation near ten-fold?

It is time for a revolution. It is time for a shift in our paradigm. It is time to apply rational thinking rather than rationing managed care. It is time to think positively about the value of our backs rather than the value of back care. Back pain has become a major problem because there are more people making a living off this problem than dying from it.

I congratulate Dr Waddell and all who have assisted him in this paradigm shifting epic. I share the hope of the author that this text will become the 'Bible of the Back Pain Revolution'.

1998   Reed B. Phillips

Acknowledgements

I claim this book my own, and I did write it, but such as this could never be a solo effort.

Most of all, I am indebted to my patients with back pain who presented their needs and posed the questions. I am acutely aware that I owe them much more than my inadequate efforts for them could ever repay. I only hope this will help future health professionals to provide a better service for future patients.

John McCulloch and the late Ian Macnab introduced me to back pain, and I have never escaped their spell. Chris Main shared the first faltering steps and has remained my trusty companion on this journey. My Fellows Emyr Morris, Mike Di Paolo, David Finlayson, Martin Bircher, Douglas Somerville, Mary Newton and Iain Henderson provided much needed support at various stages along the way.

I have tried to acknowledge the source of ideas and material as far as possible. I am particularly grateful to The Agency for Health Care Policy and Research in the US, The Clinical Standards Advisory Group, The Royal College of General Practitioners, and The Stationery Office in the UK, The National Advisory Committee on Health and Disability and The Accident Rehabilitation and Compensation Insurance Corporation in New Zealand, for permission to reproduce clinical guidelines and patient information material. Inevitably, I have gathered ideas from many papers and meetings over the years and adopted them as my own. I apologize if I have forgotten some of the original sources, and failed to acknowledge an idea. I can only say that imitation is the most sincere form of flattery.

Many friends and colleagues around the world have read draft chapters in their fields of expertise, and offered comments and suggestions: Alan Breen, Kim Burton, Peter Croft, Rick Deyo, Scott Haldeman, Craig Liebenson, Chris Main, Carol McGivern, Roger Nelson, Reed Phillips, Malcolm Pope, Clive Standen and Maurits van Tulder. I thank them all for their useful advice and accept full responsibility where I chose to ignore it. I am deeply grateful to the Medical Illustration Department, West Glasgow Hospitals University NHS Trust, who prepared most of the illustrations.

Last, and most of all, my deepest thanks go to my family. My wife Sandra spent many hours typing and pandering to my obsession. She and my three daughters, Carol, Joyce and Hazel, sacrificed much more family life than they should. Misty, my border collie, never could understand why I was not ready for her walk. I promise it will all change now, but they look at me with an air of skepticism. Thank you all, and I hope the end result makes it worthwhile.

1

The problem

Back pain is a 20th century medical disaster. We can split the atom and send men to the moon and we now have cures which past generations would literally have thought were miracles. We have vaccines to prevent polio and drugs to cure tuberculosis. We have high-tech investigations that lay bare the anatomy and pathology of the spine. We can perform bigger and better operations. Yet we have no answer for simple backache. Modern medicine has been very successful in treating many serious spinal diseases, but this traditional medical approach has failed with back pain. For all our efforts and skill, for all our resources, low back disability is getting steadily worse (Fig. 1.1). Trends of rising work loss, early retirement and state benefits all expose our failure to solve the problem. In Western society, simple back strains now disable many more people than all the serious spinal diseases put together.

There are many paradoxes about back pain. Over the past few decades we have learned much about back pain, about pain itself and about how people react to, and are affected by, pain. We should by now be able to manage back pain better, even if we still cannot offer a cure. Chronic back pain and disability should be reducing, but instead the opposite is true. Why? Why are we not delivering better and more effective health care for back pain? There are, I believe, many reasons for this. We do not seem to put our better understanding of pain into clinical practice. We are still very bad at dealing with disability. Too often, we simply

1

U.K. Sickness and Invalidity Benefit for Back Pain

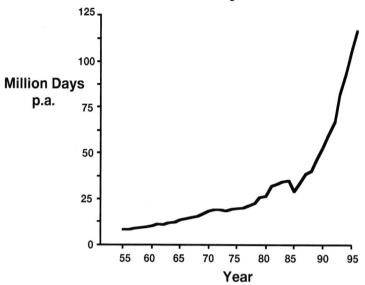

Figure 1.1 The rising trend of low back disability from 1953–54 to 1994–95. (Based on annual statistics from the UK Department of Social Security.)

ignore disability and assume that it will go away if we treat the pain. There has also been a shift in social attitudes and support. It is now socially acceptable to receive state benefits and compensation for long-term disability due to simple backache. Thus, we can already see that health care is only a part of a bigger story.

Much of this applies to all types of chronic pain. So why is back pain, in particular, such a problem? What is different about it? Part of the trouble is that back pain is only a symptom, not a disease. Most of us get back pain at some time of our lives, but most of the time we deal with it ourselves and do not regard it as a medical problem. However, back pain can also be the presenting symptom of serious spinal disease. The symptom of pain in the back is the common link between the everyday bodily symptom, serious disease and chronic disability. We get into trouble when we confuse them. It is the health care system and health care workers who label simple backache as a serious spinal disease. We do not really understand the cause of most back pain and there is often very little relation between any physical pathology and the associated pain and disability. We often

regard back pain as an injury, but most episodes occur spontaneously with normal everyday activities. Our high-tech investigations for spinal diseases tell us very little about simple backache.

So back pain is a problem. It is a problem to patients, to health professionals and to society. It is a problem to patients because they cannot get clear advice on its cause, how to deal with it, and its likely outcome. It is a problem to doctors and therapists because they cannot diagnose any definite disease or offer any real cure, so they are unsure and uncomfortable when dealing with back pain. To society, back pain is now one of the most common and fastest growing reasons for work loss, health care use and sickness benefits, yet medicine does not offer any good explanation as to why this might be.

Patients, therapists and doctors are becoming increasingly aware of the limitations of traditional medical treatment for back pain. The scientific evidence shows that most of the treatments in routine use for back pain are ineffective. Indeed, many of the things we do may actually be worse than no treatment at all. The sheer variety of treatments betrays our lack of knowledge. The variation in clinical practice suggests that many patients receive care that is less than ideal. Much of the health care offered for back pain is inappropriate. Too often, the choice of treatment reflects the skills of the professional rather than the needs of the patient. To put it simply, what treatment you receive will depend more on who you go to see than on what is wrong with your back. Many patients in the United States and in Britain are now so dissatisfied with orthodox medical treatment for back pain that they seek alternative care.

There is much agreement on the need for change. There is growing demand from patients and family doctors for improved health care services for patients with back pain. Policy makers and those who pay for health care and state benefits are in a position to enforce this demand. The health care professions, however, are conservative. We are all slow to change what we have been trained to do and to change our professional practice. Up until now, there has also been lack of a clear direction for change. There are still many gaps in our knowledge, but there is now a growing body of scientific evidence from which we can begin to draw some principles for better treatment. There is now the beginning of a consensus, and change is beginning to happen. There is still a long way to go, and a great deal of inertia and resistance to overcome. But there is now the first faint dawn of a revolution in the care of back pain.

When I completed my training as an orthopedic surgeon, I was still unhappy about treating spinal disorders, so I went to Toronto and worked for a year with Dr John McCulloch and Dr Ian Macnab. I went to learn about spinal surgery, and I had to review 103 Workmen's Compensation patients who had had repeat back operations (Waddell et al 1979). To a surgeon at the threshold of my career, the results were frightening. A first operation made 70–80% of patients better, but 15% of patients were worse after surgery and sooner or later underwent another operation. The results of repeat surgery were worse. By the third operation there was only a 25% chance of a good result and an equal chance that the patient's condition would deteriorate. It was also obvious

that the final outcome of surgery was only partly dependent on physical factors. Sixty-five per cent of these patients had psychologic problems by the time I saw them. That year changed my thinking. Ian Macnab (one of the North American kings of spinal fusion!) taught me the importance of 'knowing as much about the patient who has the back pain as about the back pain the patient has'. I will always be indebted to John McCulloch for introducing me to the non-organic signs (Waddell et al 1980). Neville Doxey taught me, to my surprise, that doctors can learn something from clinical psychologists. I went to Toronto to learn about spinal surgery and I came back a spinal surgeon, but ever since I have been intrigued by back pain, how it affects people and how they react to it. I learned that back pain is not simply a mechanical problem. Low back disability and how people react to pain and to treatment depend just as much on psychologic and social factors as on the underlying physical problem.

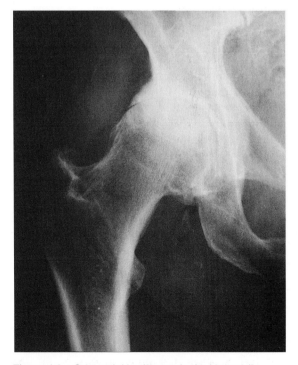

Figure 1.2 Osteoarthritic changes in the hip usually correspond reasonably well with clinical pain and disability.

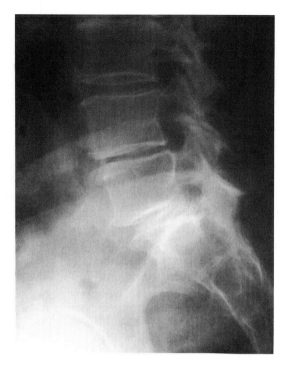

Figure 1.3 Degenerative changes in the lumbar spine bear very little relationship to clinical symptoms.

Compare a patient with back pain with one who has a hip replacement for osteoarthritis (Figs. 1.2 and 1.3) (Gray et al 1984). In back pain we often cannot find the cause or even the exact source of the pain. Patients do not understand what is wrong and cannot get clear answers to their questions. If back pain becomes chronic, patients soon realize that we do not know what is wrong. In contrast, with arthritis the problem is clear to both patient and surgeon and both can see it on X-ray. Treatment of arthritis is logical. Complications and failures do occur, but they are relatively uncommon and the reason for failure is usually obvious. Treatment for back pain is empiric and has a high failure rate. Perhaps understandably, many patients are reluctant to accept, and many doctors or therapists to admit, the limitations of treatment for back pain. So when treatment for back pain fails, the professional may look for psychologic reasons or other excuses and the patient is likely to become defensive. Both patient and professional may become angry and hostile. It should come as no surprise that some patients develop psychologic problems with their pain.

When I came back to Glasgow, I started working with Chris Main, a clinical psychologist. Soon after we started, Chris confronted me. If we were going to work together, I would need to improve my medical assessment and data to match the standard of his psychologic data. I nearly punched him! He did not have any medical qualification and appeared to me to have limited clinical experience, and yet he was trying to tell me how to do my job. The trouble was that he was right, of course. Most medical data and clinical research are not very scientific, and it was painful but instructive to apply Chris's scientific rigor to my clinical research. I learned a lot and that was the start of the closest and most productive research collaboration of my professional life.

Another paradox is that the problem of back pain is greatest in Western 'civilization'. In 1985, I visited Oman to advise on orthopedic services for back pain (Fig. 1.4). Oman is a rapidly developing Arab state. Within the previous 10 years, new oil wealth and political change had propelled Oman from a medieval state into the 20th century. In that short period, Omani health care had become as good as much of the health care in North America and Europe.

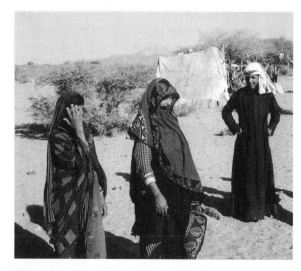

Figure 1.4 Back pain is just as common in Oman, but causes very little disability.

By 1985, health care in Oman was just beginning to reach out to the more rural areas. We held one orthopedic clinic in a desert town for children with polio, contracted before vaccination had started a few years earlier. In 1 day we saw nearly 40 severely crippled children, all under the age of 10. They had never seen a physician nor had any medical treatment. That was one of the most moving experiences of my professional life. We could only offer palliative care with splints and reconstructive surgery, but despite that, the children and their parents were grateful and uncomplaining. They accepted their fate as the will of God: *insh'allah*. Yet we needed locks and guards on the clinic doors to keep out the noisy and demanding adults with back pain. (Incidentally, all the adults who came were men, a reflection of Omani society.) Otherwise, we would never have been able to see the children with polio.

Patients with back pain flood the new orthopedic clinics in Oman. Back pain is almost universal and patients with back pain seem to crawl out from under the very stones of the desert. Or, to be more accurate, they walk out. Because the striking thing is that, although back pain is so common, it causes very little disability. People in Oman may be crippled by polio, spinal tuberculosis or spinal fractures, but no one goes to bed, no one stops their daily life and no one becomes permanently disabled by simple backache. Even the nurses do not stay off work with back pain. Two matrons in hospitals 400 miles apart each said that in 10 years they had never had a nurse off work with back pain. More careful surveys confirm this. Anderson (1984) studied a peasant community in Nepal and 'found a virtual epidemic of spinal pain': 44% of adults had back or neck pain at the time of interview, more or less the same as in Western surveys. But it was usually an incidental finding. Anderson was 'struck by the virtual absence of disability'. People expected back or neck pain as part of their lives and did very little about it.

People in less developed societies get much the same back pain as we do, but they have much less disability. Only with the introduction of Western medicine does chronic back disability

become common. Indeed, the new back cripples in Oman are those who have had the 'advantage' of treatment abroad and who have had surgery in India, Europe or the United States. Similarly, in North America and in Europe, 25–50% of patients in most pain clinics are the failures of modern treatment for back pain (Fig. 1.5). It is perhaps time to stop and ask ourselves exactly what we think we are doing for our patients with back pain.

For 17 years I ran a Problem Back Clinic for the west of Scotland. Most of these patients had a long history of chronic pain and disability. They had seen multiple medical specialists and had many investigations and treatments. They had tried alternative medicine and seen many therapists. Everyone they saw gave them a different story, but none gave lasting relief. These patients were frustrated and angry and depressed by our failure. As you would expect, I was rarely able to make any new diagnosis or

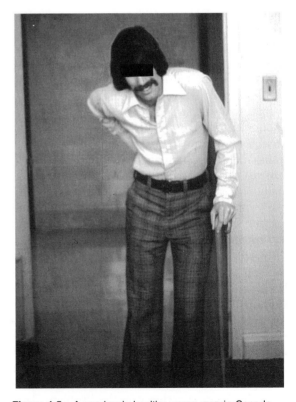

Figure 1.5 A previously healthy young man in Canada, permanently disabled by a simple back strain.

offer any miracle cure. These patients were highly selected and were not representative of all patients with back pain, but they did teach us a lot about the limitations and failures of traditional medical treatment. Listening to them, I became convinced that most of the problems were to do with our basic approach to management. Most patients with back pain do get better, but the failures of treatment may be worse than no treatment at all. Too often, I wondered if a patient might have been better if he or she had never consulted a doctor, and especially not a surgeon. It would clearly be much better to prevent these patients ever developing chronic pain and disability, rather than trying to treat their intractable pain.

Once again, the problem is that back pain is only a symptom, not a disease. Western medicine works best for acute physical diseases with clearly understood anatomy and pathology. In these cases, we can demonstrate and deal with the problem. It is much less successful in chronic and poorly understood illness, particularly if it has psychosomatic features. Back pain has all these characteristics. Most back pain is simply a mechanical disturbance of the musculoskeletal structures or function of the back. We cannot diagnose any specific pathology. We cannot even localize the source of most soft tissue pain. Some doctors and therapists do claim to be able to diagnose the site and nature of the lesion in many patients. However, that often tells us more about the health professional than about the patient's back. It is striking how these professionals disagree! To confuse the issue further, back pain is often a recurrent problem and patients are often distressed.

Another problem is that diagnosis and health care are not nearly as logical as they appear in textbooks. This is particularly obvious in studies of failed back surgery, even when we look at a clear-cut condition like an acute disc prolapse. We all know how to diagnose the nerve that requires surgical decompression. It is a logical decision based on well-known criteria. We can all reproduce the right answer in an examination. However, experience in the Problem Back Clinic shows that practice is quite different. A

careful prospective study of routine spinal surgery confirmed this (Morris et al 1986). In practice, surgical decisions depend on the severity and duration of the patient's symptoms, the patient's distress and the failure of conservative treatment more than on objective evidence of a surgically treatable lesion. 'Because it is so bad and has not got better with bed rest it must be a disc prolapse' – that is a quote from the record of a patient with nonspecific low back pain who never had any specific symptoms or objective signs of a disc prolapse. Depending on how strongly the patient demands and the surgeon feels that 'something must be done', there is a strong temptation to proceed to CT or MRI scan. We rationalize this by saying that we 'want to make sure we are not missing anything'. Alternatively, we use these tests when the clinical picture is not clear, as a short cut to differential diagnosis. We order tests instead of taking a more careful history or physical examination and using time to clarify the clinical course. If these sensitive tests show even minor changes, we forget about false-positives and the lack of matching clinical features. The trap is then complete. The patient has genuine needs and demands, we have run out of alternatives, and as surgeons we want to help. It is then very difficult to withhold the knife. Too often, in such a case, the surgical findings are unimpressive. Despite our best intentions, the brutal reality is that the patient undergoes an unnecessary operation. Not surprisingly, it does not help. But much more important, and too often forgotten even when there are no surgical complications, failed surgery may make their pain, disability and distress worse.

All my clinical experience and research have convinced me that our treatment of back pain has failed because we have lost sight of basic principles. What matters is not the technical detail but our whole strategy of clinical management. We need to rethink our whole approach. Providing that we get the basic principles right, the detail can follow. This book concentrates on these basic clinical principles:

- Why and how do some people become chronic back cripples due to simple backache?
- Why are their numbers increasing?
- What has gone wrong with our management of back pain?
- How can we stop this epidemic?
- How can we improve health care for patients with back pain?

We all agree in principle that we should treat people, not spines. Plato laid down the principle in ancient Greece: 'So neither ought you to attempt to cure the body without the soul.' All health care still has its roots in Hippocratic concepts of caring and personal obligation. We cannot separate the doctor's role as healer from his or her more ancient role as personal adviser and comforter in illness. Chiropractic and osteopathy share a similar philosophy. Physical therapists also spend their whole working life with people, helping them to regain function and get back to normal life. The problem is that in busy modern practice we all too often forget about such philosophic ideals and get on with treating pain and physical disease. We all subscribe to these ideals – the challenge is to put them into routine clinical practice.

This book presents what I have learned from 20 years of research, but it is not about academic research or scientific results. My interest has always been in the clinical care of patients with back pain, and we must apply the lessons of research to daily practice in the clinic or the office. So this is a clinical text. It starts with, concentrates on and is all about the clinical problem of back pain. Anatomy, biomechanics and pathology are often said to be the basis for clinical practice. In one sense this is true: of course we need to know this basic science. But we must also remember that these are only tools to serve our patients' needs. They cannot and must not drive our clinical practice. If we build our theories upwards from the foundation of these basic sciences, then it is too easy to select or bend the clinical facts to fit our theories. It is not surprising that such an approach to the treatment of back pain has failed. The real foundation of clinical practice is human illness and we must start from clinical reality. Only then can we select and use those basic sciences that help us to understand and explain our clinical observations.

The fascination and challenge of all health care are the variety of ways in which human beings react to illness. You cannot learn this by reading a book. You can only learn by working with patients. There is a wonderful quotation from Sir Isaac Newton:

I seem to have been only a boy playing on the sea-shore, and diverting myself in now and then finding a smoother pebble or a prettier shell than ordinary, whilst the great ocean of truth lay all undiscovered before me.

This does not do justice to a great scientist's approach to knowledge. In health care as in science, there comes a time when you have to plunge into the ocean and enter that world of experience which you cannot imagine merely standing on the shore watching the waves. So you can only truly learn about back pain from your patients. This book should serve as a companion that stimulates you to think about and learn from your clinical experience.

We are at the dawn of a revolution in back pain. Dawn is a time of light, hope and new beginnings. This book is my contribution to the new approach to back pain. It tries to develop the basic principles and describe methods to put them into clinical practice. It considers how we might improve the health care system. If you are happy with how you treat back pain and have not thought about these issues, then I hope this book will disturb you. I hope that after reading it and thinking about the questions it raises, it will change forever how you think about back pain and how you deal with these patients. This book will not give you all the answers, but I hope it will help to focus the questions and stimulate you to join the search for answers. For our patients and society rightly demand that there must be a better way of treating back pain.

REFERENCES

Anderson R T 1984 An orthopaedic ethnography in rural Nepal. Medical Anthropology 8: 46–59

Gray I C M, Main C J, Waddell G 1984 Illness behaviour and the role of psychological assessment in general orthopaedic practice. Clinical Orthopaedics and Related Research 184: 258–263

Morris E W, Di Paola M P, Vallance R, Waddell G 1986 Diagnosis and decision making in lumbar disc prolapse and nerve entrapment. Spine 11: 436–439

Waddell G, Kummel E G, Lotto W N, Graham J D, Hall H, McCulloch J A 1979 Failed lumbar disc surgery and repeat surgery following industrial injuries. Journal of Bone and Joint Surgery 61A: 201–207

Waddell G, McCulloch J A, Kummel E, Venner R M 1980 Non-organic physical signs in low back pain. Spine 5: 117–125

2

Diagnostic triage

Diagnosis is the foundation of management and is based on clinical assessment. A careful history and examination also help to build a rapport with the patient. These are basic principles of clinical practice, but they cause a problem with back pain. We can only diagnose definite pathology in about 15% of patients with back pain. Patients want a diagnosis, but we must be honest and they must be realistic about what is possible. However, we should not be too pessimistic. We can exclude serious disease, predict likely progress and provide a rational basis for management, all of which are positive and helpful. We should also present as good news the fact that we cannot find anything serious. Approximately 40% of patients with back pain worry that it might affect their job, that it might cripple them or that it is the onset of some serious disease such as cancer. We should be able to allay these fears. This chapter offers a reliable approach to diagnosis that will let you offer this reassurance with very little risk of error. It is a very simple diagnostic triage:

- simple backache
- nerve root pain
- possible serious spinal pathology.

At first sight, this approach may seem too simple. For many years I taught this to my medical students and they loved it. My surgical fellows found that it worked in the clinic, but at academic meetings experienced doctors dismissed it with the assumption that 'of course we all know and do that'. Experience in the

Problem Back Clinic (see p. 5) shows that in practice this is not true. It is the fundamentals that are most important but most difficult to get right. The Quebec Task Force first emphasized the value of such an approach (Spitzer et al 1987). Those involved in primary care are very aware of the need to deal with basics, and both American (AHCPR 1994) and British (CSAG 1994, RCGP 1996) clinical guidelines use this approach. Both guidelines also give a short list of key clinical features that should raise suspicion of spinal pathology – AHCPR (1994) called these 'red flags'. The concepts of triage and red flags also seem to have caught people's imagination and helped to sell the idea.

DIFFERENTIAL DIAGNOSIS

Textbooks often present diagnosis as a choice between a number of diseases. They then describe each disease in detail. We teach students to ask: 'Which of the diseases in my textbook most closely resembles this patient's clinical picture?' To ease the task, we hunt for pathognomonic symptoms and signs. We then seek tests to confirm our diagnosis. Medical teaching has used this approach for nearly three centuries, but it is a very inefficient way of thinking. It is a poor approach to clinical practice.

Most textbooks give long lists of diseases which cause backache, but they are all rare. Indeed, some books actually apologize that these diseases are 'rare but important'. Simple backache is at the end of the list, almost an afterthought, and diagnosis is by exclusion. Such lists do not reflect the incidence or importance of these conditions. I freely confess that I cannot think of every possible disease in my busy clinic. Also, most patients do not read medical textbooks and their symptoms and signs never quite fit the classic description. In practice, it is almost impossible to match each patient against a long list of half-forgotten thumbnail sketches. It should be no surprise that this approach often leads to misleading investigations and bad management.

Instead, I suggest that you should use a simple diagnostic triage. The concept of triage comes from battle casualties. In a busy casualty clearing station, a senior doctor assesses each casualty when he arrives. He divides them into three categories. Some have major but salvageable injuries and they receive first priority for treatment. Some have more minor injuries that need treatment, but they will not come to any harm by waiting. The third group have such major injuries that death is inevitable and they do not receive limited and over-pressed resources. The senior doctor does not attempt any more precise diagnosis or carry out any treatment, yet he makes the single most important decision in management. Everything follows from that first step. Triage decides who receives what treatment and, indeed, the final outcome. In battle casualties, triage literally decides who lives or dies.

Diagnosis determines management. Whether we make it a conscious decision, or do it without thinking, diagnostic triage of back pain is just as vital. It sets the pattern for referral, investigation and management. It very much determines the further course and final outcome of treatment. If we get it right, then the rest follows almost automatically. If we get it wrong, then the whole strategy of management goes wrong, often with a poor outcome. This is one of the basic decisions that is hardest to make but most important to get right.

I first developed this approach in a series of 900 patients with back pain (Waddell 1982). Half were routine referrals from family doctors to an orthopedic outpatient clinic and the others were at my Problem Back Clinic. The series included 35 patients with tumors, 15 with infection, 25 with osteoporosis and 23 with other pathologies. Let me hasten to say that serious spinal pathology is not nearly as common as that. This was a highly selected series that we used simply to work out the system of diagnostic triage. Deyo et al (1992) reached very similar conclusions.

Diagnostic triage

Simple backache. This term describes the common nonspecific low back pain (see Box 2.1). This is 'mechanical' pain of musculoskeletal origin in which symptoms vary with physical activities. Simple backache may be related to mechanical strain or dysfunction, although it often develops spontaneously. Simple backache may be very painful, but the severity of pain does not tell us anything about the diagnosis. Simple backache often spreads to one or both buttocks or thighs. The term simple backache also gives reassurance that there is no damage to the nerves or any more serious spinal pathology.

Box 2.1 Simple backache

- Clinical presentation usually at age 20–55 years
- Lumbosacral region, buttocks and thighs
- Pain is 'mechanical' in nature
  — varies with physical activity
  — varies with time
- Patient well

Of course, I realize that nonspecific low back pain includes a variety of different disorders. There have been a number of attempts to identify subtypes of nonspecific low back pain (Delitto et al 1993, Moffroid et al 1994, Merskey & Bogduk 1994). Unfortunately, there is a lot of overlap between the different clinical groups. There is little correlation between the anatomic identification of 'pain generators', clinical syndromes or actual pathology. Most of these findings have not been replicated and different specialists are unable to agree. Obviously, this is an important future goal, but at present we have no reliable way of subclassifying nonspecific low back pain. We will deal with a more detailed assessment of back pain in later chapters. At this stage, the first priority is to be clear that the problem is simple backache and then to direct our thinking accordingly.

Nerve root pain. This term is preferable to sciatica, since it stresses the pathologic basis and specific clinical features. Nerve root pain can arise from a disc prolapse, spinal stenosis or surgical scarring. In most patients with a low back problem, nerve root pain stems from a single nerve root. Involvement of more than one nerve root raises the possibility that there may be a more widespread neurologic disorder. Nerve root pain is well localized pain down one leg that at least approximates to a dermatomal pattern. It radiates below the knee and often into the foot or toes. There may be numbness or pins and needles in the same distribution. There may be signs of nerve irritation or neurologic signs of nerve compression, although these are not essential for the diagnosis (see Box 2.2). When present, nerve root pain is often the patient's main complaint and is greater than back pain.

Box 2.2 Nerve root pain

- Unilateral leg pain is worse than back pain
- Pain generally radiates to foot or toes
- Numbness or paresthesia in the same distribution
- Nerve irritation signs
  — reduced straight leg raising which reproduces leg pain
- Motor, sensory or reflex changes
  — limited to one nerve root

Serious spinal pathology includes diseases such as spinal tumor and infection, and inflammatory disease such as ankylosing spondylitis (see Box 2.3). Serious spinal pathology may give back pain or, less commonly, nerve root pain. The clinical presentation, diagnosis and management concern the underlying pathology.

Most back pain is simple backache. Less than 1% is due to serious spinal disease such as tumor or infection, which needs urgent specialist investigation and treatment. Less than 1% is inflammatory disease, which needs rheumatologic investigation and treatment. Less than 5% is true nerve root pain, and only a small proportion of that ever needs surgery.

Diagnosis should be a clear and logical process. A clinical history and physical examination should not be a mindless gathering of facts. Neither can you wait for these facts to fuse into a complete picture in a blinding flash of intuition. It is simpler, quicker and more efficient to start from the main presenting symptoms. The history should focus on the key items of information required for triage, and then a brief examination should supplement these key items. You may then need a few investigations to confirm or refute the diagnosis. At

---

Box 2.3 Serious spinal pathology

Red flags
- Presentation age <20 years or onset >55 years
- Violent trauma, e.g. fall from a height, RTA
- Constant, progressive, nonmechanical pain
- Thoracic pain
- Previous history
  — carcinoma
  — systemic steroids
  — drug abuse, HIV
- Systematically unwell
  — weight loss
- Persisting severe restriction of lumbar flexion
- Widespread neurology
- Structural deformity
- Investigations when required
  — sedimentation rate (ESR) >25
  — plain X-ray: vertebral collapse or bone destruction

Cauda equina syndrome/widespread neurologic disorder
- Difficulty with micturition
- Loss of anal sphincter tone or fecal incontinence
- Saddle anesthesia about the anus, perineum or genitals
- Widespread (> one nerve root) or progressive motor weakness in the legs or gait disturbance
- Sensory level

Inflammatory disorders (ankylosing spondylitis and related disorders)
- Gradual onset before age 40 years
- Marked morning stiffness
- Persisting limitation of spinal movements in all directions
- Peripheral joint involvement
- Iritis, skin rashes (psoriasis), colitis, urethral discharge
- Family history

---

each step you use symptoms, signs or investigations to confirm or modify the diagnostic process. Triage is the logical outcome from clearly identified, clinical evidence. Provided you focus on the key issues, you can cover everything that matters within the average family doctor's consultation of 7–10 minutes.

Diagnosis also depends on combining all the key facts into the decision. Individual symptoms and signs may be unreliable and no single test gives an accurate diagnosis. Diagnosis based on a combination of key symptoms and signs is more accurate and much safer.

I will present diagnostic triage as it should occur in the first clinical consultation. This is the ideal, but it is not always possible. In practice, time may play an important role in the diagnostic process. Consistent findings on several occasions may be more reliable and assume more significance. Failure to improve with time may raise the need for reassessment. The ideal is diagnostic triage on the first consultation, but there is still the opportunity to review this on subsequent visits.

PRESENTING SYMPTOMS

Patients with low back disorders present with four key symptoms:

- back pain
- leg pain
- neurologic symptoms
- spinal deformity.

More than 99% of low back problems present with back pain and it is rare to see a low back problem with no back pain. Pain always tends to radiate distally and 70% of patients with back pain also have some pain in one or both legs. Neurologic symptoms and spinal deformity are much less common but crucial to diagnosis.

These four presenting symptoms lead us on to four questions:

- Is this a low back problem and can we exclude disease elsewhere?
- Is there any major spinal deformity or widespread neurologic disorder?
- Is there any question of serious spinal pathology?
- Is there nerve root involvement?

We should direct our history and examination to answer these questions. The answers give us triage into the three broad diagnostic groups (Fig. 2.1).

Is the pain coming from the back?

The first step is to be sure that back pain is due to a low back problem. This is obvious, but we often take it for granted and sometimes forget. We must exclude back pain due to disease elsewhere in the body.

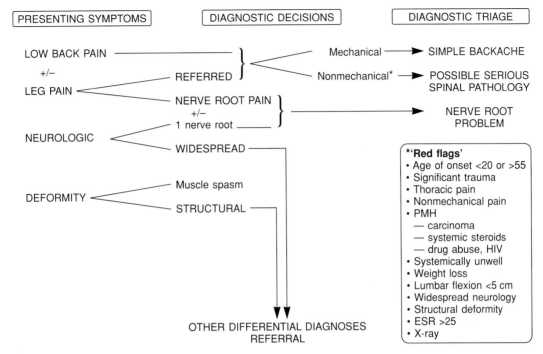

Figure 2.1 Differential diagnosis flow chart.

Back pain usually dominates the clinical picture of a low back problem and the patient often has other low back symptoms such as stiffness and tenderness.

Occasionally, back pain comes from the abdominal or pelvic organs, but these rarely present as back pain alone. There are nearly always some gastrointestinal, urinary or gynecologic symptoms. Renal lesions may give loin pain with classic radiation. If the history is suspicious, you should palpate the abdomen and perform a rectal examination, but you do not need to do so in every patient with simple backache.

Back pain may be only one part of a systemic musculoskeletal or rheumatologic problem, but this should be clear from the history. Low back pain often spreads to the buttocks and hips and you should then exclude a hip problem. The patient may describe problems with walking and hip movements. Your examination should always include the range of hip movement and gait pattern. Leg symptoms may also be due to peripheral vascular disease. Symptoms of

vascular claudication usually affect muscle groups of the leg rather than dermatomes. There are circulatory symptoms rather than sensory symptoms, and peripheral pulses and circulation may be poor.

You should usually be able to distinguish gastrointestinal, genitourinary, hip or vascular disease, *if you think about them*. We miss them when we do not think, but just assume that every patient with back pain must have a spinal problem. We must allow the patient time to present their symptoms and not focus too quickly on leading questions about their back.

Major spinal deformity and widespread neurologic disorders

Major spinal deformity and widespread neurologic disorders are rare but should be obvious – again, provided that you are aware of them.

You should not miss a major deformity such as a kyphosis or structural scoliosis *providing you get the patient to undress*. This may seem obvious, but one recent survey found that more than 50% of patients with back pain said their doctor did not examine them. In simple backache the common deformity is a list (Fig. 2.2). Muscle spasm pulls the spine to one side when the patient is standing and may also cause loss of the lumbar lordosis. In true scoliosis there is a fixed deformity with compensatory curves above and below (Fig. 2.2). A spinal list usually, but not always, improves when the patient lies prone and the muscles relax, but true scoliosis does not change. You can see early scoliosis as a rib hump when the patient reaches down to their toes.

You should not miss a widespread neurologic disorder provided you ask about a few key symptoms. Most local problems in the lower back affect a single nerve root, with dermatomal numbness or paresthesia, or muscle weakness of a single myotome. If neurologic symptoms or signs affect several nerve roots or both legs, then there may be a more widespread neurologic disorder. This may present as unsteadiness or gait disturbance. Urinary retention is an emergency. If there is loss of bladder sensation,

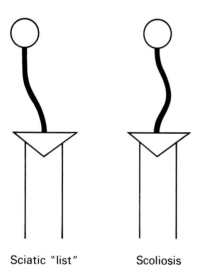

Sciatic "list"   Scoliosis

Figure 2.2 List due to muscle spasm vs. structural scoliosis. With muscle spasm the trunk is offset on the pelvis when erect, but this often corrects when the patient is prone. A structural scoliosis usually has compensatory curves above and below, so the trunk is still centered on the pelvis. A structural deformity persists at all times, even when the patient is anesthetized, and there is a rib hump when bending forward.

the patient may instead complain of difficulty passing urine or overflow incontinence. Some neurologic diseases may also give symptoms in the arms or cranial nerves. If you have any suspicion, you should do a more thorough neurologic examination, although you can still do all that is required in a few minutes (see Box 2.4).

Box 2.4 General neurologic examination when there is a question of widespread neurology

- Brief sensory testing of the arms, the trunk dermatomes and the saddle area
- Palpate the bladder
- Upper motor neurone signs in the legs include increased muscle tone, brisk reflexes, clonus, up-going plantar reflexes, loss of position sense in the toes and loss of coordination in the heel–shin test

---

The detection of serious spinal pathology

Serious spinal pathology accounts for less than 1% of all back pain. Serious pathology is rare, but one of your most important jobs is to detect it or to exclude it and reassure the patient. Indeed, some patients say that this is their only reason for coming to see a doctor. If you can assure them that there is nothing serious then they can deal with the pain themselves. That depends on confident reassurance. Bringing the patient back 'to check' raises doubt that you are not sure or, worse, that there may be something serious that you are hiding. All that we need at this point is a simple yet reliable screen to decide if there is any chance of serious spinal pathology. Diagnosing the exact nature of the pathology can come later. Triage is simply to decide if there is any need for further investigation and referral, or if there is no serious spinal pathology.

Most simple backache affects the lower back or neck. It varies with time and physical activity. It presents in the early to middle years of adult life. It does not affect general health. Serious spinal pathology presents the opposite features. In our series of 900 patients, we found that a few key features detected all 73 patients with serious spinal pathology. Deyo et al (1992) produced a similar list. AHCPR (1994) and CSAG (1994) described these as 'red flags' for possible serious spinal pathology (see Box 2.3).

Age

Most simple backache presents in the early and middle years of adult life. Patients who present for health care before the age of 20 are more likely to have serious disease or a structural problem such as spondylolisthesis. Patients who develop new or different back pain after the age of 55 are more likely to have serious disease, particularly spinal metastases or osteoporosis.

Nonmechanical back pain

Simple backache is mechanical in the sense that it varies with physical activity. Certain postures or movements may make the pain worse. A comfortable position, change of position, stretching or certain exercises may make the pain better. The pain varies over the course of a day or weeks in response to altered activities or treatment.

In contrast, nonmechanical back pain is unrelated to time or activity. It may start spontaneously and gradually. It often becomes gradually worse. Rest or exercises do not relieve it and the patient may not be able to find any position of comfort. Pain may be worse in bed at night when the patient has no distractions.

Thoracic pain

Most mechanical problems affect the lower back or the neck. Pain in the thoracic spine or between the shoulder blades is less common and when it does occur it is more likely to be due to serious pathology. In our selected series, 30% of patients referred to hospital with thoracic pain had serious spinal pathology or osteoporotic collapse of a vertebra.

Violent trauma

Only violent trauma, such as a fall from a height or a road traffic accident, is likely to fracture the normal spine. Post-menopausal women with osteoporosis or patients on systemic steroids may suffer collapsed vertebrae as a result of more minor injury.

Previous medical history

Many systemic diseases can affect the back. A history of carcinoma is most important, however long ago. A history of rheumatologic disorders, tuberculosis and any recent infection may be relevant. Drug abuse, immune suppression and HIV may predispose to infection. Systemic steroids may cause osteoporosis.

Systemic symptoms

Patients with simple backache remain well. If a patient with back pain is unwell then there is more likely to be some other disease. The most significant symptom is weight loss. General malaise, fever or simple clinical impression may all raise suspicion. However, many patients with a spinal infection do not have fever, so the absence of fever does not exclude infection. If the history raises your suspicions, your examination should include the common tumor sites – thyroid, breasts, lymph nodes, abdomen and prostrate. You may also order urine testing, an erythrocyte sedimentation rate (ESR) and a radiograph of the chest.

Limited lumbar flexion

Examination of the spine is not very good for detecting spinal pathology, apart from major spinal deformities and widespread neurologic disorders. A normal examination does not exclude serious pathology, particularly metastases.

The most important physical sign in the back itself is persistent severe restriction of lumbar flexion. In our series, 50% of patients with limited lumbar flexion had either serious spinal pathology or an acute disc prolapse. Lumbar flexion was severely restricted in 70% of patients with spinal infection. However, flexion was normal in 30% of patients with spinal infection, 81% with inflammatory disease, and 91% with spinal metastases. Spinal pathology can be present in the thoracic spine without any restriction of lumbar movement. *Remember that a normal physical examination does not exclude serious spinal pathology.*

We must also improve how we measure lumbar flexion. How close you can reach towards your toes does not test spinal movement, but depends on a combination of lumbar and hip flexion, hamstring tightness and motivation. Some patients with ankylosing spondylitis and a fused lumbar spine can still touch their toes (Fig. 2.3). If we want to measure spinal movement then we must measure the back itself. The simplest method is the Schober (1937) technique. Make two marks on the skin and see how much they move apart as the patient bends forward (Rae et al 1984; Fig. 2.4). This gives a reliable measure of lumbar flexion. We will discuss more precise methods using an inclinometer when we look at the evaluation of physical impairment in Chapter 8, but this simple method is sufficient for routine clinical use.

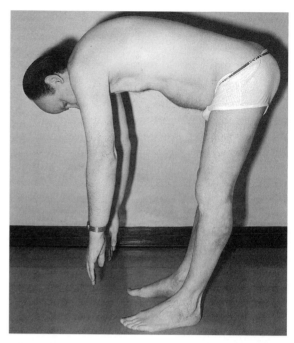

Figure 2.3 The distance from the fingers to the ground does not measure lumbar flexion. Look at the shadow on the wall showing no loss of lumbar lordosis in this patient with ankylosing spondylitis.

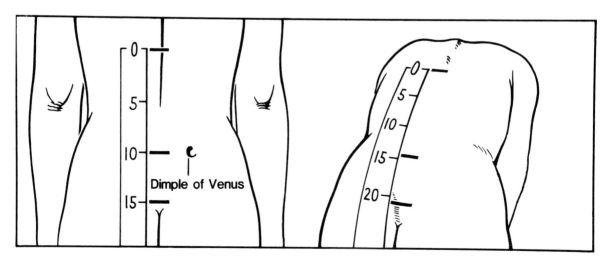

Figure 2.4 The Schober technique of measuring lumbar flexion. Make a mark at the level of the dimples of Venus, which approximates to the lumbosacral junction. Make a second mark 10 cm higher, and a third mark 5 cm lower. Ask the patient to reach down as far as they can towards their toes, and measure the increase in the distance between the top and bottom marks. The normal is at least 5 cm. (From Waddell 1982, with permission.)

Summary: possible serious spinal pathology

- The most important screen for serious spinal pathology is a careful clinical history of red flags
- A normal physical examination does not exclude serious spinal pathology
- A normal X-ray does not rule out spinal pathology.

Triage is based on red flags, but the problem is that individual red flags are not very accurate for diagnosing pathology (van den Hoogen et al 1995). There are too many false-negatives and false-positives. So it is a question of clinical judgement, combining all the clinical features. If there are no red flags on careful clinical assessment, then you can be 99% confident that you have not missed any serious spinal pathology. If there are some red flags, then it still depends on clinical judgement. With typical mechanical low back pain after a minor lifting injury in an 18-year-old, it would be reasonable to wait and see how he gets on before considering any referral or investigation. A 60-year-old who presents with several months' gradual onset of new thoracic pain and weight loss needs urgent investigation, even if the clinical examination and plain X-rays are completely normal.

The aim of triage is to decide if there is any question of possible serious spinal pathology. Exact diagnosis will come later. Triage is only to decide which patients need further investigation.

The meaning of leg pain

One of the most common mistakes is to assume that all leg pain is sciatica which must be due to a disc prolapse pressing on a nerve. This is false logic. Leg pain *may* be nerve root pain due to a disc prolapse pressing on a root, but much more often it is not. Most leg pain is not nerve root pain, and has nothing to do with a disc prolapse. There is so much confusion about the term sciatica that it is better not to use it. The classic meaning is pain in the distribution of the sciatic nerve. At present, different doctors and therapists use the word sciatica to mean anything from any leg pain to a precise description of nerve root pain. We will think and communicate more clearly if we talk about referred leg pain and nerve root pain.

It is nearly 60 years since Kellgren (1939) showed that stimulation of any of the tissues of the back can refer pain into one or both legs. Seventy per cent of patients with back pain have some radiation of pain to their legs. This referred pain can come from the fascia, muscles, ligaments, periosteum, facet joints, disc or epidural structures. It is usually a dull, poorly localized ache that spreads into the buttocks and thighs (Fig. 2.5). It may affect both legs. It usually does not go much below the knee. Referred pain is not due to anything pressing on a nerve. It is not sciatica.

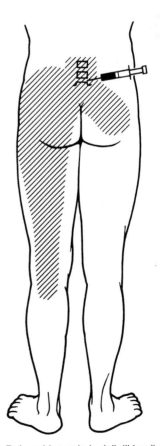

Figure 2.5 Referred leg pain is dull, ill-localized, and usually does not radiate much below the knee(s). (From Waddell 1982, with permission.)

Stimulation of the nerve root gives a quite different pain, which is sharp and well localized (Fig. 2.6). At the common L5 or S1 levels, nerve root pain usually radiates to the foot or toes. It at least approximates to a dermatomal distribution. Patients often describe the pain with sensory qualities such as pins and needles, or numbness. It usually affects one leg only and is greater than back pain. Nerve root pain is much less common than referred leg pain.

Triage must distinguish referred leg pain from nerve root pain. You can usually make a provisional decision from the patient's description of the pain. If a patient presents with back pain alone and no leg pain or neurologic symptoms, it is very unlikely that there is a nerve root problem. There is then no need for any neurologic examination. If the patient does have leg pain then you should examine their legs for signs of nerve irritation or nerve compression.

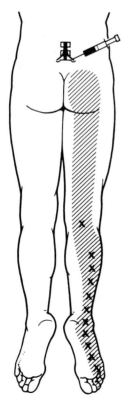

Figure 2.6 Nerve root pain usually radiates to the foot or toes and at least approximates to a dermatome. (From Waddell 1982, with permission.)

Nerve irritation and compression signs help to confirm the diagnosis of nerve root pain. Ninety-eight per cent of disc prolapses are at L4/5 or L5/S1 and affect the L5 or S1 roots, and most clinical tests look at these levels. Textbooks emphasize motor, sensory and reflex signs, but these only occur when nerve compression is sufficient to disturb the function of the nerve. Nerve irritation signs are earlier and more common, and just as important for diagnosis.

Root irritation signs

Nerve irritation signs depend on tests that stretch or press on an irritable nerve root to reproduce radiating root pain. The diagnostic finding is this *reproduction of symptomatic nerve pain*. Straight leg raising is the most widely used test for nerve irritation but many doctors and therapists misinterpret it. Limited straight leg raising in itself is not a sign of nerve irritation. The key finding is not the limitation, but the reason for it. Limitation due to back pain or hamstring spasm only shows severity and has nothing to do with irritation of a nerve. The specific sign of nerve irritation is limited straight leg raising due to reproduction of nerve pain down the leg (Edgar & Park 1974; Fig. 2.7). Pain may only radiate to the thigh and not down the full length of the dermatome. Passive dorsiflexion of the foot at the limit of straight leg raising may increase the leg pain or make it radiate more distally.

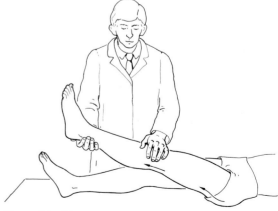

Figure 2.7 The diagnostic feature of straight leg raising is reproduction of the symptomatic root pain.

Other signs of nerve irritation also depend on reproducing nerve pain. A positive cough impulse gives pain down the leg, not back pain alone. The well-leg raising test or cross-over sign uses passive straight leg raising of the pain-free leg to give nerve pain in the symptomatic leg. The bowstring test is better known in North America than in Europe (Fig. 2.8). At the end of the straight leg raising test, slightly flex the knee to relieve pain. Then press your thumb on the nerve where it is bowstrung across the politeal fossa. With an irritable nerve, you may produce pain or paresthesia radiating up or down the leg. Local pain beneath your thumb is not diagnostic.

If the pattern of pain suggests an upper lumbar nerve root, then you should also do the femoral stretch test (Fig. 2.9). The key finding of nerve irritation is again radiating nerve pain in the anterior thigh and not back pain. You should distinguish that from hip disease or a tight quadriceps muscle.

Nerve compression signs

Compression of the nerve root interferes with its function. This may present as muscle wasting, motor weakness, sensory change or depressed tendon reflexes. Most low back problems affect a single nerve root, although they do sometimes

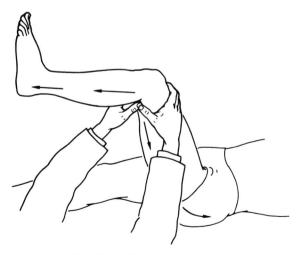

Figure 2.8 The diagnostic feature of the bowstring test is reproduction of the symptomatic root pain or paresthesia.

A

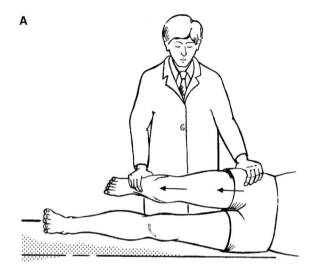

B

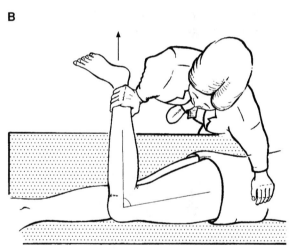

Figure 2.9 (A, B) The diagnostic feature of the femoral stretch test is reproduction of the symptomatic root pain.

affect the same nerve root to both legs. Nerve function is usually only depressed because of overlap from adjacent roots. Complete anesthesia or paralysis is rare, so you must look for minor neurologic changes. You should check each dermatome and myotome in turn (Table 2.1) and the best way to detect minor change is to compare the two legs (Figs 2.10–2.12).

The common L5 and S1 signs are weakness of the ankle and toes, sensory loss in the foot and a diminished ankle reflex (Table 2.1). You

Table 2.1 The nerve supply of the L4–S1 nerve roots

	L4	L5	S1
Distribution of pain and sensory disturbance	Anterior thigh	Dorsum of foot Great toe	Lateral border of foot Sole
Motor weakness	Quadriceps (Dorsiflexion ankle)	Dorsiflexion ankle Eversion ankle Dorsiflexion toes*	Plantar flexion ankle (Dorsiflexion great toe)
Reflex	Knee jerk	(Ankle jerk)	Ankle jerk

*An L5 lesion usually only affects some of these muscles.

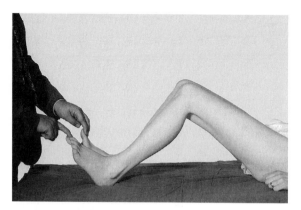

Figure 2.10 Clinical examination for motor weakness should test each myotome in turn, comparing the two legs for minor differences.

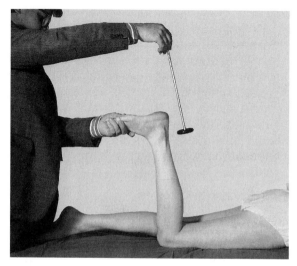

Figure 2.12 Examination for minor changes in the reflexes depends on the patient being relaxed.

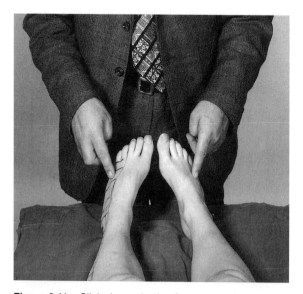

Figure 2.11 Clinical examination for sensory changes should test each dermatome in turn, comparing the two legs for minor differences.

should concentrate on these unless symptoms suggest a higher lumbar root or a widespread neurologic disorder.

The exact pattern of leg pain and a brief examination for nerve irritation and compression signs should usually allow you to diagnose a nerve root problem. Referred leg pain is simply part of more severe, but still 'simple' backache.

INVESTIGATIONS

When there are clinical red flags, the ESR and plain X-rays should form part of your routine assessment. You do not need them in every patient with recent onset of simple backache. However, you must be clear about the role and limitations of these tests. The ESR and plain

X-rays are complementary. X-rays show anatomic detail and structural problems which may not affect the ESR. The ESR may rise earlier but radiographic changes take time to develop. The ESR is also sensitive to diseases which may not affect the bones.

The erythrocyte sedimentation rate (ESR)

The ESR is nonspecific, but it is still useful as a simple screening test for disease. It is quick and easy to perform and can be ready while the patient is having X-rays or seeing a therapist.

The limitation is that the ESR is quite crude, with many false-negatives and -positives, and so a normal ESR does not exclude disease. We must also use the ESR in a way which reduces the impact of false-positives. The upper limit of normal in the standard Westergren method is variously given as 15–25 mm in the first hour. In our series only one patient with serious spinal pathology fell between these limits, so in this context it is better to use a limit of 25 mm. In our series, all the patients with a raised ESR who turned out to have serious spinal pathology also had clinical red flags. Twenty-seven patients with a raised ESR but no clinical red flags all turned out after investigation and follow-up to have no spinal pathology. I suggest, therefore, that you use the ESR selectively. If there are no clinical red flags, then do not do an ESR, because it would be more likely to mislead than to help triage. If there are clinical red flags, then perform the ESR while the patient is having X-rays. A raised ESR provides a useful check on your clinical triage and supports the need for further investigation. A normal ESR and normal X-rays mean that serious spinal pathology is less likely, but you must still judge, on the basis of the clinical red flags, whether the patient needs further referral or investigation.

Plain X-rays

The main value of plain X-rays is to show structural problems in the bones. They do not show soft tissue problems such as a disc prolapse or nerves. Most serious spinal pathology affects the vertebral body and shows up on X-rays as bone destruction. New bone formation is less common. However, these radiographic changes are nonspecific. The pattern of radiographic change may suggest a diagnosis, but this is unreliable. X-rays cannot diagnose histology or bacteriology and it is wiser not to attempt specific diagnosis from X-rays. Bone destruction must also have advanced beyond a certain point before it will show up on X-ray. Routine spinal X-rays do not detect osteoporosis until there is 30% loss of the bone mass. A lateral X-ray of the lumbar spine will only detect a focal lesion when at least 50% of the cancellous bone is destroyed, and there must be even greater destruction for it to show up on the AP view. Hence, X-rays can only detect pathology after it has been present for a certain time or reached a certain stage. The most virulent disc infection may not show any radiographic change for several weeks. Metastases may take many months to show up on X-ray. *A normal X-ray does not rule out spinal pathology.*

Nachemson claims that if there are no red flags on careful clinical assessment then X-rays only detect significant spinal pathology once in 2500 patients. The caveat is 'on careful clinical assessment'. Spinal X-rays cannot compensate for inadequate assessment.

After careful clinical assessment and plain X-rays, a bone scan may provide a better second-line screening test for serious spinal pathology.

The role of investigations

I would argue strongly that diagnostic triage should be based primarily on clinical assessment. There is a growing tendency to rely on imaging, but this is no substitute for a focused clinical history and physical examination. Deyo (1995) offers a very good introduction to understanding the accuracy of diagnostic tests.

Plain X-rays have been in routine use for most of this century, but over the last two decades there have been great advances in more sophisticated imaging. Computerized tomography (CT) and magnetic resonance imaging (MRI) now provide wonderful information about the anatomy of spinal pathology and neuro-logic compression, which is what they were designed for. For the patient who has spinal pathology or who needs surgery, this is of tremendous value, but X-rays tell us little about simple backache (with the possible exception of pain provocation techniques). Most findings on plain X-rays have very little relationship to clinical symptoms and are equally common in patients with back pain and normal asympto-matic people. Most degenerative changes are a normal age-related process. We now realize that back pain is usually due to conditions that cannot be diagnosed on plain X-rays and that most X-ray findings do not assist management. Plain X-rays are also of no value in diagnosing or assessing nerve root problems. CT and MRI may have an additional role in back pain research, but they are more likely to confuse than assist routine management of simple backache.

These investigations were not designed for differential diagnosis. Imaging has become more and more sensitive, but the more sensitive the investigation, the higher the number of false-positive findings in normal people (Table 2.2). These are very inefficient screening tools.

The unthinking use of X-rays can also do considerable harm. There is growing concern about the amount of radiation from plain X-rays. A standard set of three lumbosacral views gives 120 times the radiation dose of a chest X-ray. Some doctors argue that we can use tests to reassure patients, but this is a false argument. McDonald et al (1996) have shown that a normal test result does not reassure patients and may not outweigh the anxiety caused by ordering the test in the first place. The trouble is that modern high-quality images are seductive and the pictures almost irresistible. The greatest risk is that minor changes, and even false-positive findings, may then drive clinical management, and we fall into the trap of treating X-rays instead of patients. The more subtle danger is that these investigations are also expensive and use up health care money that could be spent in better ways for the patient with simple backache.

Diagnostic triage is a clinical decision, based on clinical assessment. When there is real doubt which might influence management, then you may use investigations to supplement the deci-sion. But you must be very clear about what information you are looking for and select the investigation which will answer that question. You must match the investigation results to the clinical findings and always remain conscious of the place and limitations of each inves-tigation. The best image is no substitute for a proper clinical assessment and diagnostic triage will always be a clinical decision.

THE MAJOR CLINICAL PROBLEM

In diagnostic triage, we start from the main presenting symptoms, carry out a clinical his-tory and a physical examination, to answer the questions described above (p. 12), and then triage into one of three major clinical problems (Figs 2.1 and 2.13). Each of these clinical prob-lems has different prognosis, investigations and treatment. Triage sets the scene for manage-ment and final outcome.

Table 2.2 The false-positive rate of radiographic investigations in normal asymptomatic people. The more sensitive the test, the higher the false-positive rate

	Degenerative and other abnormalities	Disc prolapse
Plain radiographs	0–90%	–
Myodil myelography	20%	4%
Water soluble myelography	25%	10%
CT scan	10–35%	10–20%
MRI scan	35–90%	20–35%

When there is a range, it shows the increase with age.

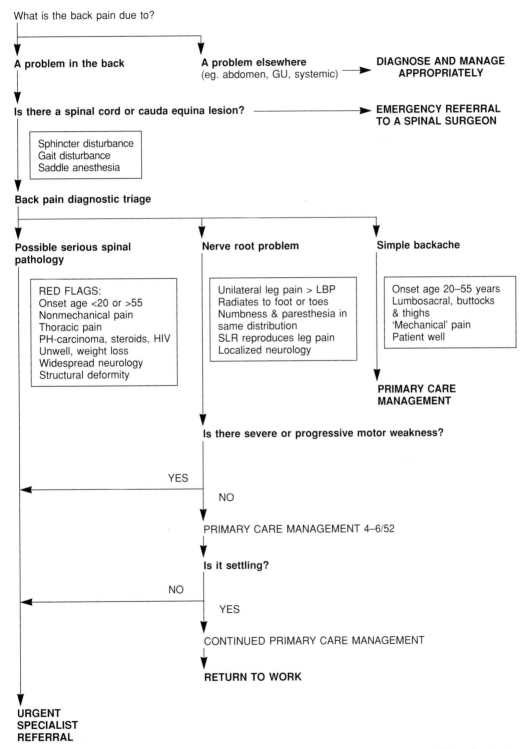

What is the back pain due to?

A problem in the back

A problem elsewhere
(eg. abdomen, GU, systemic) ——▶ **DIAGNOSE AND MANAGE APPROPRIATELY**

Is there a spinal cord or cauda equina lesion? ——————▶ **EMERGENCY REFERRAL TO A SPINAL SURGEON**

Sphincter disturbance
Gait disturbance
Saddle anesthesia

Back pain diagnostic triage

Possible serious spinal pathology

RED FLAGS:
Onset age <20 or >55
Nonmechanical pain
Thoracic pain
PH-carcinoma, steroids, HIV
Unwell, weight loss
Widespread neurology
Structural deformity

Nerve root problem

Unilateral leg pain > LBP
Radiates to foot or toes
Numbness & paresthesia in same distribution
SLR reproduces leg pain
Localized neurology

Simple backache

Onset age 20–55 years
Lumbosacral, buttocks & thighs
'Mechanical' pain
Patient well

PRIMARY CARE MANAGEMENT

Is there severe or progressive motor weakness?

YES

NO

PRIMARY CARE MANAGEMENT 4–6/52

Is it settling?

NO

YES

CONTINUED PRIMARY CARE MANAGEMENT

RETURN TO WORK

URGENT SPECIALIST REFERRAL

Figure 2.13 A differential diagnosis flow chart: diagnostic triage of a patient presenting with low back pain with or without sciatica. (After CSAG 1994, with permission.)

One of the most common fears of all health professionals working with back pain is that they will miss the patient with serious pathology. This is understandable, particularly in primary care where such pathology is rare. However, we are all so aware of that danger that with reasonable care and these screening methods the risk is very low. The most common mistake in practice is to over-diagnose nerve root problems. We must get triage into perspective. Most back pain is benign and non-specific. Less than 1% is due to serious spinal disease such as tumor or infection requiring urgent specialist investigation and treatment. Less than 1% is a systemic connective tissue disorder or inflammatory disease requiring rheumatologic investigation and treatment. Less than 5% is true sciatica due to nerve root irritation or entrapment and only a small proportion of that fails to settle and then requires consideration of surgical treatment. In the case of serious spinal pathology, it is much better to err on the side of caution and investigate further when there is any initial doubt. In the case of nerve root pain, however, over-diagnosis is likely to be much more harmful than under-diagnosis. In this case the sins of commission are much worse than the sins of omission. It may be helpful to take a legal perspective: how much real evidence do you have of a nerve root problem and how would that evidence stand up in a court of law?

I must offer one caveat. This approach is logical and has a strong clinical basis. I have found it highly successful in my clinical practice over many years, and to the best of my knowledge I have rarely missed anything serious – and practicing all that time in one tightly knit and stable community we all heard about our mistakes. All my Fellows have found it equally successful. The triage approach in the recent guidelines has also been warmly welcomed by family doctors. But as van den Hoogen et al (1995) and Little et al (1996) point out, there is very little empiric evidence as to its effectiveness in primary care. This approach was developed in hospital practice, where patients are already preselected. Clinical presentation and decisions may be subtly different in primary care. We need prospective studies in primary care on the accuracy of diagnostic triage and selection for specialist referral.

Despite that caveat about methods, triage itself is fundamental: simple backache, nerve root pain or possible serious spinal pathology. The rest of this book is about the complex and fascinating problem of 'simple backache'.

REFERENCES

AHCPR 1994 Clinical Practice Guideline Number 14. Acute low back problems in adults. Agency for Health Care Policy and Research, US Department of Health and Human Services, Rockville MD

CSAG 1994 Clinical Standards Advisory Group report on back pain. HMSO, London

Delitto A, Cibulka M T, Erhard R E et al 1993 Evidence for use of an extension-mobilization category in acute low back syndrome: a prescriptive validation pilot study. Physical Therapy 73: 216

Deyo R A 1995 Understanding the accuracy of diagnostic tests. In: Weinstein J N, Ryderik B L, Sonntag K H (eds) Essentials of the spine. Raven, New York, p 55–69

Deyo R A, Rainville J, Kent D L 1992 What can the history and physical examination tell us about low back pain? Journal of the American Medical Association 268: 760–765

Edgar M A, Park W M 1974 Induced pain patterns on passive straight leg raising in lower lumbar disc protrusion. Journal of Bone and Joint Surgery 56B: 658–667

Kellgren J H 1939 On the distribution of pain arising from deep somatic structures with charts of segmental pain areas. Clinical Science 4: 35–46

Lewis T 1942 Pain, MacMillan, New York.

Little P, Smith L, Cantrell T, Chapman J, Langridge J, Pickering R 1996 General practitioners' management of acute back pain: a survey of reported practice compared with clinical guidelines. British Medical Journal 312: 485–488

McDonald I G, Daly J, Jelink V M, Panetta F, Gutman J M 1996 Opening Pandora's box: the unpredictability of reassurance by a normal test result. British Medical Journal 313: 329–332

Merskey H, Bogduk N (eds) 1994 Classification of chronic pain. Descriptions of chronic pain syndromes and definition of pain terms, 2nd edn. International Association for the Study of Pain (IASP) Press, Seattle

Moffroid M T, Haugh L D, Henry S M, Short B 1994 Distinguishable groups of musculoskeletal low back pain patients and asymptomatic control subjects based on physical measures of the NIOSH low back atlas. Spine 19: 1350–1358

Rae P, Venner R M, Waddell G 1984 A simple clinical technique of measuring lumbar flexion. Journal of the Royal College of Surgeons of Edinburgh 29: 281–284

RCGP 1996 Clinical guidelines for the management of acute low back pain. Royal College of General Practitioners, London

Schober P 1937 Lendenwerelsaule und Kreuzschmergen. Munch Med Wschr 84: 336

Spitzer W O, Leblanc F E, Dupuis M et al 1987 Scientific approach to the assessment and management of activity-related spinal disorders. A monograph for physicians. Report of the Quebec Task Force on spinal disorders. Spine 12: 7S: s1–s59

van den Hoogen H M M, Koes B W, van Eijk J T H M, Bouter L M 1995 On the accuracy of history, physical examination and erythrocyte sedimentation rate in diagnosing low-back pain in general practice. A criteria-based review of the literature. Spine 20: 318–327

Waddell G 1982 An approach to backache. British Journal of Hospital Medicine 23: 187–219

3

Pain and disability

This book is about low back pain and disability. Before we go any further, we need to look more closely at the nature of pain and disability and the difference between them.

Pain and disability go together and we often talk about them as if they were one and the same. Unfortunately, that sloppy thinking leads to much confusion. Pain and disability are not the same, and we must make a clear distinction between them in our thinking and in clinical practice. This is equally true in assessment and in management.

Pain is a symptom, not a clinical sign, diagnosis or disease, whereas disability refers to restricted function. We cannot assess pain directly, but must always depend on the patient's report of his or her subjective experience. Hence, the report of the symptom of pain will depend on how the patient thinks and feels and how he or she communicates it. Clinical assessment of disability also usually relies on the patient's own report, so once again it is subjective and open to these same influences.

Failure to distinguish between pain and disability has a major impact on management. Many patients and health professionals assume that it is simply a question of pain causing disability and that if we treat the pain, the disability will disappear. Too often, that just does not work. This is partly because our treatment for back pain is not very effective. More fundamentally, it is because there is not a simple 1:1 relationship between pain and disability.

One of the roots of our current problem with back pain is, I believe, this assumption that pain and disability are the same. It is a basic mistake that has far-reaching consequences. Pain and disability are obviously related to each other, but they are quite different aspects of the illness. Having back pain and being disabled by it are not the same thing. Clinical experience shows that back pain does not always lead to disability, and that the amount of disability is not always proportionate to the severity of pain. We often come across patients who manage to lead surprisingly normal lives despite serious spinal pathology or severe pain; yet simple backache may totally and permanently disable other patients, despite the lack of much objective abnormality. Closer scientific study confirms that the relationship between pain and disability is weaker than we might think.

- Pain is a symptom
- Disability is restricted function
- Clinical assessment relies on the patient's *report* of pain and disability

PAIN

Pain is the main presenting symptom of 99% of patients with back trouble. Pain is the most common symptom in health care, but despite this it is one of the least understood. Lewis was one of the modern pioneers of the study of pain, yet he freely admitted the problem in the opening sentences of his classic book (Lewis 1942):

Reflection tells me that I am so far from being able satisfactorily to define pain, of which I here write, that the attempt could serve no useful purpose. Pain, like similar subjective things, is known to us by experience and described by illustration. The usage of the term in this book will be clear enough to anyone who reads its pages. To build up a definition in words or to substitute some phrase would carry neither the reader nor myself farther. But in using the undefined word it is necessary to take care that it is never allowed to confuse phenomena that may be distinct. When there is such possibility, the bare word pain is not enough; it needs and will be given qualification.

Fifty years on, we should still heed Lewis's warning! Descartes (1664), the leading philosopher of the European Renaissance, has had a major impact on thinking about pain for more than three centuries. What is commonly known as the Cartesian model is a very mechanistic view of pain; in this model pain is simply a signal of tissue damage (Fig. 3.1):

A pain, an ache, a discomfort – these are the common complaints of those who seek the doctor's help. Pain issues a warning with kindly intent. She calls to action and, pointing the way, brooks no delay. And thus the ancient cycle is served, from pain to cause, to treatment to cure. (Penfield 1969)

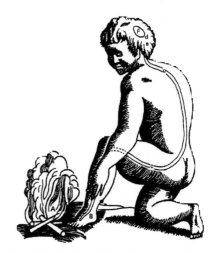

Figure 3.1 The traditional Cartesian model of specific pain pathways.

If for example fire comes near the foot, the minute particles of this fire, which as you know have a great velocity, have the power to set in motion the spot of the skin of the foot which they touch, and by this means pulling upon the delicate thread which is attached to the spot of the skin, they open up at the same instant the pore against which the delicate thread ends, just as by pulling at one end of a rope one makes to strike at the same instant a bell which hangs at the other end. (Descartes 1664, as translated by Foster 1901)

In most routine practice, doctors and therapists still consider pain in this way, i.e. 'pain-as-a-signal'. But thoughtful clinicians have always known that this does not explain many clinical observations of pain. Different patients with the same injury seem to experience very different amounts and kinds of pain, and they react in very different ways. When pain becomes chronic, it sometimes seems to become dissociated from any original tissue damage and almost develops an identity of its own. This simple approach to pain may work for acute injury, but it has been much less successful for many chronic pains.

Over the past 30 years we have begun to recognize the clinical reality that pain is much more complex. From the time of Aristotle, philosophers have distinguished pain from the five senses and classed it as one of the 'passions of the soul'. Pain has some elements in common with touch, taste, smell, vision and hearing. However, Wall (1988) pointed out that we cannot define or identify pain independently of the person who experiences it. We can measure sound waves and the electrical activity in the auditory nerve or cortex, and these correspond closely to what the listener hears. We have no such objective measure for pain. We can only know that someone is 'in pain' by his or her statements or actions. We may try to measure noxious stimuli or electrical activity in nerves, but this tells us little about the individual's experience, much less their suffering. Wall suggests that pain functions more as a basic human drive, like hunger or thirst, leading to highly predictable responses. Pain always produces some response. It also usually produces a response from those around the individual experiencing it.

Loeser (1980) described four aspects or dimensions of pain (Fig. 3.2):

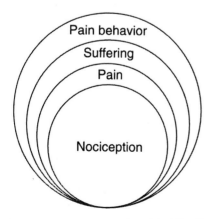

Figure 23.2 Loeser's conceptual model of the dimensions of chronic pain. (From Loeser 1980, with permission.)

- *Nociception* refers to mechanical or other stimuli that could cause tissue damage. These stimuli act on peripheral pain receptors to give activity in nerve fibers.
- *Pain* is the perception of the sensation of pain. This has two important implications. First, we must perceive nociception before it is pain. Second, it is possible to perceive pain even when no tissue damage is occurring.
- *Suffering* is the unpleasant emotional response generated in higher nervous centers by pain and other emotional situations. Suffering is not unique to pain, but also occurs with grief, stress, anxiety or depression. Indeed, we often use the language of pain to describe our suffering in these situations. But pain and suffering are different. We can have pain without suffering and suffering without pain.
- *Pain behavior* includes all acts and conduct that we commonly understand to suggest the presence of pain. Pain behaviors include talking, moaning, facial expressions, limping, taking pain-killers, seeking health care and stopping work. Note the phrase 'which we commonly understand': pain behavior is a form of communication. This does not mean it is conscious or intended. Most pain behavior is completely unconscious.

Pain and disability often involve all of these aspects of pain. Treatment of pain-as-a-signal fails to address these other dimensions of pain, which is why it is often unsuccessful.

Loeser's (1980) model begins to give us a better picture of clinical pain, but it presents a problem. It uses the word pain in two different ways: we have the one-dimensional 'pain-as-a-signal', but we also have pain as the whole experience, in all its complexity. However, this is perhaps an accurate reflection of our dilemma: we often confuse pain-as-a-signal with the whole clinical syndrome of pain.

Modern health care places great emphasis on pain, and most doctors and therapists spend much of their working life treating pain. Engel (1959) suggested that 'the relief of pain is the primary social role of the physician'. Some idealists still hanker after the unrealistic goal that medicine should provide relief for all pain. The International Pain Foundation states flatly that 'no one should have to live with pain' (Liebeskind & Melzack 1987). They then go even further: 'By any reasonable code, freedom from pain should be a basic human right, limited only by our knowledge to achieve it.' Many philosophers and theologians through history would dispute this as a narrow medical perspective on life. Of course we must improve our management of pain, but we will never abolish all pain and it is supreme medical arrogance even to try. The same muddled thinking appears in clinical practice. Some workers suggest that the patient's report of pain is the only symptom that matters. That is naive. It presents pain either as a simple physical symptom or as so complex that we cannot even try to understand it except at the most pragmatic level. I believe that we must understand pain better if we are going to improve our management of back trouble, but that we must also deal with clinical reality.

The neurophysiology of pain

Stimulation of a nociceptor produces impulses in peripheral nerves that enter the dorsal column of the spinal cord. Traditional physiology then described specific pain pathways in the spinal cord, leading to the sensory cortex. We might imagine it as a kind of giant telephone exchange. Pressing a peripheral button would ring a bell in the corresponding area of the cortex and bring the stimulus to conscious attention as pain. Unfortunately, this attractive oversimplification is inaccurate.

Modern neurophysiology provides a more complex, but much better, basis for understanding clinical pain. There are three fundamental ideas. First, pain signals do not pass unaltered into the CNS, but are filtered and modulated at every level. Second, pain is not a purely physical sensation that passes all the way up to consciousness and only then produces secondary emotional effects. Rather, the neurophysiology of pain and emotions are closely linked throughout the higher levels of the CNS. Sensory and emotional changes occur simultaneously and influence each other. Third, pain does not depend only on conscious reaction to produce motor behavior. Rather, sensory and motor elements are also closely linked at every level of the CNS, so that pain behavior is an integral part of the pain experience.

Melzack & Wall's (1965) gate control theory of pain began to crystallize these ideas. Their graphic concept of a 'gate' made it easy to understand and popularized the theory (Fig. 3.3). Stimulation of nociceptors produces impulses in peripheral nerves that then enter the dorsal column of the spinal cord. Melzack & Wall suggested that the dorsal horn then acts as a 'gate control mechanism'. Sensory information arrives in both large and small afferent fibers. Immediate, sharp pain is transmitted by large myelinated A fibers, and slow, diffuse or aching pain is transmitted by small unmyelinated C fibers. The balance of activity in these different fibers may stimulate or inhibit the next cells in the dorsal horn and so open or close the gate to transmission of impulses higher up the nervous system. Thresholds to excitation depend on preexisting levels of activity within the spinal cord. Higher CNS activity can also exert considerable influence on the gate, both by descending nerve impulses and by the release of analgesic chemicals such as endorphins.

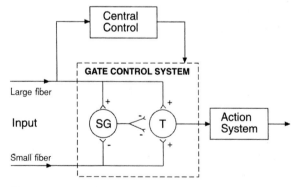

Figure 3.3 The original diagram of the gate control theory of pain in the dorsal horn of the spinal cord. SG, substantia gelatinosa; T, first central transmission neurones; +, excitation; –, inhibitory. (Reprinted from Melzack R, Wall P D Pain mechanisms: a new theory. Science 150: 971–979 copyright 1965 American Association for the Advancement of Science.)

Peripheral sensory information only triggers pain transmission after it has been modulated by both sensory feedback and higher CNS influences.

But the filtering of information at the first synapse is only the beginning of a continuous process of selection and modulation of information. It was previously thought that different parts of the CNS might serve different aspects of the pain experience. For example, the spinothalamic tract might process information about the location and sensory qualities of the pain. The brain stem, reticular formation and limbic system might be more concerned with the emotional or affective qualities of the pain. Fast dorsal column pathways and central control mechanisms at a cortical level might evaluate the sensory information, relate it to other sensory information and past experience, and then influence how all the other parts of the system deal with the incoming information. Clearly, however, there is no single pain center in the sensory cortex or in any other part of the brain. Recent studies with positron-emission tomography (PET) and functional magnetic resonance imaging have shown that many parts of the brain are active in pain states. Perhaps we are coming back to the holistic view that pain is a response of the whole human brain (Wall 1996b).

There is also a close link between afferent and efferent activity at all levels in the nervous system. Segmental reflexes can produce reflex muscle spasm or autonomic activity. Multisegmental efferents from the spinal cord and medulla may produce coordinated motor withdrawal responses. Higher CNS motor activity forms the basis of all pain behavior.

Since 1965, there have been many attacks on the neurophysiologic detail of the gate control theory, but there is now general agreement on the main events (Wall 1996a, Melzack 1996). Pain signals do not pass unaltered to the cerebral cortex, but are always and constantly modulated within the CNS before they reach consciousness. Pain, emotions and pain behavior are all integral parts of the pain experience. Both the spinal cord and the brain are best seen as a multisynaptic ascending system rather than as pain tracts. The nervous system is not like a telephone exchange, but more like a complex computer network that responds actively to incoming signals.

These concepts provide a physiologic basis for many clinical observations:

- Fundamental to all understanding of pain, they explain how the pain and suffering that we experience may diverge greatly from peripheral nociception.
- Other afferent inputs and neural activity in other parts of the CNS can greatly modify pain signals. This may explain the effects of counterirritation, acupuncture and TENS (transcutaneous electrical nerve stimulation).
- Pain transmission may be modulated by endorphins. These are chemical substances in the cerebrospinal fluid that act as analgesics like morphine. These and a number of similar substances are produced by certain cells in the CNS. The concentration rises in the cerebrospinal fluid after exercise.
- The complex neurophysiology of pain explains why surgical division of a nerve or pain tract is unlikely to give long-term relief of pain. Pain soon recurs and associated sensory disturbance may make it even more unpleasant. This kind of ablative surgery is rarely, if ever, indicated for simple backache.

There may also be neurophysiologic changes in chronic pain. The CNS is not a set of rigid electrical circuits, but rather is plastic in nature. We are all familiar with axon injury and regrowth, but there is little evidence of nerve damage in most cases of simple backache. Chronic pain may involve more functional changes in the nervous system (Devor 1996). Tissue damage or inflammation can cause peripheral sensitization of peripheral nociceptors, so that normal stimuli produce pain. Sensory neurones can become hyperexcitable and cause neuropathic pain. Central sensitization may occur in the spinal cord and higher levels of the CNS. But, crucially, in many normal people the CNS seems to adapt to continued pain and reduce its sensitivity.

Chemical and morphologic changes in the dorsal horn of the spinal cord may *either raise or lower* receptor thresholds. Summation or habituation may occur in the spinal cord. There may be abnormal electrical and chemical activity in the brain itself. The neural networks themselves can change and may be altered by neural activity itself over time. There is experimental evidence for all of these events. These changes may be lasting and could explain how pain may persist after the original peripheral stimulus has stopped. They could also account for spread, so that pain seems to come from a wider area.

However, neurophysiology alone cannot fully explain human pain. If that were all there was to it, then pain behavior would be largely a reflex response, even if modern theories of neurophysiology would let that response be quite complex. Clinical experience shows that we must also allow for mental events and psychologic influences on how people react and what they do. Modern neurophysiology explains how physiologic and psychologic events can interact, not only to influence afferent input but also to influence the pain we feel, suffering and pain behavior. But it only explains the mechanisms by which these events take place.

Modern neurophysiology certainly helps us to understand that pain is much more complex than the old Cartesian model of pain-as-a-signal. But clinical pain is a complex and subtle experience in a thinking, feeling human being. To fully understand the pain experience we must also look at emotions, psychology and human behavior. We might draw an analogy with grand prix racing: of course we must understand the internal combustion engine and the chemistry of high-octane fuel if we are to compete, but we need to know a lot more than that if we are to win the race.

Definition

Let us return to clinical pain and try to integrate these clinical and neurophysiologic ideas (Anand & Craig 1996).

- *Pain is a complex, sensory and emotional experience. It is much more than just a signal of tissue damage*
- Pain signals do not pass unaltered to the cerebral cortex. They are always and constantly modulated within the CNS before they reach consciousness
- The sensation of pain, emotions and pain behavior are all integral parts of the pain experience
- The CNS is plastic in nature, and there may be neurophysiologic changes over time with the development of chronic pain

We all know what pain is from our own experience. But if we try to define it in words it is surprisingly difficult. Most people start with examples of what causes pain rather than describing pain itself. Even when we get beyond that stage, it is difficult to define pain precisely and comprehensively. From a clinical perspective, I believe the best definition of pain is still that from the International Association for the Study of Pain (Merskey 1979):

… an unpleasant sensory and emotional experience associated with actual or potential tissue damage, or described in terms of such damage.

This is a profound statement that is the outcome of much thought and debate. Read it several times. Stop and think it through. It has many clinical implications:

- Stimulation of peripheral receptors and activity in neural pathways is not pain. Pain is always a mental state, even if we most often associate pain with such physiologic events. We experience, assess and act upon pain at a conscious level. A dentist once examined Bertrand Russell and asked: 'Where does that hurt?' 'In my mind, of course. Where else could it hurt?' replied the philosopher.
- This definition avoids tying pain to the stimulus. All pain is real to the person who suffers. It feels just the same to them whether or not we can identify tissue damage. If they regard their experience as pain and if they report it as pain, then we should accept it as pain. Attempts to separate mental and physical pain, organic and nonorganic, betray a fundamental misunderstanding of the problem. They do not help to understand the

clinical problem and will destroy our relationship with the patient. We should simply accept that pain is real to the patient and direct our efforts to understanding their pain.

- The definition lays equal weight on the sensory and emotional aspects of pain. Pain is unquestionably a sensation about a part of the body but it is also unpleasant and therefore always an emotional experience.
- Pain is a subjective and personal experience. The way in which each of us deals with and expresses our pain varies. It will depend on our experience of pain in general and this pain in particular. It will also depend on our current mental and emotional state.
- The definition allows for actual events, anticipation of possible future events, and the patient's interpretation of the pain. Anticipation and fear of pain may be as potent as pain itself.
- Because pain is so subjective, it is difficult to communicate across the barriers of language. The *way the patient reports the pain* will always be influenced by how they think and feel and by their ability and style of communication. There is a major gap in communication about pain between patients and health professionals.

Acute and chronic pain

Clinicians traditionally classify low back pain as acute or chronic. Acute pain is usually defined as being of less than 3 months' duration. Many patients have recurrent attacks, but these often continue to be like acute pain. In the past, the definition of chronic pain involved a duration of more than 6 months, which stressed its intractable nature. But 6 months may be too late to begin thinking about and dealing with chronic pain, and most workers now classify chronic pain as being of more than 3 months' duration. In terms of clinical progress and the risk of chronicity, 6 weeks may actually be a better cut-off. The key distinction is not the duration of the pain, but the persistence of chronic pain beyond expected recovery times and the intractable nature of chronic pain.

There are marked clinical differences between acute and chronic pain, which too many doctors and therapists ignore at their patients' peril. Loeser once exclaimed that 'acute and chronic pain have nothing in common but the four letter word pain'. Acute and experimental pains usually have a simple relation to nociception and tissue damage. There may be some anxiety about the meaning and future effects of acute pain, but that is easy to understand and it is not usually a major problem. Acute pain and disability are usually in proportion to the physical findings. The natural tendency of most acute pain is to recover, and physical treatment is relatively effective. Management *should* be easy.

The clinical presentation of chronic pain is very different. Chronic pain and disability often seem to become dissociated from the original physical problem. There may indeed be very little evidence of any remaining tissue damage or nociception. Instead, chronic pain and disability seem to become self-sustaining and intractable to treatment. Continued attempts to treat tissue damage do not relieve symptoms, but may actually reinforce pain and perpetuate the problem. Clinical patterns of chronic pain become complex and varied. Management is far from easy, and indeed is one of the most difficult challenges of health care.

Sternbach (1974, 1977) was one of the first to explore the differences between acute and chronic pain. He compared acute pain to the sympathetic reaction of 'fight or flight'. There is release of adrenaline; heart rate, blood pressure and blood flow increase; breathing becomes faster; palms sweat; pupils dilate. Acute pain has biologic meaning and value as a warning of tissue damage. But these changes are also characteristic of anxiety states. Sternbach argued that pain and anxiety are closely related. Treatment of acute pain tries to deal with the cause, but it should also deal with anxiety, as this can help to reduce pain. We can reduce anxiety by *repeated* explanations and reassurances. With the passage of time these autonomic responses habituate and disappear. A pattern of 'vegetative changes' now emerges. Patients often develop sleep and appetite disturbance, loss of libido and irritability. There is gradual withdrawal from social activities, and feelings of helplessness and hopelessness. Chronic pain loses its biologic meaning and purpose, and becomes counter-productive. These changes are also characteristic of depression. Sternbach believed that chronic pain is almost always accompanied by depression. We can best treat depression by rehabilitation with increasing activity, retraining and giving reasons to be hopeful.

These various observations allow us to begin to see the problem of chronic pain, but we should not overstate the distinction between acute and chronic pain. There is no absolute cut-off in time – acute pain merges into chronic pain. Only a very small proportion of back patients develop chronic intractable pain, and the rate and the manner at which this happens may vary greatly.

We will consider many of these issues in greater depth throughout this book. Suffice it to say, at this point, that we cannot understand or treat chronic back pain like the acute pain of tissue damage. We may treat acute back pain with simple physical measures and reassurance and expect early recovery. But chronic back pain persists, and is almost by definition a failure to recover properly or to respond to treatment. Hence we cannot treat it simply by continuing the management that has already failed, but must now deal with the whole pain syndrome.

Assessment of pain

Assessment of pain is a routine and basic part of clinical practice (Turk & Melzack 1992). Yet once we recognize the complexity of pain, it should be no surprise that assessment is difficult and often inadequate.

For all the reasons that we have discussed, only the patient can really assess his or her pain. Clinical assessment is only an attempt to put the patient's report into medical terms. It always remains the patient's report of his or her own symptoms, and so is open to subjective influences (Main & Burton 1995). However, the report of pain is not as straightforward as it may seem. It varies with the level of distress. It may also depend on previous encounters with health professionals, and social or cultural influences on consulting behavior. Previous failed treatment may have a profound effect on the report of pain, as may expectations about further treatment. These are not only of theoretic importance, but they also have a direct effect on how patients respond when asked about their pain. Doctors and therapists who are not aware of these issues may easily misunderstand the patient's report of pain. This is also why we must always look at pain in the context of the whole clinical picture, and not base diagnosis and management on the report of pain alone.

Anatomic distribution

We generally define low back pain as being between the lowest ribs and the inferior gluteal folds. The simplest and most reliable classification is from the Quebec Task Force (Spitzer et al 1987):

- low back pain alone
- low back pain with radiating pain into the thigh but not below the knee
- nerve root pain, with or without neurologic deficit.

Many workers feel this is too simple, but it is one of the few classifications of back pain on which different specialists and therapists can agree. It reflects the diagnostic triage in Chapter 2 and is a very practical working classification.

Selim et al (1998) tested this in practice. They found a clear clinical gradient across four groups:

- group 1 – back pain alone
- group 2 – back pain with radiating leg pain above the knee
- group 3 – back pain with leg pain below the knee
- group 4 – back pain with leg pain below the knee and a positive straight leg raising test.

Intensity of pain, level of disability, and analgesic consumption all increased from group 1 to group 4. Group 4 patients were more likely to have an MRI scan and surgery. Selim et al suggested that this simple method may be useful in assessing case mix in epidemiologic and clinical studies.

Time pattern – acute, subacute or chronic

The traditional clinical classification is (Spitzer et al 1987):

- acute: less than 6 weeks.
- subacute: 6–12 weeks.
- chronic: more than 3 months of continuous pain.

This classification rests on the assumption that patients start with an episode of acute pain that then either recovers after a varying period of time, or fails to get better and continues indefinitely. But when we look at the epidemiology, we will see that is not an accurate picture. One of the main characteristics of back pain is that it often runs a fluctuating or recurring course. An isolated acute attack with no previous history and complete recovery is rare. Most people have some previous history and many have some persisting or recurring symptoms. Each 'attack', or episode of health care, may be against a background of recurrent attacks or persisting minor symptoms. Even chronic pain usually fluctuates in intensity. The most important feature of chronic pain, perhaps, is not its duration but its impact on the patient's life and its intractable nature.

We will expand upon this classification when we consider disability, and consider further the course of back pain over time in Chapter 7.

So back pain is often neither acute nor chronic in the traditional sense of these terms, and the duration of each episode or time to remission may not give a true picture of its outcome. Von Korff et al (1993) suggested that it may be better to assess either the total days in pain over a period of time, or the characteristic severity of the episodes. For example, in one study they classified low back pain as:

- occasional – pain present on less than 30 days in the past 6 months
- frequent – pain present on more than 50% of days for the past 6 months.

Measuring pain

The real difficulty comes when we try to measure the severity of low back pain (Jensen et al 1986, Jensen & McFarland 1993). Despite the emphasis on *diagnosis* of the pathologic cause of pain, our training and practice pay little attention to the actual assessment of pain. We usually rely on clinical impressions or observer judgements of pain, but these correlate poorly with the patient's own report of pain. They are unreliable and prone to observer bias.

We can assess pain on some form of scale, by drawings or by the words patients use to describe their pain. Some form of scale is the best and probably the most widely used method for both clinical practice and research (see Figs 3.4 and 3.5). It is simple to give and to score, and most patients find it easy to use. The scale is exactly 100 mm long. To use it, ask the patient to put a mark on the scale and then measure that mark in millimetres to give a

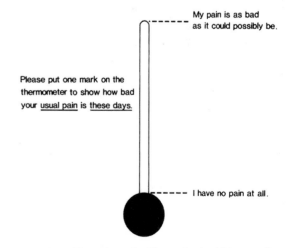

Figure 3.4 The pain scale. The scale should be exactly 100 mm long and the level marked by the patient is scored as a percentage. Some patients find it easier to mark this on a thermometer scale, but you must make sure they do not mistake this for an anatomic diagram of the back! (From Waddell 1987, with permission).

result from 0 to 100%. A diagram of a thermometer may help patients who do not understand the concept of a scale, but make sure they do not mistake this for a diagram of the spine (Fig. 3.4). The difficulty is how to interpret what the pain scale means. It is not an objective measure of pain and does not match any physiologic or pathologic change. It is still the patient's report of pain, and reflects all the influences that we have discussed. It is not clear to what extent the pain scale measures pain or distress, as the two are closely linked in clinical practice. We must not over-interpret the pain scale, but simply accept it as a measure of how bad this patient reports his or her pain to be. The pain scale may be most useful for following an individual patient's progress over time, rather than for comparing different patients.

We have little epidemiologic data about the severity of back pain. Table 3.1 presents US data from the *Nuprin Pain Report* (Taylor & Curran 1985) and Table 3.2 presents UK data from the Consumers' Association survey (1985). These findings illustrate the problem of how to interpret the pain scale. They simply tell us how these people scored their pain. Does this really tell us much more about back pain in the United States or in Britain?

The adjectives that patients use to describe their pain can assess the quality of the pain in a very crude way. The most widely used

Table 3.1 Duration and severity of back pain in American adults (based on data from Taylor & Curran 1985)

Duration (days in year)		Percentage of adults
1–5		22
6–10		7
11–30		12
31–100		6
101 or more		9

Severity	Scale (1–10)	Percentage of those with back pain
Slight	1–3	16
Moderate	4–6	44
Severe	7–9	23
Unbearable	10	14

Table 3.2 Severity of back pain in British adults (based on data from the Consumers' Association 1985)

Severity of back pain in the last 12 months on a scale of 0–10	Percentage of those who reported back pain
0 (minimal)	1
0–1	2
1–2	7
2–3	10
3–4	14
4–5	17
5–6	12
6–7	9
7–8	8
8–9	6
9–10	5
10 (intolerable)	8

method is the McGill Pain Questionnaire (Melzack 1975). There is now a shorter version (Melzack 1987) which is more practical for routine use (Fig. 3.5). The adjectives are divided broadly into those that describe the sensory qualities and those that describe the emotional qualities of the pain (Table 3.3).

Pain drawings may provide information about the anatomic distribution of the pain and a very crude estimate of the 'amount' of pain. However, they mainly provide a different kind of information that is more appropriate to consider at a later stage.

Table 3.3 Sensory and emotional adjectives for pain (from the McGill Pain Questionnaire)

Sensory	Emotional
Throbbing	Tiring
Shooting	Exhausting
Stabbing	Sickening
Sharp	Fearful
Cramping	Punishing
Gnawing	Cruel
Hot and burning	
Aching	
Heavy	
Tender	
Splitting	

Assessment of pain
- Anatomic distribution
- Time course
- Severity
- Quality

McGill Pain Questionnaire
Please tick those adjectives that describe your pain, as mild, moderate or severe.

	None	Mild	Moderate	Severe
Throbbing				
Shooting				
Stabbing				
Sharp				
Cramping				
Gnawing				
Hot – burning				
Aching				
Heavy				
Tender				
Splitting				
Tiring – exhausting				
Sickening				
Fearful				
Punishing – cruel				

Visual analog scale

No pain |————————————————————————————| Worst possible pain

Present pain intensity
0 – no pain
1 – mild
2 – discomforting
3 – distressing
4 – horrible
5 – excruciating

Scoring
Adjectives 1–11 are 'sensory' and adjectives 12–15 are 'emotional'. Score each adjective: none = 0, mild = 1, moderate = 2, severe = 3. Add the sensory and emotional scores separately.
  The visual analog scale and present pain intensity scale are also included to provide overall pain intensity scores. The visual analog scale is exactly 100 mm long and the score is measured by ruler.

Figure 3.5 The short form of the McGill Pain Questionnaire. (From Melzack R, The short-form McGill Pain Questionnaire, Pain 30; 191–197, 1987, with kind permission from Elsevier Science, NL, Sara Burgerhartstraat 25, 1055 KV, Amsterdam, the Netherlands.)

DISABILITY

I have tried to emphasize that pain and disability are not the same (see Table 3.4). This is so fundamental and important that I will repeat it without apology.

Definition

Disability is restricted activity. Martinat (1966) defined disability as 'diminished capacity for everyday activities and gainful employment'.

Garrad & Bennett (1971) compared it with normal: the 'limitation of a patient's performance compared to a fit person of the same age and sex'. The most comprehensive definition is by the World Health Organization (WHO) (1980):

A disability is any restriction or lack (resulting from an impairment) of ability to perform an activity in the manner or within the range considered normal for a human being.

There are a number of assumptions in the WHO definition. It assumes that the normal is to have

Table 3.4 Low back disability among those with back pain for at least 2 weeks (based on data from Deyo & Tsui-Wu 1987)

Self-rated pain	Percentage who reduced activities	Mean days work loss per annum	Mean days in bed per annum
Mild	40	11	4
Moderate	54	18	7
Severe	55	34	13

no disability or restriction of any kind, which is not completely true. It assumes that disability is 'due to an impairment' and is often taken to imply that disability is a health problem, which is not always true. We will come back to that later. The core of all the definitions is that disability is restricted activity.

Administrative definitions for the purpose of compensation are mainly about capacity for work. The US Social Security Administration (US Bureau of Disability Insurance 1970) defines disability as 'inability to engage in any substantially gainful activity by reason of a medically determinable physical or mental impairment'. But incapacity for work is only one aspect of disability. Unfortunately, every official body seems to feel the need to introduce its own terms and definitions for disability. These do not help us to understand the problem, although you must obviously learn and use the terms where you work.

WHO (1980) also defines handicap, as follows:

A handicap is a disadvantage for a given individual, resulting from an impairment or a disability, that limits or prevents the fulfilment of a role that is normal (depending on age, sex, social and cultural factors) for that individual.

The WHO definitions apply best to an objective physical impairment such as a fused knee due to a fracture or infection. The resulting disability is then loss of flexion of the knee and inability to squat or kneel, and the handicap is, for example, the individual's inability to work as a plumber. This fits the WHO scheme of cause and effect:

Physical impairment → disability → handicap

Unfortunately, this approach does not work well for pain. As we have already stressed, pain is a symptom, not an objective impairment. Chronic back pain, disability and handicap are

all subjective and difficult to measure. They depend on many influences as well as pain. In this context, the distinction between disability and handicap is more philosophic than real. 'I have backache. I avoid bending. I cannot walk more than 50 yards. I cannot work. And I have lost my job.' Is that disability or handicap? Which is which? In clinical practice we cannot distinguish what the patient is unable to do from what he or she does not do. All that we can assess is his or her performance, not capability. This person does not bend or walk more than 50 yards and he or she attributes these restrictions to back pain. He or she is restricted bending, walking and working. Disability is restricted activity and that is his or her disability; or, to be more precise, that is their report of his or her disability.

Clinical assessment of disability

We have already seen the problems of measuring pain, and to some extent we encounter the same problems with disability. Once again we depend largely on the patient's own report, which is subject to the same influences. Despite that, we can define and assess disability better than pain. Measures of disability are more reliable and give a more valid account of what we are trying to measure. This is perhaps because reports of disability simply require a description of concrete events, while reports of pain depend on complex evaluation of subjective experiences. Many research groups around the world now agree that the best way to assess low back disability is to base the assessment on activities of daily living, which gives a direct measure of basic activity. Back pain may affect many daily activities, such as bending and lifting, sitting, standing, walking, traveling, socializing, sleeping, sex and dressing. A few simple questions can give an accurate picture of the impact of back pain on the patient's life.

When asking about disability, you must focus on limited activity rather than pain. Your questions should be clear and precise. The key question is 'Are you actually restricted in that activity?' rather than 'Is that activity painful?' Other useful questions are: 'Does your back limit how much you do?' and 'Do you now require help with that activity?' Any restriction must be from the onset of back pain and must be due to back pain. You should note the common or usual effect, not occasional effects or special efforts. Our studies (Waddell & Main 1984) have shown that the clinical interview can give a reliable assessment of disability in activities of daily living. We found that the following limits are most useful for low back pain:

- Bending and lifting – help required or avoids heavy lifting (30–40 pounds, a heavy suitcase or a 3- to 4-year-old child)
- Sitting – sitting in an ordinary chair generally limited to less than 30 minutes at a time before needing to get up and move around
- Standing – standing in one place generally limited to less than 30 minutes at a time before needing to move around
- Walking – walking generally limited to less than 30 minutes or 1–2 miles at a time before needing to rest
- Traveling – traveling in a car or bus generally limited to less than 30 minutes at a time before needing to stop and have a break
- Socializing – regularly miss or curtail social activities and normal social mobility (not sports which are a very different level of disability)
- Sleeping – sleep regularly disturbed by pain, i.e. two or three times per week
- Sex life – reduced frequency of sexual activity because of pain
- Dressing – help regularly required with footwear (tights, socks or shoelaces).

Simple yes or no answers about each of these activities give a basic disability score out of nine that is sufficient for clinical purposes.

This may seem over-simplified, but the scale is robust and useful in clinical practice. Despite, or because of, its simplicity, it compares well with more elaborate disability questionnaires (Beurskens et al 1995). If you wish, you can build up a complete disability evaluation on the basic scale. You can explore the exact limit in each of the nine basic activities and how that affects the patient's work, home and leisure activities. You obtain and record this information but you must always remember that it is the patient's own subjective report of disability.

Disability questionnaires

Patients can give the same information on a disability questionnaire. These questionnaires are suitable for routine clinical use, but also give high-quality information for research. They are more consistent and reliable than interviews because they present the questions in exactly the same way to every patient, every time. Millard & Jones (1991) looked at four different questionnaires and found that they all gave comparable, though slightly different, measures of low back disability.

The two most widely used measures of low back disability are the Oswestry (Fairbank et al 1980) and Roland questionnaires (Roland & Morris 1983). The Roland questionnaire (Box 3.1) was developed from the Sickness Impact Profile, which is a widely used, general disability questionnaire. Several independent studies have confirmed the value of the Roland questionnaire. Deyo (1986) and Jensen et al (1992) compared the Roland questionnaire with the original Sickness Impact Profile. They found that it was simpler, quicker and easier to use, but that it gave very similar results in both acute and chronic low back pain. It gave a sensitive measure of change both during recovery from the acute attack and following treatment of chronic pain.

Roberts (1991) directly compared the Roland and Oswestry questionnaires. He found that the Roland questionnaire was simpler, faster and more acceptable to patients. He agreed with Deyo that it provides a more sensitive

---

Box 3.1 The Roland disability questionnaire (from Roland & Morris 1983, with permission)

When your back hurts, you may find it difficult to do some of the things you normally do.

This list contains some sentences that people have used to describe themselves when they have back pain. When you read them, you may find that some stand out because they describe you *today*. As you read the list, think of yourself *today*. When you read a sentence that describes you today, put a tick against it. If the sentence does not describe you, then leave the space blank and go to the next one. Remember, only tick the sentence if you are sure it describes you today.

1. I stay at home most of the time because of my back.
2. I change position frequently to try and get my back comfortable.
3. I walk more slowly than usual because of my back.
4. Because of my back I am not doing any of the jobs that I usually do around the house.
5. Because of my back, I use a handrail to get upstairs.
6. Because of my back, I lie down to rest more often.
7. Because of my back, I have to hold on to something to get out of an easy chair.
8. Because of my back, I try to get to get other people to do things for me.
9. I get dressed more slowly than usual because of my back.
10. I only stand for short periods of time because of my back.
11. Because of my back, I try not to bend or kneel down.
12. I find it difficult to get out of a chair because of my back.
13. My back is painful almost all the time.
14. I find it difficult to turn over in bed because of my back.
15. My appetite is not very good because of my back pain.
16. I have trouble putting on my socks (or stockings) because of the pain in my back.
17. I only walk short distances because of my back pain.
18. I sleep less well because of my back.
19. Because of my back pain, I get dressed with help from someone else.
20. I sit down for most of the day because of my back.
21. I avoid heavy jobs around the house because of my back.
22. Because of my back pain, I am more irritable and bad tempered with people than usual.
23. Because of my back, I go upstairs more slowly than usually.
24. I stay in bed most of the time because of my back.

---

measure of early and acute disability. It gives the best measure of recovery or the early development of chronic pain and disability. Its main disadvantage is that it is less able to measure very severe levels of chronic disability. I believe that the Roland low back disability questionnaire is the best that is available at present, for most clinical use and research.

Classification of chronic pain and disability

Chronic low back pain is not the same as chronic pain-related disability. It may be better to classify by pain and functional outcome over time.

Von Korff et al (1992) have developed a simple method of grading the severity of chronic pain and disability. They originally designed this for population studies and tested it on 2389 American patients. They used pain intensity, disability, duration and persistency to give a simple grading into:

- grade I: low disability – low intensity back pain.

- grade II: low disability – high intensity back pain.
- grade III: high disability – moderately limiting back pain.
- grade IV: high disability – severely limiting back pain.

Cassidy et al (1997) studied 1133 adults in the general population in Canada. Seventy-two per cent reported some back symptoms during the past 6 months: 48.2%, grade I; 12.4%, grade II; 7.2%, grade III; and 4.7%, grade IV.

This takes us back to our classification of acute, recurring and chronic pain. The importance of chronic pain is not simply the duration of the pain but its impact on the patient's life. Von Korff's classification reflects the severity and impact of chronic pain and the importance of both pain and disability.

Functional capacity evaluation (FCE)

All of these clinical methods, whether interviews or questionnaires, are limited by their dependence on the patient's own subjective report of his or her disability. In principle, we should be able to get a more objective measure of disability by independent observation of the patient's performance.

Functional capacity evaluation (FCE) attempts to do this (Blankenship 1986, Hart et al 1993, Yeomans & Liebenson 1996). FCE measures whole body ability and limitations such as cardiovascular fitness, lifting capacity and fitness for work. It puts the patient through a standard protocol of physical tasks while a trained observer records their performance and limitations. It is simple, safe, and 'low-tech' and gives reliable results. It contains tests and checks that try to determine if the patient is cooperating fully and exerting maximum effort. The report is in a standard format, and contains normal population values for comparison. It can be used to describe clinical progress and outcomes, to prescribe rehabilitation needs and goals, and for vocational assessment.

Unfortunately, despite these advantages, FCE also has limitations. Although it is standardized and much better than 'clinical impression', it is not as wholly objective as some of its advocates claim. There are many competing systems of FCE. Reducing clinical observations to numbers sometimes gives a spurious impression of accuracy. FCE is also misnamed: it is an evaluation not of capacity, but of performance, so it still depends on effort. I also have doubts about some of the methods used in FCE to assess effort and symptom magnification which will become clearer in later chapters.

Harding et al (1994) developed a simple functional capacity evaluation for severely disabled patients with a variety of chronic pain problems. A simplified version they now use in routine clinical practice (VR Harding, personal communication) is shown in Box 3.2. They showed that these tests are reliable and are sensitive to change after a chronic pain management program. Other patient groups may be fitter and show different values.

Several studies in back pain are now using the *shuttle walk test* alone (Box 3.3). This is

---

Box 3.2 A simple clinical functional capacity evaluation

The test area should be quiet and free of passing people. Put up warning signs for staff and other patients when tests are taking place. The patient should not need to walk a long distance to reach the test area or between the different tests. Ask the patient to wear comfortable shoes and loose clothing.
- *Five minutes of walking.* The distance walked up and down between marks 20 m apart in 5 min. Choose a quiet, empty corridor with a non-slip surface or hard carpet. There should be walls or doors on either side that can be used if necessary for support, but not handrails. Patients should not use walking aids but can use the walls for support or can sit down for a rest. Inform the patient of the time at the end of each lap or every minute if they are slower (mean, 185 m).
- *One minute of stair climbing.* Climbing up and down a straight flight of standard stairs with one handrail and an opposite wall within easy reach. Have a chair available for resting if the patient needs it. Count the number of steps up and down, e.g. 20 up + 15 down = 35 steps (mean, 48 steps).
- *One minute of stand-ups.* The number of times the patient can stand up from a chair in 1 min. Use a firm, upright chair with a padded seat and back rest but no arm rests. The seat height should be about 45 cm, or 18 inches. There should not be any wall or other furniture within reach that the patient could use for support (mean, 11 stand-ups).

Standardization of test instructions. The tester should have written instructions. The tester must respond neutrally at all times and maintain a 'test' atmosphere. Do not give the patient any advice or encouragement during the tests as feedback influences their performance. Only give information on the time to help patients to pace themselves if they are able. Tell the patient this is a test of current performance. It is a measure of how much they can manage, bearing in mind the journey home after their assessment. These instructions are designed to prevent anxiety and over-exertion.

Box 3.3 The shuttle walk test

The patient walks up and down a 10 m course, round two cones inset 0.5 m from either end to avoid the need for abrupt changes in direction. On the first test the patient has to walk 30 m in 1 min. The speed of walking is increased by 10 m each minute, so that in the 12th minute they have to walk 140 m. The end of the test is either when the patient decides to stop due to fatigue or back symptoms, or when the observer finds they have not met the target speed. The observer then simply counts the total number of meters the patient has managed to walk in that time.

again a general measure of fitness or disability (Singh et al 1992). Fogg & Taylor (1997) found the shuttle walk test to be simple, reliable and to give a sensitive measure of response to treatment for back pain.

Such assessments can give a more objective measure for comparison with the patient's own subjective report. They can measure the patient's performance at a particular point in time in a structured setting, but they cannot overcome the basic limitation that we can only observe what the patient does, and this does not tell us what he or she is able to do or what he or she should be able to do. Capacity may be limited by physiology, but performance is limited by psychology. What the patient does or does not do will always depend on effort and motivation. Even the most 'objective' assessment is not of actual capacity but of the patient's performance.

Work loss

Most health care focuses on relief of symptoms. The most important health outcome, however, is not any clinical measure of pain or disability, but rather how the illness affects the patient's life. The single most crucial impact of low back pain is on ability to work, which pervades all other aspects. For working patients, time off work, loss of earnings and loss of their job have the greatest ill-effects on them and their family. It is also the most important measure of the social impact of back pain on employers, the economy and social costs. This is the reason for political interest in back pain. For all these reasons, work loss is the most important measure of low back disability.

Work loss does have limitations as a measure of disability and outcome. Work loss is only weakly related to clinical measures of pain or disability. It only applies to the working population. It misses low back disability in the young, the elderly, housewives and those with other disabilities. Work loss only measures more severe disability and only one aspect of disability due to back pain. It misses lesser degrees of disability and finer aspects of work such as limited duties, lower productivity, loss of overtime and

loss of promotion. The greatest problem is that work loss and return to work depend on other influences as well as pain and disability – many of which have nothing to do with illness or health care. These influences include the demands and conditions of the person's job, ability to modify the job, and job satisfaction. They also include job availability, local economic conditions, alternative sources of income, compensation and closeness to retirement age.

We can measure loss of time from work easily and accurately. We can check sickness records. Work loss, sick certificates and receipt of state benefit, however, are not the same thing. Most people with work loss of more than a few days do also get some form of medical sick certification. Payment of benefit, however, depends on entitlement to benefit. As a result, many people may lose time from work yet not be entitled to benefits and therefore are not included in official statistics. On the other hand, patients may get sick certificates and benefits without work loss, e.g. if they are unemployed.

Despite these limitations, there is growing agreement that work loss is the single most important social measure of low back disability and health care (Spitzer et al 1987, Fordyce 1995). That is not to argue that pain does not matter, or that we should relabel back pain as 'activity intolerance'. It does mean, however, that we must look at both pain and disability.

Assessment of disability
• Activities of daily living • Questionnaires • Functional capacity evaluation • Work loss • Capacity for work

CONCLUSION

Pain, disability and work loss are inextricably linked, but the relationship between them is subtle and complex and influenced by many factors. We must make a clear distinction between pain and disability, and assess each separately. We may ask patients to keep a pain diary linking pain severity, medication use, sleep and activity patterns over a week or two, and this may give insight into how these are related. Understanding the other influences that link low back pain and disability will take us a long way toward understanding the clinical problem and our present epidemic.

REFERENCES

Anand K J S, Craig K D 1996 New perspectives on the definition of pain. Pain 67: 3–6

Beurskens A J, de Vet H C, Koke A J, van der Heijden G J, Knipschild P G 1995 Measuring the functional status of patients with low back pain: assessment of the quality of four disease-specific questionnaires. Spine 20: 1017–1028

Blankenship S K 1986 Functional Capacity Evaluation: the procedure manual. American Therapeutics, Macon, GA

Cassidy J D, Carroll L, Cote P, Senthilselvan A 1997 The prevalence of graded chronic low back pain severity and its effect on general health: a population based study. Presented to the International Society for the Study of the Lumbar Spine, Singapore: 8

Consumers' Association 1985 Back pain survey. Consumers' Association, London

Descartes R 1644 L'homme (transl. by Foster M). Cambridge University Press, New York

Devor M 1996 Pain mechanisms and pain syndromes. In: Pain – an updated review. International Association for the Study of Pain Refresher Course. IASP Press, Seattle, p 103–112

Deyo R A 1986 Comparative validity of the sickness impact profile and shorter scales for functional assessment in low back pain. Spine 11: 951–954

Deyo R A, Tsui-Wu Y-J 1987 Functional disability due to back pain. Arthritis and Rheumatism 30: 1247–1253

Engel G L 1959 Psychogenic pain and the pain prone patient. American Journal of Medicine 26: 899–918

Fairbank J C T, Mbaot J C, Davies J B, O'Brien J P 1980 The Oswestry low back pain disability questionnaire. Physiotherapy 66: 271–273

Fogg A J B, Taylor A E 1997 The usefulness of the shuttle walk test in a population of low back pain patients. Presented to the International Society for the Study of the Lumbar Spine, Singapore: 21

Fordyce W E 1995. Back pain in the workplace: management of disability in nonspecific conditions. IASP Press, Seattle, p 1–75

Foster M 1901 Lectures on the history of physiology during the sixteenth, seventeenth and eighteenth centuries. Cambridge University Press, Cambridge (translated from Descartes R 1664 L'homme)

Garrad J, Bennett A E 1971 A validated interview schedule for use in population surveys of chronic disease and disability. British Journal of Preventive and Social Medicine 25: 97–104

Harding V R, Williams A C, Richardson P H, et al 1994 The development of a battery of measures for assessing physical functioning of chronic pain patients. Pain 58: 367–375

Hart D L, Isernhagen S J, Matheson L N 1993 Guidelines for functional capacity evaluation of people with medical conditions. Journal of Orthopedic and Sports Physical Therapy 18: 682–686

Jensen M P, Karoly P, Braver S 1986 The measurement of clinical pain intensity: a comparison of six methods. Pain 27: 117–126

Jensen M P, McFarland C A 1993 Increasing the reliability and validity of pain intensity measurement in chronic pain patients. Pain 55: 195–203

Jensen M P, Strom S E, Turner J A, Romano J M 1992 Validity of the Sickness Impact Profile Roland scale as a measure of dysfunction in chronic pain patients. Pain 50: 157–162

Lewis T 1942 Pain. Macmillan, New York

Liebeskind J C, Melzack R 1987 The International Pain Foundation: meeting a need for education in pain management (Editorial). Pain 30: 1–2

Loeser J D 1980 Perspectives on pain. In: Turner P (ed) Clinical Pharmacy and therapeutics. Macmillan, London, p 313–316

Main C J, Burton A K 1995 The patient with low back pain: who or what are we assessing? An experimental investigation of a pain puzzle. Pain Reviews 2: 203–209

Martinat E H 1966 Evaluation of permanent impairment of the spine. Journal of Bone and Joint Surgery 48A: 1204–1210

Melzack R 1975 The McGill pain questionnaire; major properties and scoring methods. Pain 1: 277–299

Melzack R 1987 The short-form McGill Pain Questionnaire. Pain 30: 191–197

Melzack R 1996 Gate control theory: on the evolution of pain concepts. Pain Forum 5: 128–138

Melzack R, Wall P D 1965 Pain mechanisms: a new theory. Science 150: 971–979

Merskey R 1979 Pain terms: a list with definitions and notes on usage. Pain 6: 249–252

Millard R W, Jones R H 1991 Construct validity of practical questionnaires for assessing disability of low back pain. Spine 16: 835–838

Penfield W 1969 Foreword. In: White J, Sweet W H (eds) Pain and the neurosurgeon. CC Thomas, Springfield, Illinois

Roberts A 1991 The conservative treatment of low back pain. MD thesis, University of Nottingham

Roland M, Morris R 1983 A study of the natural history of back pain. Part I: development of a reliable and sensitive measure of disability in low back pain. Spine 8: 141–144

Selim A J, Ren S R, Fincke G, Deyo R A, Rogers W, Miller D R, Linzer M, Kazis L 1998 The importance of radiating leg pain in assessing health outcomes among patients with low back pain: results from the Veterans Health Study. Spine 23: 470–474

Singh S J, Morgan M D L, Scott S, Walters D, Hardman A E 1992 Development of a shuttle walking test of disability in patients with chronic airways obstruction. Thorax 47: 1019–1024

Spitzer W O, Leblanc F E, Dupuis M, et al 1987 Scientific approach to the assessment and management of activity-related spinal disorders. A monograph for physicians. Report of the Quebec Task Force on spinal disorders. Spine 12: 7S: s1–s59

Sternbach R A 1974 Pain patients: traits and treatment. Academic Press, New York

Sternbach R A 1977 Psychological aspects of chronic pain. Clinical Orthopaedics and Related Research 129: 150–155

Taylor H, Curran N M 1985 The Nuprin pain report. Louis Harris and Associates, New York, p 1–233

Turk D C, Melzack R (ed) 1992 Handbook of pain assessment. Guilford Press, New York

US Bureau of Disability Insurance 1970 Disability evaluation under social security. A handbook for physicians. US Government Printing Office, Washington DC

von Korff M, Ormel J, Keefe F, Dworkin S F 1992 Grading the severity of chronic pain. Pain 50: 133–149

von Korff M, Deyo R A, Cherkin D, Barlow W 1993 Back pain in primary care: outcomes at one year. Spine 18: 855–862

Waddell G, Main C J 1984 Assessment of severity in low back disorders. Spine 9: 204–208

Waddell G 1987 Clinical assessment of lumbar impairment. Clinical orthopaedics and related research 221: 110–120

Wall P D 1988 The John J Bonica distinguished lecture: stability and instability of central pain mechanisms. In: Dubner R, Gebhart G, Bond M (eds) Proceedings of the Vth world congress on pain. Elsevier, Amsterdam, p 13–24

Wall P D 1996a Comments after 30 years of the gate control theory. Pain Forum 5: 12–22

Wall P D 1996b The mechanisms by which tissue damage and pain are related. In: Pain 1996 – an updated review. International Association for the Study of Pain Refresher Course. IASP Press, Seattle: 123–126

WHO 1980 International classification of impairments, disabilities and handicaps. World Health Organization, Geneva

Yeomans S G, Liebenson C 1996 Quantitative functional capacity evaluation: the missing link to outcomes assessment. Topics in Clinical Chiropractic 3: 32–43

4

Back pain through history

Gordon Waddell   David B. Allan

Back pain is not new. Human beings have had back pain throughout recorded history, and probably long before. So what has changed? How did back pain become such a problem? Let us try to put our present epidemic into historic perspective (Allan & Waddell 1989).

UNDERSTANDING AND MANAGEMENT OF BACK PAIN

The symptom of pain in the back is the common link between the simple backache that most people have at some time in their life, a number of serious spinal diseases and low back disability. We should try to keep these different perspectives in mind as we look at the history of back pain.

The oldest surviving surgical text is the Edwin Smith papyrus from about 1500 BC (Fig. 4.1). It is a series of 48 case histories, the last of which is an acute back strain (Breasted 1930):

Examination. If thou examinest a man having a sprain in a vertebra of his spinal column, thou shouldst say to him: extend now thy two legs and contract them both again. When he extends them both he contracts them both immediately because of the pain he causes in a vertebra of the spinal column in which he suffers.
   Diagnosis. Thou shouldst say to him: One having a sprain in the vertebra of his spinal column. An ailment I shall treat.
   Treatment. Thou shouldst place him prostrate on his back; thou shouldst make for him...

At this tantalizing point the unknown Egyptian scribe died and the papyrus lay in his

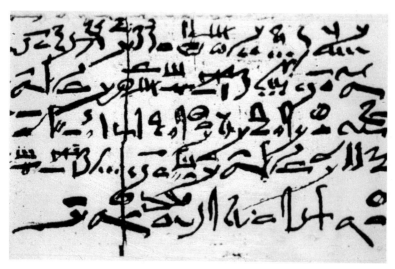

Figure 4.1 The oldest surviving description of back pain. The Edwin Smith papyrus (c. 1500 BC). (From Breasted 1930, with permission.)

tomb for almost 3500 years. This is an early 20th century translation that reflects thinking at that time, but the accuracy of the clinical description only adds to our frustration. We do not know what the ancient Egyptians thought about back pain or how they treated it. The ambiguity of the last sentence is particularly frustrating when we look at the modern debate about rest or staying active. From the contemporary evidence, however, it is unlikely this was a prescription of rest. It is more likely to have been the start of some form of local application or manual therapy.

The *Corpus Hippocraticus* (c. 400 BC) is the collected writings of the Greek library at Cos and Cnidus. It includes reports of spinal deformities and fractures, and discusses pain in the back in that context. Back pain itself received little attention.

The writings of Galen (c. 150 AD) and his disciples dominated medicine for the next 1200 years. Galen thought that disease was due to disturbed 'humors' and treatment was empiric. Back pain was a symptom of many illnesses but also one of the 'fleeting' pains affecting joints and muscles. Treatment was symptomatic with spas, soothing local applications and counterirritants. When the Graeco-Roman Empire fell,

exiled Christians took medical learning to Persia. The Arab world preserved that knowledge and reintroduced it to Europe after the Dark Ages, but Islamic laws banned dissection and frowned on surgery, which largely limited them to the preservation of the ancient writings.

Medical thought almost ceased during the Dark Ages as patient care moved into the hands of the church. Monks saved the ancient writings but only in degenerate forms. Back pain was a matter for folk medicine. The Welsh 'shot of the elf' and the German 'witch's shot' reflected beliefs that pain was due to external influences.

Modern Western medicine began with the Renaissance. The scientific method used careful observation to unlock Nature's secrets by the power of human reason rather than by religious revelation. Studies of anatomy, physiology and pathology laid the foundation. Paracelsus (1493–1541) was one of the leaders of the rebellion against the ancient writings. He began clinical freedom by treating each patient on the basis of his own observation and diagnosis. Sydenham (1624–1689) made a clear distinction between illness and underlying disease, and introduced our present concept of clinical syndromes. They should be 'reduced to certain and determinate kinds with the same exactness as we see it done by botanic writers in the treatises of plants'. Diagnosis depends on 'certain distinguishing signs which Nature has particularly affixed to every species'. Sydenham classified back pain or lumbago with the rheumatic diseases. The word rheumatism came from the Greek *rheuma*, a watery discharge or evil humor that flowed from the brain to cause pain in the joints or other parts of the body.

Modern use of the term rheumatism started in the 17th century. At that time it included what we now recognize as many musculoskeletal disorders ranging from acute rheumatic fever to arthritis. The only common feature was pain in the joints or muscles. Doctors at that time thought that rheumatism was due to cold and damp. They did not relate it to trauma. Gradually, different workers identified a number of diseases within this group. Sydenham, who himself suffered from gout, distinguished gout from acute rheumatism and described lumbago as a third form of rheumatism.

By 1800, physicians began to look for a cause for back pain. They suggested that it was due to a build-up of rheumatic phlegm in the muscles, so they used both local and systemic treatment to remove the phlegm. Scudamore (1816) published the first systematic treatise on chronic rheumatism. He blamed inflammation of the white fibrous tissue of the body 'unaccompanied by fever but aggravated by motion'. They still thought the inflammation was due to cold and damp. Throughout the 19th century, treatment of back pain was by general measures against rheumatism such as relief of constipation, counter irritants, blistering and cupping. The theory was now to remove the rheumatic exudi from the affected area. Surgeons removed septic foci in the teeth, toenails and bowel.

Two key ideas in the 19th century laid the foundations for our modern approach to back pain: that it comes from the spine and that it is due to trauma. In 1828 a physician called Brown in Glasgow Royal Infirmary published a paper on *spinal irritation* (Fig. 4.2). Brown suggested for the first time that the vertebral column and the nervous system could be the source of back pain. He also described local

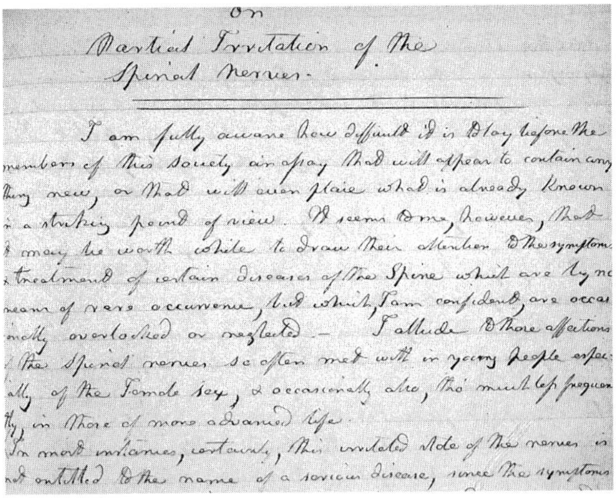
On
Partial Irritation of the
Spinal Nerves.

I am fully aware how difficult it is to lay before the members of this Society an essay that will appear to contain any thing new, or that will even place what is already known in a striking point of view. It seems to me, however, that it may be worth while to draw their attention to the symptoms & treatment of certain diseases of the Spine which are by no means of rare occurrence, but which, I am confident, are occasionally overlooked or neglected — I allude to those affections of the Spinal nerves so often met with in young people especially of the Female sex, & occasionally also, tho' much less frequently, in those of more advanced life.
In most instances, certainly, this irritated state of the nerves is not entitled to the name of a serious disease, since the symptoms

Figure 4.2 Spinal irritation. The copper plate minutes of Brown's original presentation to the Glasgow Medical Society in January 1923. (With thanks to the Royal College of Physicians and Surgeons of Glasgow.)

spinal tenderness. The concept of spinal irritation swept the US and Europe, and held sway for about 30 years. For a time, nervous 'irritability' got a kind of spurious legitimacy because it was compared with inflammation. However, inflammation was a local condition with objective features; irritation was only a hypothesis based on distant, subjective complaints. Spinal irritation had a profound effect on medicine. Neither Brown nor his followers ever demonstrated its pathology and the diagnosis gradually fell into disrepute. But spinal irritation introduced the idea that the spine is the source of back pain; and the idea that a painful spine must somehow be irritable lingers in our subconscious to this day.

It is difficult for us to believe that all through history neither doctors nor patients thought that back pain was due to injury. This idea only came in the latter half of the 19th century. The industrial revolution, and particularly the building of the railways, led to a spate of serious injuries. Violent trauma could cause spinal fractures and paralysis, so perhaps less serious injuries to the spine might be the cause of simple backache. There might be cumulative or repetitive trauma. Some people even thought that the speed and nature of early railway travel could damage human health.

Erichsen (1866) described the condition and named it *railway spine* (Fig. 4.3; Keller & Chappell 1996). He suggested that severe jarring or shaking of the spine and nervous system could disturb spinal cord function, and compared it to disturbed mental function after concussion of the brain. It might be a form of molecular derangement, so it was impossible to demonstrate. Alternatively, there might be an insidious and even more ominous disorder. A slight blow to the spine could lead to meningitis or myelitis with back pain, motor or sensory disturbance in the arms or legs, and mental symptoms of confusion and lassitude. Railway spine was a syndrome of subjective weakness and disability. As you might expect, noone ever confirmed its pathology and this diagnosis also eventually fell into disrepute. Railway spine, like spinal irritation, was a key act in this story that we will see again. Suffice it to say that, for the first time, it linked back pain to trauma. Most health professionals and patients still regard back pain as an injury.

Sciatica

The word sciatica has been in use from Greek times, and is derived from ischias or pain around, or coming from, the hip and thigh. Before modern ideas of pathology, it did not mean pain in the distribution of the sciatic nerve.

Hippocrates (460–370 BC) noted that 'ischiatic' pain mainly affected men aged 40–60 years. In younger men it usually lasted 40 days. Radiation of pain to the foot had a good prognosis but they dreaded pain that stayed in the hip (this was probably tuberculosis or another serious disease of the hip joint). Areteus (150 AD) first distinguished nervous and arthritic 'schiatica'. He blamed nervous sciatica on an excess of cold and suggested that the remedy was local heat. They again used spas, soothing ointments and counter irritants. This theory culminated in the use of cautery (Fig. 4.4).

ON

RAILWAY AND OTHER INJURIES

OF THE

NERVOUS SYSTEM.

BY

JOHN ERIC ERICHSEN,

FELLOW OF THE ROYAL COLLEGE OF SURGEONS,

Professor of Surgery and of Clinical Surgery in University College;
Surgeon to University College Hospital;
Examiner in Surgery at the University of London;
and formerly so at the
University of Durham, and the Royal College of Physicians.

"JE RACONTE, JE NE JUGE PAS."
MONTAIGNE.

LONDON:
WALTON AND MABERLY,
137, GOWER STREET; AND 27, IVY LANE, PATERNOSTER ROW.
1866.

Figure 4.3 Erichsen's classic description of railway spine. (With thanks to the Royal College of Physicians and Surgeons of Glasgow.)

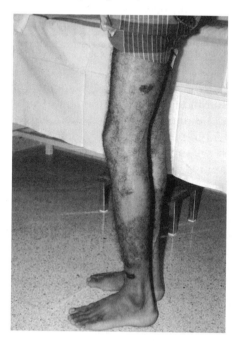

Figure 4.4 Cautery with a red hot iron is still in use in parts of the world today. See the S1 distribution.

Hippocrates first mentioned cautery and it appears throughout the ancient writings. 'Dung cautery' was in use from 100 AD and probably came from Arabic cauterization with goat's dung. Albucasis (1100 AD) described local and wrist cautery for sciatica and drew a number of the instruments.

Domenico Cotugno (1765) wrote the first book on sciatica (Boni et al 1994). He combined new knowledge of anatomy and pathology with clinical observation. He separated nervous and arthritic sciatica and divided nervous sciatica into anterior and posterior types. He knew that the condition could be continuous or intermittent. He noted that sometimes the continuous became intermittent but never the other way around. Apart from Hippocrates' note that most attacks recover in 40 days, this was one of the first observations on the natural history of recovery. Cotugno thought that sciatica was due to an excess of fluid surrounding the nerve, which is not surprising as he also gave the first description of the dural sac and cerebrospinal fluid. His treatment was to remove the excess fluid by cupping, blistering and aquapuncture (sic) which put needles into the nerve itself to draw off the excess fluid. For many years sciatica was known as Cotugno's disease.

In the 19th century, sciatica, like back pain, was thought to be a kind of rheumatism. There was inflammation of the sciatic nerve that was either primary or secondary. Primary causes included gout, rheumatism, syphilis, neuromata, poisons, trauma and cold. Secondary causes included pelvic tumors, a distended rectum and bone disease, especially hip joint disease. This shows the new emphasis on identifiable pathology. But they still did not understand sciatica itself. In 1852 Fuller wrote a book on rheumatism, rheumatic gout and sciatica. He felt that 'the history of sciatica is, it must be confessed, the record of pathologic ignorance and therapeutic failure'.

Orthopedic principles

Modern medical treatment for back pain is closely linked to the emergence of the specialty of orthopedics.

Early orthopedics was mainly about childhood deformities, and orthopedics first took an interest in sciatica because of sciatic scoliosis. From these roots, orthopedics expanded in the second half of the 19th century to include all musculoskeletal problems. Interest in spinal deformities extended to sciatica and back pain, and focused on the spine. Previously, back pain and sciatica were regarded as separate diseases. From now on they were linked in the spine. Since that time, failure to distinguish our concepts and treatment of back pain and sciatica has caused much confusion which continues to this day.

There was no precedent for the scale of casualties in World War I. For the first time, medical concern with trauma matched previous concern with disease. It also brought the treatment of fractures within the scope of orthopedics. Between the two world wars orthopedic surgeons struggled to gain control of fractures and trauma and so expand their professional practice. They also stressed that back pain was an injury and hence within the growing province of orthopedics.

The discovery of X-rays opened up a whole new perspective on back pain. For the first time it was possible to visualize the spine during life. Soon, every incidental radiographic finding became a cause of back pain and sciatica. They blamed lumbosacral anomalies, facet joint degeneration and sacroiliac disease. The 1920s and early 1930s saw operations to correct these anomalies by sacroiliac fusion, lumbosacral fusion, transversectomy and facetectomy. The problem of back pain remained intractable.

In Britain, the father of modern orthopedics was Hugh Owen Thomas, who was a qualified medical practitioner from Liverpool (Fig. 4.5). He came from a long line of Welsh bone setters but worked with his father for less than a year before separating from him. There was an inevitable conflict of interest between the new orthopedic doctors and lay bone setters. Thomas (1874) incorporated many of the bone setters' manipulative skills into orthopedic treatment of fractures and dislocations, but

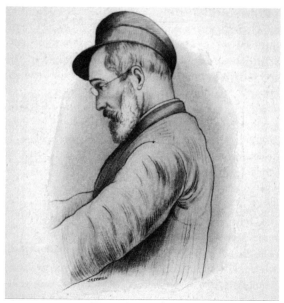

HUGH OWEN THOMAS,

Figure 4.5 Hugh Owen Thomas (1834–1891), the father of English speaking orthopedics. (From a sketch made about 1884 [Keith 1919], with thanks to the Royal College of Physicians and Surgeons of Glasgow.)

rejected many of the bone setters' principles. In particular, he would have nothing to do with manipulation for musculoskeletal symptoms. Instead, Thomas proposed rest as one of the main orthopedic principles for the treatment of fractures, tuberculosis and arthritis. This was actually quite reasonable in the days before internal fixation, antibiotics and joint replacement. Therapeutic rest, suggested Thomas, must be 'enforced, uninterrupted and prolonged'. Orthopedics used bracing, bed rest or later surgical fusion. The idea of rest is so fundamental to the whole management of back pain that it merits a chapter to itself (Ch. 15). Thomas' pupil and nephew Sir Robert Jones (1857–1933) later spread Thomas' teaching across the English speaking world.

Bone setters treated back pain by manipulation and mobilization. They did this in the context of daily life and their patients continued with their normal activities. Medicine now moved back pain into a medical context – back pain was now a disease and the sufferer became a patient. Medical treatment often required the patient to stop normal activities and actually prescribed disability.

The dynasty of the disc

Vesalius (1543) drew the anatomy of the intervertebral disc. In the 19th century there were a number of postmortem reports of major trauma and disc damage causing paraplegia. Luschka (1858) first described two cases of prolapsed intervertebral disc. He actually showed a connection from the nucleus pulposus through the posterior longitudinal ligament to the protrusion. Later Schmorl (1929) and Andrae (1929) made postmortem studies of large series of spines. They described both posterior disc protrusions and protrusions into the vertebral bodies (Schmorl's nodes). They thought that most were asymptomatic in life (!). However, although pathologists saw these disc lesions, no one related them to the clinical symptoms of sciatica.

Despite these reports, clinicians remained unaware of the disc. Middleton & Teacher (1911) reported a case of fatal paraplegia from a central disc prolapse. They related it to the 'sprains and racks of the back' and did a crude experiment to produce a disc prolapse. Goldthwait (1911) described a case of paresis after manipulation of the back for a 'displaced sacroiliac joint'. Harvey Cushing carried out a laminectomy and found nothing apart from 'narrowing of the canal' at the lumbosacral junction. In an anguished search for the cause of this iatrogenic disaster, Goldthwait and Cushing considered compression of the nerve at the lumbosacral joint. They suggested the disc as the cause of 'many cases of lumbago, sciatica and paraplegia'. Dandy (1929) gave the first complete account of disc surgery, a description of two cases with beautiful illustrations. They had paraplegia, myelographic evidence of complete block, a presumptive diagnosis of spinal cord tumor and histologic proof of a sequestrated disc. There was clinical recovery in both cases. Dandy's only mistake was to compare it to osteochondritis in the knee – and so he missed his place in surgical history.

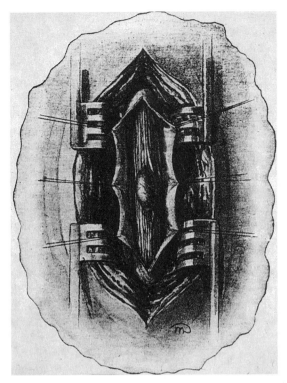

Figure 4.6 Surgery for 'the ruptured disc'. (From Mixter & Barr 1934, with permission.)

Mixter & Barr (1934) were the real discoverers of 'the ruptured disc' as the cause of sciatica. Mixter was a prominent neurosurgeon and Barr a young orthopedic surgeon. Mixter had a patient with recurrent sciatica after a skiing accident. They thought he might have a spinal tumor, but a myelogram did not show a block and so was reported normal. Despite that, they went ahead with laminectomy and the operative diagnosis and pathology report were of enchondroma. Barr wondered if this might not be similar to Schmorl's pathologic description of posterior disc protrusion. Mixter & Barr then reviewed the histology of previous cases and compared them with normal discs. They had to make special sections as no one had been interested in the disc before. Of 16 surgical specimens of 'enchondromas', they found that 10 were normal disc cartilage. Mixter & Barr then began to look for patients, and on December 19 1932 operated on the first

patient with a preoperative diagnosis (Fig. 4.6). Their classic paper (Mixter & Barr 1934) gave the first complete clinical, pathologic and surgical description of disc prolapse as the cause of sciatica. It also showed that surgical treatment was possible.

Mixter & Ayer (1935) wrote a much more radical paper the following year. This was very influential, although few authors quote it now. It added several key ideas to the concept of disc prolapse. It suggested that disc rupture might cause back pain, even when there were no objective neurologic signs. It started modern myelography by describing the use of large quantities of dye and subsequent identification of an indentation of the dye column rather than a complete block. Even at that early stage, they admitted that the results of disc surgery were less than ideal. Surgery cured leg pain in all but one case, but 'some patients complain subsequently of lame back'. Most important was their idea that the lesion was traumatic, although only 14 of their 23 cases reported even minor trauma. Disc lesions were now 'injuries to the spine'. The authors admitted that this concept 'opens up an interesting problem in industrial medicine'. This paper was the real start of the 'dynasty of the disc'.

Disc rupture brought together the 19th century ideas that back pain was an injury, an injury to the spine, and a mechanical problem that should be treated according to orthopedic principles. If the worst came to the worst, it could be fixed surgically. Disc rupture made this into a marketable package. For the next 50 years the disc dominated medical thinking about back pain.

The first surgeons made the diagnosis of disc prolapse on hard neurologic signs. Their successors soon relied on symptoms alone, partly because of the risks and costs of early myelography. These moves away from the early strict criteria unleashed on an unsuspecting public a wave of surgical enthusiasm held back only by World War II. Key caused a furor at a meeting of the Southern Surgical Association in 1945 by claiming that 'inter vertebral disc lesions are the most common cause of low back pain with or without sciatica'. Even the published discussion (Key 1945) was heated. Magnuson retorted that this was no more logical than saying that 'all kittens born in an oven are biscuits!'

From the 1950s there was an explosion of disc surgery, closely related to the growth of orthopedics and neurosurgery. Indeed, it was claimed at one time that the average US neurosurgeon made half his income from disc surgery. But the rapid growth of disc surgery soon exposed its limitations. Even the enthusiasts admitted it was difficult to assess the results: 'The question of liability, compensation and insurance loom large on the horizon and add complications compounded to an already knotty problem.' By 1970, spinal surgery was accused of 'leaving more tragic human wreckage in its wake than any other operation in history'. Surgeons gradually came to realize that disc surgery only helps the few patients with a surgically treatable lesion and that success depends on careful selection.

Undaunted, orthopedic surgeons then extended the concept of 'disc lesions'. If sciatica is caused by disc prolapse, then back pain might be caused by disc degeneration. They ignored the normal age-related nature of these radiographic changes and their poor relation to symptoms. They used biomechanical studies to support the hypothesis, despite the lack of clinical correlation. Once again, they could blame the disc for most back pain. The answer was spinal fusion, and this reestablished the role of surgery in back pain. It also reinforced the influence of orthopedics in the management of simple backache. This approach has gravely distorted health care for the 99% of people with back trouble who do not have or need surgery. It caused us to see back pain as a mechanical or structural problem, and therefore patients expect to be 'fixed'. Just as when they take their car to a mechanic to be fixed, it is the doctor's or therapist's responsibility to fix their backs. By the time they discover that there is no such magic cure for back pain, they are trapped. They no longer have simple backache, but have become patients with a serious back injury or irreversible degeneration. This has led to unrealistic expectations and has

diverted resources from attacking the real problem of back pain.

There have been great medical advances over the past two centuries. Since World War II, an explosion of material resources and medical technology has given us powerful tools, and we now deal confidently with many serious spinal diseases. Disc surgery has survived the test of time for more than half a century because 80–90% of carefully selected patients get rapid relief of pain. This rational physical approach to health care reached its apogee in unraveling the mystery of life itself in the DNA molecule, and in our ability to replace artificial hip joints and even to transplant hearts. In this mood of medical achievement and euphoria it was possible to assert confidently that the primary role of the physician is the control, and even ideally the relief, of all pain. Sadly, this medical technology has not solved the problem of simple backache.

A HOLISTIC APPROACH

Most philosophers and many doctors stress the relationship between mind and body. It is fundamental to human existence and to medicine. Plato encapsulated this:

So neither ought you to attempt to cure the body without the soul, and this is the reason why the cure of many diseases is unknown to the physicians of Hellas, because they are ignorant of the whole which ought to be studied also, for part can never be well unless the whole is well.

In 100 AD, Rufus of Ephesus saw the need for a complete clinical assessment:

And I place the interrogation of the patient first, since in this way you can learn how far his mind is healthy or otherwise; also his physical strengths and weaknesses, and get some idea of the part affected.

Stahl (1660–1734), writing at the time of the Renaissance, felt that the new physical sciences were not enough in themselves to explain human behavior. He was one in a long line of doctors since Hippocrates who took this view. His work has a surprisingly modern ring, emphasizing:

- the essential unity of the organism
- the personal element in liability to illness

- the part played by mental conditions in mental and physical disease
- emotional life is important in treating patients and is independent of reason.

Sadly, the mechanistic approach of orthodox medicine soon swamped such holistic ideas. The Cartesian model of pain has had a major influence on medicine to this day. Descartes himself was actually less mechanistic than most people now believe, but his followers divided human existence rigidly into mind and body. In this dichotomy, medicine dealt with the body, and pain was a simple warning signal of disease. It took another two centuries to develop the tools to turn this into practical reality. Haller (1707–1777) founded modern physiology, so illness could become a matter of disordered physiology. Perhaps the most dramatic example was when Pasteur (1822–1895) showed that infections are caused by microbes, and paved the way for modern treatment with antibiotics. At about the same time, the German pathologist, Virchow (1858), put forward the concept of cellular pathology, which led to the disease model of human illness:

- Recognize patterns of symptoms and signs – *history and examination*
- Infer underlying pathology – *diagnosis*
- Apply physical therapy to that pathology – *treatment*
- Expect the illness to recover – *cure*.

Orthodox medicine became a matter of physical disease. We have already seen how the disease model changed medical thinking about back pain. Haller's concept of nerve excitability or irritability led to Brown's spinal irritation and Charcot's *grande hysteria*. So began our modern approach to the spine. But by concentrating entirely on physical disease it also introduced a bias that has continued to the present day. Brown (1828) described the syndrome of spinal irritation in young women. They had spinal tenderness, pain in the left breast and many vague bodily symptoms. But these patients were unaware of their spinal tenderness until medical examiners drew it to

their attention! The beauty of the diagnosis was that there was nothing physically wrong with the spine. But the more dramatic the treatment, the more effective it was for psychosomatic symptoms: 'The ensuing orgy of blistering, leeching and cupping of the spine probably represents the first (unwitting) use of placebo therapy in modern surgery' (Shorter 1992). During the 1820s an increasing number of young women presented with spinal complaints in response to medical suggestion.

Railway spine is one of the most distressing episodes in the history of back pain (p. 48). Erichsen (1866) brought together the spate of railway accidents, the new compensation laws and Brown's concept of spinal irritation (Fig. 4.7). He suggested that minor railway injuries to the spine could have long-term effects. Controversy raged over the nature and indeed the existence of railway spine for many years in both medical and legal circles. In Europe, Valleix (1841) suggested that many of these symptoms were hysteric. In the US, Page (1885) denounced railway spine as little more than traumatic lumbago, or a nervous disturbance with overtones of simulation or hysteria,

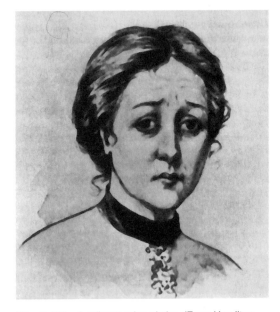

Figure 4.7 A railway spine victim. (From Hamilton 1894, reproduced with permission from *Spine*.)

combined with the deleterious effects of law suits. This view that the psychic shock of the accident produced 'neurasthenia' gradually prevailed. This 'exhaustion of the nervous system' or disease of civilization related to industrialization was in vogue by the end of the 19th century. At about the same time, the great French neurologist Charcot developed his theories of hysteria. Shortly before his death in 1896, Erichsen himself agreed that railway spine was probably a form of traumatic neurasthenia. As the diagnosis of railway spine fell into disrepute, doctors, lawyers and claimants shifted their focus to this new diagnosis. The condition spread from the railways to other work, road and domestic accidents. With the acceptance of high speed travel, better clinical examination and the new X-rays, the diagnosis of railway spine slowly faded. But Erichsen's railway spine caused a great deal of trouble before it was extinguished, and, like spinal irritation, some of its concepts endure to this day. Both medico-legal and lay circles came to accept that back pain is an injury and that minor trauma can lead to severe and permanent low back pain and disability.

The striking aspect of the stories of spinal irritation and railway spine is that vague clinical features gained such ready medical acceptance as a physical disease. This is not unique to back pain. Even today, many health professionals seem uncomfortable dealing with psychosomatic problems. They search desperately for a purely physical or neurophysiologic explanation, however unlikely, for the vaguest symptoms.

Medicine's struggle with these problems coincided with the growth of psychology and psychiatry. Heinroth first coined the term 'psychosomatic' in 1818. He did not imply a psychologic cause but simply wanted to describe the mutual interaction between psychologic and physical events. It is now nearly a century since Freud reaffirmed the importance of psychologic factors in medicine. He showed how doctors could assess psychoneurotic symptoms and gain insight into emotional processes. Meyer, one of the founders of American psychiatry, recognized that psycho-logic factors affect the course and outcome of every illness, physical as well as mental.

People have always had psychosomatic or stress-related symptoms, but the form they take varies depending on what each culture accepts as legitimate. They must be acceptable to the patient's family, health professionals and society. What is acceptable changes over time and the history of psychosomatic disorders is of 'ever-changing steps in a pas-de-deux between doctor and patient' (Shorter 1992). Up to the 18th century, psychosomatic symptoms were largely related to folklore beliefs about external influences on health. In the 19th century, medical ideas focused on the nervous system and irritability. Psychosomatic symptoms changed to hysteric paralysis, then neurasthenia and traumatic neurosis. As medical ideas changed in the 20th century, so did psychosomatic systems. Now we focus on pain and fatigue. They are not only symptoms, but have even become accepted as syndromes. People are also now much more aware of their health. From 1928–1931, a survey of US adults reported 82 episodes of illness per 100 people per annum. By 1982 that had risen to 212 illnesses per 100 people. People are now much more prone to regard themselves as 'ill' and to seek health care, despite vast advances in nutrition, health care and public health. At the same time medicine has lost much of its authority, and patients develop their own fixed beliefs about disease.

MANUAL THERAPY

The value of massage to soothe pain has been known since the fifth century (Schiotz & Cyriax 1975). It is still a common lay remedy today (Fig. 4.8).

Manual therapy is use of the hands to mobilize, adjust, manipulate, apply traction, massage, stimulate or otherwise influence joints and muscles. In back pain, the basic idea is to *influence* spinal motion and so relieve pain and dysfunction. It may also produce change in neurophysiologic function and reduce muscle spasm. However, we still do not have a clear

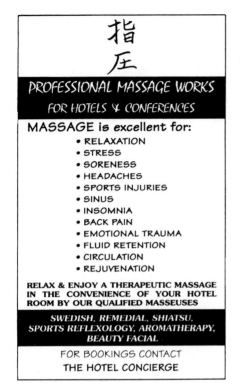

指
圧

PROFESSIONAL MASSAGE WORKS

FOR HOTELS & CONFERENCES

MASSAGE is excellent for:

- RELAXATION
- STRESS
- SORENESS
- HEADACHES
- SPORTS INJURIES
- SINUS
- INSOMNIA
- BACK PAIN
- EMOTIONAL TRAUMA
- FLUID RETENTION
- CIRCULATION
- REJUVENATION

RELAX & ENJOY A THERAPEUTIC MASSAGE IN THE CONVENIENCE OF YOUR HOTEL ROOM BY OUR QUALIFIED MASSEUSES

SWEDISH, REMEDIAL, SHIATSU, SPORTS REFLEXOLOGY, AROMATHERAPY, BEAUTY FACIAL

FOR BOOKINGS CONTACT
THE HOTEL CONCIERGE

Figure 4.8 Massage is still in widespread use. An advert in an international hotel, 1997.

understanding of *how* manipulation works (McClune et al 1997). Manual therapy includes manipulation and mobilization. Manipulation is generally defined as the application of a high-velocity, low-amplitude thrust to the spinal joint slightly beyond its passive range of motion. Mobilization is the application of force within the passive range of the joint, without a thrust. However, the term 'manipulation' is often used very loosely to describe a wide range of procedures. There are striking similarities in the techniques developed by different professions, yet it is surprising how unaware the various practitioners seem to be of these similarities.

Ancient medical texts, from Hippocrates and Galen to Pare in the 16th century, describe manipulation. These were powerful spinal manipulations usually combined with traction and were probably for fractures and dislocations, or deformities of the spine (Fig. 4.9).

Spinal manipulation appears in folk medicine over many centuries from places as far apart as Norway, Mexico and the Pacific Islands. The most common form was 'trampling' for lumbago. For several hundred years, professional

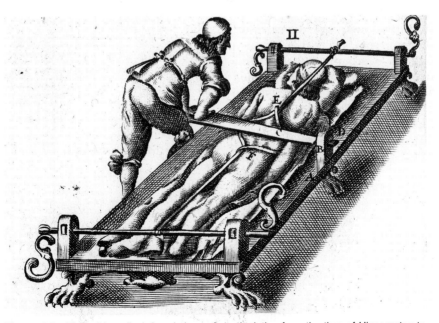

Figure 4.9 Most old medical descriptions of manipulation from the time of Hippocrates to the 17th century were for fracture-dislocation or deformity. (From Sculteti 1662, with thanks to Glasgow University library.)

'bone setters' or 'sprain rubbers' also developed skilled manual manipulation. This was usually a family business handed down from one generation to the next by apprenticeship. St Bartholomew's Hospital in London had bone setters on its staff in the 17th century, and one was even knighted.

They were called bone setters because they attributed the pain to 'a little bone lying out of place'. Manipulation *reset* the bone to relieve the pain. The relationship between orthodox medicine and bone setters varied from respect and cooperation to outright hostility. Paget gave a lecture to medical students in St Bartholomew's Hospital in 1866 on 'cases that bone-setters cure': 'Few of you are likely to practice without having a bone-setter as an enemy ...' He cautioned against 'the mischief that they do', but also admitted that 'it sometimes does some good', with lumbago as an example: 'Learn then to imitate what is good and avoid what is bad in the practice of bone-setting.' The success of bone setters was partly due to their practical skill and experience, but also to medical ignorance and neglect of musculoskeletal symptoms (oh, how little has changed today!).

Although orthopedics took over the manipulation of spinal fractures and dislocations, orthodox medicine in the 19th century rejected manual therapy for symptomatic relief. This reflected its focus on identifiable pathology and 'science'. As medicine struggled for professional status, it was happy to leave such hands-on therapy to others. In the UK, the Medical Act of 1858, which registered medical practitioners, made it unethical to refer patients to unregistered practitioners. The result was to leave a vacuum, to be occupied by alternative health care, for people with spinal pain for whom orthodox medicine had little interest or help.

In the US, osteopathy and chiropractic developed to meet this need.

Osteopathy

On June 22 1874, Dr Andrew T Still 'flung to the breeze the banner of osteopathy' (Fig. 4.10). Still was an old school physician in Kansas and

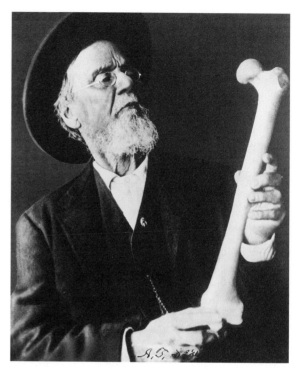

Figure 4.10 Dr Andrew T Still (1828–1917), the founder of osteopathic medicine. (From the British School of Osteopathy, with thanks.)

Missouri. He had little formal medical education but learned his trade by apprenticeship, as was normal practice for the time. He had an MD from the Kansas City Medical School, and practiced as a physician for a few years. Still lost three of his children in an epidemic of meningitis, and orthodox medicine could not save them. His brother was also a morphine addict through medical treatment. Still then started a campaign against orthodox medicine and 'the indiscriminate use of drugs'. He sought a better alternative, so he combined ancient principles of holistic medicine with the bone setters' art, and based osteopathy on two main principles (Still 1899):

• The body has within itself the power to combat disease. Hippocrates had argued that 'it is our natures that are the physicians of our diseases. We must not meddle with or hinder Nature's attempt towards recovery. First, do no harm.'

- The human framework is a machine, subject to the same mechanical principles and disturbed function as a steam engine. The cause of disease is 'dislocated' bones, abnormal ligaments and contracted muscles – especially in the back – that cause pressure on blood vessels and nerves, that also leads to ischemia and necrosis, in part due to a disturbance of the life force traveling along nerves. This dislocation was the original 'osteopathic lesion'.

Manipulation did not in itself cure the problem. Rather, it allowed the body to heal the osteopathic lesion. The 'structure–function' concept was of an intimate bond between the framework and the workings of the human body. Still combined his holistic approach to health and the healing power of nature with a practical approach to mechanical factors in health and disease. This provided a unified philosophy for manipulative therapy. But osteopathic medicine is more than just manipulation. It is a whole system of diagnosis, assessment, therapy and prophylaxis. It is 'a therapeutic system based on the belief that the body, in normal structural relationship and with adequate nutrition, is capable of mounting its own defences against most pathologic conditions' (DiGiovanna & Schiowitz 1991). Even if used primarily to treat symptoms, it also aims to help restore the individual to a more nearly ideal physiologic state of well-being.

DiGiovanna & Schiowitz (1991) give a succinct modern summary of osteopathic principles:

- Osteopathic physicians … are primarily interested in the achievement of normal body mechanics as central to good health.
- The neuro-musculo-skeletal system is salient to the full expression of life.
- Structure governs function.
- The heart of osteopathy is the recognition of the body's ability to heal itself, with some external help, of most pathologic conditions.

Martinke (1991) and Seffinger (1997) present the same ideas in a slightly different way:

- The body is a unit. It does not function as a collection of separate parts but is an integrated unit. The person is a single entity of body and mind.
- Structure and function are reciprocally interrelated.
- The body is capable of self-regulation, self-healing and health maintenance.
- Rational treatment is based upon an understanding of the basic principles of body unity, self-regulation and the inter-relationship of structure and function.

Chiropractic

D D Palmer (Fig. 4.11) carried out the first chiropractic treatment in Iowa on September 18 1895. Palmer was a magnetic healer, who knew the early medical literature well and the methods of the bone setters. He was probably also acquainted with osteopathic techniques in use in neighboring Missouri. There are many similarities between chiropractic and osteopathy, but they have always had distinct professional identities and philosophies.

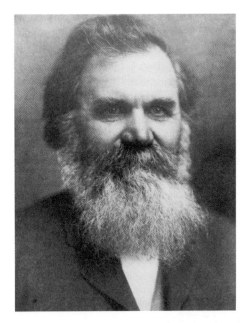

Figure 4.11 D D Palmer (1845–1913), the founder of chiropractic. (Courtesy of Palmer College of Chiropractic Archives, David D Palmer Health Sciences Library.)

Chiropractic dealt with *subluxations* – reduced mobility and slight malposition of a vertebral segment. It laid more emphasis on the resulting pressure on nerves and ignored the flow of blood or body fluid. Palmer (1910) also placed more stress on the method of manipulation or *adjustment*:

I do claim … to be the first to replace displaced vertebrae by using the spinous or transverse processes as levers whereby to rack displaced vertebrae into normal position, and from this basic fact, to create a science, which is destined to revolutionize the theory and practice of the healing art…

Chiropractic also had, and still has, a strong philosophic base (Haldeman et al 1992). Palmer founded chiropractic on the twin pillars of science and vitalism, with strong emphasis on the mind–body relationship (Box 4.1). The mechanical side was the manipulation of subluxations. Vitalism gave an equally strong metaphysical and spiritual side. Palmer saw this as a life force, expressed in the individual as innate intelligence that controls and coordinates bodily activity and influences health and illness. It is the fundamental ability of the body to heal itself. Vitalism is holistic and naturopathic. Holism integrates body, mind and spirit. It considers that health depends on obeying certain laws and adopting a certain lifestyle, and that deviation can lead to illness. The 'innate intelligence' gives purpose, balance and direction to all biologic function. The naturopathic approach is the opposite of orthodox or allopathic medicine. The allopathic approach considers that disease is due to an external cause overcoming the body's resistance. Orthodox medicine's answer is to counter the external cause, e.g. antibiotics

for infection. The naturopathic approach considers that illness is largely due to the person's lowered resistance, and so the answer is to strengthen the person, regardless of the external cause. Healing depends on mobilizing the innate recuperative powers within the patient.

The emphasis of chiropractic is on natural remedies. It restores musculoskeletal integrity and neurophysiologic function. It stresses a proper diet, lifestyle and a healthy environment. It uses conservative, safe treatments and avoids drugs and surgery. It helps the patient to understand that his or her illness is the result of the body's failure to maintain a healthy state. Manipulation may stimulate healing, but the patient also has to change and return to more healthy living. It is a patient-centered, hands-on approach that depends on good communication between doctor and patient. Touch and physical contact between doctor and patient help to mobilize this internal healing power. It is wellness-oriented rather than sickness-oriented, and is concerned with the person who is ill rather than the illness that the person has.

Rereading these two sections, I may have given the impression that chiropractic is more holistic than osteopathic medicine. That is not the case. Both have strong holistic roots, and, today, both emphasize a biopsychosocial approach. There are, however, widely differing views in both professions. At one extreme are those practitioners who see themselves as musculoskeletal specialists. At the other extreme are those with an almost evangelic faith in the benefits of their treatment for the human condition. There is also some variation between views in the US and the UK.

There is a danger, of course, that if this philosophy is carried to extremes it may become dogma. We must balance the holistic and the mechanistic approaches, i.e., 'first do no harm' (Hippocrates), but at the same time remember that 'it ill behoves the skilled physician to mumble charms over ills that crave the knife' (Sophocles). Modern osteopathic medicine and chiropractic have a holistic approach but incorporate and use knowledge from the mechanistic, scientific approach.

Box 4.1 A humanistic philosophy

- Vitalism – recognize the patient's own capacity for self-healing
- Holism – focus care on the whole patient, in the context of his or her life
- Humanistic – recognize and respect the patient's point of view
- Egalitarian – share responsibility for care with the patient

The reaction of orthodox medicine

We must see the origins of osteopathy and chiropractic in the context of their time (Northup 1966). In the late 19th century, Kansas, Missouri and Iowa were still the American frontier. This was an age of heroic medicine. The primitive state of medical science meant that some of the new invasive treatments for disease did as much harm as good, which led to public outrage and a search for safer alternatives. The medical reform movement in the US stressed the need for personal responsibility for health, lifestyle recommendations and professional alternatives to orthodox medicine. Osteopathy and chiropractic also sought to preserve some of the ancient principles that orthodox medicine seemed to be abandoning. This was the Bible belt, and the medical reform movement had strong evangelic overtones. That philosophic base has helped to sustain the professional identity of osteopathic medicine and chiropractic to this day.

This background also helps us to understand the reaction of orthodox medicine. These were direct competitors at a time when orthodox medicine was struggling to establish its own professional status. Alternative medicine also vehemently accused orthodox medicine of abandoning ancient medical principles. It is little wonder that orthodox medicine met the new health professions with outright hostility and persecution. From 1896 and as late as 1949, hundreds of chiropractors went to jail in the US for giving 'unlawful treatment' and for the unlawful practice of medicine. Despite that, osteopathic medicine and chiropractic survived, supported by patients who continued to choose them in preference to orthodox medicine.

They also developed professional education, the equal of orthodox medicine, with virtually no external funding. Andrew Still founded the American School of Osteopathy in 1892 and D D Palmer founded the first school of chiropractic in 1896. During the 20th century, osteopathic training in the US gradually became very like medical training, though with more emphasis on musculoskeletal disorders and manual therapy. By 1968 the American Medical Association finally withdrew its opposition and proposed eventual amalgamation of orthodox and osteopathic medicine. By the 1980s osteopathic medicine was fully recognized in every state. A DO is now equivalent to an MD. Osteopathic physicians are once again part of mainstream medicine and they practice in every medical specialty. Chiropractic stayed completely independent and recognition as a health profession was slower. There are now 15 colleges of osteopathy and 13 of chiropractic in the US. Progress in Europe has been much slower. The British School of Osteopathy opened in 1917, but the Anglo-European College of Chiropractic did not open until 1965. In Britain, the Act of Parliament to register and regulate osteopaths was not passed until 1993, and the corresponding Act for chiropractors was not passed until 1994. Even today, most osteopaths and chiropractors practice independently, and quite separately from orthodox medicine. They are just beginning, very gradually, to treat a few NHS patients.

Manual medicine

Orthodox medicine has been slow to learn anything from osteopathy and chiropractic. Early enthusiastic claims that spinal manipulation could cure distant diseases ranging from diabetes to goiter laid osteopathy and chiropractic open to medical ridicule. There is still a major problem of communication and scope for misunderstanding. For example, subluxation means different things to a chiropractor and an orthopedic surgeon. Patients still frequently misinterpret osteopathic and chiropractic explanations of segmental dysfunction as 'discs out' which orthodox physicians then deny.

But orthodox medicine never wholly abandoned manual therapy. In the 19th century physicians stopped doing manipulation themselves, but medicine was still interested in physical therapies. Magnetism, electrotherapy and hydrotherapy were all in vogue. In Europe this was the age of the spa, where new wealth and ease of travel let the middle classes, mainly women, congregate to indulge in these therapies.

In the mid-20th century, there was also a re-emergence of an orthodox specialty of 'manual medicine'. Cyriax (1969) in England led the fight to restore the place of manipulation in the treatment of musculoskeletal disorders. At the same time he strongly rejected osteopathic and chiropractic theories and philosophies as quackery. Instead, he tried to reintegrate manipulation as a purely physical modality. However, there are still few physicians who have learned these skills, and musculoskeletal medicine has remained a tiny specialty. Orthodox medicine has largely delegated manual therapy to physiotherapists.

Physical therapy

Physiotherapy in Britain, Europe and the rest of the English speaking world is the same as physical therapy in the US.

'Physiotherapy is a health care profession that emphasizes the use of physical approaches in the prevention and treatment of disease and disability' (CSP 1991). The *Standards of physiotherapy practice* (CSP 1993) expands on this:

Physiotherapy is a health care profession with an emphasis on analysis of movement based on the structure and function of the body and the use of physical approaches to the promotion of health, and the prevention, treatment and management of disease and disability. ... The aim is to identify and diagnose the specific components of movement or function responsible for the patient's physical problems.

This 'is based on an assessment of movement and function' and also 'takes account of the patient's current psychologic, cultural and social factors'.

In 1894, a group of British nurses started the *Society of Trained Masseuses* for women practicing massage or 'medical rubbing' (Wickstead 1948). Their original aim was 'to make massage a safe, clean and honorable profession for British women'. At first, the society and its examinations were entirely about massage. By 1920, it got a Royal Charter 'to promote a curriculum and standard of qualification for the persons engaged in the practice of massage, medical gymnastics, electro therapies and kindred

methods of treatment'. In 1994, a writer in the centennial issue of *Physiotherapy* wrote:

while not wanting to enter into the debate about their use, misuse or disuse in every day practice, suffice it to say that these remain, in one form or another, the basis of practice today.

Manual therapy has always played an important part, but since the 1970s, there has been increasing interest in mobilization and manipulation, largely led by therapists in Australia and New Zealand. Over the last decade or so, in the face of growing competition from chiropractic and osteopathy, they have also become more involved in manipulation.

Physical therapy in the US started officially during World War I (Murphy 1995). The Surgeon General of the US army saw the need for a core of young women to assist the 'reconstruction' of maimed and disabled soldiers (Fig. 4.12). They were led by Mary MacMillan, who had qualified in physical education and had then done postgraduate physiotherapy and orthopedic studies in England. By the end of the war there were 1200 'reconstruction aides' with valuable clinical experience. They also had the respect and support of orthodox medicine, and

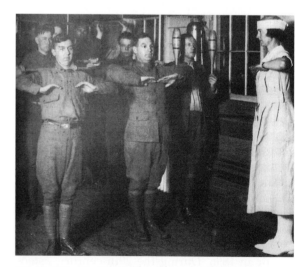

Figure 4.12 A rehabilitation class in a 'reconstruction center' in 1919. (Reprinted with permission of the American Physical Therapy Association from Murphy W. Healing the generations: A history of physical therapy and the American Physical Therapy Association. Alexandria, VA: American Physical Therapy Association 1995.)

in 1921 they set up the American Physical Therapy Association (APTA).

There have always been close links between US and UK physiotherapy. However, from the first, physical therapy in the US had a strong emphasis on exercise and rehabilitation. This partly reflects the different background of its early leaders, and its whole *raison d'etre* for rehabilitation of the injured. Its work with polio and then in World War II, the Korean war and the Vietnam war reinforced its focus on neuro-muscular and musculoskeletal disabilities.

The APTA (1997) *Guide to physical therapist practice* puts this first. Physical therapy is about 'the preservation, development and restoration of maximum physical function'. It is 'the examination, evaluation, treatment and prevention of neuromuscular, musculoskeletal, cardiovascular and pulmonary disorders that produce movement impairments, disabilities and functional limitations'. This includes:

- examining patients with impairments, functional limitations and disability or other health-related conditions in order to determine a diagnosis, prognosis and intervention
- alleviating impairments and functional limitations by designing, implementing and modifying therapeutic interventions that include, but are not limited to, the following (note the order):
  - therapeutic exercise (including aerobic conditioning)
  - functional training in self-care and home management (including activities of daily living)
  - functional training in community or work reintegration activities
  - manual therapy techniques (including mobilization and manipulation)
  - prescription, fabrication and application of assistive, adaptive, supportive, and protective devices and equipment
  - physical agents and mechanical modalities
  - electrotherapeutic modalities
  - patient-related instruction

- preventing injury, impairments, functional limitations and disabilities, including the promotion and maintenance of fitness, health, and quality of life.

This continues an ancient Greek tradition of physical culture and remedial exercises, and draws on the 'Swedish movements' of the early 19th century. In Britain, also, experience in two world wars, and close links with orthopedics, increased the emphasis on remedial exercises and reeducation. This changing role led to a change of name, to the Chartered Society of Physiotherapy (CSP), with passionate debate. Some therapists felt that to reduce the role of massage was to forfeit the birthright of the profession. However, the change of name did recognize the increasing role of 'restoration of function by active work on the part of the patient'. That dilemma is still not fully resolved on either side of the Atlantic. A more critical writer in the centennial edition of *Physiotherapy* still had reservations in 1994:

Most current treatments are really only dealing with symptoms and giving short-lived relief. They are usually received by a passive patient, from a therapist who very much *gives* a treatment.

Physiotherapy has always been closely allied to orthodox medicine. At the end of the 19th century, like the nursing profession from which it arose, it was subservient. The CSP's first rule of professional conduct stated: 'no massage to be undertaken except under medical direction'. Not until the 1970s did physicians in the UK stop prescribing the modalities and course of physiotherapy treatment. The current rules of the CSP date from 1987, following a major revision in collaboration with the British Medical Association: 'Chartered physiotherapists shall communicate and cooperate with registered medical practitioners in the diagnosis, treatment and management of patients.' It still assumed that patients would make first contact with a physician but did accept that the therapist was now properly involved in clinical assessment and diagnosis. By 1993, the *Standards of physiotherapy practice* were much more confident (CSP 1993): 'Physiotherapists, where appropriate, are members of the multi-disciplinary team caring for the patient.' However, 'this role does not restrict chartered physiotherapists who so wish from accepting the responsibility of independent professional practice'.

There has been a similar but faster trend in the US. The American Medical Association accredited schools of physical therapy until 1980, when the APTA finally took over. Academic standards have steadily risen. Four-year bachelor degrees had become standard by the early 1950s. By the mid-1960s, physical therapy programs were part of Schools of Allied Health. During the 1960s and 1970s there was a rapid expansion of research activities and increasing numbers of physical therapists gained PhDs.

THE HISTORY OF LOW BACK DISABILITY

There is little mention of low back disability in ancient times, although, in fairness, medical writing did not show much interest in any form of disability. Seriously ill people who took to the sick bed usually did not survive long. Chronic disability depends on some form of social support. Some cripples became beggars, but that was always a precarious existence. Early codes of compensation dealt only with serious bodily mutilation, and did not mention a minor problem like back pain. It seems unlikely that simple backache was accepted as a reason for chronic disability in the harsh conditions of earlier times. Chronic low back disability was probably not possible, apart from rare exceptions in privileged social classes.

Our modern concept of disability hinges on our present pattern of work. After the industrial revolution there were radical changes in the whole social structure, including work to earn a living. This also led to the need for financial support for those who were unable to work.

The first report of work-related back pain was by Ramazzini (1705), who wrote *A treatise on the diseases of tradesmen*. He found that servants at court who stood for long periods

and weavers because of the violent action of their looms were liable to 'pains in the loyns'. Fowler (1795) noted that 'the lumbago is a very common disease among labouring farmers from their frequent exposure to cold and hardships'. However, these were solitary reports and they did not mention disability.

The first report of low back disability was on the railways. A Lancet Commission (Lancet 1862), *The influence of railway travel on the public health*, found that railway workers had more sickness than seamen, miners or laborers. Lumbago was one of the most common causes. Railway spine became an increasing problem between 1860 and 1880. The first reports of prolonged low back disability were in the 1880s and 1890s in the context of compensation.

There was growing interest in low back pain and disability in an industrial context during the first two decades of the 20th century. King (1915) in New Orleans wrote one of the first papers about industrial back pain and by the early 1920s there were many articles. The medical answer was better diagnosis, better treatment and the detection of malingering. The industrial answer was better selection of employees and better working practices. The US Draft Board in the First World War supported this. They examined conscripts and rejected many because of 'static problems' that they thought might lead to back pain. Despite this, many recruits broke down with back pain during training. The alarmed authorities set up special training battalions and the results were striking. They quickly made 80% of these 'derelicts' fit for service. They suggested that back pain might be 'a fitness problem' rather than a medical problem.

Early epidemiology was about mortality, infectious disease and child health. Not until 1921 did the UK Ministry of Health commission a report on rheumatic diseases. This found that 16% of all disabilities were due to rheumatism, and more than half of these were due to lumbago, muscular pain and undefined rheumatism.

The Department of Health for Scotland gathered some of the first detailed morbidity data in the world during the 1930s. They made a national survey of people who had been sick-listed continuously for 12 months. Rheumatism caused 12.6% of all chronic disability, and three-quarters of these cases were lumbago, muscular and undefined rheumatism. Rheumatism was now a more common cause of long-term disability than tuberculosis, even though TB was still rife. Only mental diseases were more common (21.4%). They made the important point that rheumatic disability was mainly found in younger adults. They also found that chronic disability due to rheumatism was growing faster than any other form of disability.

There were similar changes in low back disability in the British Forces between the two world wars. Lumbago caused 0.23% of 'medical admissions' in 1914–1918, and 1.07% in 1939–1945 (this military term is closer to sick certification than hospitalization). This increase in back pain contrasts with sciatica which caused 0.2% of medical admissions in both wars. In World War I, back pain was still usually diagnosed as either 'fibrositis' or other rheumatic conditions. By World War II, it was more likely to be a 'strain'. The outcome also changed. In World War I, 50% were back to duties within 2 weeks, but in World War II the average period off duty was 2 months and 'the men are often reconciled to being a chronic case'. By World War II, 'fibrositis and mild referred sciatica pain has ousted dyspepsia, diarrhea and headache as the chief cause of withdrawal from army duties'.

There is one fascinating footnote. The above history of low back disability is almost entirely about men. There was very little mention of low back disability in women. In this respect, women lagged behind men for many years, which may reflect the different social roles of men and women, particularly in work. Only recently have trends of sexual equality allowed women to have low back disability as well.

Compensation

The history of low back disability and compensation go together, and most definitions of disability imply the need for compensation. But it is wrong to say that compensation causes disability. Indeed, the converse is true. It was recognition of the need that led to legislation. However, it is also true that social support does make chronic disability possible. The prospect of compensation undoubtedly does attract claims, and not all claims are of equal merit. By 1924, one writer felt that 'the compensation dole has made a lazy hibernation possible'.

Our present form of social support for sickness dates from the social, industrial and medical revolutions of the 19th century, but compensation itself is much older. Indeed, compensation seems to be one of the earliest social and legal hallmarks of civilization.

Ancient compensation codes predate written history. The most primitive was that of 'ius Taliones' of which the best known example is the Law of Moses (c. 800 BC): 'An eye for an eye; tooth for tooth; hand for hand; foot for foot.' This may at first appear to be simply a form of retribution, but it is much more than that. The Code of Hammurabi (c. 1750 BC) only applied these penalties to those of equal social rank. Financial compensation was given between different ranks. If a freeman destroyed the eye of a freeman, he also lost an eye. If the victim was a plebeian, the freeman paid one mina of silver. If the victim was a mere slave, he paid the owner half the slave's value. The slave got nothing. Financial compensation gradually applied between social equals also.

During the early stages of the industrial revolution, a worker could claim compensation from an employer or fellow employee for accidental injury. It depended on proving that someone was to blame for the accident. But these legal rights were limited, and in practice it was difficult and expensive. The first case of a worker successfully suing his employer for a work injury in England was not until 1836. No claim was possible if the accident was due to 'ordinary risk' in the course of employment or to an Act of God. Nor could a worker claim if he had been even partly to blame for the accident: that was 'contributory negligence'. The 'fellow-servant' doctrine meant that the employer was not responsible for negligence by another worker. Even more unjust, any legal case stopped with the death of the worker, and his dependants then had no claim.

During the 19th century, there was growing acceptance of society's responsibility to provide care for the sick and disabled. There had been war pensions for disabled soldiers since Greek times. Now, society also began to care for 'the wounded soldiers of industry' (Fig. 4.13). The start was again the building of the railroads. The world's first railway line opened in England in 1825 and the carriage bore the legend 'a public service free of danger'. But rapid and uncontrolled growth of the railways led to casualties on a scale unprecedented except in war. In a single year, 1145 people died and 3038 were injured either working or travelling on the railways in Britain. Public anxiety led to legislation. When the Berlin–Potsdam railway opened in 1838, the Prussian government made the railway companies legally responsible for any accidents. In England, the Fatal Accidents Act of 1846 first gave the right of compensation to the family of a person killed in an accident. The Employers' Liability Act of 1880 went some way to abolish the 'fellow-servant' doctrine, and started compulsory insurance, but it was still necessary to prove fault and this limited its value. By 1886, the Employers Liability Assurance Corporation recorded 10 217 accidents, but only 24% made any claim and only 12% got any compensation.

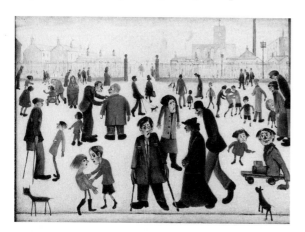

Figure 4.13 The 'wounded soldiers of industry'. ('The Cripples' by L S Lowry, courtesy of City of Salford Museums and Art Gallery.)

The new laws led to a spate of legal and medical activity. Many of the injuries were severe and fully justified compensation, but there was soon a problem of many claims for trivial injuries. Some of these claimants had subjective symptoms without much objective evidence of injury. 'Sprains and strains' of the back were soon a leading example. The limitations of medical examination made the problem worse: 'Lawyers and judges appear to have a pretty generally formed opinion that a doctor's statement concerning disability of the lower back is largely a matter of guesswork' (Wentworth 1916). As legislation extended the scope of compensation, so the scale of the problem grew. By 1915, 'pain in the back as a result of injury is the most frequent affection for which compensation is demanded from the casualty company'. King (1915) summed up the dilemma neatly: 'Lumbago is a condition of most frequent occurrence. The laborer however seldom suffers from the pain of lumbago but is a frequent victim of pain in the back due to injury'. He did not imply that the worker was always lying. Conn (1922) stated:

It is easy to trace the mental process of a patient who, after a hard previous day's work, honestly concludes that the lumbago of today had its origin in the employment of yesterday. Such an individual is scarcely a malingerer, but rather the victim of a false conception, the more deep rooted often because of tactless disputes at previous examinations.

Wentworth (1916) summed up what many doctors still feel: 'Exaggeration is as common as malingering is rare.'

The limitations of civil litigation led to schemes for compensation without going to the courts. The first Workman's Compensation Act in Britain was passed in 1897. It made insurance compulsory for large groups of workers regardless of fault. By 1906 it covered all workers and also included industrial disease as well as accident. In 1911, Lloyd George introduced the first compulsory state insurance scheme to cover sickness. From that time the state has provided a growing proportion of support for the sick and disabled in all Western countries. The right to civil litigation for further compensation remains, but few sick or injured people now

Table 4.1 The historic parallels between low back pain, sciatica, disability and compensation

Date	Backache	Sciatica	Disability	Illness behavior	Compensation
2000					≈1750 Code of Hammurabi
1500	1500 Edwin Smith papyrus — case presentation				
1000 / 500 (BC)		≈400 **Hippocrates** — clinical description		**Hippocrates**	≈800 ius Taliones Military pensions Roman Law
BC 100 / 0 / AD 100					
150	150 **Galen** — symptom of disease — fleeting pains of joints and muscles	≈150 **Aretaeus** — nervous — arthritic			
500 / 1000				Arabian medicine — isolated case presentations	
1500					
1681 / 1765 / 1705	1681 **Sydenham** — rheumatism	1765 **Contugno** — modern clinical entity	1705 **Ramazzini** – occupational back pain		
1800	1828 **Brown** – spinal irritation			1816 **Heberden** 1828 Spinal irritation	1836 First personal injury case in English High Court 1846 Fatal Accident Act
1850 / 1866	1866 **Erichsen** — railway spine 1874 **Thomas** — orthopedic surgery therapeutic rest		1866 Railway spine	1866 Railway spine 1880 **Freud** — psychologic medicine	1880 Employers' Liability Act 1897 Workmen's Compensation Act — compulsory insurance
1900			1900–20 Industrial back pain	1910 Medicolegal assessment	1911 National Health Insurance Act — state insurance for injury and sickness
1930 / 1934	1934 **Mixter & Barr** — disc rupture — disc surgery		1930 First population morbidity statistics Post-WWII epidemic of low back disability Chronic pain syndrome		
1950	Degenerate disc disease Chronic pain syndrome			1960 Mechanic-illness behavior	1948 National Health Service and comprehensive social security

depend mainly on civil litigation. Post-war legislation in Britain during 1946–1948 created a comprehensive National Health Service and Social Security for all sick and disabled people. The United States was slow to follow the European example in workmen's compensation. The first legislation was passed in New York State in 1910, but it was not until 1949 that all states had workmen's compensation legislation. The US still does not have a universal system of health care and sickness benefits.

AN HISTORIC PERSPECTIVE

- Human beings have had back pain all through history, and it is no more common or severe than it has always been

- What has changed is how we understand and manage the symptom of pain in the back. Three key ideas in the 19th century laid the foundation for traditional 20th century management:
  — back pain comes from the spine and involves the nervous system
  — it is due to injury
  — the back is irritable and should be treated by rest

- The discovery of the disc brought these ideas together and made them into a marketable package. Since World War II, orthopedic surgeons have come to dominate orthodox medical thinking and the treatment of back pain and sciatica

There is nothing new about back pain. What is new is the scale of chronic disability attributed to simple backache. Apart from rare cases, this began in the late 19th century and has increased dramatically since World War II. It is closely linked to a changed understanding and management of back pain. Better social support makes rest possible and may even encourage chronic disability due to simple backache. Health care has certainly not solved the problem, and may even have contributed to it.

There is another side to this story. Osteopathic medicine, chiropractic, physical therapy and manual medicine all have much in common as musculoskeletal specialties. Although in some ways they seem very different, they all share ancient traditions. They all have distinct professional identities, and to some extent compete for the same patients. The politics of their relationships vary in each country and I do not wish to take sides. Let me simply nail my colors to the mast, and say as an independent observer that they seem to me to have more in common than otherwise. We can all potentially learn from each other, but first we must be willing to communicate. We must develop a common language. The desperate needs of patients with back pain should override our professional dignities. I recognize the political obstacles to achieving this, but I have no doubt about the goal.

History shows that chronic low back disability is not an inevitable consequence of simple backache. If we can create such an epidemic, then we can also stop it. We cannot turn back the clock. Instead, we must learn from our past mistakes to reach a better understanding of the problem and its management (see Table 4.1).

REFERENCES

Allan D B, Waddell G 1989 An historical perspective on low back pain and disability. Acta Orthopaedica Scandinavica (suppl 234) 60: 1–23

Andrae A 1929 Ueber Knorpelknotchen am hinteren Ende der Wirbelbandscheiben im Bereich des Spinalkanals. Beitr z path Anat u z allg Path 82: 464–474

APTA 1997 Guide to physical therapist practice: a description of patient management, 2nd edn. American Physical Therapy Association, Alexandria, VA, vol I

Boni T, Benini A, Dvorak J 1994 Historical perspectives: Domenico Felice Antonio Cotugno. Spine 19: 1767–1770

Breasted J H 1930 The Edwin Smith papyrus: published in facsimile and heiroglyphic transliteration with translation and commentary in two volumes. University of Chicago Press, Chicago

Brown T 1828 On irritation of the spinal nerves. Glasgow Medical Journal 1: 131–160

Conn H R 1922 The acute painful back among industrial employees alleging compensation injury. Journal of the American Medical Association 79: 1210–1212

Cotugno D 1765 De ischiade nervosa commentarius. Neapoli apud frat Simonios (A treatise on the nervous sciatica or nervous hip gout). English translation 1775 Wilkie, London

CSP 1991 Curriculum of study. Chartered Society of Physiotherapists, London

CSP 1993 Standards of physiotherapy practice. Chartered Society of Physiotherapists, London

Cyriax J 1969 Textbook of orthopaedic medicine. Williams & Wilkins, Baltimore

Dandy W E 1929 Loose cartilage from intervertebral discs simulating tumour of the spinal cord. Archives of Surgery 19: 660–672

DiGiovanna E L, Schiowitz S (eds) 1991 An osteopathic approach to diagnosis and treatment. Lippincott, Philadelphia

Erichsen J E 1866 On railway and other injuries of the nervous system. Six lectures on certain obscure injuries of the nervous system commonly met with as a result of shock to the body received in collisions in railways. Walton & Maberly, London

Fowler T 1795 Medical reports of the effects of blood letting, sudorifics and blistering in the cure of acute and chronic rheumatism. Johnstone, London

Fuller H W 1852 On rheumatism, rheumatic gout and sciatica: the pathology, symptoms and treatment. Churchill, London

Goldthwait J E 1911 The lumbosacral articulation. An explanation of many cases of 'lumbago', 'sciatica' and paraplegia. Boston Medical and Surgical Journal 164: 365–372

Haldeman S 1992 History, philosophy and sociology of chiropractic. In: Haldeman S (ed) Principles and practice of chiropractic, 2nd edn. Appleton & Lange, Norwalk Ca, p 1–59

Hamilton A M 1894 Railway and other accidents. William Wood, New York, p 15–44

Keith A 1919 Menders of the maimed. Oxford Medical Publications, London

Keller T, Chappell T 1996 Historical perspective: the rise and fall of Erichsen's Disease (railway spine). Spine 21: 1597–1601

Key J A 1945 Intervertebral disc lesions are the most common cause of back pain with or without sciatica. Annals of Surgery 121: 534–544

King H D 1915 Injuries of the back from a medical legal standpoint. Texas State Journal of Medicine 11: 442–445

Lancet Commission 1862 The influence of railway travelling on public health. Lancet 1: 15–19, 48–53, 79–84

Luschka H 1858 Die Halbgelenke des menschlichen Korpers. G Reimer, Berlin

McClune T, Clarke R, Walker C, Burton K 1997 Osteopathic management of mechanical low back pain. In: Giles L G F, Singer K P (eds) Clinical anatomy and management of low back pain. Butterworth-Heinemann, Oxford, p 358–368

Martinke D J 1991 The philosophy of osteopathic medicine. In: DiGiovanna E L, Schiowitz S (eds) An osteopathic approach to diagnosis and treatment. Lippincott, Philadelphia, p 3–6

Middleton G S, Teacher J H 1911 Injury of the spinal cord due to rupture of an intervertebral disc due to muscular effort. Glasgow Medical Journal 76: 1–6

Mixter W J, Ayer J B 1935 Herniation or rupture of the intervertebral disc into the spinal canal. New England Journal of Medicine 213: 385–395

Mixter W J, Barr J S 1934 Rupture of the intervertebral disc with involvement of the spinal canal. New England Journal of Medicine 211: 210–215

Murphy 1995 Healing the generations: A history of physical therapy and the American Physical Therapy Association. American Physical Therapy Association, Alexandria, VA

Northup G W 1966 Osteopathic medicine: an American reformation. American Osteopathic Association, Chicago

Page H W 1885 Injuries of the spine and spinal cord. Churchill, London

Paracelsus (Bombastus A B Hohenheim – Aureolus Philipus Theorastus) 1493–1541 Samtliche Wenke Harausg (14 vols). von K Sudhoff und W Mathiessen (1922–23), Munchen, Berlin, Barth und Oldenburg

Palmer D D 1910 The science, art and philosophy of chiropractic. Portland Printing House, Oregon

Ramazzini B 1705 A treatise on the diseases of tradesmen. Bell, London

Schiotz E H, Cyriax J 1975 Manipulation past and present. Heinemann, London

Schmorl G 1929 Ueber Knorpel knoten an der Hinterflache der Wirbelbandschieben. Fortschr a.d Geb.d Rontgenstrahlen 40: 629–634

Scudamore C 1816 A treatise on the nature and cure of gout and rheumatism. Longmans, London

Sculteti I 1662 Armamentarium Chirurgicum. Amstellodami

Seffinger M A 1997 Development of osteopathic philosophy. In: Ward R C (ed) Foundations of osteopathic medicine. Williams & Wilkins, Baltimore, p 3–12

Shorter E 1992 From paralysis to fatigue: a history of psychosomatic illness in the modern era. Free Press, New York

Still A T 1899 Philosophy of osteopathy. A T Still, Kirksville Mo

Sydenham T 1734 The whole works of that excellent physician Dr Thomas Sydenham (translated by John Pechey), 10th edn. W Feales, London

Thomas H O 1874 Contributions to medicine and surgery. Lewis, London

Valleix F L I 1841 Traite des neuralgies ou affections douloureuses des nerfs. J B Baillière, Paris

Vesalius A 1543 De humani corporis fabrica. Basileae ex off Ioannis Oporini

Virchow R 1858 Die Cellular pathologie in Ihrer Begrundug auf physiologische und pathologische. A Hirschwald, Berlin

Ward R C (ed) 1997 Foundations of osteopathic medicine. Williams & Wilkins, Baltimore

Wentworth E T 1916 Systematic diagnosis in backache. Journal of Bone and Joint Surgery 8: 137–170

Wickstead J H 1948 The growth of a profession. Being the history of the Chartered Society of Physiotherapy 1894–1945. Edward Arnold, London

5

The epidemiology of low back pain

What is the impact of back pain today? There is no doubt that it is a common problem, however we try to measure it. We may look at low back pain as a symptom in the general population, as a cause of disability, as a reason for health care, or as a cause of short- and long-term work loss. By any of these measures, back pain is a major problem. But is it true that we now have an epidemic of low back pain? Is it an increasing problem? As we saw in Chapter 3, we must look at pain and disability separately. First, we will look at the occurrence of back pain today. Then we will look at the present scale of low back disability. Finally, we will see how they are changing.

Defining the problem

To understand the epidemiology of low back pain, we must first consider what we are trying to measure and how we can measure it. Most recent surveys define low back pain between the costal margins and the gluteal folds. Some surveys now include a diagram (Fig. 5.1).

We should also remind ourselves about common epidemiologic terms:

- *Prevalence* is the proportion of people in a known population who have the symptom over a particular period of time.
- *Point prevalence* is the percentage who have pain now, on the day of interview.
- *One month* or *1 year prevalence* is the percentage who have pain at some time during that period.

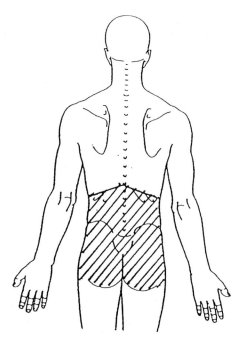

Figure 5.1 The diagram of low back pain used in all recent British surveys. (From the *South Manchester Study,* with thanks.)

- *Lifetime prevalence* is the percentage who can remember pain at some time in their life, whether or not they have it now.
- *Incidence* is the percentage of a known population who develop new symptoms within a given time. It is commonly applied to those who report injuries or present for health care.

There is a major problem in defining what constitutes 'low back pain'. Do we include any low back symptoms, no matter how mild or how brief their duration? How do we draw the line between symptoms, trouble, ache and pain? Many surveys ask about pain that lasts for a certain time, often a day or week(s). Is the pain severe enough to stay off work? But then we are talking about disability rather than pain. Is the pain severe enough to seek health care? We must make a very clear distinction between back pain, back disability and health care for back pain. We have already seen that pain and disability are not the same thing. The epidemiologic rates of low back pain, low back disability and health care use for back pain are very different.

There is another major limitation to the information we can obtain. We depend largely on peoples' own report of pain and disability, which is open to all the errors of subjective bias. There is a problem of recall bias: the longer the time we ask about, the more unreliable the answers. If we try to overcome this by asking about a shorter period, such as 1 month or 1 year, someone who has had more severe trouble may be more likely to include earlier information. We can get data about work loss, health care use, sick certification and sickness benefits from official statistics, but these usually give lower rates than self-reports of these events from population surveys.

Also, there may be bias from the particular sample we study. Many surveys look at a particular group of workers or patients, who may not be typical of the general population. Most data on the epidemiology of back pain comes from North America, Britain and Europe. Raspe (1993) and Shekelle (1997) have reviewed nearly 40 studies. Many of these, particularly the earlier studies, looked at particular groups, at 'clinical' back pain, or at work loss. Many of the surveys are not directly comparable. For example, there is a misconception that back pain is less common in the United States than in Europe. Many authors quote Deyo & Tsui-Wu (1987) for a 1 year prevalence of 10.3% and a lifetime prevalence of 13.8% in the United States, compared with the usual 40–60% in Europe. But this does not compare like with like. Many American surveys try to pick out 'significant' or 'disabling' back pain. Deyo & Tsui-Wu used the Second National Health and Nutrition Examination Survey (NHANES II) which only included back pain that lasted 'most days for at least two weeks'. Another American survey only looked at back pain that caused days in bed or that led to health care. Such questions will only include the more severe cases of back pain. Those US studies that ask more open questions about back pain get very similar results to those found in Europe.

The best evidence on the epidemiology of back pain is from large, representative population surveys (Table 5.1). Most recent surveys have used similar wording for their questions, and

Table 5.1 Recent population surveys

Survey	Country	Population	Size	Definition of low back pain (LBP)
Consumers' Association (1985)	UK	Random population survey, age 16+	2000	Some sort of back trouble, or discomfort in your back that has inconvenienced you
Nuprin Pain Report, Taylor & Curran (1985)	US	Random population survey by telephone, age 18+	1254	How many days in the past year have you had LBP?
Von Korff et al (1988)	US	Enrolees large HMO in Seattle	1016	Pain lasting 1 day or more
Walsh et al (1992)	UK	Adults in family practices in eight areas	2667	LBP lasting more than 1 day
Mason (1994)	UK	Random population survey, age 16+	6032	LBP lasting more than 1 day
South Manchester Study 1992–1993	UK	Adults in two family practices, Manchester	7699	LBP lasting more than 1 day
Skovron et al (1994)	Belgium	Random population sample, age 15+	4208	Do you ever have pain in the lower part of your back?

many have asked about pain lasting more than 24 hours, to exclude minor or passing symptoms.

The South Manchester Study

I will describe the *South Manchester Study* because it is one of our best sources of information, and appears frequently in the next three chapters. It may also help us to understand such surveys. This was a longitudinal, community survey to investigate patterns and predictors of back pain and health care use. It looked at 7699 adults aged 18–75 who were registered with two family practices. One was in a large housing project with high social deprivation and unemployment. The other was in a well established, residential area with a broad social mix. An initial postal survey in March 1992 got a 59% response – 4500 subjects (Papageorgiou et al 1995). Health care utilization for back pain was studied prospectively over the next 12 months from medical records (Croft et al 1994). Those who were free of back pain at baseline had a repeat postal questionnaire 12 months later, with a 60% response – 1540 subjects (Papageorgiou et al 1996). An overlapping cohort of 1412 who were free of back pain and employed at baseline underwent a more detailed assessment of work-related psychosocial factors and distress, to find predictors of back pain over the next 12 months (Croft et al 1995, Papageorgiou et al 1997, Macfarlane et al 1997).

THE FREQUENCY OF BACK PAIN

Most people probably get some back symptoms at some time in their lives, but by no means do all these symptoms pose a real health problem. Those who present for health care are sometimes described as 'the tip of an iceberg' which implies that there is a hidden reservoir of disease awaiting treatment. That is a poor analogy. Rather, they form an island of health care amidst a sea of bodily symptoms.

A large number of international studies show that 17–31% of people report some back symptoms on the day of interview; 19–43% report back pain in the last month; and about 60–70% report back pain at some time in their life. The exact figures in different studies appear to depend mainly on the wording of the question rather than on differences among the people studied.

About 70% of Americans have back pain at some time in their life. The *Nuprin Pain Report* (Taylor & Curran 1985) found that back pain was the second most common pain after headache. 56% of American adults said they had had at least 1 day of back pain in the previous year; 34% had pain for 6 days or more; and 14% had pain for more than 30 days in the year. Most back pain was mild and short-lived and had very little effect on daily life, but recurrences were common.

Von Korff et al (1988) found that 41% of American adults aged 26–44 years had back pain in the previous 6 months. Most people had occasional short attacks of pain over a long period. Their pain was usually mild or moderate and did not limit activities. However, about a quarter of those with any back pain said they had it on more than half the days and that it did cause some limitation of their activities.

Recent British surveys give similar figures. Mason (1994) found a point prevalence of 14%. The *South Manchester Study* found a 1 month prevalence of 39% (Papageorgiou et al 1995).

Both Walsh et al (1992) and Mason (1994) found a 1 year prevalence of 36–37%. Both Walsh et al (1992) and Papageorgiou et al (1995) found a lifetime prevalence of 58%, while a large Belgian survey (Skovron et al 1994) found an almost identical lifetime prevalence of 59%. The similarities between the results are striking, despite the differences in the surveys. Mason (1994) and Skovron et al (1994) interviewed national population samples. Walsh et al (1992) and the *South Manchester Study* in Britain, like von Korff et al (1988) in the United States, used questionnaire data from a sample of adult patients at family practices. All the British surveys, like von Korff et al (1988), asked about pain that lasted 24 hours or more and used a diagram to define the lower back. The Belgian survey did not define any duration of pain, but the similarity of the results suggests that people made some sort of judgement themselves and only reported back pain they considered to be 'significant'. The Belgian interviewers did not use a diagram but pointed out the same area of the lower back. Figure 5.2 shows the distribution of back pain in British adults. Walsh et al (1992) obtained similar results.

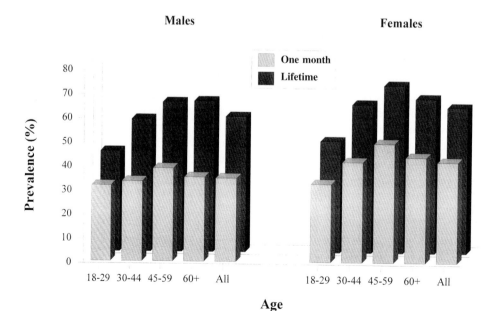

Figure 5.2 Age distribution of 1 month and lifetime prevalence of back pain lasting more than 24 hours in British adults. (From Papageorgiou et al 1995, with permission.)

Table 5.2 Total duration of pain during the previous year as a percentage of those reporting back pain (from Mason 1994, with permission from the Office of National Statistics)

Duration of pain	Male	Female
<1 week	19%	13%
1–4 weeks	38%	28%
1–3 months	15%	18%
3–12 months	10%	16%
Complete year	17%	22%

Mason (1994) asked how long people had had back pain during the previous year (Table 5.2). Nearly half the people with back pain said that it had lasted less than 4 weeks in the year. However, for 19% it lasted the whole year, suggesting that about 6–7% of all adults have back problems throughout the year. The Consumers' Association (1985) had similar findings.

The General Household Survey in Britain (1988–89) found that back problems are one of the most common causes of 'chronic sickness'. About 3–4% of the population aged 16–44 years and 5–7% of those aged 45–64 years report back problems as a 'chronic sickness'. Back trouble is the most common cause of chronic sickness in both men and women under the age of 45 and one of the most common between the age of 45 and 65. Only in women aged over 45 years and men aged over 65 years do 'arthritis and rheumatism' become more common than back trouble. Other bone and joint problems also become more common in both sexes over the age of 65.

The traditional clinical classification of back pain is:

- acute – current attack less than 3 months
- recurrent – current attack less than 3 months, but experienced previous attacks
- chronic – current attack more than 3 months.

This may be a convenient clinical division, but the epidemiology shows that it is not a true picture. Back pain is usually a recurrent, intermittent and episodic problem (Fig. 5.3). Croft et al (1997) suggested that the most important epidemiologic concept is the pattern of back pain over long periods of the individual's life. They base this on four observations:

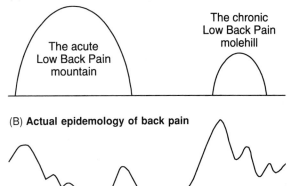

(A) **Traditional clinical concept**

The acute Low Back Pain mountain

The chronic Low Back Pain molehill

(B) **Actual epidemology of back pain**

Figure 5.3 The time course of back pain. (A) The assumed clinical course of acute low back pain. (B) The real course of low back pain. (From Croft et al 1997, with permission.)

- 60–80% of people get low back pain at some time in their lives
- most acute clinical attacks settle rapidly, but residual symptoms and recurrences are common
- 35–40% of people report low back pain lasting 24 hours or more each month and 15–30% of people have some low back symptoms each day
- the strongest known predictor of a further episode of low back pain is the history of previous episodes.

These authors suggested that we should summarize the back pain experience in terms of the total days of pain over 1 year. They also looked at patterns of prevalence and incidence of new episodes over a 1 year period (Papageorgiou et al 1996). At the start of the year, the adult population fits into three groups (Fig. 5.4):

- group 1 – those who have been free of back pain for the previous 12 months (62%)
- group 2 – those who have had intermittent or less disabling low back pain during the previous 12 months (32%)
- group 3 – those who have had long-standing or serious disabling low back pain during the previous 12 months (6%).

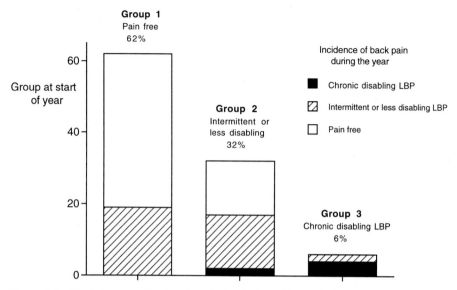

Figure 5.4 The incidence of back pain episodes in the adult population during the course of a year. (Based on ideas and data from Croft et al 1997.)

Over the course of the following year, about one-third of those in group 1 will develop a new episode of low back pain. Hence the 1 year incidence of 'new' episodes among previously pain-free adults is 19%. However, few of them are really experiencing their first ever episode of low back pain. Almost half of group 2 will have further episodes during the following year. Although we often assume that severe and chronic low back pain will continue indefinitely, that is not true. One-third of those in group 3 will improve and have less severe problems during the following year. However, they will be replaced by a comparable number of people from groups 1 and 2 who develop more severe problems during the year. These figures all balance out and the size of each group remains the same. The incidence of new episodes is balanced by the number of people who improve. So the annual prevalence stays at about 38%, and the pool of chronic disabling back pain stays at about 6% of the adult population. Individuals move in and out of the different groups.

Sciatica

Few surveys use strict criteria for sciatica. A number of reports give a lifetime prevalence of

leg pain of 14–40%, but they do not distinguish true nerve root pain from the more common referred leg pain. In the US, Deyo et al (1992) estimated the lifetime prevalence of 'surgically important disc herniation' to be about 2%. In the UK, Lawrence (1977) found the prevalence of 'sciatica suggesting a herniated lumbar disc' to be 3.1% in men and 1.3% in women. Neither of these studies gave their diagnostic criteria. Heliovaara et al (1987) reported the only large population survey with acceptable clinical criteria of nerve root pain: the lifetime prevalence of back pain was 77% in men and 74% in women over the age of 30 years; 35% of men and 45% of women reported some leg pain. Applying strict diagnostic criteria, however, the lifetime prevalence of true sciatica was only 5.3% in men and 3.7% in women.

Comorbidity

Back pain is the third most common bodily symptom, after headache and tiredness. So it is not surprising that people with back pain often report other complaints. The *Nuprin Pain Report* found that 90% of those with frequent back pain had multiple pains, but 50% of them said that back pain was the 'most troublesome'. Clinical and epidemiologic studies show that up to 60% of people with low back pain also report some neck symptoms. Makela (1993) found that many chronic musculoskeletal pains go together. The association was particularly strong between back pain, neck pain and osteoarthritis of the hips and knees. However, inflammatory joint disorders were quite separate.

From an epidemiologic perspective, back pain is not an isolated clinical problem but is often part of general pain complaints. The *South Manchester Study* confirmed the close association between the presence of other pains and the likelihood of developing new back pain (Table 5.3).

Men and women who attend their family doctor with back pain also attend more frequently with other problems. Porter & Hibbert (1986) found that 17% of men who consult their family doctor with back pain also consult about neck pain at some time. Patients who consult with back pain and neck pain, but not sciatica, are also more likely to consult with stress and mental disorders; or, at least, they may be more likely to get a diagnosis of stress and mental disorders.

In Britain, 53% of new recipients of invalidity benefit report more than one long-term health problem (Erens & Ghate 1993).

- About 35–40% of adults report low back pain each year
- This is commonly associated with other bodily symptoms
- The lifetime prevalence of true sciatica is <5%

Table 5.3 Back pain as part of general pain complaints (from the *South Manchester Study*, personal communication)

No back pain at baseline Number of other pains at baseline	Percentage who develop new back pain in next 12 months
0	23.6%
1 area	38.7%
2 areas	37.8%
3 areas	40.5%

LOW BACK DISABILITY

The most important characteristic of low back pain is its impact on the individual's life. It may impact on general health and well-being, activities of daily living, and work.

Remember that all surveys give people's own report of their disability. This report is purely subjective and most surveys only ask about disability in the most general terms. There is no objective evidence or pathologic basis for these figures.

The *Nuprin Pain Report* (Taylor & Curran 1985) found that 14% of adult Americans said that back pain interfered with their routine activities, work or sleep for one or more days in the year. Andersson (1991) found that back problems were the most common cause of activity limitation in people below the age of 45 and the fourth most common in those aged 45–64 years. Seven per cent of adults reported a disability due to their back or due to both their back and other joint problems. On average, this limited their activities for about 23 days each year.

These various figures suggest that 7–14% of adults in the US have some disability due to back pain for a least 1 day each year, i.e. about 15–25 million people. Just over 1% of Americans are permanently disabled by back pain, and another 1% are temporarily disabled by back pain at any one time, i.e. 5 million people.

There are several detailed surveys of low back disability in Britain. Mason (1994) found that 11% of adults said that back pain had restricted their activities during the last 4 weeks. Almost all those aged 16–24 years only had restrictions for a few days. However, there was surprisingly little difference between the ages of 25 and >65 years. About one-third had restrictions for 1–5 days and about one-third had them for the whole 4 weeks. The effect on their lifestyle varied, but mainly involved restriction of normal activities in the home and garden, and restriction of sporting activities or mobility.

Walsh et al (1992) reported the only population survey to use clinical measures of low back disability. They assessed eight activities of daily living to give a total disability score from 0 to 16. Table 5.4 shows the 1 year and lifetime prevalence of low back disability by age and sex.

Mason (1994) found that about 3% of adults in Britain said they had lain down all day or most of the day for at least 1 day during the previous 4 weeks because of back pain. The proportion was similar in men and women and in most age groups. Lying down was most commonly for 1 or 2 days in the past month, although it varied from 1 to 28 days. The *South Manchester Study* found that 8% of adults said they had bed rest for back pain at some time during the previous 12 months. Again, remember that all of these figures reflect what adults in the general population say they do about back pain, not what treatment they receive.

Work loss

It is surprisingly difficult to get accurate information on the amount of work loss associated with back pain. Work loss may vary greatly in different countries and under different social security or compensation systems. Quite apart from the actual differences in work loss, each system also collects different data and has different obstacles to getting an accurate picture.

In most countries, data about work loss is held by individual employers and there are no national statistics. Health care systems do not keep any data on patients' work loss. Social security and compensation systems only keep data about claims and the payments they make. For example, many US authors quote figures for workers' compensation, but this is only a selected part of the whole picture. Many British authors misquote figures for sickness benefits paid, but that is quite different from work loss. The Clinical Standards Advisory Group (CSAG 1994) showed this most clearly. They estimated that work loss due to back pain in 1993 was about 52 million days, while 106 million days' benefits were paid in respect of back pain. However, there was only 7 million days overlap between these two groups. Most of the workers who had short periods off work were paid by their employers and did not receive any state sickness benefit or appear in the Department of Social Security (DSS) statistics. Most of the benefits went to people who were not working anyway.

Guo et al (1995) provided the best estimate of work loss due to back pain in the United States, using data on 30 074 workers from the National Health Interview Survey. In 1988, about 22.4 million people, i.e. 17.6% of all US workers, lost 149 million working days due to back pain. This is the best available estimate, although it is difficult to cross-check, and it is now considerably out of date.

CSAG (1994) estimated that there were about 52 million days of work loss in the UK in 1993, but this was a very rough estimate. It was based on small samples and there was a large range of possible error. Mason (1994) provided data from a sample of 1136 working people with back pain. In total, 6% of workers with back pain said that they had lost some time from work because of back pain during the previous 4 weeks. That is about 2% of all working people, and includes about 0.3% of all workers who were off for the entire 4 weeks (see Table 5.5).

Table 5.4 One year and lifetime prevalence of back pain, disability and time off work (from Walsh et al 1992 with permission from the BMJ Publishing Group)

Prevalence (%)	Age (years)				
	20–29	30–39	40–49	50–59	Total
Male					
Back pain					
1 year	35.4	37.1	38.2	40.5	37.6
Lifetime	52.0	60.4	64.2	70.5	61.3
Disability score >8/16					
1 year	4.1	5.8	6.6	5.3	5.4
Lifetime	8.2	12.6	20.8	23.1	15.9
Time off work					
1 year	9.5	13.5	9.4	9.5	10.6
Lifetime	22.4	31.3	38.2	46.2	34.1
Female					
Back pain					
1 year	27.0	33.6	43.7	35.7	34.8
Lifetime	45.2	53.8	62.3	63.7	55.8
Disability score >8/16					
1 year	2.1	4.7	5.7	5.6	4.5
Lifetime	7.7	13.1	16.4	15.8	13.1
Time off work					
1 year	6.1	5.1	9.8	6.5	6.8
Lifetime	16.9	18.4	29.8	29.8	23.3

Table 5.5 Days off work in the past 4 weeks attributed to back pain in working people with back pain (from Mason 1994, with permission from the Office of National Statistics)

Days off work due to back pain	Number of persons Male	Female
None	547 (95.6%)	521 (92.4%)
1	6	3
2	6	9
3	–	5
4	1	1
5	2	5
6	–	2
7	2	3
8–14	2	4
15–20	2	4
Entire 4 weeks	4	7

Watson et al (1998) provided the most recent UK data from the island of Jersey. The Jersey data is unique, because all work loss of more than 1 day requires medical certification, and all sick pay is by the state, not the employer. Jersey records all individual sickness, incapacity and accident benefits on a computer database. Benefits are paid at a fixed rate and are not related to wages lost. Unique among Western countries, there is no unemployment benefit in Jersey, but the true unemployment rate is less than 3%. In economic terms, the island has virtually full employment. All of these differences mean that the Jersey data may not be typical of the rest of the UK. Despite this, the findings are actually quite close to the CSAG estimates. In 1994, the 1 year incidence of new claims for back pain causing more than 1 day's work loss was 5.6%. Including those still off work from the previous year, the 1 year prevalence of work loss due to back pain was 6.3%. Other surveys suggest that about 35% of those who take time off work are only off for 1 day, and so would not be included in these statistics. If we adjust for this, the 1 year prevalence of back pain in Jersey could be 8.2%. For comparison, Walsh et al (1992) found a 1 year prevalence of work loss of about 6.5% in women and 9.5% in men. By age 50, the lifetime prevalence of any work loss due to back pain was about 30% in women and over 40% in men.

About half the total days lost are by the 85% of people who are off work for short periods, most commonly for less than 7 days. The other half is by the 15% of people who are off work for more than 1 month. This is reflected in the social costs of back pain. It is widely known that 80–90% of the health care costs of back pain are for the 10% of patients with chronic low back pain and disability. The Jersey data shows that the same is true for the costs of wage compensation. In 1994, back pain accounted for 10.5% of all sickness absence in Jersey. Only 3% of those off work with back pain were off for more than 6 months, but they accounted for 33% of the benefits paid (Fig. 5.5).

Work-related back injuries

Back injuries make up almost one-third of all work-related injuries in the United States. There are now about 1 million compensation claims for work-related back injuries each year.

In the UK, the Health & Safety Executive records all work injuries that cause at least 3 days off work. It recorded 34 720 nonfatal back injuries in 1990/91. Only 469 (1.4% of back injuries) were 'major injuries' severe enough to need hospital admission and 48% of these

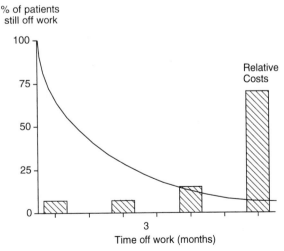

Figure 5.5 The large percentage of wage replacement costs accounted for by a small percentage of claimants. (Based on data from Watson et al 1998.)

major spinal injuries were due to a fall from a height. Major spinal injuries comprised only 3% of all major injuries needing hospital admission. Most back injuries were less serious 'sprains or strains', but they accounted for 23% of all minor work injuries.

Minor back injuries lead to longer time off work, and to higher health and compensation costs than other minor injuries. Table 5.6 combines data from a number of US workers' compensation sources.

Table 5.6 The relative severity of back and other sprains and strains (based on data from various US workers' compensation sources)

	Back sprains and strains	Other sprains and strains
Days off work	38	23
Days of medical treatment	21	8
Total costs (1984 US$)	$308	$167

Sickness benefits

There are many sources of sickness benefits in the US and it is not possible to get total national figures.

There is better data in the UK, although it still has major limitations. The DSS records benefits paid rather than sickness or work loss, and the amount depends on eligibility for benefit. The statistics omit all short spells of sickness lasting 1–3 days. For most workers, sickness lasting anything up to 28 weeks is now covered by statutory sick pay from their employer and does not appear in the DSS statistics. Because of these large omissions, the DSS statistics no longer provide a measure of disability due to back pain. Instead, they are now only a measure of benefits paid for chronic back incapacity.

Table 5.7 shows the DSS statistics for back incapacities for the latest available year, 1995–1996. Remember that these diagnoses reflect what doctors put on certificates rather than actual pathology.

Table 5.7 UK sickness and invalidity benefit for back incapacities during 1995–1996 (based on statistics from the Department of Social Security)

	Spells		Days	
	Males	Females	Males	Females
Ankylosing spondylitis and other inflammatory spondylopathies	38 700	15 100	12 547 900	4 964 400
Spondylosis and allied disorders	30 400	21 100	8 470 800	6 293 100
Intervertebral disc disorders	23 700	11 000	6 863 800	3 072 900
Dorsalgia	180 700	101 700	45 387 600	26 961 000
Sprain and strain of neck	2400	2500	250 800	494 700
Sprain and strain of lumbar spine and pelvis	3700	2300	794 600	592 500
Sprain and strain of unspecified parts of back	6300	2400	592 600	273 800
Total back incapacities	286 100	156 100	74 908 100	42 652 400
All incapacities	2 237 700	1 135 500	599 524 300	297 647 100

Spells are the number of periods of sickness benefits.
Days are the total number of days benefit was paid.

Each year:
- About 35–40% of adults get back pain
- About 5–10% report some low back disability
- Possibly 5–10% lose some time off work, the majority for <7 days
- About 1% are permanently disabled by back pain
- About 6–10% seek health care for back pain

TRENDS OVER TIME

Pain

There is no evidence of any change in the prevalence of back pain. Most surveys for the past 40 years show very similar figures, and apparent differences are mainly due to the wording of the questions. Leboeuf-Yde & Lauritsen (1995) compared 26 Nordic studies from 1954 through 1992 and could not find any definite trend. Leino et al (1994) in Finland reported the only longitudinal study that has used the same questions each year from 1978 to 1992. The prevalence of back pain stayed the same over this time.

Both the historic review and modern epidemiologic surveys agree. All the evidence is that back pain is just the same as it has always been. Back pain is no more common, no different nor any more severe than it has always been; nor is there any evidence of any change in the pathologic basis of simple backache.

Low back disability and sickness benefits

We simply do not have any accurate data on whether there has been any change in clinical disability due to back pain.

There has certainly been a major rise in sickness benefits paid for back incapacities in all Western countries. Again, because of the many sources of sickness benefits in the US, it is difficult to get national figures. Many authors still quote the 2000% rise in SSDI awards from 1957 through 1975. This is a figure from the Social Security Administration, but it gives a completely wrong impression. It refers to the single diagnosis of 'displacement of the inter vertebral disc'. It reflects medical fashion for that particular diagnosis rather than the total impact of back pain. There was then a fall of 42% from 1977 through 1984 that few authors quote. More generally, the National Health Interview Survey showed that more than 1 million adults in the US felt they were 'chronically and totally disabled by back pain' in 1987. This had increased by 21% from 1983. However, we should be cautious when drawing any conclusions about trends from two figures over such a short period. The National Council on Compensation Insurance (NCCI 1992) reported a gradual rise in the proportion of workers' compensation claims due to back injuries from 1981 to 1990 (Fig. 5.6). However, look at the scale of the vertical axis in Figure 5.6 – the change is actually quite small; and it is only illustrating the proportion of claims.

There are much better figures on state sickness benefits for back pain in the UK. Since 1953–1954 the DSS have kept national statistics for sickness and invalidity benefits. Again, remember the limitations of this data. These are benefits paid; they are not trends of back pain or even of low back disability. They are certainly not statistics of work loss, although they are often quoted as such. More specifically, they are statistics of state benefits paid for chronic incapacity attributed by medical certification to some form of back trouble. Over this period, repeated changes in the DSS rules have excluded many people from benefits, so the real increase is probably greater.

We have already seen the dramatic rise in DSS benefits for back incapacity in the UK up to 1994–1995 (Fig. 1.1). Figure 5.7 shows the rates for men and women separately, expressed as days per 1000 members of the population at risk. We saw in the history review that low back disability was for many years a male problem. Over recent years, women are catching up, which probably reflects social trends toward sexual equality.

Table 5.8 compares the change in back incapacities with that of other major diseases over a specific period. Musculoskeletal disorders are now the most common cause of chronic incapacity. Back pain accounts for more than half of

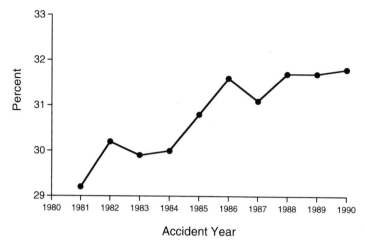

Figure 5.6 Back claims as a percentage of total workers' compensation claims in the United States. (From NCCI 1992, with permission.)

all musculoskeletal incapacity. Table 5.8 also shows the percentage increase from 1978–1979 to 1994–1995, the longest period with comparable statistics. Back incapacities are rising faster than any other incapacity.

These trends in Britain are comparable to other Western countries. For many years, Sweden appeared to be the worst affected. Sweden has a working population of 4.5 million people. There was a dramatic increase in the number of people staying off work with back pain, and in

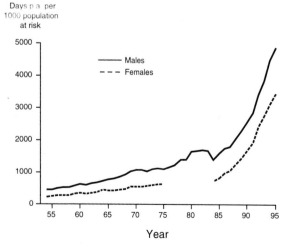

Figure 5.7 Male and female sickness and invalidity benefits for back incapacities in the UK, expressed as the rate per 1000 members of the eligible population. (Based on statistics from the DSS.)

the average time taken off, from the early 1970s to the early 1990s (Table 5.9).

CONCLUSION

The conclusions may be surprising. Despite popular belief, there is no epidemic of back pain. Back pain has not changed. Instead, all the evidence is of an epidemic of disability associated with simple backache. More specifically, all Western countries show a dramatic increase in sick certification and in benefits paid for chronic disability attributed to nonspecific low back pain.

You may notice that throughout this review of the epidemiology I have carefully written about disability *attributed to* or *associated with* back pain rather than *due to* or *caused by* back pain. From a clinical point of view, we have already stressed that pain and disability are not the same. The epidemiology shows the same thing. The real change is not in pathology or even in clinical symptoms, but in patterns of sick certification and sickness benefits. This is very much a social phenomenon.

Up to this point, these statistics show a trend of escalating disability that may seem irreversible. They are a matter of public and political concern. In Sweden, by the early 1990s, there was a cataclysmic forecast that at some time early in the next century, there would not be enough

Table 5.8 A comparison of UK sickness and invalidity benefit for back and other incapacities (based on statistics from the Department of Social Security)

	Days (% of total)		Percentage increase, 1978–1979 to 1991–1992
	1978–1979	1994–1995	
All incapacities	371 041 500 (100%)	745 386 300 (100%)	101%
Musculoskeletal diseases	60 103 600 (16.2%)	223 633 100 (30%)	–
Back incapacities	26 380 000 (7.1%)	115 971 100 (15.6%)	340%
All other musculoskeletal incapacities	33 723 600 (9.1%)	107 622 000 (14.4%)	219%
All circulatory diseases	56 655 100 (15.3%)	123 034 100 (16.5%)	117%
All mental disorders	57 586 200 (15.5%)	153 644 200 (20.6%)	167%
All respiratory diseases	53 746 100 (14.5%)	46 212 200 (6.2%)	–14%

people still working to pay for those with back pain. Fortunately, there are now the first tentative hints that the situation may be beginning to improve.

Concern about these trends in Sweden led to a government report on back pain (Nachemson 1991), which got considerable professional and political attention. It probably had some impact on health care attitudes and practice, although this is difficult to measure. Whether or not due to this report, the proportion of all primary health care visits for back pain in Sweden has fallen from 3.2% in 1990 to 2.2% in 1994. There were also changes in state benefits. Up to 1990,

sickness benefits in Sweden were 90% of salary from day 1. From March 1991, this was reduced to 65% of salary for the first 3 days, 80% from day 4 and 90% from 3 months. From April 1993, it was reduced further to no benefits for the first day, 75% for days 2–3, and 80% from day 4. Over this period there has been a dramatic fall in all sickness. For back pain, the annual prevalence of sick leave has fallen from 6.2% in 1992 to 3.9% in 1996. Total sick leave for back pain has fallen from 28 million days in 1987 to 19.2 million days in 1995. Figure 5.8 shows the reversal in the trend of early retirement due to disability. There is also a slight fall of 10% in the total societal cost of back pain from 1987 to 1995, after adjusting for inflation. However, the current cost of about 30 billion Swedish kroner in 1995 is still 1.5% of Swedish GDP; that is about 2000 SEK (US$250) per inhabitant, which is probably about the same as in most European countries.

It is difficult to tell how much of these Swedish statistics reflect changes in social attitudes, health care or the sickness benefit system. They probably all act together. Indeed,

Table 5.9 Low back disability in Sweden (based on data from the Swedish Council for Technology Assessment in Health Care)

Year	Percentage losing time off work with back pain	Average days lost per annum
1970	1	20
1975	3	22
1980	4	25
1987	8	36
1992	8	39

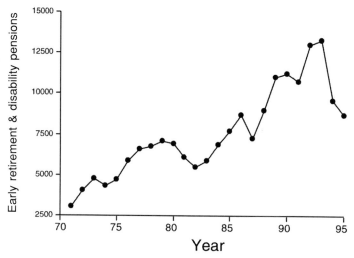

Figure 5.8 The reversal of the trend of the number of people starting early retirement with disability pensions for back pain in Sweden. (Based on data from the Swedish Council on Technology Assessment in Health Care (SBU).)

it may be difficult to change one without the others.

In the UK, a new incapacity benefit was introduced in place of the old sickness and invalidity benefit in April 1995. This changed the regulations for entitlement. Probably more important, it also made major changes in the method and administration of assessment. It is now based on independent medical assessment, which includes a form of functional capacity evaluation, and considers fitness for any form of work. During 1995, the DSS studied a sample of 1200 claimants using the new *all work test* (Swales & Craig 1997). Almost half had a musculoskeletal problem and the majority of these had low back pain. They had all been certified as unfit to work by their own family doctor. When these claimants filled in a detailed questionnaire about their disabilities, only 84% reported themselves as unfit to work. Independent medical assessment suggested that 54% were fit for some form of work (Table 5.10).

The DSS Social Research Branch is continuing to follow a cohort of claimants. The preliminary results suggest that since the changes in 1995, there has been a fall in the number of new claims, and the number starting benefit has plateaued (Dr M Aylward, personal communication). Figure 5.9 shows that for the first time in a generation, the number of days benefit paid for back incapacities did not rise during 1995–1996. We await impatiently the detailed DSS statistics for the next few years!

Some clinicians object that this is all just tinkering with the sickness benefit system and does not do anything about the real clinical problem. Even worse, they suggest that this approach denies benefits to some patients. There is certainly some truth in this view, but this goes to the heart of the current dilemma. We have already seen that we cannot understand or deal with these trends purely as a clinical or health care problem. There is no epidemic of spinal pathology nor even of low back pain. The dramatic increase in benefit claims and

Table 5.10 DSS study of fitness for work using the new *all work test* (based on data from Swales & Craig 1997)

Claimed functional limitation	No significant problems found on independent examination
Walking	65%
Rising from sitting	62%
Sitting	55%
Bending and kneeling	52%
Standing	44%

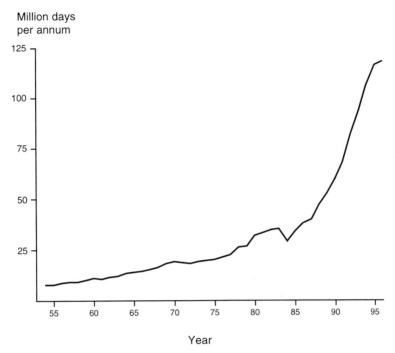

Million days
per annum

Figure 5.9 Trends in UK sickness and invalidity benefits for back pain, showing the apparent levelling off during 1995–1996. (Based on statistics from the DSS.)

payments is for self-reported, nonspecific, low back symptoms. It has been supported by a change in the pattern of sick certification, without any clear pathologic basis. If this is really a social rather than a disease epidemic, then it is entirely proper to address it at least partly by social measures.

The epidemiology, like the clinical analysis, shows that we must distinguish low back pain from disability. We should make a very clear distinction between the epidemiologic sea of those with low back symptoms and the small proportion who become a health problem or receive sickness benefits. We must also consider low back disability and sickness benefits in their social context.

A back pain epidemic?

- There is no evidence of any change in low back pathology
- The prevalence of low back pain has not changed
- There is an exponential increase in chronic disability, medical certification and sickness benefits associated with nonspecific low back pain
- Recent changes to sickness benefit systems may be altering these trends

---

REFERENCES

Andersson G B J 1991 The epidemiology of spinal disorders. In: Frymoyer J W (ed) The adult spine: principles and practice. Raven Press, New York, vol 1 p 107–146

Clinical Standards Advisory Group (CSAG) 1994 Epidemiology review: the epidemiology and cost of back pain. Annex to the CSAG report on back pain. HMSO, London, p 1–72

Consumers' Association 1985 The Which report on back pain. Consumers' Association, London

Croft P, Joseph S, Cosgrove S et al 1994 Low back pain in the community and in hospitals. A report to the Clinical

Standards Advisory Group of the Department of Health. Arthritis & Rheumatism Council, Epidemiology Research Unit, University of Manchester.

Croft P R, Papageorgiou A C, Ferry S, Thomas E, Jayson M I V, Silman A J 1995 Psychologic distress and low back pain: evidence from a prospective study in the general population. Spine 20: 2731–2737

Croft P, Papageorgiou A, McNally R 1997 Low back pain. In: Stevens A, Rafferty J (eds) Health care needs assessment, 2nd series. Radcliffe Medical Press, Oxford, ch 3, p 129–182

Deyo R A, Tsui-Wu Y-J 1987 Functional disability due to back pain. Arthritis and Rheumatism 30: 1247–1253

Deyo R A, Rainville J, Kent D L 1992 What can the history and physical examination tell us about low back pain? Journal of the American Medical Association 268: 760–765

Erens B, Ghate D 1993 Invalidity benefit: a longitudinal study of new recipients. Department of Social Security Research report no. 20. HMSO, London, p 1–127

Guo H-R, Tanaka S, Cameron L L et al 1995 Back pain among workers in the United States: national estimates and workers at high risk. American Journal of Industrial Medicine 28: 591–602

Heliovaara M, Impivaara O, Sievers K, Melkas T, Knekt P, Korpi J, Aromaa A 1987 Lumbar disc syndrome in Finland. Journal of Epidemiology and Community Health 41: 251–258

Lawrence J S 1977 Rheumatism in populations. Heinemann, London

Leboeuf-Yde C, Lauritsen J M 1995 The prevalence of low back pain in the literature: a structured review of 26 Nordic studies from 1954 to 1993. Spine 20: 2112–2118

Leino P L, Berg M A, Puschka P 1994 Is back pain increasing? Results from national surveys in Finland. Scandinavian Journal of Rheumatology 23: 269–276

Macfarlane G F, Thomas E, Papageorgiou A C, Croft P R, Jayson M I V, Silman A J 1997 Employment and work activities as predictors of future low back pain. Spine 22: 1143–1149

Makela M 1993 Common musculoskeletal syndromes. Prevalence, risk indicators and disability in Finland. Publications of the Social Insurance Institution, Finland (ML 123)

Mason V 1994 The prevalence of back pain in Great Britain. Office of Population Censuses and Surveys, Social Survey Division (now Office of National Statistics). HMSO, London, p 1–24

Nachemson A 1991 Ont i Ryggen. Back pain – causes, diagnosis, treatment. SBU Report. Swedish Council on Technology Assessment in Health Care, Stockholm, p 19

NCCI 1992 Workers compensation back claim study. National Council on Compensation Insurance, Florida, p 1–25

Papageorgiou A C, Croft P R, Ferry S, Jayson M I V, Silman A J 1995 Estimating the prevalence of low back pain in the general population. Evidence from the South Manchester back pain survey. Spine 20: 1889–1894

Papageorgiou A C, Croft P R, Thomas E, Ferry S, Jayson M I V, Silman A J 1996 Influence of previous pain experience on the episode incidence of low back pain: results from the South Manchester Back Pain Study. Pain 66: 181–185

Papageorgiou A C, Macfarlane G F, Thomas E, Croft P R, Jayson M I V, Silman A J 1997 Psychosocial factors in the workplace – do they predict new episodes of low back pain? Spine 22: 1137–1142

Porter R W, Hibbert C S 1986 Back pain and neck pain in four general practices. Clinical Biomechanics 1: 7–10

Raspe H 1993 Back pain. In: Silman A J, Hochberg M C (eds) Epidemiology of the rheumatic diseases. Oxford University Press, Oxford, ch 14, p 330–374

Shekelle P 1997 The epidemiology of low back pain. In: Giles L G F, Singer K P (eds) Clinical anatomy and management of low back pain. Butterworth Heinemann, London, ch 2

Skovron M L, Szpalski M, Nordin M, Melot C, Cukier D 1994 Sociocultural factors and back pain. A population-based study in Belgian adults. Spine 19: 129–137

Swales K, Craig P 1997 Evaluation of the incapacity benefit medical test. In-house report 26. Social Research Branch, Department of Social Security, London

Taylor H, Curran N M 1985 The Nuprin pain report. Louis Harris and Associates, New York, p 1–233

Von Korff M, Dworkin S F, Le Resche L A et al 1988 An epidemiologic comparison of pain complaints. Pain 32: 173–183

Walsh K, Cruddas M, Coggon D 1992 Low back pain in eight areas of Britain. Journal of Epidemiology and Community Health 46: 227–230

Watson P J, Main C J, Waddell G, Gales T F, Purcell-Jones G 1998 Medically certified work loss, recurrence and costs of wage compensation for back pain: a follow-up study of the working population of Jersey. British Journal of Rheumatology 37: 82–86

6

Risk factors for low back pain

Who gets back pain? The simple answer, of course, is that most of us get back pain at some time, but there is obviously much more to it than that. Let us consider personal and occupational risk factors in more detail. Box 6.1 lists those factors that are generally considered in relation to work-related back pain.

Box 6.1 Risk factors that have been associated with work-related back pain

---

Physical work factors
- Heavy manual work
- Lifting and twisting
- Postural stress
- Whole body vibration

Psychosocial work factors
- Monotonous work
- Lack of personal control
- Low job satisfaction

Physiologic factors
- Low physical fitness
- Inadequate trunk strength

Health behavior
- Smoking

PERSONAL RISK FACTORS

Heredity

Genetic factors influence certain spinal disorders, such as spondylolisthesis, scoliosis and ankylosing spondylitis. A few clinical studies suggest that there may sometimes be a familial or genetic predisposition to disc prolapse. However, this is of little relevance to nonspecific back pain.

The Finnish twin study (Battie et al 1995) found that identical twins showed very similar MRI changes in their spines, despite different occupational histories. This is frequently misquoted as showing that genetic factors largely determine degenerative changes in the spine. However, these findings are hardly surprising, considering that identical twins, by definition, have the same body build and metabolism, and share their early lives. The main message of this study was that genetics, body build and make-up, and early environment are more important than occupational factors in determining the pattern of degenerative changes with aging. The authors are quick to point out that this kind of study cannot separate genetic, anthropometric and metabolic factors, and the effect of shared early environment and lifestyle influences (personal communication). Furthermore, these findings still left a great deal of degenerative changes unexplained, particularly at the lower lumbar levels which are most important clinically. We must also remember that there is very little correlation between MRI changes and symptoms. In an earlier and rarely quoted study, Heikkila et al (1989) compared more than 9000 pairs of identical and non-identical twins. Only about 10% of 'sciatica' could be explained by constitutional similarity. As most of us get back trouble anyway, because we are human, this statistic is not very meaningful.

Most importantly, there is no evidence whatsoever that genetic or constitutional factors determine who is going to become a back cripple.

Sex

Men and women get more or less the same back pain.

Table 6.1 shows data from all the recent large population surveys in the UK. Most of these surveys show a slightly higher prevalence of back pain in women than in men. We should, however, interpret this against a background that women report a slightly higher level of most symptoms. This could be due as much to bodily awareness, pain perception and style of reporting, as to any physical difference in their backs.

The evidence on low back disability is conflicting. Women report most long-standing sickness slightly more frequently than men, yet 'chronic sickness' due to back trouble is slightly lower in women. Mason (1994) found that 9% of men and 13% of women said that back pain had restricted their activities in the previous 4 weeks. Walsh et al (1992) found 1 year prevalences of more severe low back disability of 5.4% in men and 4.5% in women. The lifetime prevalences were 15.9% in men and 13.1% in women.

Mason (1994) found that 2.5% of men and 3.4% of women said they had laid down for all or most of the day at least once in the previous 4 weeks. Again, remember the difference in how women report symptoms. Overall, there does not appear to be any major difference in low back disability between men and women.

The evidence on work loss is also conflicting. Almost all workers' compensation figures show more work-related back injuries and

Table 6.1 Prevalence of back pain by sex

Prevalence	Study	Male (%)	Female (%)
Point prevalence	Mason (1994)	12	15
1 month prevalence	Consumers' Association (1985)	34	42
	Papageorgiou et al (1995)	43	48
1 year prevalence	Walsh et al (1992)	38	35
	Mason (1994)	36	38
Lifetime prevalence	Consumers' Association (1985)	43	48
	Walsh et al (1992)	61	56
	Papageorgiou et al (1995)	56	60

claims in men, although in some series women stay off work longer. However, we cannot draw general conclusions because this data only covers work-related back pain in selected groups of workers. Men and women often do very different jobs, with different physical demands and different psychosocial conditions. To see the effects of gender, we must look at population surveys. Mason (1994) found that 4% of working men and 6% of working women had time off work with back pain in the previous 4 weeks. The Consumers' Association (1985), in contrast, found that 21% of working men and 18% of working women had time off work in the previous year with back pain. In that survey, 8% of men and 3% of women said they had changed their job because of back pain, while 7% of men and 5% of women said they had given up work because of back pain. In the UK, the social security benefits paid for chronic back incapacity have always been higher in men than in women, although women do now seem to be catching up (Fig. 5.7). Mason (1994) found that 26% of men and 15% of women who are not employed blame their not working at least partly on back pain.

All of these figures may reflect the social settings of each survey more than any biologic difference between men and women.

Sciatica does appear to be more common in men than in women. Heliovaara et al (1987) found lifetime prevalences of 5.3% in men and 3.7% in women. Lawrence (1977) found prevalences of 3.1% in men and 1.3% in women. Clinical reports all show more men coming to spinal surgery, although this may also be due to different referral patterns and different selection for surgery in men and women.

Many women have back pain during the later stages of pregnancy, possibly an effect of altered posture and hormonal changes in ligaments. This does not, however, appear to have any lasting effect. Several early reports suggested that women with multiple pregnancies might continue to have a higher prevalence of back pain. More detailed studies do not seem to confirm this. Recent studies by Ostgaard et al (1996) suggest that there may have been confu-

sion between posterior pelvic pain and lumbosacral pain. The main problem in pregnancy may be pelvic pain, which usually settles after delivery. When they distinguished this, pregnancy did not appear to influence future back pain.

Back pain in men and women

- There is very little evidence of much biologic difference in back pain between men and women
- Women report a slightly higher prevalence of back pain than men, as is the case for most other bodily symptoms
- Sciatica is more common in men
- There is conflicting evidence and probably little difference in low back disability
- Back injuries at work, time off work, sickness benefits, and compensation claims may reflect different social and work patterns rather than any biologic difference

---

Age

Most clinical series suggest that the peak incidence of back pain and sciatica is at about 40 years of age, but this only tells us about presentation for health care, and most of these series are about selected groups of patients attending specialists.

Population surveys show a slightly older and much flatter peak prevalence. Papageorgiou et al (1995) found that the 1 month prevalence of back pain rose with age, but then fell slightly over the age of 60 (Fig. 5.2). Walsh et al (1992) found that the 1 year prevalence rose steadily with age in men. In women, it rose with age but then fell slightly over the age of 50 (Table 5.4). Mason (1994) found that the 1 year prevalence rose with age but fell over the age of 65 in both men and women. The Consumers' Association (1985) and Croft et al (1994) found that lifetime prevalence increased from the late teens up to 45–55 years and then remained more or less constant. These studies all suggest that the peak prevalence of back pain is somewhere between 40 and 60 years. There is probably a slight fall in later life. There is one exception to these findings. Mason (1994) found a steady increase in point prevalence with age in both men and women, from 26% under 35 years to

48% over 65 years. This raises the possibility that older people under-report their past history of back pain because of poorer memory.

Population surveys of adults suggest that age of onset is spread evenly from 16 to the early 40s. It is uncommon to develop simple backache for the first time after the mid-50s. However, several recent studies of children show a higher prevalence of back pain than we previously realized. Burton et al (1996a) prospectively studied 216 adolescents aged between 11 and 15 years. Only 12% of 11-year-olds said they had ever had back pain, but by age 15 this rose to 50%. Their back pain was usually recurrent but did not deteriorate with time. Adolescents appear to have about the same prevalence of back pain as adults, but it is rarely disabling and few seek health care. Burton et al (1996a) suggested that we should consider most adolescent back trouble to be a normal life experience and not attach undue significance to it. We have no evidence that it leads to more severe low back trouble in adult life.

The Consumers' Association (1985) and Mason (1994) both found that the amount of back pain experienced during the year increased with age. Twenty-four per cent of those aged 16–24 with back pain said it lasted less than 1 week and

only 6% said it lasted the whole year. In contrast, only 12% of those aged over 65 with back pain said it lasted less than 1 week, whereas 27% said it lasted the whole year.

All forms of chronic disability increase with age, and particularly affect the elderly. Mason (1994) found that restricted activities attributed to back pain rose with age in both men and women (Fig. 6.1).

We have already seen that Walsh et al (1992) presented the best data on low back disability. They found a rise between the ages 20–29 and 30–39, but disability then remained constant up to age 50–59. Mason (1994) found that 8–9% of those with back pain had lain down for all or most of the day at least once in the previous 4 weeks. There was little change from age 16 to 64. If anything, it fell slightly to 6% in those over 65, but these were all small samples.

None of these surveys found much difference in the number of days off work with back pain between the ages of 16 and 64. This does not, however, allow for those who retire early because of back pain and who are no longer employed. Mason (1994) found that older people who were not employed were more likely to give back pain as their reason for not working (Table 6.2).

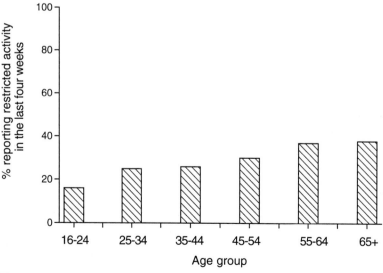

Figure 6.1 Age variation of restricted activity due to back pain. (Based on data from Mason 1994, with permission from the Office for National Statistics.)

Table 6.2 Relation between age and back pain as reason for not working (based on data from Mason 1994, with permission from the Office for National Statistics)

Age	Percentage of those not employed giving back pain as the reason
16–24	2%
25–44	16%
>45	21%

Back pain and age

- Back symptoms generally start between adolescence and early adult life
- The prevalence of back pain increases from our teens to our late 40s or early 50s, but may fall slightly above the age of 60 years
- In those who do continue to have back pain, it is likely to be more frequent or more constant with increasing age
- There is conflicting evidence as to whether low back disability and work loss increase much between our late 20s and mid- to late 50s

Body build

Many studies have looked for possible relationships between body build and back pain. Some studies suggest that taller people may have slightly more back trouble, but more studies disagree. Contrary to popular belief, most studies show that body weight, and even obesity, does not increase the risk of back pain. There is also no evidence that weight loss is an effective treatment for back pain. Doctors and therapists frequently comment on unequal leg length, but most studies fail to prove any significant relation to back pain.

Overall, the data is conflicting but generally shows that there is no strong relation between height, weight, body build and back pain.

Physical fitness

There is now considerable interest in the role of physical fitness in back pain. There is clinical evidence that people with chronic back pain are less fit, but this could be an effect rather than the cause. Some authors suggest that people who are physically active and take

regular exercise have less back pain, but this rests mainly on a single classic study. Cady et al (1979) found that physically fit firefighters got fewer back injuries than those who were less fit. Noone has replicated that study, and it may be unique to a very select population in a high-risk situation. Gyntelberg (1974) and Troup et al (1987) found that aerobic capacity did not predict future back pain. The *Boeing study* (Battie et al 1989a) and Ready et al (1993) also found that physical fitness did not predict future work-related back injuries.

Leino (1993) carried out a prospective, 10-year study of the effect of leisure time physical activity on low back disorders. People who took regular physical exercise had fewer low back symptoms and better physical condition of the back, as assessed by a physiotherapist. This effect was statistically significant, but only in men. There was no effect in women, and even in men the effect was very weak, about 1–2%. In any event, it is not clear to what extent this reflected more general aspects of lifestyle.

There are many health advantages to being physically fit. There are strong theoretic reasons and some clinical evidence to suggest that physically fit patients may make a more rapid recovery from acute back pain and be less likely to develop chronic pain and disability.

In summary, physical fitness may help to reduce the likelihood of developing new episodes of back pain, but is probably more relevant to dealing with back pain once it has occurred.

Smoking

Many studies link back trouble with smoking. Battie et al (1991) looked at various theories. Smoking varies with social class, education and occupation. Hence, smoking may simply reflect a complex set of demographic, psychosocial and lifestyle factors that alter the risk of back pain. Smoking also seems to be linked to how people report pain and may be related more strongly to pain in the limbs than to pain in the neck or back. Smoking could also have a more direct physical effect. There may be some relation between smoking, physical fitness and body weight. In theory, smoking may cause chronic cough, which may affect disc prolapse and sciatica, although there is no direct evidence on the relationship between smoking and sciatica. In animal experiments, smoking causes changes in disc nutrition. Battie et al (1991) found degenerative changes on MRI in the discs of smokers compared with their nonsmoking identical twins.

Deyo & Bass (1989) made a careful analysis of a very large population sample in the United States. They found a threshold effect between smoking and back pain, with a higher risk in people who smoke three or more packs per day. This was true even after allowing for exercise and obesity. Those who had stopped smoking more than 10 years previously had no higher risk of back pain than nonsmokers.

In summary, there is consistent evidence of a higher prevalence of back pain associated with smoking, but it may not be simple cause and effect – and the effect is quite weak.

Social class

There are many social influences on back pain and disability. As a very crude starting point, we might look at variation with social class. Most British surveys use a classification of social class based mainly on occupation:

I: professional groups such as doctors, lawyers and scientists
II: 'intermediate' groups such as teachers, nurses and self-employed shopkeepers
III: skilled occupations
    — IIINM: skilled nonmanual, such as clerical workers
    — IIIM: skilled manual, such as tradesmen
IV: partly skilled, such as process workers in industry or transport workers
V: unskilled, such as laborers and cleaners.

This classification is really twofold. It is partly occupational, with a major division between manual and nonmanual, and that may be why it usually shows more effect in men than in women. It is also partly socioeconomic, and serves as a proxy for all facets of social disad-

vantage, such as education, housing and income, in both men and women.

Walsh et al (1992) provided most detail on the relation between back pain and social class (Table 6.3). In men, the prevalences of back pain, disability and work loss all rose between social classes I–II and IV–V. In women, however, there was very little correlation, and only the 1 year prevalence of disability showed a similar pattern to men. In complete and unexplained contrast, however, there was no trend in lifetime disability in either men or women. Croft & Rigby (1994) tried to disentangle the socioeconomic influences. In men, the only correlation seemed to be with unskilled manual labor. Women in the lowest income category and those with less formal education also had more back pain, and in these cases it seemed to be a question of social disadvantage. We simply do not know what aspects of social environment, lifestyle, or attitudes and behavior account for this.

Mason (1994) found little relation between the prevalence of back pain or disability and social class. However, there was a clear relation with work loss, generally between the nonmanual social classes I–IIINM and the manual classes IIIM–V. A higher proportion of both men and women in the manual classes blamed their back pain on work. They were also more likely to lie down with back pain. In employed people with back pain, about 4% in the

Table 6.3 Relation between back pain and social class (from Walsh et al 1992, with permission from the BMJ Publishing Group)

	Social class			
	Men		Women	
Prevalence	I–II	IV–V	I–II	IV–V
Back pain				
1 year	23%	42%	No trend	
Lifetime	51%	65%	No trend	
Low back disability				
1 year	2.9%	8.1%	1.9%	6.2%
Lifetime	No trend		No trend	
Work loss due to back pain				
1 year	5.6%	13.9%	No trend	
Lifetime	22.3%	38.5%	No trend	

nonmanual classes and 8.7% in the manual classes were off work for at least 1 day in the previous 4 weeks with back pain. The Consumers' Association (1985) also found corresponding figures of 14 and 23%, respectively, for the number who had lost any time off work in the previous year. There was a clear social gradient in those who had given up work and said that it was because of back pain (Table 6.4).

Many international studies show a similar relationship between lower education level and a higher prevalence of back pain, although a few studies disagree. Several studies show, without exception, a relationship between lower education and more work loss due to back pain. Many of these studies emphasize the interrelation between social class, education and heavy manual work, but few try to unravel this.

In a very careful analysis, Makela (1993) concluded that education was simply an indirect measure of heavy work, work stress and work injury. In an equally careful study, Deyo & Tsui-Wu (1987) found that education did have an independent influence. Viikari-Juntura et al (1991) made one of the few longitudinal studies and found no link between intelligence or socioeconomic status in adolescence and low back symptoms in adult life. Dione et al (1995) carried out a much shorter 2-year study of education and back-related disability in adults. Like most previous studies, they found that people with less than 13 years of schooling had more disability. More important was what happened over the next 2 years. Disability tended to improve, particularly in those with more education, but it did not improve as much in those with less education. These authors also considered possible mechanisms to explain the relationship, and suggested that occupational

and psychologic factors are most important. They did not think it was a question of health care access or use.

In summary, there is conflicting evidence concerning the relationship between the prevalence of back pain and lower social class, and the effect is probably weak. There is good evidence that back pain leads to more work loss in people of lower social class. The relationship to social class is fairly consistent in men but less clear in women. The problem is what this means. Social class is a very crude index to a host of social, educational, occupational, economic, lifestyle and psychosocial influences, any of which could affect work loss associated with back pain. It is probably partly a matter of manual work, particularly in men. It is probably also a matter of social disadvantage in both men and women, although we do not know exactly which aspects of this disadvantage are important or how they affect back pain.

The influence of social class on back pain

- Social class reflects occupation, particularly manual vs. nonmanual, and social disadvantage
- The prevalence of back pain may be slightly greater in those from a lower social class
- There is a clear and marked increase in work loss due to back pain with lower social class
- It is not clear what aspects of work, social disadvantage, lifestyle, or attitudes and behavior influence this

---

OCCUPATIONAL RISK FACTORS

Our present ideas about work-related back pain are largely based on the concept of injury (Pope et al 1991). Biomechanical theory suggests that direct trauma, a single 'overexertion', and repetitive or sustained loading could all cause damage to the back. Musculoskeletal strength may vary with sex, age, body build, physical fitness or fatigue, so the load that may cause injury will vary with the individual and with time.

Various studies suggest that there are five job-related factors that load the spine which may relate to back pain, back injury and work loss:

Table 6.4 Social class and giving up work (based on data from the Consumers' Association 1985)

Social class	Number who said they gave up work because of back pain
I–II	2%
III	4%
IV–V	11%

- heavy manual work
- lifting
- twisting
- sitting
- driving.

Many jobs involve several of these factors, so it is difficult to sort out their relative importance.

There are many pitfalls to this kind of research and we should interpret the findings with caution. Most studies are cross-sectional or retrospective in design, and only show *associations*. That does not necessarily mean cause and effect – look again at the discussion about smoking (p. 89). Back symptoms, back injury and work loss due to back pain are all quite different. Most studies focus on reported work injury, time off work and claims for compensation, which introduces possible bias in self-reports. Most of the early reports were retrospective studies looking at small groups of workers and matched controls. These groups were often highly selected and not at all typical of the general population. Most studies depend entirely on subjective self-reports, with all the associated potential for bias. The history of back pain and of work exposure to physical load both depend on memory over many years, which may be selective and biased. Several studies have shown that such reports can be wrong. People with back pain overestimate the physical demands of their work compared with their fellow workers who do not have back pain. It is difficult to assess objectively the physical demand of many jobs. Different people in the same job may actually have different duties, and jobs change considerably over a working life. The 'healthy worker effect' may mean that people with back pain change to lighter work or retire, so only the healthier workers are left. Asking people about the onset or cause of their back pain may tell us about what they believe to be the cause, but that may have no pathologic basis. The workers' compensation system and civil litigation may actually encourage workers to blame their job.

The American Academy of Orthopedic Surgeons (AAOS) has recently reviewed the scientific evidence on work-related back pain (Bigos et al 1998). They carried out a systematic review of nearly 1400 abstracts looking for prospective cohort studies and case–control studies, and found very few acceptable studies before 1990. Most of the earlier studies had major weaknesses in methodology, severe bias and inadequate statistics. In this whole field up to 1994, they found only 12 prospective cohort studies and five case–control studies that they considered to be acceptable. Five of the cohort studies looked at the influence of work factors on back symptoms; the other seven cohort studies and all the case–control studies looked at back injuries and claims.

We should keep these problems and that critical review in mind as we consider the occupational risk factors for back pain.

Heavy manual work

Many earlier studies, reviewed by Troup & Edwards (1985), suggested that back trouble is more common in people with heavy manual jobs. Let us look, in turn, at degenerative changes, low back pain, work injuries and work loss.

A number of early radiographic studies showed more frequent signs of severe disc degeneration in men with heavy manual jobs. Most of these studies compared selected groups of workers known to have back trouble with matched controls in lighter jobs. Many of these studies were completely invalid; for example, the frequently quoted study by Lawrence (1977) used small, highly selected groups, failed to allow for X-ray changes with age, and had faulty statistics. However, Riihimaki et al (1989) made a more careful radiographic comparison and found that concrete reinforcement workers had slightly more disc space narrowing and osteophytes than house painters. There are three large population studies which were carried out when it was still ethically acceptable to take radiographs of normal people. Two showed a clear relationship between heavy manual work and radiographic degeneration (Hult 1954b, Biering-Sorensen et al 1985), but the third did not (Hult 1954a). Videman et al (1990) studied 86 male cadavers and found that vertebral osteophytes were more common in those with a history of heavy manual jobs. In contrast, however, symmetrical disc degeneration was more common in those with a history of sedentary work, which casts some doubt on their findings. Battie et al (1995) carried out an MRI study of identical twins and found that occupational exposure to spinal loading had very little effect on degenerative changes.

Many earlier studies showed that people with heavy manual jobs report more back pain. A rough average of these studies suggests that the lifetime prevalence may increase from about 55–60% in workers in light manual occupations to about 70% in workers in heavy manual occupations. However, there are exceptions to these findings. Several studies found little or no relation between back pain and heavy manual work. Housewives get just as much back pain as working women.

Heliovaara et al (1987) found no relation between the prevalence of sciatica and heavy manual work whereas Riihimaki et al (1989) did. Frequently quoted studies by Kelsey et al (1984a,b) suggested a relation between disc prolapse and heavy manual work, but this was a highly selected, clinical series.

Most workers' compensation data suggests that men with heavy manual jobs suffer more back injuries at work. The Labor Force Survey (Hodgson et al 1993) found that manual workers report all musculoskeletal complaints more than nonmanual workers. They also had more persistent symptoms 3 years after stopping work.

There is almost unanimous agreement that people with heavy manual jobs lose more time from work with back pain than other workers. Mitchell (1985) found that people with heavy manual jobs do not stay off work with back pain any more frequently than other workers, but when they do, they stay off longer. Andersson et al (1983) showed that time off work is longer among blue collar workers than among white collar workers (Fig. 6.2). Perhaps surprisingly, however, they found that the same proportion do finally get back to work.

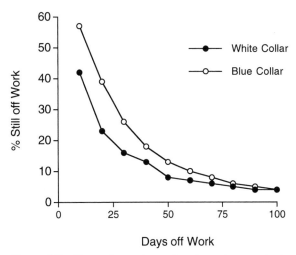

Figure 6.2 Blue collar workers return to work more slowly than white collar workers after an attack of back pain. (Based on data from Andersson et al 1983.)

In summary, then, people with heavy manual jobs do seem to experience more back trouble, but we must be careful about how we interpret this.

Back pain and heavy manual work

- Some early, poor-quality studies suggested that heavy manual work is associated with more degenerative changes in the spine. Better, recent studies do not show any consistent effect
- There is conflicting evidence that people in heavy manual jobs report slightly more back pain. Bigos et al (1996) did not find any scientifically acceptable studies on this fundamental point
- People in heavy manual jobs report more low back injuries
- Back pain does have a greater impact on people in heavy manual jobs. They are more likely to stay off work and they stay off longer. This may, however, be largely the effect of their back pain rather than the cause. It may also reflect medical advice

Lifting

Ideally, we should be able to identify which physical activities in heavy manual work may affect back pain. From biomechanical studies, lifting and twisting are the most likely to damage the spine; these activities are also the ones that have been studied the most in the work place.

Certainly, workers and patients identify lifting as the most common cause of acute back pain. However, this raises all the usual questions about back pain as an injury and whether the lifting is the actual cause of the problem or merely the trigger for symptoms. Many of these reports are of recurrence or aggravation of existing symptoms and not necessarily of lifting as the primary cause. It is the person's own attempt to seek an explanation, which is further confounded by the question of work injury and compensation. Nevertheless, industrial accident and workers' compensation statistics show that back injuries are reported more commonly in jobs that involve:

- heavy lifting
- lifting objects which are bulky or must be held away from the body
- lifting from the floor
- frequent lifting.

The role of frequent heavy lifting over long periods of time is much less clear. Kelsey & Golden (1987) combined several studies and reviewed the biomechanical evidence. They concluded that jobs with frequent lifting of 25 pounds or more have an increased risk for back pain. Lifting less than 25 pounds does not cause a detectable risk. Frymoyer & Cats-Baril (1991) felt that there is little relation between heavy lifting and simple backache, but that people who repetitively lift more than 40 pounds are more likely to seek health care for back pain. Walsh et al (1991) found that both men and women lifting or moving weights of more than 50 pounds are more likely to report back symptoms. None of these studies resolves the question of whether frequent lifting actually causes back pain, or whether back pain simply has more impact if you have a heavy manual job.

In theory, ability to lift and the risk of injury will also vary with the person's strength. Heavy lifting that exceeds the individual's ability may carry greater risk. However, Bigos et al (1998) found no acceptable scientific evidence to confirm this. Moreover, it is difficult to set safe limits. In addition to the weight, we must also consider the frequency and rate of lifting, the level of the lift and the position of the body. The distance between the load and the body greatly increases the forces on the back. Sudden unexpected loads may also increase the risk of injury. Lifting standards set by the US National Institute for Occupational Safety and Health (Waters et al 1993) or the UK Health and Safety Executive (HSE 1992) are simply based on consensus.

Bigos et al (1998) found no acceptable scientific studies on the effect of lifting on the occurrence of back pain itself. The *South Manchester Study* looked at this in their prospective study of working people who were initially free of back pain (Macfarlane et al 1997). They found very little difference in the incidence of back pain during the following year in people in different occupations. People who stood and walked more than 2 hours per shift, and those who lifted or moved weights of more than 25 pounds, developed more low back symptoms. Those who sat for more than 2 hours per shift developed less back pain. However, these effects were only in women and they were relatively weak. In men, none of these job activities had any significant effect on the development of new back pain. Surprisingly, these effects did not increase with age, and occupational history had no cumulative effect.

Twisting

Several studies and strong biomechanical evidence suggest that the risk of back injury is greater when lifting is combined with bending and particularly twisting. The risk of disc prolapse is especially high with combined heavy lifting and twisting. Twisting alone, without lifting, is probably not much risk. Once again, this is all quite different from the risk of back pain.

Stretching and reaching may also be risk factors for back injury but there is little evidence. There is again little data specifically on pushing and pulling, although heavy manual jobs often involve these activities as well.

Bigos et al (1998) found no acceptable studies on twisting.

Sitting

Some studies suggest that prolonged sitting in one position may increase the risk of backache, but the whole debate seems unconvincing to me. Disc pressure at L3 is greater when sitting compared with standing, but this is static loading and the pressure is very low compared with that required to cause experimental damage. There is no other biomechanical evidence that sitting may damage the spine. The epidemiologic evidence is equally unconvincing. Some studies suggest that people who sit in one position for prolonged periods have an increased prevalence of back trouble, but other studies disagree. Some studies suggest that both people who do heavy manual work and those who sit doing very little have an increased prevalence of back trouble, and that only those who do moderate activity experience fewer problems. That makes little sense. Once again, the problem may be that prolonged sitting in one position aggravates back pain that is already present.

We all sit nowadays and back pain is so common that any association may be coincidental; it is very difficult to prove cause and effect. Bigos et al (1998) found no acceptable scientific studies on the effect of sitting.

Driving and exposure to vibration

Many jobs expose workers to vibration, most commonly in vehicles. The dominant frequency of vibration in many vehicles is 4–6 Hz, which is also the resonating frequency of the spine (Pope et al 1991).

Many studies show a higher prevalence of back pain, early degeneration of the spine and disc prolapse with driving. The key physical event seems to be exposure to whole body vibration. Hulshof & van Zanten (1987) reviewed these studies. Troup (1978) estimated that people who spend more than half their working lives driving are particularly likely to suffer from back trouble.

Even Bigos et al (1998) accepted that there is some evidence that driving leads to more back symptoms. Hulshof & van Zanten (1987) concluded cautiously that there is a link between driving and back pain, but we still do not have sufficient data to establish how strong it is.

Repetitive strain

Repetitive strain occurs as a result of repeated voluntary movements or activities, which is quite different from passive exposure to vibration.

Repetitive strain injury (RSI) is currently fashionable, particularly in a medico-legal context. RSI usually affects the upper limb, although the pathology and the diagnosis itself are now hotly disputed. More recently, legal claims about back pain have explored the same concept.

It is certainly possible to produce fatigue failure due to repetitive strain in the laboratory. There are, however, major differences between such experiments and clinical back pain. Most of the biomechanical studies are on bones and discs, which are probably not the site of any work-related back pain. There are some hypotheses about how this might apply to soft tissues but there is little experimental data. The many thousands of rapid cycles required to produce failure are quite different from the pattern of repeated everyday movements in work. In vitro experiments also fail to allow for biologic adaptation and healing in response to repeated strain.

There is little clinical evidence to support the idea of repetitive strain injury to the back. Most claimants have already done the same tasks over long periods without symptoms. There is nothing new or changed in their job when back pain develops. The symptoms are subjective and are the same as the common, simple backache. Noone has defined any specific clinical syndrome or objective pathology with repetitive strain injury. When back pain is present, such repetitive activities may aggravate symptoms, but yet again this is not proof of cause and effect. Finally, there is no epidemiologic evidence of any specific relationship between back pain and repetitive activities at work.

In conclusion, repetitive strain injury seems to be more of a medico-legal concept than a clinical or pathologic reality.

Psychosocial factors

Several early Scandinavian studies from the 1970s suggested that psychosocial aspects of work are important. People with monotonous work, little control over their job, and low job satisfaction have more sickness absence, report more back injuries and stay off work longer with back pain. However, it is not clear whether this tells us more about their back pain or their work.

Krause et al (1997a,b) have recently looked at this more closely in San Francisco urban transit drivers. As expected, they confirmed a dose–response relationship between the number of years of driving plus current hours driving each week and reported back pain. Ergonomic factors such as problems adjusting the driving seat properly modified the relationship. Even after allowing for these physical factors, they found that psychosocial job factors had an independent effect on reported back pain. Frequent job problems, high psychologic demands, low job satisfaction, and poor supervisor support were all important.

Most important, however, are population studies that look at normal people and follow them to see who develops low back pain. The *Boeing Study* followed 3000 aircraft workers over 4 years (Bigos et al 1991) and found that psychologic distress and dissatisfaction with work were the best predictors of low back injury. Indeed, these were more important than any physical factors. The study also showed that physical examination and strength testing did not predict back injury (Battie et al 1989b, 1990a,b). However, these psychosocial factors predicted *reporting* of work-related, low back injury – not actual injury or even low back pain – and the effect was quite weak. Because of the large numbers in the study, it reached a high level of statistical significance, but these psychosocial factors only accounted for about 3% of the findings. The real message of the

Boeing Study was that traditional biomedical measures do not predict back pain. The psychosocial findings only received as much attention as they did because this mammoth study showed so little.

In contrast, Hansen et al (1995) found that distress did not predict back pain on 20-year follow-up from age 50 to 70 years. Instead, they felt that these psychologic changes were a consequence of the pain. von Korff et al (1993) found that people with clinical symptoms of depression were not any more likely to develop back pain over the next 3 years. Manninen et al (1995) carried out a 10-year study of disability pensions in more than 8000 Finnish farmers. Those with mental stress at the start of the study were slightly more likely to get a disability pension for nonspecific low back pain. Mental stress was a stronger predictor of other musculoskeletal injuries, cardiovascular disability and depression. The problem with these three studies is that they did not consider pre-existing back pain that might have caused distress at the start of the study, and might also have led to recurrent back pain. Hence, they do not fully distinguish cause and effect.

There are three excellent, recent studies that try to disentangle these influences. The *South Manchester Study* found that people who were free of back pain but more distressed were more likely to report a new episode of back pain in the next 12 months (Croft et al 1995). They were also more likely to consult a doctor. From the same study, Papageorgiou et al (1997) found that people who were dissatisfied with their work were also more likely to report a new episode of back pain, although the effect was not as strong.

Mannion et al (1996) also tried to distinguish cause and effect between low back pain and psychologic factors. They studied 403 female nurses and health workers aged 18–40 who had no previous history of 'serious' low back pain, by which they meant no medical attention or work loss. Thirty-five per cent did have some previous back pain that did not require medical attention or work loss. At the start of the study, they found that those with more distress were more likely to report previous back pain. They also had lower experimental pain tolerance. Over 18 months of follow-up, 40% reported some low back pain but this was not associated with any rise in levels of distress; 20% reported serious back pain and sought health care or took time off work. The latter group showed slightly greater levels of distress. The initial physical assessment did not predict those who would develop any back pain or serious back pain. Work load also had little effect, whether judged by the job description or by the workers' own perception of their jobs. The best predictor was psychologic distress, but the effect was again weak and explained less than 3% of future back pain.

Burton et al (1996b) looked at the problem from a different angle. Like Croft et al (1995), they made a careful distinction between the prevalence of existing low back symptoms and the incidence of first onset low back trouble. Their results suggested that physical loading on the spine led to first onset back pain with a dose–response relationship. However, continued exposure to physical stress did not lead to chronic problems. Chronic pain and work loss seemed instead to depend mainly on psychosocial factors.

Many, but not all, of these studies do suggest that people with distress are more likely to develop, or at least report, back pain; but in most of the studies the effect is weak. Croft et al (1995) calculated that 16% of new episodes of low back pain might be linked to psychologic factors, and this is by far the largest estimate. Most other studies estimate that it is closer to 3%. This also appears to be part of a more general finding. The effect of distress on back pain is weaker than the effect on other musculoskeletal injuries, cardiovascular disability and clinical depression. We must be careful about the conclusions we draw from these studies. There is no evidence linking psychologic factors to the development of physical pathology in the spine. Manninen et al (1995) found that mental stress only predicted nonspecific low back pain, and not spinal pathology such as disc prolapse and stenosis. These studies show that psychologic factors predict the *report* of back pain or, as in the *Boeing Study,* the report of back injury at work. Reports of pain depend on thresholds of awareness, recall, and the decision that a symptom is worth reporting. Distress also influences decisions to seek health care.

We will consider psychosocial factors in more detail in later chapters. Suffice it to say at this point that they are of fundamental importance to the experience and reporting of back pain.

CONCLUSIONS

What do these risk factors mean in practice?

The review of personal risk factors suggests that most of us are going to get back pain at some time in our lives. It does not make much difference if we are male or female, young or old, tall and thin, or small and fat. There is not a lot we can do about these personal characteristics in any event, but we do not need to worry about them. We may all be fated to have some back pain, but there is nothing in our genes that dictates it must inevitably lead to chronic pain and disability.

It is good general health advice to stop smoking, avoid excess weight and be physically fit. This will probably only slightly reduce the chances of getting back pain, although we will see later that it may help us to deal with it better.

The question of heavy manual work is vital, although the answer is not as clear as commonly believed. Many patients and health professionals believe that heavy manual work may cause back injury or wear and tear, and that further exposure might then cause further damage and so hinder recovery or lead to chronic pain and disability. There is little evidence to support this. Bigos et al (1998) were very critical of the scientific evidence on occupational risk factors and cautious in their conclusions (Table 6.5).

Back pain is certainly work-related to the extent that people of working age commonly get back pain and it impacts on their work.

Table 6.5   Scientific evidence on risk factors for work-related back pain (from Bigos et al 1998)

Study	Findings	Evidence
Prospective cohort studies		
Reported symptoms		
Riihimaki et al (1994), construction workers	History of back pain	Adequate
Leino et al (1987), metal manufacture	*Not* strength	Adequate
Riihimaki et al (1989), construction workers	History of sciatica	Adequate
	Prior compensation	Weak
Pietri et al (1992), drivers	Drive motor vehicle	Weak
Harber et al (1994), nurses	History of back pain	Weak
Claims		
Rossignol et al (1993), aircraft manufacture	Prior compensation	Strong
Bigos et al (1992), aircraft manufacture	Job satisfaction, distress > physical	Adequate
Cady et al (1979), firefighters	Low fitness	Weak
Ready et al (1993), nurses	*Not* fitness, prior compensation, smoking, job satisfaction	Weak
Chaffin & Park (1973), electronics manufacture	Spine load	Weak
Duecker et al (1994), steel mill	*Not* strength	Weak
Mostardi et al (1992), nurses	*Not* history of LBP, *not* isokinetic strength	Weak
Case–control studies		
Claims		
Tsai et al (1991), mixed hourly	Non-work factors	Some
Ryden et al (1989), hospital employees	History of back pain	Some
Daltroy et al (1991), postal employees	History of back pain	Some
Nuwayhid et al (1993), firefighters	Life-threatened duty	Some
Zwerling et al (1993), postal employees	History of back pain	Some

Detailed references to these studies are in Bigos et al (1998).

People with heavy manual jobs do report more back symptoms, but the relation between such jobs and back trouble is complex (Troup & Edwards 1985, Burton et al 1998). General clinical experience and a few reasonable studies do show that physical loading at work may have a short-term effect on low back symptoms. However, the size of this effect is quite modest, and it is short term. Persistent symptoms and disability do not seem to be related to physical stress or occupational exposure. Any physical effect is soon swamped by stronger psychosocial influences on the reporting of symptoms, claims, work loss and, as we shall see in the next chapter, the development of chronic pain and disability.

In summary, there is little convincing evidence that work is physically harmful to the back. On the contrary, as we will see in later chapters, work is generally good for people with back pain.

This has major implications for what we tell our patients. Too often, we tell patients that they have back pain because they are too tall, too fat, the wrong build or their legs are of unequal lengths. This is nonsense, and it is a dangerous message because it implies that their back pain is inevitable and there is nothing that they, or we, can do about it. It is time to stop advancing the myth that obesity causes back pain. There may be other health reasons for advising patients to lose weight but it will probably not make any difference to their back pain. We should probably tell people with back pain to stop smoking, although unfortunately this is still not a widely known or publicized message. We will see in Chapter 16 the argument for advising people to stay active and physically fit, but we should not pretend that this will prevent them ever getting back pain. Indeed, if we say that and they do then get back pain, it is likely to undermine the message.

All too often, doctors and therapists tell patients that their back pain is due to their job and that they should stay off work until they are better. Advice to change to lighter work, give up their job and even to retire early all follows from this fundamental belief. This review shows that there is very little good evidence to support such advice. It is usually not possible to say with any certainty that a patient's back pain is due to his or her job, or that the job is bad for his or her back. Too often, we give such advice glibly without adequate thought for the impact on our patients and their families. Just imagine if someone casually told you to give up your job, for no very good reason – saying only that it might be good for you. How would that affect you? Education, knowledge and insight would probably allow you to discount such advice. Your patients may not be so lucky – they may trust you.

It is too important a matter to make these decisions lightly on such flimsy evidence. It is rarely justified to advise patients to stay off work, change their job or give up work completely because of simple backache. Advice such as that can easily become self-fulfilling.

Summary of risk factors

- Most people get back pain. Heredity, gender and body build make little difference
- It is good general health advice to stop smoking, avoid excess weight and get physically fit. This may help to reduce the likelihood of developing new episodes of back pain, but such advice is more relevant to dealing with back pain after it occurs
- Social class is probably the strongest personal predictor of back trouble. This is partly related to heavy manual work, especially in men; and partly to social disadvantage, in men and women
- Heavy manual work leads to slightly more short-term back pain, but this effect is soon swamped by stronger psychosocial influences on the reporting of symptoms, claims, work loss, and the development of chronic pain and disability

FURTHER READING

A recent review by Andersson (1997) gives an extensive list of references on personal and occupational risk factors. The American Academy of Orthopedic Surgeons provides a more critical review of the scientific evidence and full references for the 'acceptable' scientific evidence in Table 6.5 (Bigos et al 1998). Burton et al (1998) offer a thoughtful discussion on the relative role of biomechanical and psychosocial factors in work-related back pain.

REFERENCES

Andersson G B J 1997 The epidemiology of spinal disorders. In: Frymoyer J W (ed) The adult spine: principles and practice. Lippincott-Raven, Philadelphia, 2nd edn, ch 7: p 93–141

Andersson G B J, Swensson H-O, Oden A 1983 The intensity of work recovery in low back pain. Spine 8: 880–884

Battie M C, Bigos S J, Fisher L D et al 1989a A prospective study of the role of cardiovascular risk factors and fitness in industrial back pain complaints. Spine 14: 141–147

Battie M C, Bigos S J, Fisher L D et al 1989b Isometric lifting strength as a predictor of industrial back pain complaints. Spine 14: 851–856

Battie M C, Bigos S J, Fisher L D et al 1990a Anthropometric and clinical risk measures as predictors of back pain complaints in industry: a prospective study. Journal of Spinal Disorders 3: 195–204

Battie M C, Bigos S J, Fisher L D et al 1990b The role of spinal flexibility in back pain complaints within industry. A prospective study. Spine 15: 768–773

Battie M C, Videman T, Gibbons L E, Fisher L D, Manninen H, Gill K 1995 Determinants of lumbar disc degeneration. A study relating lifetime exposures and MRI findings in identical twins. Spine 20: 2601–2612

Battie M C, Videman T, Gill K et al 1991 Smoking and lumbar intervertebral disc degeneration: an MRI study of identical twins. Spine 16: 1015–1021

Biering-Sorensen F, Hansen R R, Schroll M, Runeborg O 1985 The relation of spinal x-ray to low back pain and physical activity among 60 year old men and women. Spine 10: 445–451

Bigos S J, Battie M C, Spengler D M et al 1991 A prospective study of work perceptions and psychological factors affecting the report of back injury. Spine 16: 1–6

Bigos S J, Holland J, Webster M et al 1998 Reliable science about avoiding low back problems at work. Springer-Verlag, In press

Burton K A, Clarke R D, McClune T D, Tillotson K M 1996a The natural history of low back pain in adolescents. Spine 21: 2323–2328

Burton A K, Tillotson K M, Symonds T L, Burke C,

Mathewson T 1996b Occupational risk factors for first-onset and subsequent course of low back trouble. A study of serving police officers. Spine 21: 2612–2620

Burton A K, Battie M C, Main C J 1998 The relative importance of biomechanical and psychosocial factors in low back injuries. In: Waldemar Karwolski Morris (eds) A handbook of occupational ergonomics. CRC Press, Boca Raton, in press

Cady L, Bischoff D, O'Connel E 1979 Strength and fitness and subsequent back injuries in firefighters. Journal of Occupational Medicine 21: 269–272

Consumers' Association 1985 The Which report on back pain. Consumers' Association, London

Croft P, Joseph S, Cosgrove S et al 1994 Low back pain in the community and in hospitals. A report to the Clinical Standards Advisory Group of the Department of Health. Arthritis & Rheumatism Council, Epidemiology Research Unit, University of Manchester

Croft P R, Papageorgiou A C, Ferry S, Thomas E, Jayson M I V, Silman A J 1995 Psychologic distress and low back pain: evidence from a prospective study in the general population. Spine 20: 2731–2737

Croft P R, Rigby A S 1994 Socioeconomic influences on back problems in the community in Britain. Journal of Epidemiology and Community Health 48: 166–170

Deyo R A, Bass J E 1989 Lifestyle and low-back pain: the influence of smoking and obesity. Spine 14: 501–506

Deyo R A, Tsui-Wu Y-J 1987 Functional disability due to back pain. Arthritis and Rheumatism 30: 1247–1253

Dione C, Koepsell T D, Von Korff M, Deyo R A, Barlow W E, Checkoway H 1995 Formal education and back-related disability: in search of an explanation. Spine 20: 2721–2730

Frymoyer J W, Cats-Baril W L 1991 An overview of the incidences and costs of low back pain. Orthopedic Clinics of North America 22: 263–271

Gyntelberg F 1974 One year incidence of low back pain among male residents of Copenhagen age 40–59. Danish Medical Bulletin 21: 30–36

Hansen F R, Biering-Sorensen F, Schroll M 1995 Minnesota multiphasic personality inventory profiles in persons with or without low back pain: a 20-year follow-up study. Spine 20: 2716–2720

Heikkila J K, Koskenvuo M, Heiovaara M et al 1989 Genetic and environmental factors in sciatica. Evidence from a nationwide panel of 9365 adult twin pairs. Annals of Medicine 21: 393–398

Heliovaara M, Impivaara O, Sievers K, Melkas T, Knekt P, Korpi J, Aromaa A 1987 Lumbar disc syndrome in Finland. Journal of Epidemiology and Community Health 41: 251–258

Hodgson J T, Jones J R, Elliott R C, Osman J 1993 Self-reported work-related illness. The Labour Force Survey 1990. Health and Safety Executive, Research Paper 33. HMSO, London

HSE 1992 Health and Safety Statistics 1990–91. Health and Safety Executive, Employment Gazette. Occasional Supplement No 3: 1–103

Hulshof C, van Zanten B V 1987 Whole body vibration and low back pain. A review of epidemiologic studies. Internal Archives of Occupational and Environmental Health 59: 205–220

Hult L 1954a The Munkfors investigation. Acta Orthopaedica Scandinavica (supplement) 16: 1–76

Hult L 1954b Cervical, dorsal, and lumbar spinal syndromes. Acta Orthopaedica Scandinavica (supplement) 17: 1–102

Kelsey J L, Githens P B, O'Connor T et al 1984a Acute prolapsed lumbar intervertebral disc: an epidemiologic study with special reference to driving automobiles and cigarette smoking. Spine 9: 608–613

Kelsey J L, Githens P B, White A A et al 1984b An epidemiologic study of lifting and twisting on the job and risk for acute prolapsed lumbar intervertebral disc. Journal of Orthopaedic Research 2: 61–68

Kelsey J L, Golden A L 1987 Occupational and workplace factors associated with low back pain. Spine: State of the Art Reviews 6: 2–7

Krause N, Ragland D R, Greiner B A, Syme S L, Fisher J M 1997a Psychosocial job factors associated with back and neck pain in public transit workers. Scandinavian Journal of Environmental Health 23: 179–186

Krause N, Ragland D R, Greiner B A, Fisher J M, Holman B L, Selvin S 1997b Physical workload and ergonomic factors associated with prevalence of back and neck pain in public transit workers. Spine 22: 2117–2122

Lawrence J S 1977 Rheumatism in populations. Heinemann, London

Leino P L 1993 Does leisure time physical activity prevent low back disorders? Spine 18: 863–871

Macfarlane G J, Thomas E, Papageorgiou A C, Croft P R, Jayson M I V, Silman A J 1997 Employment and physical work activities as predictors of future low back pain. Spine 22: 1143–1149

Makela M 1993 Common musculoskeletal syndromes. Prevalence, risk indicators and disability in Finland. Publications of the Social Insurance Institution, Finland, ML 123

Manninen P, Riihimaki H, Heliovaara M, Makela P 1995 Mental distress and disability due to low back and other musculoskeletal disorders – a ten year follow up. Presented to the International Society for the Study of the Lumbar Spine, Helsinki, p 37

Mannion A F, Dolan P, Adams M A 1996 Psychological questionnaires: do 'abnormal' scores precede or follow first-time low back pain? Spine 21: 2603–2611

Mason V 1994 The prevalence of back pain in Great Britain. Office of Population Censuses and Surveys Social Survey Division (now Office for National Statistics). HMSO, London, p 1–24

Mitchell J N 1985 Low back pain and the prospects for employment. Journal of Social and Occupational Medicine 35: 91–94

Ostgaard H C, Roos-Hansson E, Zetherstrom G 1996 Regression of back and posterior pelvic pain after pregnancy. Spine 21: 2777–2780

Papageorgiou A C, Croft P R, Ferry S, Jayson M I V, Silman A J 1995 Estimating the prevalence of low back pain in the general population. Evidence from the South Manchester back pain survey. Spine 20: 1889–1894

Papageorgiou A C, Macfarlane G F, Thomas E, Croft P R, Jayson M I V, Silman A J 1997 Psychosocial factors in the workplace – do they predict new episodes of low back pain? Spine 22: 1137–1142

Pope M H, Wilder D G, Krag M H 1991 Biomechanics of the lumbar spine: A. Basic principles. In: Frymoyer J W (ed) The adult spine: principles and practice. Raven Press, New York, p 1487–1501

Ready A E, Boreskie S L, Law S A et al 1993 Fitness and lifestyle parameters fail to predict back injuries in nurses. Canadian Journal of Applied Physiology 18: 80–90

Riihimaki H, Wickstrom G, Hanninen K, Mattson T, Waris P, Zitting A 1989 Radiographically detectable lumbar degenerative changes as risk indicators of back pain. A cross-sectional epidemiologic study of concrete reinforcement workers and house painters. Scandinavian Journal of Work and Environmental Health 15: 280–285

Troup J D G 1978 Driver's back pain and its prevention. A review of the postural vibratory and muscular factors, together with the problem of transmitted road-shock. Applied Ergonomics 9: 207–214

Troup J D G, Edwards F C 1985 Manual handling: a review paper. Health and Safety Executive. HMSO, London

Troup J D G, Foreman T K, Baxter C E, Brown D 1987 The perception of back pain and the role of psychophysical tests of lifting capacity. Spine 12: 645–657

Videman T, Nurminen M, Troup J D G 1990 Lumbar spinal pathology in cadaveric material in relation to history of back pain occupation and physical loading. Spine 15: 728–740

Viikari-Juntura E, Vuori J, Silverstein B A, Kalimo R, Kuosma E, Videman T 1991 A life-long prospective study on the role of psychosocial factors in neck-shoulder and low back pain. Spine 16: 1056–1061

von Korff M, Deyo R A, Cherkin D, Barlow W 1993 Back pain in primary care: outcomes at one year. Spine 18: 855–862

Walsh K, Cruddas M, Coggon D 1991 Interaction of height and mechanical loading of the spine in the development of low back pain. Scandinavian Journal of Work and Environmental Health 17: 420–424

Walsh K, Cruddas M, Coggon D 1992 Low back pain in eight areas of Britain. Journal of Epidemiology and Community Health 46: 227–230

Waters T R, Putz-Anderson V, Garg A, Fine L J 1993 Revised NIOSH equation for the design and evaluation of manual lifting tasks. Ergonomics 36: 749–776

7

The clinical course of low back pain

Let us now return to the clinical picture. The last chapter was about predicting who gets back pain. This chapter is about what happens to them after they get it:

- What is the clinical course of nonspecific low back pain?
- How does it start?
- How does it progress and recover?
- Can we predict which patients will do well and who is at risk of developing chronic pain and disability?

THE ONSET OF BACK PAIN

We asked more than 500 British patients how their back pain started (Fig. 7.1). There was little difference between patients who saw their family doctor and those who came to a routine hospital clinic, or between men and women.

About 60% said that their first attack began suddenly and the others said that the pain came on gradually. Of those whose pain began suddenly, almost two-thirds said it was an 'accident'. The other one-third said that the pain began spontaneously and they could not think of any precipitating event. For most people, however, the 'accident' was an everyday activity such as bending or lifting. They had done the same thing many times before and had done nothing different on this occasion. At most, it was what some authors describe as 'over-exertion'.

Fewer of these patients could identify the cause of their present attack, despite it being

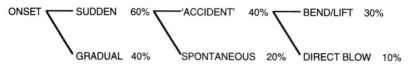

ONSET ⟨ SUDDEN 60% ⟨ 'ACCIDENT' 40% ⟨ BEND/LIFT 30%

GRADUAL 40% SPONTANEOUS 20% DIRECT BLOW 10%

Figure 7.1 Onset of back pain in a personal series of 500 patients.

more recent. That is surprising. Usually, patients can give more detail of recent events and are less sure about their earlier medical history. Furthermore, only about one-third were able to say what usually caused recurrent attacks. Two-thirds felt their attacks came on spontaneously or unpredictably. This inability to identify the cause of present and recurrent attacks casts doubt on their description of the first attack.

Troup and colleagues looked at back pain in an occupational health setting (Troup et al 1981, Lloyd & Troup 1983). They studied nearly 1000 people when they returned to work after an episode of back pain or sciatica. In 50%, the current attack was spontaneous with no question of any kind of injury. In 18%, the pain began unexpectedly at work with normal activity, most often lifting or handling. Thirty-one per cent described what these authors accepted was a true accidental event leading to injury (Table 7.1). Remember, however, that this was a selected series of work-related cases of back pain.

The perceived causes of back pain

Population studies show a different picture. The *Nuprin Pain Report* (Taylor & Curran 1985)

found that 27% of Americans with back pain thought it was due to an injury. In the UK, Mason (1994) also looked at factors that people thought were related to the onset of their back pain (Table 7.2). The most common single factor they mentioned was work, either a work-related injury or simply the nature of their work. However, the reasons varied with sex and age: two-fifths of men aged 18–34 said sports injuries; over a third of women of that age said pregnancy or childbirth; about a fifth of women over 35 blamed housework; about a quarter of men and a third of women over 55 mentioned arthritis or rheumatism. A third of the respondents gave a host of other reasons. Many gave more than one reason. Obviously, the factors people blame must vary at different stages of their lives!

The Labour Force Survey in the UK in 1990 showed the importance of the context in which we ask these questions (Hodgson et al 1993). It found that back pain was by far the most common 'illness, disability or other physical problem caused or made worse by work'. This occupational survey estimated that 460 000 people had work-related back trouble

Table 7.1 Onset of work-related backache and sciatica (based on data from Lloyd & Troup 1983)

Type of onset	Percentage of patients
Spontaneous	51%
Sudden, during normal activity	
Lifting and handling	14%
Other	3%
Accidental event leading to injury	
Slips and falls	12%
Handling	9%
Blow on the back	4%
Other	7%

Table 7.2 Factors people think are related to the onset of back pain (based on data from Mason 1994, with permission from the Office of National Statistics)

Factors related to start of back pain	Percentage of those with back pain	
	Men	Women
Accident/injury at work	21	9
Type of work done	35	18
Accident/injury at home	6	9
Accident/injury playing sport	16	5
Accident/injury elsewhere	5	9
Doing housework/garden	11	18
Pregnancy or childbirth	–	18
Arthritis and rheumatism	13	17
Other reasons	31	35

in the UK each year: 61% said that their work caused the pain, and 39% said that work made it worse. The only remotely comparable problem was 'stress and depression' in 180 000 people. However, this survey recognized that many people over-estimate the role of work in musculoskeletal problems. Only a small minority make any formal legal claim, and even fewer have sufficient evidence to win in court. A study of nearly 8000 people who attended the Canadian Back Institute may help to explain some of these apparently contradictory reports (Hall et al 1998). Two-thirds of people who were responsible for their own health care expenses and had no litigation could not identify any cause for their back pain. In contrast, 91% of people with compensation or litigation blamed a specific event.

We must always remember that these are simply patients' own attempts at an explanation for their pain. These answers probably tell us more about what people think about back pain than about cause and effect. Most of the above answers seem to reflect the normal activities of the different age groups and their circumstances when back pains started. They tell us little about the physical cause or pathology of back pain. The truth is that we have very little information about what causes or even triggers back pain. Most back pain probably starts spontaneously or while doing an everyday activity that we have done many times before.

THE COURSE OF A CLINICAL EPISODE

Remember the epidemiologic background. Most people have back symptoms at some time in their lives, and about 40% have back pain each year and each month. Back pain is a recurrent and fluctuating problem and we must view any clinical episode against that background of symptoms.

Traditional clinical teaching is that 75–90% of acute attacks of low back pain recover within about 4–6 weeks. This figure is quite consistent in clinical series over the past 40 years. Vernon

(1991) looked closely at a small group of chiropractic patients. He found 25% improvement in pain, disability and lumbar flexion in 7–10 days; 50% improvement took 2–3 weeks; 75% improvement varied from 4–6 weeks; and 100% improvement took 6–9 weeks or more. Disability and lumbar movement lagged behind improvement in pain. This is a typical clinical picture of an episode of health care. However, it is a limited view of a single episode, and it emphasizes the end of health care and return to work.

In contrast, Lloyd & Troup (1983) found that 70% of people still had residual symptoms when they returned to work. Moreover, when we view back pain as a recurrent problem, the outcome of a clinical episode appears less favourable. Perhaps we should say more cautiously that up to 90% of acute attacks presenting for health care settle sufficiently to stop health care and return to work within 6 weeks.

Clearly, we need to look at what happens over a longer period of time. We now have a wonderful set of primary care studies from the United States (von Korff et al 1993), the UK (Roland et al 1983, Klenerman et al 1995, Papageorgiou et al 1996), France (Coste et al 1994), the Netherlands (Chavannes et al 1986, van Tulder et al 1996), Belgium (Szpalski et al 1995) and Denmark (Hansen et al, personal communication, 1997).

The *South Manchester Study* investigated patients who consulted family doctors with back pain (Papageorgiou et al 1996). Sixty-nine per cent presented with a new attack, and 20% presented with an acute exacerbation of a more chronic or persistent complaint. For 8%, the consultation was simply part of a continuing problem. At 3 months follow-up, 27% reported complete recovery and 28% were improved; 30% remained the same and 14% had become worse.

Burton (personal communication) looked at recurrent attacks in osteopathic patients over 4 years. Quite apart from the success of treatment, the natural history was that 79% of patients still had some symptoms at 1 year. Table 7.3 shows what happened to them from year 1 through 4 after the initial presentation.

Table 7.3 Recurrent back pain 1–4 years after initial presentation for osteopathic treatment (from Burton, personal communication, 1997)

Recurrent back pain between years 1 and 4	Initial presentation		
	Acute	Subacute	Chronic
No further attacks	29%	20%	5%
1–5 further attacks	57%	35%	15%
Many attacks (>5)	10%	33%	40%
Never got better	4%	12%	40%

Klenerman et al (1995) studied a more select group of 123 British patients who saw their family doctor within the first week of a new episode. They looked at patterns of pain, disability and work loss when they presented and 2 and 12 months later. At follow-up, 26 patients had no pain, 88 continued to have intermittent pain, and nine had constant pain. These three types of patients showed very different progress over the year. In patients with no pain or intermittent pain at follow-up, their pain, disability and work loss had all improved by 2 months. Those with no pain showed further improvement in disability and had no further work loss between 2 and 12 months, while those with intermittent pain continued to have comparable levels of pain, disability and work loss in the same period. Patients with constant pain showed a slight improvement in pain by 2 months, but their pain then increased again by 12 months. They did not show any improvement in disability or work loss over the entire 12-month period.

von Korff et al (1993) studied 1128 American patients presenting to a large health maintenance organization. Only 17% of these patients had back pain of recent onset and a first ever attack within the previous 6 months. One year later, 70–80% of patients still said they had some back pain in the previous month. von Korff et al distinguished patients with only occasional back pain (<30 days in the previous 6 months) from those with frequent pain (>90 days in the previous 6 months). Patients with only occasional pain when first seen usually continued to have only occasional pain at 1 year; those who pre-sented with frequent pain usually continued to have frequent pain. About 90% of patients who presented with low-intensity nondisabling back pain had a similar good outcome at 1 year. For patients with severe pain and severe disability at first presentation, the outcome depended on the duration of the problem. If the initial duration was less than 30 days in the previous 6 months, they had a two-thirds chance of a good outcome at 1 year; but if it was more than 90 days out of the previous 6 months, they had only had a one-third chance of a good outcome.

von Korff et al (1993) summed up the likely course of an acute episode of back pain pre-senting for health care as follows:

- *Short-term outcomes*: Most primary care patients who seek treatment for back pain will improve considerably over the first 4 weeks, but only 30% will be pain-free. At 1 month, one-third will continue to experience back pain of at least moderate intensity, while 20–25% will still have substantial activity limitations.
- *Long-term outcomes*. At 1 year, 70–80% will still report some recurrent back symptoms, one-third will continue to have intermittent or persistent pain of at least moderate intensity, and about 15–20% will have a poor functional outcome.

Back pain is a recurrent problem, and the best predictor of future progress is past history.

von Korff et al (1993) also considered how patients should be told about the likely course of their back pain (see Box 7.1).

Box 7.1 Information for patients

- We can reassure them honestly that their pain is likely to improve
- Most people either stay at work or can return to work quickly, even if they still have some pain
- Back pain often recurs. Attacks may settle over several years, but back pain sometimes becomes chronic. However, even chronic back pain does not inevitably continue forever, and about one-third of people improve spontaneously each year
- It may also help to tell them that most people with back pain do manage to continue most activities and to work despite their pain

---

Long-term clinical follow-up

There have been two 10-year follow-up studies in a primary care setting. Barker (personal communication) studied 150 patients who presented with back pain in 1979. One hundred and thirty had only one attack in that year, 14 had two attacks and four had three attacks. Barker followed up 85 of his patients 10 years later: 80% had further problems, and more than half of these had frequent recurrences. Of those with recurrent problems, 40% were free of pain between attacks, 40% said that the pain did not go away completely between attacks, and 20% had back pain most days. Acute attacks or exacerbations lasted a few days in 52%, about a week in 16% and 2 or 3 weeks in 26%. Caldwell & Glanville (1993; quoted in Frank et al 1996) also made a 10-year follow-up of 373 patients under the age of 40 who consulted with back pain. Most attacks lasted less than 2 weeks, but 89% of patients had at least one recurrence.

Hasue & Fujiwara (1979) studied the very long-term prognosis of acute attacks in orthopedic surgeons aged 50 years or over. This is a very small and atypical sample of people with back pain! The study was retrospective but follow-up ranged from 5 to 50 years. Only 14% were completely free of symptoms after the first attack. Thirty-four per cent had some continuing symptoms but these were generally not disabling. Fifty-two per cent had a second attack, 30% went on to a third attack, and 15% continued to have frequent attacks. Only 26% sooner or later became completely symptom-free.

There is some tendency for recurrences to diminish over several years. Biering-Sorensen (1983) showed that the longer the time since the last attack, the lower the chance of recurrence (Table 7.4).

RETURN TO WORK

Table 7.5 and Figure 7.2 each combine data from several large American and Scandinavian series to show the duration of work loss due to an acute attack of back pain. Patients with nerve root pain are off work longer, but there are no good figures.

Table 7.4 The likelihood of further attacks diminishes with the time since the last attack (based on data from Biering-Sorensen 1983)

Time since last attack	Likelihood of further attack(s) in the next year
Less than 1 week	76%
1–4 weeks	63%
1–12 months	52%
1–5 years	43%
More than 5 years	28%

At a population level:

- Most acute exacerbations settle in days or a few weeks without work loss or health care
- Most people return to work in days or a few weeks, with or without health care
- Most episodes requiring health care settle sufficiently to allow return to work within a matter of weeks
- However, that is often against a background of continuing or recurring symptoms (not necessarily requiring health care) over long periods of our lives

There is little doubt about the overall shape of the graph (Fig. 7.2), but this version is based on early series from the 1960s and 1970s which are now really only of historic interest. More recent series show great variation in how quickly people return to work and, perhaps most importantly, how many go on to chronic disability. Coste et al (1994) found that 90% of patients who presented within 3 days of onset

Table 7.5 Return to work after an acute attack of back pain as a percentage of those who lose any time off work (based on various Scandinavian and US series)

Time off work	Percentage return to work	Percentage remaining off work
1 day	35	65
1 week	67	33
2 weeks	75	25
4 weeks	84	16
2 months	90	10
3 months	93	7
6 months	96	4
1 year	97	3

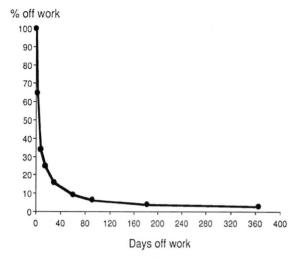

% off work

Days off work

Figure 7.2 Return to work after an acute attack of back pain. Based on collected Scandinavian and US series.

completely recovered, both pain and disability, within 2 weeks. Coste et al (1994), Watson et al (1998) and Hansen et al (personal communication, 1997) all found that only about 1–2% of patients were still off work at 1 year. Other clinical studies in Britain (Klenerman et al 1995) and Sweden (Lindstrom et al 1992) suggest that

as many as 5–10% may still be off work at 1 year, although these may be selected groups of patients at higher risk. Disability trends certainly suggest that the number eventually going on to chronic disability has increased greatly in most Western countries.

Let us look more closely at some of the factors that seem to influence this trend. Watson et al (1998) showed a marked difference between the rate of return to work after a first attack and that after a recurrent attack (Fig. 7.3). Most importantly, they found that only 1% were still off work 1 year after a first attack, compared with 4.5% after a recurrent attack.

We might expect marked differences in selected clinical groups of patients, but large population series also show surprising variation. Figure 7.4 compares the general population of Jersey (Watson et al 1998) with two workers' compensation series in British Columbia (Hrudey, personal communication) and Ontario (Frank, personal communication). This is not just an effect of work-related injury and compensation, because the Jersey data in this graph also includes selected claims

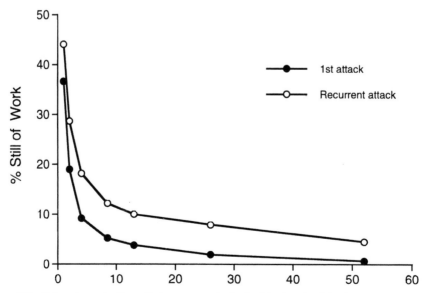

% Still of Work

- ●— 1st attack
- ○— Recurrent attack

Figure 7.3 Return to work after a first or recurrent attack of back pain. Based on data from Watson et al (1998).

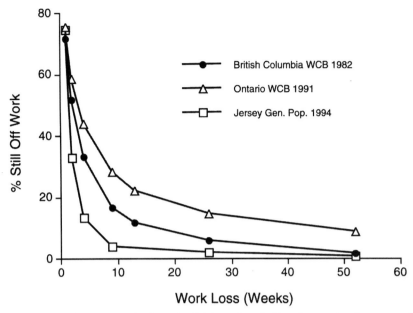

Figure 7.4 Return to work after a back injury at work. Based on workers' compensation data from British Columbia (Hrudey, personal communication), Ontario (Frank, personal communication), and Jersey (Watson et al 1998).

about back injury at work. Nor is it simply a changing pattern over the years. If we look more closely at what happens during the first month, there are even more fascinating differences (Fig. 7.5). The initial plateau in the Jersey data seems to reflect the fact that no sickness benefit is paid for the first day. It appears that if people claim benefits at all, they are then likely to stay off for a working week. The Danish data (Hansen et al, personal communication, 1997) shows a somewhat similar pattern for recurrent attacks.

We may speculate that the rate of return to work and the number going on to chronic disability seem to vary with different socio-economic settings. Return to work is generally delayed in the following cases:

- if back pain is due to nerve root pain or specific spinal pathology
- if it is a recurrent attack (as opposed to a first attack)
- manual workers
- those from a lower social class
- the longer the patient is off work.

This also shows the limitations of this kind of perspective on a single acute attack. If back pain is more of a recurrent problem, it may be a rather artificial view of what happens. Just as it may be more meaningful to consider the number of days of back pain over 12 months, so it may be better to look at total days of work loss in a year. von Korff et al (1993) showed that up to two-fifths of primary care patients who present with back pain may still be taking at least the occasional day off work at 1 year. Hansen et al (personal communication) also found that, although 90% of their patients returned to work within 1 month and only 2% remained off work for 1 year, 15% did have some further sick leave.

Probability of return to work

We can look at this graph of return to work in another way, i.e. as probability of return to work vs. time off work (Fig. 7.6). It was McGill (1968) who first pointed out that the longer anyone is off work with back pain, the lower

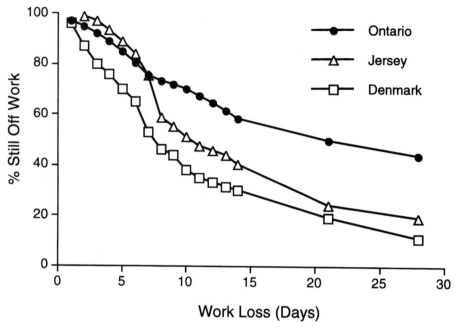

Figure 7.5 Return to work in different settings in the 1990s. Based on data from Ontario WCB (Frank, personal communication), Jersey (Watson et al 1998) and Denmark (Hansen et al, personal communication, 1997).

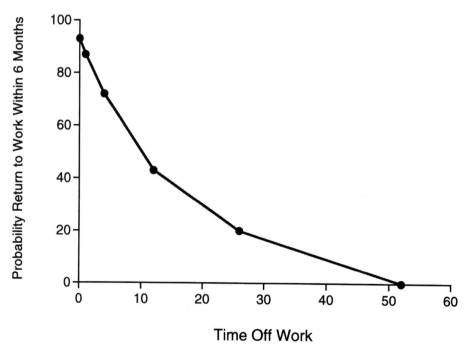

Figure 7.6 The probability of returning to work within the next 6 months with 'usual care'. Based on Canadian workers' compensation data. (Frank, personal communication.)

their chance of returning to work. Recent data from larger series and clinical experience confirms this. It is equally true today and it is fundamental to management. This may seem obvious, but many health professionals caring for back pain still seem oblivious to the disastrous impact of prolonged time off work.

Most people recover from an acute attack and return to work quite rapidly, so the initial prognosis is good. However, we should not be too sanguine. Depending on the particular health care and benefits system, the day someone stops work with back pain they have a 1–10% chance of still being off work a year later. And this prognosis soon deteriorates (see Table 7.6). Once they are off work for a month, they have a 20% risk of long-term disability. Once they are off work for 6 months, they have only a 50% chance of ever returning to their previous job. Once they have been off work for 2 years or have lost their job, *which may be much earlier*, then they are unlikely to work again in the foreseeable future. The further a patient slides down that slippery slope, the harder it is for them to escape, almost irrespective of the physical condition of their back or health care.

Both recovery from the acute attack and the development of chronic pain and disability are processes that take place over time. Health professionals are certainly aware of the importance of the patient's clinical progress. However, this epidemiologic view stresses that the passage of time, *in itself*, changes the patient's whole situation. This is so simple and obvious that we often dismiss it as a truism, to our patients' peril.

Frank et al (1996) pointed out another implication: the factors that influence recovery vary over time, and the course and duration of the illness itself may play a role in the process. As time passes we must consider other factors that may not have been important, or even present, at onset but that only develop over time. These may include not only physical changes in the patient's back, but also the patient's reaction to 'failure to recover as expected', the health care he or she receives, and changes in his or her work situation. Those factors at onset that predict chronic pain and disability may differ from those at 3–4 weeks, or at 3 months. The influence of many of these factors may reduce over time, while other factors may become more important. For example, age, the type and circumstances of injury, and severity of symptoms may all be important predictors of recovery initially, but their effects diminish over the first few months. Conversely, the patient's psychological reaction to failure to recover as expected only develops with the passage of time.

There may also be a threshold effect. The simplistic assumption that this whole sequence of events starts from the *initial onset* of pain is not true for most patients with chronic disability. Most of these patients have had previous, recurrent or chronic pain before this episode. It may be more appropriate to consider this as a sort of equilibrium. Stopping work may then be more of a threshold when the patient is no longer able to tolerate more pain. This may be due to a more acute exacerbation of pain, but it also may be simply that they are worn down by months of chronic pain and no longer able to cope, that they are overwhelmed by changed circumstances, or that demands at work or at home are increasing. Return to work may involve tilting the equilibrium to cross the threshold in the opposite direction. The change from working to being off sick is a dramatic social threshold. A person's whole social situation is very different when he or she goes off sick, not only in such obvious ways as changes in his or her finances or how he or she spends his or her time, but also in the employer's attitudes to the patient and the patient's attitudes

Table 7.6 Probability of return to work as a function of time off work

Time off work	Odds of still being off work one year later
Day 1	1–10%
1 month	20%
6 months	>50%
2 years (or lose job, which may be much earlier)	Up to 100%

to work. Return to work then depends partly on the physical state of the patient's back and his or her pain. But it also depends partly on whether those factors in the worker's life and his or her feelings that encourage return to work outweigh those that make it easier to stay off.

THE DEVELOPMENT OF CHRONIC PAIN AND DISABILITY

Let us relate this to clinical progress. After we rule out serious pathology, there are basically two kinds of patients with nonspecific low back pain. Most patients with acute low back pain get better quite rapidly, no matter what we do. They need little more than analgesics, reassurance and advice. The other 10–20% are at risk of developing chronic pain and disability. They present complex clinical and occupational problems for which we have no easy answer.

Frank et al (1996) pointed out that, from the moment they stop work, every patient must pass through various phases on the way to chronic disability. They propose a three-phase model (Fig. 7.7): acute, subacute and chronic.

The acute phase lasts from stopping work to about 3–4 weeks. There is ample evidence that the natural history of back pain should be benign and self-limiting. For most patients in this phase the prognosis is good, irrespective of health care.

The subacute phase lasts from 3–4 weeks through about 12 weeks off work. By 1 month most patients have returned to work, even if they still have some pain. Those who are still off work in the subacute phase have a 20% risk at least of going on to chronic pain and disability. By this phase, natural history alone is not enough. This is the phase at which we want to intervene more actively to control pain and help patients restore activity levels. This is also the phase when treatment is likely to be most effective.

The chronic phase is beyond about 3 months. Any patient who is still off work now has a chronic pain syndrome. Simple backache has become a source of major suffering and chronic disability. These chronic patients become trapped in a vicious circle of pain, disability and failed treatment. It has major impact on their whole lives, their family and their work. This small

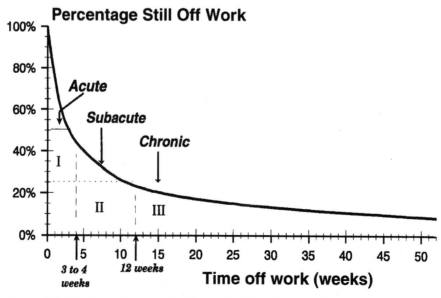

Figure 7.7 The three-phase model of back pain. (From Frank et al 1996, with permission.)

minority has a disproportionate effect, in terms of the total cost to society of back pain. Mason (1994) showed that 15% of patients account for more than half of all working days lost with back pain. Less than 10% of patients account for more than 90% of social costs for chronic back incapacity. This 10–15% of patients account for more than 80% of health care use for back pain. These chronic patients have a poor prognosis for recovery. Treatment is more difficult and has a lower success rate. Successful rehabilitation is difficult and becomes less likely with time.

Predicting chronic pain and disability

We clearly want to distinguish those patients who are likely to get better from those who are likely to go on to chronic pain and disability. The sooner we can do this, the better – ideally soon after onset or at the first consultation. Most patients will recover rapidly and need minimal investigation and treatment. It is unnecessary and wasteful to provide intensive and expensive health care to patients who are going to recover anyway. They do not need it, and indeed may be better off not having it. The main priority for them is to make sure that health care does not delay or hinder natural recovery. However, we do want to identify as early as possible those few who are at risk of developing chronic pain and disability. In principle, prevention is better than cure both for the patient and for society. It is also easier to prevent chronic disability than it is to reverse it once it is established. If we can identify those patients at risk, we should direct more intensive resources to them. This would direct treatment where it is needed and would likely do the most good, and also the least harm. It would also be the most effective and cost-effective use of finite resources. At the other extreme, we may be able to identify some patients who are never going to return to work whatever we do. For them, we should choose more realistic goals and treatments.

The ability to identify patients at risk of chronic pain and disability clearly depends on identifying the risk factors. In the same way that we had red flags for possible serious spinal pathology, we might consider 'yellow flags' for risk of chronic pain and disability (Kendall et al 1997). There have been considerable efforts to do this and it has become almost a kind of holy grail in back care. Unfortunately, most studies have only considered a few possible factors and have used much too simplistic an approach to analysis. We are still completely unable to identify individual patients at risk on day 1. We do now have some evidence on 'yellow flags' for those at risk by the subacute stage (Box 7.2). However, Frank et al (1996) pointed out that many of these markers may in fact be early manifestations of chronic pain and disability, rather than true predictors. They may simply be means of identifying the problem early, but in practice this does not matter.

Box 7.2 Predictors of chronicity within the first 6–8 weeks ('yellow flags')

- Nerve root pain or specific spinal pathology
- Reported severity of pain at the acute stage
- Beliefs about pain being work-related
- Psychologic distress
- Psychosocial aspects of work
- Compensation
- Time off work

The longer someone is off work with back pain, the lower the probability that they will return to work

---

Past history and clinical course of back pain

Because back pain is a recurrent problem, the single best predictor of future progress is the previous history, as illustrated in von Korff et al's (1993) study:

- At what stage are they already?
- How many previous attacks?
- How many days of pain in the last year?
- Previous medical consultations – number of doctors consulted; previous admissions to hospital; and most important of all, any previous low back surgery?
- Any loss of time from work – how often? how much? how long off work at present and how many days off in the last 12 months?

- Work-related back injuries and claims for compensation?

Similarly, observation of progress over time may be better than assessment at any one point in time. The simplest and surest way of identifying those who are developing chronic pain and disability is the passage of time. Those who are still off work after 4–6 weeks are at risk of chronic pain and disability. Unfortunately, if we simply 'wait and see', it may then be too late to do anything about it. The key is to identify what is happening as early as possible.

Physical factors

The nature and severity of the original injury seems to have remarkably little effect on future progress (Lloyd & Troup 1983, Gatchel et al 1995). However, this may to some extent merely reflect our inability to measure a simple back strain.

A series of studies in the early 1980s (Pedersen 1981, Biering-Sorensen 1983, Roland et al 1983, Lloyd & Troup 1983, Chavannes et al 1986) identified physical predictors of chronic pain and disability:

- gradual onset of pain
- radiating leg pain
- limited straight leg raising (SLR)
- root irritation signs
- weak trunk muscles.

Certainly, patients with a nerve root problem progress more slowly and are at higher risk of chronic pain and disability than those with simple backache. The physical findings are less helpful when it comes to the patient with simple backache. These studies suggest that referred leg pain without nerve root involvement may be significant. However, none of these studies looked specifically at referred leg pain as distinct from nerve root pain and they do not give a clear answer. It is the same with straight leg raising. None of the studies distinguished SLR limited by back pain alone from SLR as a specific sign of nerve irritation.

These early studies do suggest that patients with more severe physical findings are likely to recover more slowly, which makes clinical sense. Several more recent studies have looked at non-specific back pain and at severity of pain. Coste et al (1994) found that severity of pain within the first 3 days was the best predictor of symptomatic recovery but not of return to work. Burton et al (1995), Gatchel et al (1995) and Klenerman et al (1995) all found that persisting pain intensity at 3–6 weeks was one of the best predictors of pain and work status at 1 year. Other studies have failed to show this or have shown that severity of pain predicts slow recovery of symptoms but does not help to predict return to work. We are beginning to get back to the question of what influences the patient's report of pain. Frank et al (1996) suggested that severity of pain may be a useful predictor at the acute stage, but as time passes it becomes a much weaker predictor. This may be because of the increasing influence of psychologic and other factors on the report of pain and disability, and because of the increasing divergence of pain and disability.

None of these studies showed that severity of the initial injury (Gatchel et al 1995) or mechanical findings in the back (Coste et al 1994, Burton et al 1995) were useful guides to clinical progress or return to work.

Frank et al (1996) reviewed more than 150 recent articles on the natural history of back pain. They considered that only six studies were well enough designed to give reliable evidence on prognostic factors. They found scant evidence on early risk factors within the first 3–4 weeks. The overwhelming message is that the initial medical history and examination are a poor guide to how a patient with simple backache is likely to progress.

Psychosocial factors

Almost all of the more recent studies show that by the subacute stage, non-medical and psychosocial factors are stronger predictors of chronic pain and disability than any biomedical information.

Cats-Baril & Frymoyer (1991) asked a panel of experts to use their clinical experience to list what factors predict chronic pain and disability. They included demographic, injury, medical, psychosocial, health behavior and work factors. The authors then followed 250 patients to see which of these factors best predicted who was still off work after 6 months. They found that the best predictors, in order of decreasing accuracy, were:

1. job characteristics – whether or not working initially, work history, occupation, job satisfaction, satisfaction with retirement policies and benefits
2. Beliefs about whether back pain was compensable, who was at fault and legal involvement
3. past hospitalization for back pain
4. educational level.

Work and social factors were by far the most powerful influences on chronicity. These factors were 84% accurate in predicting who became chronically disabled. A standard medical assessment was only 42% accurate.

This led to the Vermont Disability Prediction Questionnaire (Fig. 7.8; Hazard et al 1996). This is a simple questionnaire for routine use. The more yellow flags it picks up, the higher the score, and the higher the risk of disability. This questionnaire has so far only been tested in a selected group of workers in Vermont, and we do not know how it will perform in other clinical situations. You must learn how it works with your patients and in your clinical situation before you can draw any clinical conclusions.

We saw in the last chapter that psychosocial factors are probably stronger than physical risk factors for predicting who will report back pain. There is now overwhelming evidence that psychosocial factors are more important than physical factors in the development of chronic pain and disability.

Patients who report poor general health, general bodily symptoms and 'always feeling sick' are more likely to develop chronic low back disability (Biering-Sorensen & Thomsen

Figure 7.8 The Vermont Disability Prediction Questionnaire. Templates permit easy scoring of each question as 0, 1 or 4 and all the scores are added together. The final score is the total score divided by the total possible score. If the answer to question #1 is 'yes', the total possible score is 19. If the answer to question #1 is 'no', the total possible score is 17. So a patient who answers question #1 as 'yes', with a total score of 8, will have a final score of 8/19 = 0.42. Another patient who answers question #1 as 'no', with a total score of 8, will have a final score of 8/17 = 0.47. The higher the score, the higher the risk of chronic disability. As a rough guide, a score of more than about 0.50 indicates a risk of disability, but you are probably better to develop your own cut-off for your patients and your needs. (From Hazard et al 1996, with permission.)

1986, Deyo & Diehl 1986). These symptoms appear to reflect psychologic dysfunction rather than the severity of physical illness.

Several recent studies show that psychologic factors are the best predictors of clinical progress, pain and disability at 1 year, and of return to work (Burton et al 1995, Gatchel et al 1995, Klenerman et al 1995, Dione et al 1996). This is certainly true by 6–8 weeks, and possibly within the first 3 weeks. Patients' beliefs about the pain, their level of psychologic distress and depression all appear to be important.

Social factors are also important, including work-related and socioeconomic factors (Lehmann et al 1993, Coste et al 1994, Ohlund et al 1994, Gatchel et al 1995, Klenerman et al 1995). One of the most powerful influences on return to work and work status at 6–12 months is patients' own beliefs about their pain. These include their beliefs about what has happened to their backs, beliefs that their back pain is work-related, and fear of re-injury. Indeed, Lehmann et al (1993) concluded that any patient who believes that their back pain is work-related and who is still off work after 2 weeks is at risk of chronic pain and disability. Socioeconomic influences such as compensation are also important. Perhaps surprisingly, these psychosocial factors appear to have more influence on return to work than do the physical demands of the job.

CONCLUSION

All of these studies suggest that back pain starts with a physical problem in the back, but that psychosocial factors soon become more important in the development of chronic disability. This is a dynamic process, and the first 6–12 weeks are probably the critical period. Gatchel et al (1995) suggested that clinical management and future research should focus on 'emotional vulnerability' and psychosocial events in that first critical period.

REFERENCES

Biering-Sorensen F 1983 A prospective study of low back pain in the general population. I – occurrence, recurrence and aetiology. Scandinavian Journal of Rehabilitation Medicine 15: 71–80

Biering-Sorensen F, Thomsen C 1986 Medical, social, and occupational history as risk indicators for back trouble in the general population. Spine 1: 720–725

Burton A K, Tillotson M, Main C J, Hollis S 1995 Psychosocial predictors of outcome in acute and subchronic low back trouble. Spine 20: 722–728

Cats-Baril W L, Frymoyer J W 1991 The economics of spinal disorders. In: J Frymoyer J W (ed) The adult spine: principles and practice. Raven Press, New York, ch 7, p 85–105

Chavannes A W, Gubbels J, Post D, Rutten G, Thomas S 1986 Acute low back pain: patient's perceptions of pain four weeks after initial diagnosis and treatment in general practice. Journal of the Royal College of General Practitioners 36: 271–273

Coste J, Delecoeuillerie G, Lara A C, Le Parc J M, Paolaggi J B 1994 Clinical course and prognostic factors in acute low back pain: an inception cohort study in primary care practice. British Medical Journal 308: 577–580

Deyo R A, Diehl A K 1986 Patient satisfaction with medical care for low back pain. Spine 11: 28–30

Dione C, Koepsell T D, von Korff M, Deyo R A, Barlow W E, Checkoway H 1997 Predicting long term functional limitations among back pain patients in primary care settings. Journal of Clinical Epidemiology 50: 31–43

Frank J W, Kerr M S, Brooker A-S et al 1996 Disability resulting from occupational low back pain. Spine 21: 2908–2929

Gatchel R J, Polatin P B, Mayer T G 1995 The dominant role of psychosocial risk factors in the development of chronic low back disability. Spine 20: 2702–2709

Hall H, McIntosh G, Wilson L, Melles T 1998 The spontaneous onset of back pain. Clinical Journal of Pain 14: 2

Hasue M, Fujiwara M 1979 Epidemiologic and clinical studies of long-term prognosis of low back pain and sciatica. Spine 4: 150–155

Hazard R G, Haugh L D, Reid S, Preble J B, MacDonald L 1996 Early prediction of chronic disability after occupational low back injury. Spine 21: 945–951

Hodgson J T, Jones I R, Elliott R C, Osman J 1993 Self-reported work-related illness. The Labour Force Survey 1990. Health and Safety Executive, Research Paper 33. HMSO, London

Kendall N A S, Linton S J, Main C J 1997 Guide to assessing psychosocial yellow flags in acute low back pain. Accident Rehabilitation and Compensation Insurance Corporation and National Advisory Committee on Health and Disability. Wellington, NZ

Klenerman L, Slade P D, Stanley I M et al 1995 The prediction of chronicity in patients with an acute attack of low back pain in a general practice setting. Spine 20: 478–484

Lehmann T R, Spratt K F, Lehmann K K 1993 Predicting long-term disability in low back injured workers presenting to a spine consultant. Spine 18: 1103–1112

Lindstrom I, Ohlund C, Eek C et al 1992 The effect of graded activity on patients with sub-acute low back pain: a randomized prospective clinical study of an operant conditioning behavioural approach. Physical Therapy 72: 279–291

Lloyd D C E F, Troup J D G 1983 Recurrent back pain and its prediction. Journal of Social and Occupational Medicine 33: 66–74

McGill C M 1968 Industrial back problems: a control program. Journal of Occupational Medicine 10: 174–178

Mason V 1994 The prevalence of back pain in Great Britain. Office of Population Censuses and Surveys Social Survey Division, HMSO, London

Ohlund C, Lindstrom I, Areskoug B, Eek C, Peterson L-E, Nachemson A 1994 Pain behavior in industrial subacute low back pain. Part I. Reliability: concurrent and predictive validity of pain behavior assessments. Pain 58: 201–209

Papageorgiou A C, Croft P R, Thomas E, Ferry S, Jayson M I V, Silman A J 1996 Influence of previous pain experience on the episode incidence of low back pain: results from the South Manchester Back Pain Study. Pain 66: 181–185

Pedersen P A 1981 Prognostic indicators in low back pain. Journal of the Royal College of General Practitioners 31: 209–216

Roland M O, Morrell D C, Morris R W 1983 Can general practitioners predict the outcome of episodes of back pain? British Medical Journal 286: 523–525

Szpalski M, Nordin M, Skovron M L, Melot C, Cukier D 1995 Health care utilization for low back pain in Belgium. Influence of sociocultural factors and health beliefs. Spine 20: 431–442

Taylor H, Curran N M 1985 The Nuprin Pain Report. Louis Harris and Associates, New York

Troup J D G, Martin J W, Lloyd D C E F 1981 Back pain in industry: a prospective survey. Spine 6: 61–69

van Tulder M W, Koes B W, Bouter L M (eds) 1996 Low back pain in primary care: effectiveness of diagnostic and therapeutic interventions. Institute for Research in Extramural Medicine, Amsterdam

Vernon H 1991 Chiropractic: a model incorporating the illness behaviour model in the management of low back pain patients. Journal of Manipulative and Physiological Therapy 14: 379–389

von Korff M, Deyo R A, Cherkin D, Barlow W 1993 Back pain in primary care: outcomes at one year. Spine 18: 855–862

Watson P J, Main C J, Waddell G, Gales T F, Purcell-Jones G 1998 Medically certified work loss, recurrence and costs of wage compensation for back pain: a follow-up study of the working population of Jersey. British Journal of Rheumatology 37: 82–86

8

Physical impairment

What is the physical basis of nonspecific low back pain? Let us start by looking at the clinical findings, and try not to prejudge them against any theoretic ideas about pathology. What are the objective physical findings in patients with back pain? What do they tell us about the physical problem? What does this tell us about low back disability?

ASSESSMENT OF SEVERITY

One of the most important characteristics of any illness or disease is its severity, which affects the impact of the problem on the patient, their family, the health care system and society. Severity of symptoms and their interference with lifestyle are most important to the patient. Health care also depends on severity. Treatment, outcomes, prognosis and social support all depend to some extent on severity, particularly in a nonspecific condition such as back pain. Fair and consistent rating of permanent impairment is an important part of assessing the injured worker and determining compensation. For all these reasons we want to be able to assess the severity of low back trouble.

We can assess severity of any illness in terms of diagnosis, pain, disability, physical impairment and ability to work. In most chronic disorders with clear pathology – such as osteoarthritis of the hip – we can assess all these aspects. Our assessment is reliable and different experts will agree. The patient's report of pain, disability and work loss is usually in proportion to the diagnosis and the physical findings. This is not the case in chronic back pain. Here we often cannot diagnose any pathology, and traditional medical assessment may not even be able to find any clear physical basis for the patient's continuing symptoms. It should not surprise us that we cannot agree on how to assess low back disability. Yet in view of the human, health care and social impact of back pain, and despite the practical problems, we must try.

It is an instructive discipline to regard clinical assessment as evidence. How well would it stand up to cross-examination in a court of law? In health care, as in science or in law, we should be able to substantiate our findings.

Apply this test to diagnosis. Diagnosis gives a broad classification of the severity of an injury or disease. Diagnosis of pathology is the usual basis for treatment and prognosis. It also determines when rehabilitation is complete and what abnormality or loss we should consider as permanent. At first sight, diagnosis looks like an important and useful measure of severity. In a spinal fracture, this is true. There is an obvious range between a minor fracture of a transverse process and a severe T10/11 fracture dislocation with paraplegia. Now try to apply this diagnostic approach to nonspecific low back pain. The first and insurmountable problem is that we cannot make any real diagnosis in most patients. We can diagnose injury to the bones or nerves of the spine and our assessment of nerve root dysfunction is accurate and reliable, but none of this helps with simple backache. Clinical examination of the spine itself is much less helpful. X-rays tell us about fractures, but the common radiographic changes of degeneration tell us nothing about a patient's back pain. Even when we can make a diagnosis, different patients with the same diagnosis may have very different degrees of pain and disability. It is illogical to give every patient with a particular diagnosis the same rating. Unfortunately, diagnosis and X-rays offer little help in assessing the severity of back pain.

Definitions

The key concepts are physical impairment and disability, which are fundamentally different.

WHO (1980) defines impairment as 'any loss or abnormality of psychologic, physiologic or anatomic structure or function'. This covers all kinds of impairment, and we need a more practical clinical definition. *Physical impairment* is 'pathologic, anatomic or physiologic abnormality of structure or function leading to loss of normal bodily ability' (Waddell & Main 1984). In the UK, impairment is sometimes called 'loss of faculty'. We should be clear about what kind of evidence we can use, and we must assess impairment on the basis of objective observations. We must make a clear distinction between the health professional's assessment of impairment and the patient's report of pain and disability:

- pain
- disability } subjective
- physical impairment – objective.

Most jurisdictions in the US do make this clear distinction between the assessment of impairment and disability. Impairment is medically determined loss of structure or function of part of the body. Disability is the degree to which the individual is affected by that impairment and is an administrative or legal decision. Medical evidence on impairment is only one factor that the legal or compensation system takes into account in determining disability. Other factors include the claimant's own evidence, his or her circumstances and needs, and his or her credibility. Consider a laborer and a pianist who each suffer amputation of their little finger. Medical assessment of impairment will be the same, but a court may rate their disability very differently. The court will take into account the physical demands of their job. The court may also allow for the person's report of his or her pain and suffering. Social support and compensation place greatest value on incapacity for work. Assessment of impairment is a professional responsibility. The final decision on disability rating and compensation is a legal or administrative responsibility. All parties have found this to be a useful division of responsibility.

Both in clinical practice and in law, we need objective assessment of physical impairment, in order to provide an essential check on the patient's own report.

Returning to our wish to assess the severity of back trouble, let us now consider physical impairment in more detail. The definition could include two different kinds of impairment:

- pathologic or anatomic loss or abnormality of structure
- physiologic loss or limitation of function.

The main demand of many jurisdictions is that impairment should be objective. Some social security systems, such as the US Bureau of Disability Insurance (1970), insist that it should be 'demonstrable by medically acceptable, clinical and laboratory diagnostic techniques'. From this point of view, medical evaluation has always stressed structural impairment, which reflects tissue damage. However, in the context of pain, physiologic loss of function may be just as important and would still meet the definition. The main proviso is that we should be able to demonstrate any such loss of function objectively.

Compare back pain with other forms of physical impairment. We all agree about impairment in an amputee and we do not argue in court about the degree of impairment or disability. In cases of back pain, on the other hand, we cannot even agree on how to assess lumbar impairment, never mind agreeing on the result. Clinical assessment is often based on the examiner's impression, and different 'experts' offer different findings. Due to these problems, some research workers decry objective assessment of lumbar impairment. However some form of objective check on the patient's report of pain and disability is essential in logic, in practice and in law.

These criticisms mean that we must stop and rethink how we assess lumbar impairment. First, we must by definition base it on objective physical characteristics. Second, we must use reliable clinical methods. Third, these clinical methods should provide a real and valid measure of the particular physical characteristic. Some clinical tests meet all these criteria, like nerve compression signs. Many routine methods of examination are not very reliable (Waddell et al 1982, McCombe et al 1989), e.g. posture, deformity, tenderness, palpation, sacroiliac tests and spinal movements. We must develop better techniques for routine clinical examination. We must also make sure that our tests are valid: that we really do measure what we intend to measure. The best example of this is lumbar flexion (Ch. 2): how well the fingers reach the toes tells us about total body movement, but if we want a valid measure of lumbar flexion we must look at the back.

Also, we must use objective measures of physical findings. As far as possible, we must exclude behavior from our assessment. Many physical tests deliberately elicit pain, so the way the individual reacts will vary with their response to pain. How they respond may also vary due to conscious or unconscious exaggeration related to a claim for compensation. We must make a clear distinction between objective physical findings and behavior, and build cross-checks into our examination.

Finally, the aim of the exercise is to look for the objective physical basis of low back pain and disability. As an example of a physical attribute that is not useful, consider lordosis. Lordosis varies widely in normal people, and has little to do with low back pain or disability. Hence the degree of lordosis tells us nothing about impairment, and lordosis should not be part of how we assess impairment. We are looking for physical characteristics that *lead to loss of normal bodily ability*. That means they should relate to low back disability and should distinguish patients with back pain from people who are free of pain.

METHODS OF RATING PHYSICAL IMPAIRMENT

We may agree on the principles of assessing lumbar impairment, but it is more difficult to put this into practice. In the United States there has been considerable effort to standardize impairment ratings. The American Medical Association's (AMA 1993) *Guides to the evaluation of permanent impairment* is now the standard for most musculoskeletal conditions. It is in its fourth edition and has been adopted as the official guidelines in 80% of states. It is also used in Canada and Australia. However, it has been attacked in court for having no scientific basis, and that is certainly true. It is a consensus document based on agreement about what is 'reasonable' impairment from clinical experience. There is no scientific proof of the reliability or validity of the guidelines, but they do give a more consistent rating than relying only on an expert's opinion. When it comes to back pain, however, the AMA guidelines are much less satisfactory. It may be worth reviewing the problems of various systems of rating lumbar impairment.

McBride

McBride (1936) made the first attempt to assess musculoskeletal impairment. He developed a comprehensive rating of quickness, coordination, strength, severity, endurance, safety and physique (McBride 1963). These are all difficult to define, and this system depends entirely on subjective judgements by the examiner. Many of McBride's concepts are clinically important, but his system does not give reliable ratings. It is almost impossible to apply to back pain and has never gained wide acceptance.

AMA and AAOS

More practical methods of rating lumbar impairment began about 40 years ago. Both the American Medical Association (AMA 1958) and the American Academy of Orthopedic Surgeons (AAOS 1962) produced guides to the evaluation of permanent impairment. These are now the most widely used methods of rating in low back disorders. Brand & Lehman (1983) found that 60% of US surgeons used the AMA scale, 30% used the AAOS scale, and 5% used the McBride system. But the AMA and AAOS scales suffer similar problems. They depend on diagnosis and radiographic findings and work best in the few patients with objective bone or nerve damage.

We can demonstrate this with the most recent, fourth edition of the AMA guidelines (1993). It now recognizes these problems, and suggests a two-stage evaluation of impairment. In the first stage, it is suggested that you try the 'diagnosis-related estimates' (DRE) model, if the patient's condition fits one of those listed in Table 8.1. This needs clinical diagnosis, neurologic findings or radiographic demonstration of instability. The guidelines then compare this with a number of specific pathologic diagnoses, such as fractures, disc lesions, spondylolisthesis and spinal operations. It is a very orthopedic view of the spine. Unfortunately, none of this is relevant to most patients with nonspecific low back pain. The AMA guidelines recognize this, and suggest that if this DRE model fails, you should then use the 'range of motion model'. Previous editions of the guidelines used invalid methods of

Table 8.1 AMA guides to lumbosacral impairment: diagnosis-related estimates model (AMA 1993)

DRE category	Whole person impairment
I – complaints or symptoms, no objective findings	0%
II – minor impairment	5%
III – radiculopathy	10%
IV – loss of motion segment integrity	20%
V – radiculopathy and loss of motion segment integrity	25%
VI – cauda equina-like syndrome without bowel or bladder signs	40%
VII – cauda equina syndrome with bowel and bladder signs	60%

measuring spinal movement, but the new edition now uses a valid and reliable method with a goniometer. The measured ranges of lumbar flexion, extension and lateral flexion are then graded and converted using a table to 'per cent whole-person impairment'. There is little scientific basis for this method, which depends entirely on the observed range of movement during clinical examination. We will discuss the meaning and limitations of this later.

Waddell and Main

In the early 1980s, we made a first attempt to identify 'objective physical characteristics' and to develop a clinical method of assessing lumbar impairment (Waddell & Main 1984). We looked at disability in 480 patients with various chronic low back problems. We used reliable methods of clinical examination and discounted behavioral reactions to examination. We then tried to find the physical characteristics that explained low back disability (Box 8.1). The problem is that this is a very mixed group of physical characteristics, many of which only apply to patients with particular spinal pathologies. This reflects the patients in our study. In this series, the findings were dominated by patients with serious spinal damage, nerve root problems and previous surgery. Despite this, the study does provide some useful lessons. Only fractures, nerve compression signs and previous surgery are true structural impairments, but none of these apply to the patient with nonspecific low back pain. In practice, the patient's reports of the anatomic and time pattern of pain had most influence on this score, but these do not meet the definition of physical impairment. The final problem was that we could not combine these characteristics statistically into a homogeneous scale. This study helped to show us the principles and the problems of assessing physical impairment in back pain, but it did not give us the answer.

NIOSH

The US National Institute for Occupational Safety and Health (NIOSH) also tackled this problem. Their approach was to put a great deal of effort into developing reliable methods of physical examination (Nelson & Nestor 1988). They used a literature review and an expert panel to find 105 clinical tests for back pain. They carried out extensive reliability studies in different centers. Their final 'low back atlas' had 19 well-defined tests (NIOSH 1988), but unfortunately their only criterion was a very high level of reliability. This led to a rather bizarre group of tests. Six of the 19 tests were measures of pelvic tilt, and four were of lordosis. Yet pelvic tilt and lordosis have little or nothing to do with low back disability. The atlas did not include any form of palpation and the only movement was lateral flexion. It included a few measures of strength but they were all of doubtful reliability. That original set of tests may be reliable but they give a limited view of lumbar impairment.

Moffroid et al (1992) modified the NIOSH atlas slightly and confirmed its reliability. They then compared the tests in 115 patients with nonspecific low back pain and 112 matched controls. About half the tests discriminated between the patients and asymptomatic people. The most powerful single test was pain on initiation of prone press-up. Box 8.2 presents the group of tests they considered as providing the best discrimination.

Moffroid et al (1992, 1994) also used the same data to try to separate four different symptom clusters. This was quite successful statistically, but clinically the clusters had a lot of overlap and it is difficult to see any clear clinical syndromes. As far as I know, this work has not gone any further yet.

Box 8.1 Our first attempt at a clinical method of assessing lumbar impairment in a mixed group of patients (Waddell & Main 1984)

- Anatomic pattern of pain
- Time pattern of pain
- Lumbar flexion
- Straight leg raising
- Nerve compression signs
- Previous lumbar surgery
- Spinal fractures

Box 8.2 The NIOSH atlas tests discriminating patients with back pain from normal people (after Moffroid et al 1992)

- Pain at initiation of press-up
- Lumbar mobility on forward bend
- Total range of hip rotation
- Whether the prone press-up test produces changes in the pattern of pain
- Pelvic tilt sitting
- Lower abdominal muscle strength

Other approaches

Ideally, we might try to combine pain, physical impairment and disability into a single scale. That might give us an overall measure of severity for clinical, legal and compensation purposes. Several research groups have tried to produce such a score (Lehman et al 1983, Clark et al 1988, Greenough & Fraser 1992). This approach works for patients whose pain and disability are in proportion to the diagnosis and physical impairment. Often, however, that is not the case. This approach fails to address the common problem where the patient's report of pain and disability does not match the objective physical findings. The statistics reflect this basic problem: these different measures do not fit well into a single score, and the scales and the loading on each measure are arbitrary. The basic problem is that these combined scales fail to distinguish the different concepts of pain, disability and physical impairment. The results have little clinical meaning.

Other groups have tried to overcome this difficulty by falling back on a panel of experts. This approach starts with a literature review, and then a panel of experts selects, based on experience, the most useful tests for impairment. Statistical analysis of the experts' opinions allows us to put a weight on each item to produce a scale. This does give a comprehensive scale that looks reasonable, as in the California Disability Rating Schedule (Clark et al 1988). Frymoyer & Cats-Baril (1987) also used this approach to predict chronic disability, and in their study it gave a useful starting point. However, the expert scale did not predict the outcome as accurately as the raw clinical data. Moreover, I believe there is a basic flaw in this approach. No matter how sophisticated the methodology, it only gives a consensus of current clinical opinion. Statistical scoring of the experts' votes is only an illusion of science. It cannot replace hard clinical data or real understanding of the problem. In the past, such a committee would probably have *proved* that boiling tar was the best possible treatment for amputation stumps!

ASSESSMENT OF PHYSICAL IMPAIRMENT

There are problems associated with all of the methods described above, so we tried to develop a new method of assessing lumbar impairment, starting from basic principles (Waddell et al 1992). Our study had three aims:

- to investigate physical impairment in patients with chronic low back pain
- to develop a method of clinical evaluation suitable for routine use
- to study the relation between pain, disability and physical impairment.

Our study was on patients with chronic low back pain, with or without referred leg pain. We excluded patients with nerve root involvement, previous surgery or structural problems like fractures and spondylolisthesis. This in effect excluded the permanent structural impairments that we found in our earlier study (Waddell & Main 1984).

From the definition of physical impairment, we limited our assessment to objective findings on physical examination. We used reliable clinical tests and excluded behavioral responses. We looked at 27 physical signs that might apply to simple backache, and did three pilot studies to develop reliable tests for 23 of the signs (Box 8.3), excluding four tests because they were unreliable. We had to exclude a further nine tests because they were too behavioral in nature. Most of these were tests that reproduced pain and depended on how patients responded to pain.

Box 8.3   Possible physical tests for lumbar impairment

- Lumbar lordosis and thoracic kyphosis
- Pelvic tilt and leg length
- Lumbar list
- Tenderness
  - lumbar
  - paravertebral
  - buttock
- Flexion
  - lumbar
  - pelvic
  - total
- Extension
- Lateral flexion
- Straight leg raising
- Passive knee flexion and pain*
- Passive hip flexion and pain*
- Hip flexion strength and pain*
- Hip abduction strength and pain*
- Prone extension
- Sit-up
- Bilateral active straight leg raising

*Reproduction of pain was subsequently excluded because it is too behavioral.

Table 8.2   Our final physical impairment scale (from Waddell et al 1992, with permission)

Physical test	Cut-off
Total flexion	<87°
Total extension	<18°
Average lateral flexion	<24°
Average SLR	
— female	<71°
— male	<66°
Spinal tenderness	Positive
Bilateral active SLR	<5 seconds
Sit-up	<5 seconds

Each scored 0/1 to give a total score out of 7.

Pre-examination procedure

The first step is to find the anatomic landmarks (Fig. 8.1). You will find it easiest to palpate these with the patient lying prone and relaxed. Make horizontal marks on the skin in the midline at S2 and T12/L1. The posterior superior iliac spines lie at the bottom of the posterior part of the iliac crest. They are just below and

We then looked at the remaining signs in 70 pain-free, normal subjects and 120 patients with chronic low back pain. We wanted to find those signs that told us about physical impairment, so we went back to the definition. They should relate to back pain, so they should discriminate the patients from the normal subjects. Physical findings are only an impairment if they cause disability, so they should also correlate with low back disability. Only the results will be considered here; the detailed statistics can be found in our article (Waddell et al 1992).

We did manage to find a group of physical signs that combine into a scale of physical impairment, as detailed in Table 8.2. This final scale could discriminate patients with back pain from normal people, and also correlated well with disability. Simple cut-offs made the scale simple and quick to use, with very little loss of accuracy. This scale is suitable for routine use in patients with simple backache.

Examination technique

Accurate assessment depends on careful and standard methods of examination.

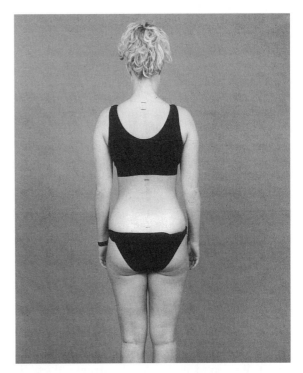

Figure 8.1   Reliable evaluation of physical impairment depends on a warm-up, a standard starting position, and careful marking of the anatomic landmarks.

lateral to the dimples of Venus and correspond to S2. You can then find T12/L1 by counting up the spinous processes. Check that the iliac crests are at about the L4/5 level. Then make further vertical marks in the midline over the spinous processes of T12 and T9.

Next, get the patient to perform warm-up exercises. They should flex and extend twice, rotate to the left and right twice, lateral flex to either side twice and then flex and extend once more. Therapists routinely use a warm-up before measuring any physical function, because it makes quite a difference to the results. A warm-up should now be standard before testing lumbar impairment.

You must then standardize the examination positions with care. We had considerable difficulty getting a consistent *erect* position, but reliable measures of movement depend on a standard starting point. It took a lot of trial and error to produce the following method. Have the patient stand in bare feet, with heels together, knees straight, and weight supported evenly on both legs. They should look straight ahead, with arms hanging at their sides. They should not hold themselves tense, but should relax without slumping. If a patient has severe muscle spasm, you should ask them to get as close to that position as they can hold comfortably for a few minutes. The *supine* position is with the patient lying flat on their back with their head on the couch without a pillow. They should relax with their arms by their sides, and extend their hips and knees as fully as possible without tension. The *prone* position is with the patient lying flat on their front on the couch without a pillow. They should relax with their arms by their sides.

The only equipment that you need is a ball-point pen and some kind of inclinometer. We found an electronic inclinometer more convenient, but it is not vital.

Tests

You can perform the tests in any order you prefer. We found it simplest to arrange them in sequence in the erect, prone and supine positions.

Flexion. Measure flexion with the inclinometer (Fig. 8.2). Stand the patient in the erect position, and record at S2 (Fig. 8.2A) and then at T12/L1 (Fig. 8.2B). Hold the inclinometer on T12/L1, and ask the patient to reach down with the fingertips of both hands as far as possible towards their toes. Check that the knees are straight. While the patient is fully flexed, make the third reading at T12/L1 (Fig. 8.2C). Tell the patient to hold that position and make the fourth reading at S2 (Fig. 8.2D). These four readings permit simple calculation of total flexion, pelvic flexion, and by subtraction, lumbar flexion (Fig. 8.3).

Extension. Measure extension at T12/L1 (Fig. 8.4). Take the first reading with the inclinometer while the patient is in the erect position. Then ask the patient to arch backwards as far as possible, looking up to the ceiling. Use one hand on the patient's shoulder as a support. This helps them to maintain their balance and gives them some feeling of security. Then take the second reading. Subtraction gives the measure of total extension.

Lateral flexion. To measure lateral flexion, use the longer bar on the inclinometer. While the patient is in the erect position, line up the bar between the spinous processes at T9 and T12 (Fig. 8.5). Take the first reading. Then ask the patient to lean straight over to the side as far as possible and to reach their fingers straight down the side of their thigh. Use one hand to support the patient's shoulder. Make sure that the patient does not flex forwards or twist round and that both feet are flat on the floor. Measure lateral flexion to both sides.

Tenderness. Reliable testing for tenderness depends on particularly careful technique (Fig. 8.6). The patient should lie prone and you should make sure that they relax their muscles. Palpate the spine slowly without sudden pressure. Tenderness depends on eliciting pain, but do not hurt the patient unnecessarily. We will look at behavioral responses to examination in Chapter 10. It is enough at this point to note that widespread superficial or nonanatomic tenderness is behavioral. If these are present, you cannot examine for physical tenderness.

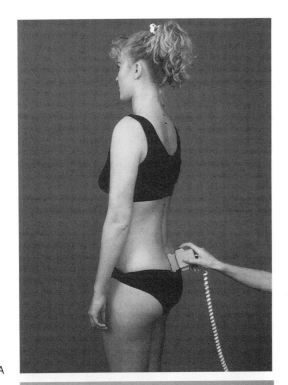

A

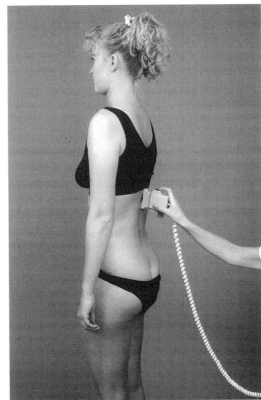

B

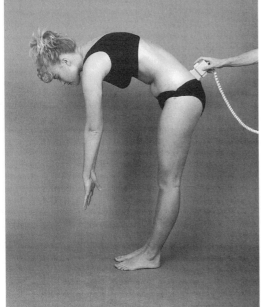

C

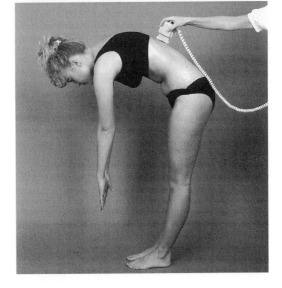

D

Figure 8.2 A–D: Measurement of flexion.

Look for local tenderness over the spinous processes and interspinous ligaments at each level from T12 to S2. Spinal tenderness is within 1 cm of the midline. You should use exact wording: 'Is that painful?' You should take *all* responses other than 'no' to be positive, i.e. a response such as 'only a little bit' should be taken to mean 'yes'. If the patient is doubtful or does not answer, then repeat the question: 'Is that painful when I do that?'

Straight leg raising (SLR). Test SLR with the patient lying supine (Fig. 8.7). Make sure that they stay relaxed and do not lift their head to watch what is happening. Hold their foot with one hand and make sure that the hip is in neutral rotation. Use the other hand to hold the inclinometer on the tibia just below the tibial

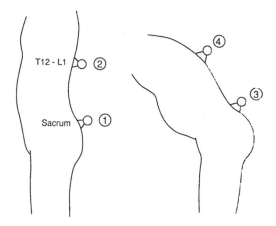

Figure 8.3 The inclinometer technique of measuring flexion: 3 – 1 = pelvic flexion; 4 – 2 = total flexion. The difference between them is lumbar flexion. In this diagram, pelvic flexion = 35°, total flexion = 60°, and therefore lumbar flexion = 25°.

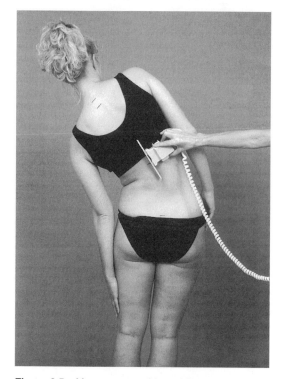

Figure 8.5 Measurement of lateral flexion

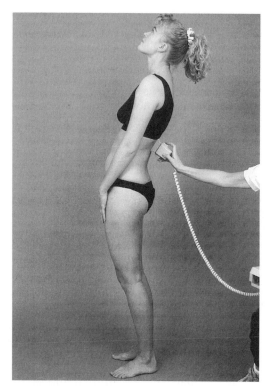

Figure 8.4 Measurement of extension.

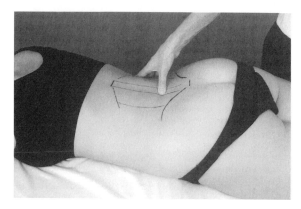

Figure 8.6 Lumbar spinal tenderness.

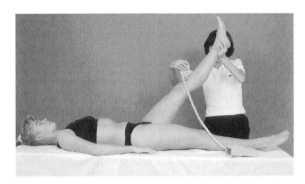

Figure 8.7   Straight leg raising

tubercle. Set the inclinometer to zero. Then raise the leg passively, using your other hand to hold the inclinometer in place and also to hold the patient's knee fully extended. Raise the leg slowly to the highest SLR that the patient will tolerate, not just to the onset of pain. Record the highest reading in degrees. If SLR is limited, you should always check this while you distract the patient at a later stage (see Ch. 10). If distraction SLR is positive, then you should discount SLR on formal examination.

Bilateral active SLR.   This is a strength test, which should be carried out in the supine position (Fig. 8.8). Ask the patient to lift both legs together six inches off the couch and hold that position for five seconds. They should raise both heels and calves clear of the couch. You should not count aloud or give any verbal encouragement. Do not allow the patient to use their hands to lift their legs. Only if the patient manages to hold their legs clear for the full 5 seconds should you count the test as successful. If they fail to lift their legs clear of the couch, or lift them clear but lower them again in less than 5 seconds, that is a positive impairment.

Active sit-up.   Like bilateral active SLR, this is also a strength test, and should also be carried out in the supine position (Fig. 8.9). Ask the patient to bend their knees to 90° and to place the soles of both feet flat on the couch. Use one hand to hold down both feet. Then ask the patient to reach up with the fingertips of both hands to touch their knees. They should rest their fingers on their knees and not hold on. They should hold that position for 5 seconds. Again, you should not count aloud or give verbal encouragement. If the patient fails to reach the fingertips of both hands to their patellae, or does not hold the position for 5 seconds, that counts as a positive impairment.

Interpretation of physical impairment

This is a comprehensive group of clinical tests for physical impairment in nonspecific low back pain. It includes spinal movement, SLR, spinal tenderness and strength tests. It is somewhat similar to the AMA guidelines and to Moffroid's scale. In our study, it discriminated patients with back pain from normal subjects and helped to explain low back disability.

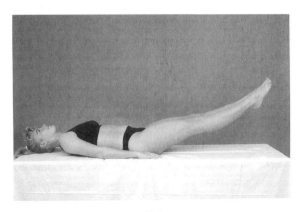

Figure 8.8   Bilateral active SLR.

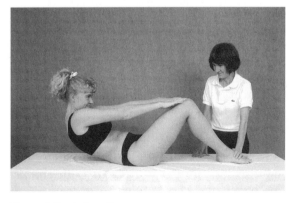

Figure 8.9   Active sit-up.

To interpret this scale we must look carefully at the definition of impairment. This is a pragmatic method based on clinical findings. It does not depend on pathologic or clinical diagnosis. Our previous study showed that the only permanent lumbar impairments were structural deformities, fractures, surgical scarring and neurologic deficits. None of these apply to the patient with nonspecific low back pain, and they do not appear in this scale. This method does provide an objective clinical evaluation, but it is not a measure of anatomic or structural impairment. Instead, the tests in our scale are all measures of physical function. They are 'functional limitations' associated with pain or disuse. More graphically, they are measures of 'inability to do' because of pain. They provide an objective check on the patient's own report of disability. It is a matter of perspective whether we regard these findings as physiologic impairment as in the WHO definition. Alternatively, they are clinical observations of performance. In any event, performance in these tests will depend on how the patient reacts to pain and on the patient's effort, just as much as on the physical or physiologic disorder. We cannot interpret 'inability to do' only in terms of physical impairment.

One of our most surprising findings was that these patients with chronic low back pain did not have significant loss of lumbar flexion. Many studies suggest that lumbar flexion may be the most specific measure of true lumbar impairment. It is the most useful test of clinical severity and progress in serious spinal pathology such as infection, and for disc prolapse and nerve root problems (Ch. 2). It is also the most useful measure of recovery from an acute attack of back pain. Direct measurement of lumbar flexion includes distraction and is hard to fake. It is the test that is least behavioral. For all these reasons, lumbar flexion may be the most valid single measure of true lumbar impairment.

Despite this, we found that lumbar flexion is more or less normal in patients with chronic low back pain. This may surprise many clinicians. The reason may be that we looked only at patients with simple backache. Most previous clinical studies, like our 1984 study, included patients with fractures, nerve root problems or spinal surgery. Our normal subjects were also from the entire age range, whereas many previous studies used young and athletic normal subjects as controls. However, we are not alone in our findings. Burton et al (1989) measured lumbar movement in nearly 1000 people aged 10–84 years. They compared those with no history of back pain, those with a previous history, and those with current pain. They found relatively minor differences in flexion in each group. Age and sex had a much greater effect. A recent study by Esola et al (1996) found changes in the *pattern* of lumbar flexion, but no restriction in the range of flexion in adults with a history of back pain. Gronblad et al (1997) also looked at spinal movements, pain, disability assessments and physical performance tests in patients with chronic low back pain. They found very little relation between spinal movements and any of these measures of severity. These findings again make us question the nature of impairment in chronic low back pain. There may be physiologic change in the pattern of movement and reduced total body performance, rather than any structural impairment of the lumbar spine.

We made every effort to separate our assessment of physical impairment from how patients respond to examination. Despite our efforts, we were only partly successful. All the tests in our scale still correlated to some extent with pain behavior. Our final scale was still more closely related to the emotional than to the sensory scale of the McGill pain questionnaire. It correlated more with measures of illness behavior than with pain itself. By their very nature, all of these tests may also be open to exaggeration. It is never possible to separate clinical examination of pain wholly from such influences. Ultimately, this is a measure of physical performance.

By the nature of these tests, they can only be measures of current impairment. In practice, we assess a patient at one point in time. We cannot know what was previously normal function for that individual; we can only compare our findings with the average for normal people. We can try to allow for age, sex and build. Ultimately, however, these tests only tell us about the current state. This is an objective clinical evaluation of current functional limitation in patients with back pain.

Objective clinical evaluation of physical impairment in simple backache

- There is no clinical evidence of any permanent anatomic or structural impairment
- These are findings of current physiologic impairment or functional limitation associated with pain
- These clinical findings are a measure of performance, and depend on effort
- This physical impairment has the potential to recover

IMPAIRMENT AND DISABILITY

Back pain, impairment and disability go together in clinical practice (see Fig. 8.10). The very definitions of impairment and disability relate them to each other. Impairment is that which causes disability; disability is that which results from impairment. Both are associated with back pain and we attribute them to pain, but it is not a 1:1 relationship. We often see patients with severe pain and disability, in whom we can find little impairment. Other people have severe pain or impairment, yet refuse to admit to much disability. Disability must depend on other influences, as well as pain and impairment. Before we look at these other influences in the following chapters, we should stop and

reflect further on impairment and disability (Fordyce 1995).

WHO (1980) defines impairment as a medical matter. Assessment requires an objective observer, standard tests and a cooperative patient. Without all three, assessment may not be valid. The problem is that we cannot assess back pain: we can only assess the person with back pain. Pain, suffering and pain behavior all confound our assessment of impairment.

The problem is that we cannot separate body and mind. Physical defects affect the person's beliefs and expectations about his or her situation. On the other hand, beliefs and expectations help to shape the impact of physical defects on function. There are also powerful social influences. Concepts of impairment and disability must allow for this dynamic interaction. We must not under-estimate the extent to which psychologic and social processes influence physical function, and vice versa. Disability is not only a question of physical impairment or medical assessment; nor is it only to do with functional capacity. It is a question of performance. To assess disability we must look at physical impairment and also at how the person copes with that impairment. We must consider all the possible influences on that person's performance.

Performance depends on anatomic and physiologic abilities, but also on psychologic and social resources. It depends on effort. Testing itself may cause pain and inhibit performance. Capacity may be set by physiologic limits; performance is set by psychologic limits. Medical assessment of impairment tries to

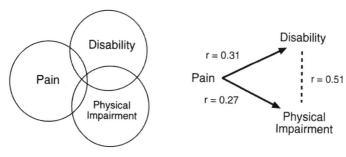

Figure 8.10 The relation between pain, disability and impairment. *r* is the correlation coefficient, where 0 is no relation at all and 1 is complete identity. *r* = 0.30 is about 10% overlap in common, and *r* = 0.50 is about 25%.

provide an objective basis to aid decisions about social support, but it can never be independent of these aspects. Concepts of disability are really at the interface between medicine and social issues.

We use the word disability to mean either loss of capacity for activity or actual reduction of activity, but we often blur and confuse these two meanings. We assume that disability means loss of physical capacity, but we assess disability either from the person's report or by our observation of reduced activity (Ch. 3). In fact, what we are assessing is performance. This may be due to loss of capacity; or it may be that the person stops before reaching his or her physical limits; or that he or she may not even attempt the activity. Fordyce (1995) defines a 'state of disability ... as ... when the person prematurely terminates an activity, under-performs or declines to undertake it'. Our concept and measure of disability cannot be independent of performance.

Disability has even wider meanings. It may imply the presence of illness, reduced capacity, actual reduction in activity, or handicap. Impairment does not always cause disability. At first, minor dysfunction may not even cause any symptoms. If it gets worse, it may give symptoms and become an illness, but that person may still have no disability. He or she may draw on his or her resources and make greater effort to maintain activity. Even once he or she no longer has the physical capacity for activity as before, he or she may modify his or her approach to maintain activity. If the patient's hand is injured, he or she may use the other hand. He or she may split a load and make smaller lifts. He or she may even buy a wheelbarrow. Only when no alternative remains, or when the person gives up the effort, is he or she actually disabled.

From a limited disease perspective, physical impairment causes disability. This simple view may be adequate for a structural impairment such as an amputated limb, but it does not provide an adequate basis to explain or assess disability associated with pain. In that case, physiologic impairment is again simply a mea-sure of performance. Impairment may be the expression of the patient's 'inability to do' in the context of clinical examination, whereas disability is the patient's report of 'inability to do' in daily activities. Pain itself does not fulfil the definition of impairment. But if activity aggravates pain and the person then avoids or reduces that activity, then pain leads to disability. The question then is how and why there is so much variation in the amount of disability resulting from back pain.

We recognize that pain involves emotional or psychologic disturbance. We may then ask whether this is a psychologic impairment. It is very easy to get into a circular argument, and the simplest and most logical solution is to define the level of psychologic disturbance. If it meets standard criteria for a psychiatric disorder, then it would be a separate psychologic impairment. More often, we are talking about 'suffering' or the emotional component of pain, which does not meet the criteria of a primary psychiatric illness. In that case, we should regard it as part of pain, and it may only confuse the issue to try to apply a psychiatric label.

In addition to these problems, assessment at one point in time suffers from major limitations. Impairment and disability are not static or passive. Both can vary with time, disuse and rehabilitation. We have not found any physical basis for permanent disability in simple backache, and physiologic impairments at least have the potential to recover. Psychologic, behavioral and social impairments may all be remediable. Functional limitation may persist as long as pain lasts, and there is good clinical and epidemiologic evidence to suggest that the chances of successful rehabilitation of chronic pain reduce over time. But, in principle, this kind of impairment always has the potential to improve. Mayer and colleagues have proved this, even in chronic low back cripples (Cox et al 1988).

In practice, we must judge disability within a broad clinical framework. We start with diagnosis or at least attempt to recognize symptom clusters. We look for objective evidence of impairment. We must allow for effort and for the coexistence of physical and psychologic dysfunction. The patient gives us their account of symptoms and disability and the impact on their life and work. This may be in the context of a claim for compensation and we must try to discount exaggeration or observer bias. We must distinguish temporary and permanent disability. We must assess the potential for recovery and how much of current impairment is likely to be permanent. The final judgement of severity depends on the balance between the patient's report of pain and disability and the examiner's diagnosis and assessment of impairment. Together these give a comprehensive picture. When all are in proportion, we can combine them into an unequivocal assessment of severity. The objective clinical evidence then supports the patient's report of symptoms and disability. Sometimes, however, there may be

a real discrepancy between the patient's claim of pain, disability and incapacity for work and the examiner's assessment of pathology and impairment. We must then try to discover the reasons why. To understand disability, we must look at the entire clinical picture in more detail.

Assessment of severity

- Diagnosis
- Patient report
  - pain
  - disability
- Professional assessment
  - physical impairment
  - functional capacity evaluation
- Judicial decision
  - working capacity
  - compensation

REFERENCES

AAOS 1962 Manual for orthopedic surgeons in evaluating permanent physical impairment. American Academy of Orthopedic Surgeons, Chicago.

AMA 1958 A guide to the evaluation of permanent impairment of the extremities and back. Journal of the American Medical Association (Supplement) 166: 1–122

AMA 1993 Guides to the evaluation of permanent impairment, 4th edn. American Medical Association, Chicago, p 94–138

Brand R A, Lehmann T R 1983 Low-back impairment rating practices of orthopedic surgeons. Spine 8: 75–78

Burton A K, Tillotson K M, Troup J D G 1989 Variation in lumbar sagittal mobility with low back trouble. Spine 14: 584–590

Clark W L, Haldeman S, Johnson P et al 1988 Back impairment and disability determination. Another attempt at objective reliable rating. Spine 13: 332–341

Cox R, Keeley J, Barnes D, Gatchel R, Mayer T 1988 Effects of functional restoration treatment upon Waddell impairment/disability ratings in chronic low back pain patients. Presented to the International Society for the Study of the Lumbar Spine, Miami

Esola M A, McClure P W, Fitzgerald G K, Siegler S 1996 Analysis of lumbar spine and hip motion during forward bending in subjects with and without a history of low back pain. Spine 21: 71–78

Fordyce W E (ed) 1995 Back pain in the workplace: management of disability in non-specific conditions. International Association for the Study of Pain (IASP) Press, Seattle, p 1–75

Frymoyer J W, Cats-Baril W 1987 Predictors of low back disability. Clinical Orthopaedics and Related Research 221: 89–98

Greenough C G, Fraser R D 1992 The assessment of outcome in patients with low back pain. Spine 17: 36–41

Gronblad M, Hurri H, Kouri J-P 1997 Relationships between spinal mobility, physical performance tests, pain intensity and disability assessments in chronic low back pain patients. Scandinavian Journal of Rehabilitation Medicine 29: 17–24

Lehmann T, Brand R A, O'Gorman T W O 1983 A low back rating scale. Spine 8: 308–315

McBride E D 1936 Disability evaluation and principles of treatment of compensable injuries, 1st edn. Lippincott, Philadelphia

McBride E D 1963 Disability evaluation and principles of treatment of compensable injuries, 6th edn. Lippincott, Philadelphia

McCombe P F, Fairbank J C T, Cockersole B C, Pynsent P B 1989 Reproducibility of physical signs in low back pain. Spine 14: 908–918

Moffroid M T, Haugh L D, Henry S M, Short B 1994 Distinguishable groups of musculoskeletal low back pain patients and asymptomatic control subjects based on physical measures of the NIOSH low back atlas. Spine 19: 1350–1358

Moffroid M T, Haugh L D, Hodous T 1992 Sensitivity and specificity of the NIOSH low back atlas. NIOSH Report RFP 200–89–2917 (P). National Institute Occupational Safety & Health, Morgantown, West Virginia

Nelson R M, Nestor D E 1988 Standardized assessment of industrial low-back injuries: development of the NIOSH low-back atlas. Topics in Acute Care and Trauma Rehabilitation 2: 16–30

NIOSH 1988 National Institute for Occupational Safety and Health low back atlas. US Department of Health and Human Services, Morgantown, West Virginia

US Bureau of Disability Insurance 1970 Disability evaluation under social security. A handbook for physicians. US Government Printing Office, Washington, DC

Waddell G, Main C J 1984 Assessment of severity in low back disorders. Spine 9: 204–208

Waddell G, Main C J, Morris E W, Venner R M, Rae P S, Sharmy S H, Galloway H 1982 Normality and reliability in the clinical assessment of backache. British Medical Journal 284: 1519–1523

Waddell G, Sommerville D, Henderson I, Newton M 1992 Objective clinical evaluation of physical impairment in chronic low back pain. Spine 17: 617–628

WHO 1980 International classification of impairments, disabilities and handicaps. World Health Organization, Geneva

9

The physical basis of back pain

Let us pose the question again. What is the physical basis of nonspecific low back pain? Structure and function are intimately related, and we must consider them together. Let us now look at the basic science.

Most books about back pain start with chapters on the anatomy and pathology of the spine. Macnab described this as a form of Brownian movement: it seems very busy, but is really mindless and serves no useful purpose. Having made that comment, he went ahead and started with that chapter anyway! You already know that I resisted that temptation. This was deliberate. I firmly believe that we must start with the clinical problem, and only then look for the basic science that helps to explain our clinical observations. The danger of starting from anatomy, biomechanics or pathology is that they set the agenda. We too easily become prisoners of theory and then select or twist the clinical facts to fit that theory. Instead, I will try to take a very clinical perspective of the basic science.

Clinical characteristics

Back pain is a mechanical problem. It is mechanical in the sense that symptoms arise from the musculoskeletal system and vary with physical activity.

Fiddler (1980) surveyed the members of the International Society for the Study of the Lumbar Spine (ISSLS). They described a mechanical syndrome for nonspecific back pain without

135

nerve root involvement (see Box 9.1). Different authors describe these mechanical characteristics as movement disorders or activity-related spinal disorders.

Box 9.1 'Mechanical' low back pain

- Pain is usually cyclic
- Low back pain is often referred to the buttocks and thighs
- Morning stiffness or pain is common
- Start pain is common
- There is pain on forward flexion and often also on returning to the erect position
- Pain is often produced or aggravated by extension, lateral flexion, rotation, standing, walking, sitting and exercise in general
- Pain usually becomes worse over the course of the day
- Pain is relieved by a change of position
- Pain is relieved by lying down, especially in the fetal position

---

These clinicians obviously focused on what made the pain worse. However, most people with back pain actually say that various activities make their pain either better or worse (Table 9.1). We also looked at patterns of activity-related back pain (Table 9.2). Many patients made a distinction between the immediate effects of activity on their symptoms and what seemed to be the best long-term management for their problem. Disability varied with these mechanical characteristics. Patients who said that physical activity, walking and physical therapy made their pain worse were more severely disabled. They also responded worse to treatment.

Pain receptors

Pain can only arise from structures that contain nerve endings. Most nociceptors are unmyeli-

Table 9.1 Effect of physical activities on back pain in 200 osteopathic patients (from Dr K Burton, with thanks)

	Aggravates	Relieves
Sitting	30%	23%
Walking	22%	12%
Movement	17%	16%
Lying	9%	35%

nated, free nerve endings. More specialized nerve endings in tendons, ligaments and joint capsules are sensitive to mechanical stimuli. These normally serve proprioception, but can also give pain under certain conditions.

Kellgren (1938, 1939) performed a classic experiment to find possible sources of low back pain. He injected hypertonic saline into various low back structures to produce different patterns of pain. Later studies had more accurate placement of stimuli, used different types of stimuli and relieved the pain by local anesthetic, but they broadly confirmed Kellgren's work. On the basis of such studies, we now believe that the following low back structures can give rise to pain (Bogduk & Twomey 1991, Merskey & Bogduk 1994):

- *Facet joint capsules* – these have a rich supply of nociceptors
- *Ligaments and fascia* – these also have rich innervation
- *Intervertebral disc* – histology of the normal disc suggests that only the most peripheral annulus is innervated; however, granulation or scar tissue may grow into the degenerate disc, and the new blood vessels in this tissue may contain nociceptors
- *Vertebrae* – there are nociceptors in periostium and with blood vessels in cancellous bone

Table 9.2 Patterns of activity-related low back pain in 500 primary care patients

	Male	Female
Pain aggravated by certain positions and relieved by moving about or changing position	17%	35%
Pain unrelated to physical activity	10%	3%
Pain aggravated by certain activities and relieved by changing or stopping activities	74%	62%

- *Dura and nerve root sleeves* – this is quite separate from stimulation of the actual lumbar nerve root
- *Muscle* – there is considerable anatomic debate about muscle as a site of back pain. There are mechanoreceptors in tendons and muscle insertions that may give rise to pain. There are nociceptors in the region of blood vessels and in fascia. It is doubtful if muscle fibers themselves can produce pain, but muscle spindles are sensitive to mechanical stimuli. If a muscle contracts under ischemic conditions, pain develops within 1 minute. Muscle use may lead to lowered oxygen tension, acidity and local build-up of metabolites. These cause increased sensitivity to stretch and increased muscle tone. Disuse makes these physiologic events more marked, while training reduces them. The question has been raised of increased muscle pressure in back pain, but this is unconfirmed. The paraspinal muscles are unique in that they are innervated by the posterior primary rami, while all other voluntary muscles in the body are innervated by the anterior primary rami. In clinical experiments, painful stimuli to muscles give local pain and tenderness but not referred pain.

The posterior primary rami of the lumbar nerve roots supply all these structures, with overlap between several adjacent levels. There are also links with sympathetic and parasympathetic nerves. Stimulation of most of these structures gives pain in the lower back. Referred pain may also radiate down the leg in a sclerotome pattern. The distribution of pain depends on the lumbar level that we stimulate.

A STRUCTURAL BASIS FOR BACK PAIN?

For more than a century, workers in orthodox medicine, orthopedics and biomechanics have looked for a structural basis for back pain. They have sought a mechanical cause, an injury or a disease that will fit the disease model.

We should interpret this evidence with care. The source of pain is quite different from the cause of pain. The anatomic site and pathologic nature of any disorder are separate questions. Finding a painful site does not diagnose the pathology. Conversely, even when we cannot localize the exact site we may still be able to understand the nature of the disorder. Further, the various structures at one segmental level are closely linked, share common innervation and function together. So even when we localize pain to one level, that may not tell us which of the structures at that level is the cause of the problem. Even if one part of the segment seems to be most sensitive now, the initial cause of the disturbance may be in other linked parts of the segment. We have often blurred these issues in our search for the cause of back pain.

Radiologic anomalies

The historic review (Ch. 4) described how early X-rays led to the temptation to blame back pain on every incidental radiologic finding. But anatomic coincidence is not proof of cause and effect. That would be like saying: 'Red hair is not normal in the sense that it is quite uncommon. It is close to the site of headache. So your red hair must be the cause of your headache. Maybe, we should think about shaving your hair to cure your head pain.' That is clearly absurd, but it is the same kind of logic. We must be more critical. Back pain is very common and so are many X-ray findings. First, we must show that the finding is more common in people with back pain than in those without. We should be able to establish a causal link. Anesthetic blocks or treatment of the abnormality should relieve the pain. When we apply these tests, most radiologic anomalies turn out to be incidental findings (Box 9.2).

Disc prolapse

The discovery of the disc prolapse (Fig. 9.1) seemed at first to end the long search for the cause of back pain. In Chapter 4, we saw how early enthusiasts claimed that it was the cause of most, if not all, back pain. One reason for this was the natural history of disc prolapse.

> **Box 9.2** Radiographic anomalies that appear to be incidental findings in back pain (Wiltse 1971, Nachemson 1975, van Tulder et al 1997)
>
> - Transitional vertebra
> - Lumbarization, sacralization
> - Spina bifida occulta
> - Accessory ossicles
> - Schmorl's nodes
> - Disc calcification
> - Height of sacrum in pelvis
> - Lumbosacral angle
> - Lumbar lordosis
> - Mild–moderate scoliosis
> - Spondylolysis
> - Spondylolisthesis
> - Scheuermann's disease

Many patients with disc prolapse have a previous history of recurrent back pain over the years. The acute episode may also start with back pain that, over a period of days or weeks, changes to nerve root pain. Hence back pain may be part of the natural history of disc prolapse. We know that stimulation of the posterior longitudinal ligament and dura can produce back pain, and that disc prolapse can irritate these structures. So there is a possible pathologic mechanism. However, it is an enormous and illogical jump to claim that disc prolapse is a common cause of most back pain. Sixty per cent of adults have back pain each year, but only 3–5% ever have a disc prolapse in their whole lives. No one can dispute that disc prolapse may cause back pain, but it is a rare cause.

Disc degeneration

Few of us now believe that disc prolapse is the usual cause of back pain, but the lure of the disc is still strong. Many doctors, therapists and patients find radiographic or MRI changes of degeneration almost irresistible. Look at the X-ray in Figure 9.2. This is the end result of spinal degeneration. The discs are severely worn, there is loss of alignment of the spine, and there is osteoarthritis in the facet joints. It looks terrible and must be painful. There is only one snag to this story, and the clue is the distended stomach. This is an abdominal X-ray of an 80-year-old lady with acute intestinal obstruction. She has never had back pain in her life.

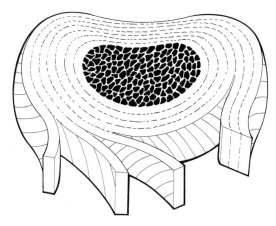

Figure 9.1 The dynasty of the disc. The disc is most accessible to experiment and investigation, but this has led to the neglect of 'soft tissues' which may be more important in simple backache. (Drawing by Stewart Wood, with thanks.)

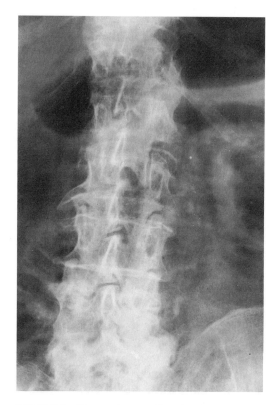

Figure 9.2 Severe degenerative changes – an incidental radiographic finding.

We now know a great deal about the gross changes, histology, biochemistry and biomechanics of disc degeneration (Buckwalter 1995). However, this information has mainly come from cadaver and laboratory studies, and most of the changes are normal and age-related, and bear little relationship to clinical symptoms. Van Tulder et al (1997) reviewed the clinical evidence. They found 12 studies of reasonable quality that compared X-ray findings in people with or without symptoms. These do show a consistent association between degenerative changes and nonspecific low back pain. The relationship is statistically significant, but weak. A large proportion of the asymptomatic people show the same radiographic changes. van Tulder et al also pointed out a number of weaknesses to these studies. In particular, many of the studies compare present X-ray changes with past history of back pain. They concluded that they could not establish a cause and effect relationship between degenerative changes and clinical symptoms.

Most disc degeneration is a normal age-related process, like grey hair.

Facet joints

The facet joints are another potential source of pain. These are synovial joints and so they can develop true osteoarthritis.

Fiddler (1980) tried to distinguish syndromes of disc, facet and instability pain. Unfortunately, the members of ISSLS could not agree. One-third of the experts freely admitted that they could not separate these syndromes. The others thought that they could, but their descriptions were all different. Scientific studies have been just as inconclusive. Jackson et al (1988) found no relation between pain on extension and pain relief by local anesthetic injection into the facets. Lilius et al (1989) found no link between initial pain relief by local anesthetic and lasting relief from cortisone injection. In a controlled trial, injections into or around the facet were no better than placebo. Both groups felt that they could not identify a facet joint syndrome. The review by van Tulder et al (1997) did not link X-ray changes in the facet joints to back pain.

Sprains and strains

The most common clinical diagnosis for nonspecific low back pain, especially an acute episode with sudden onset, is a sprain or strain. We often simply assume it is an injury, even if any 'accident' is usually a normal, everyday activity. We rarely specify the exact site or tissue, but assume it is muscle or connective tissue. The diagnosis seems plausible and may even be likely in some cases, but there is little direct evidence.

Most minor limb injuries are to the soft tissues, mainly the connective tissues. Structural damage to a muscle is quite rare, although muscle symptoms associated with use are common. By analogy, there may be similar injuries in the back, but they are more difficult to assess because the tissues are deeply placed. It is possible that we simply do not have the clinical ability or investigations to demonstrate soft tissue injuries in the back. These cases do not come to autopsy or surgery, so we have no tissue studies. Nevertheless, for a clinical problem which is so common, we have surprisingly little direct evidence. There is still considerable doubt as to whether there is any true soft tissue injury with structural damage, either in general or in the individual patient. At present, I would advance the old Scots verdict of 'not proven'.

Conclusion

So, are we dealing with spinal anomalies, disc prolapse, disc degeneration or soft tissue injury? For more than 100 years, workers in orthodox medicine, orthopedics and biomechanics have searched for a structural cause for back pain. They have focused on tissue damage or mechanical failure, whether due to single injury or fatigue failure as a result of repetitive loading. Early osteopathic concepts of displacement and early chiropractic concepts of subluxation to some extent reflected the same approach. Surgeons and engineers have focused research on the spine and discs, but this may simply reflect their professional interests and skills.

The spine may simply be more accessible than other structures to medical investigations and laboratory experiment. This approach has been very informative for spinal injury, disc prolapse and nerve root problems, but has failed to find the cause of back pain. Perhaps after so much fruitless search we should question our starting assumption that nonspecific low back pain is due to injury and structural damage. The 'soft tissues' of the back may be at least as important, or even more important, in back pain. There is an extensive knowledge of these soft tissues in alternative medicine that needs to be integrated into medical and biomechanical research.

BIOMECHANICS*

Most biomechanics starts from the concept of injury or mechanical failure, usually of the spine (Adams & Dolan 1995). In theory, musculoskeletal damage may be caused by direct trauma, by a single 'overexertion' or by repetitive or sustained loading. Tissue strength varies with sex, age, body build, physical fitness and fatigue. Damage may be to one or more of the musculoskeletal structures. Direct trauma may injure many tissues at the same time. Overexertion, such as lifting, usually only damages one tissue. Repetitive or sustained loading is also likely to lead to fatigue failure at one site. In life, a single injury is followed by healing. However, with repetitive or sustained loading, continued damage and healing may occur simultaneously.

We must always remember the fundamental limitations of our present biomechanical knowledge. We perform most studies in the laboratory on cadaver material, and most studies are of a single 'motion segment' of the spine (Fig. 9.3). Many studies are on one or two specimens only. The tissues are no longer alive and are completely inert; there is no nutrition or neuromuscular activity, and there is no biologic response or inflammation and certainly no

*I am indebted to Pope et al (1991) for much of the material in this section.

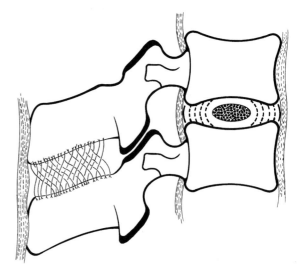

Figure 9.3 The motion segment – two adjacent vertebrae with the disc, facet joints, ligaments and muscles between them. (Drawing by Stewart Wood, with thanks.)

healing. Testing segments of the spine to failure tells us about the mechanics of spinal fracture and disc prolapse but is of doubtful relevance to simple backache. The earliest in vivo experiments measured the pressure in the intervertebral disc, and showed the load on the spine in different activities (Fig. 9.4). However,

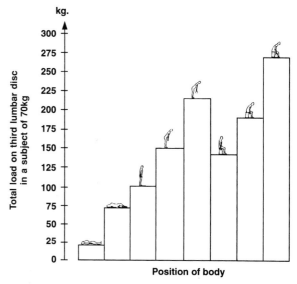

Figure 9.4 The load on the spine with different activities. (From Nachemson & Morris 1964, with permission.)

once again, the disc was simply the most suitable site to measure these loads. Actually, this reflects comparable loads on various parts of the musculoskeletal system. More studies now include the facet joints and the ligaments of the spine, but they usually consider ligaments, muscles and soft tissues mainly for their influence on the spine, rather than as being of interest in their own right. This is a fundamental bias that may not reflect clinical reality.

The spine

The spine is mechanically complex because it has to serve different functions (Box 9.3). The demands on the spine are conflicting but it has to meet them all simultaneously.

Box 8.3 The functions of the spine

- Support
  — body
  — loads
- Movement
  — flexion–extension
  — lateral bending
  — axial rotation (twisting)
- Protection
  — CNS and nerve roots

In biomechanics, as in embryology and mythology, the spine forms the backbone of the body. It supports the head and the trunk and the limbs. Even the internal organs are suspended from the spine. If support were its only function, a rigid spine would be simplest and strongest. It is the need for mobility at the same time which causes the problem. So, instead of being rigid, the spine is a flexible column of bony blocks joined by discs. The demands of support and those of mobility are always in conflict, and achieving a balance between them requires good control mechanisms. We must maintain an equilibrium between the load on the spine and the tension in discs, ligaments and muscles. If we are to stay upright, there must be a balance between the moments of all the forces acting. When we lift, the load on the back will depend on the weight and the

distance from the body. Pregnancy also alters posture and the loads on the back.

Panjabi (1992) suggested that stability of the spine depends on three subsystems (Fig. 9.5). The passive system is the spinal column, made up of the vertebrae, discs, facet joints, ligaments and joint capsules. The active system is the muscles and tendons that surround and can apply forces to the spinal column. The neurologic or control system monitors the position, loading and demands on the spine, and directs the active system to provide the required stability and actions. Dysfunction in any one system leads to a response in one or both of the other systems, which may or may not compensate, or lead to long-term adaptation or failure.

The spine is a flexible column with multiple curves. The thoracic spine is splinted by the ribcage. The sacrum is more or less fixed in the pelvis and the coccyx has no mechanical function. The lumbar and cervical spines are flexible, but, of the two, the lumbar spine has to carry greater loads. The transitional regions between fixed and flexible parts of the spine have greater functional demands, which might explain why these are the areas of most symptoms.

The anterior and posterior elements of the spine serve different mechanical functions. The main anterior column of the spine is made up of the vertebral bodies and discs. These provide support and in life carry 75–80% of the load. The discs allow flexion, extension and lateral

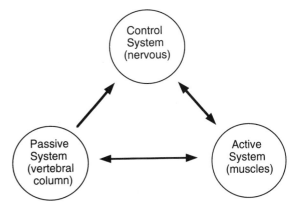

Figure 9.5 The three subsystems of spinal stability. (From Panjabi 1992, with permission.)

bending and also a limited amount of rotation and glide. The flexibility of the spine, with the spinal curves and discs, allows it to act as a shock absorber so that we do not suffer concussion every time we jump down on to our heels. The posterior half of each vertebra is an arch of bone to surround and protect the spinal cord and nerves. Each arch articulates with the arch above and below by two small facet joints. Bony processes project backwards and to each side as levers for ligaments and muscles.

Movement of the spine never occurs as pure flexion or extension in one plane. The spine is flexible, and must be controlled in three dimensions. In practice, there is always some movement in the other planes. Even a simple axial load causes such a 'coupled response'. In real life we subject our backs to complex movements and loads. Consider a simple lift at work. We may start with flexion and axial loading, and when we turn to lay the load down, there may be axial rotation, lateral bending and shear forces. Each of these demands occurs at different stages of the lift and in varying combinations.

Vertebral body

The vertebral body is a honeycomb of cancellous bone that gives a high strength-to-weight ratio. There is a roughly linear relationship between the mineral content of the bone and the load at which it fails, as in osteoporosis. The trabeculae develop to withstand the forces acting on the bone, so their pattern reveals the common forces on the vertebrae. In life the vertebrae are full of blood, which may add hydraulic strength. The vertebrae are stronger lower down the spine where the load of the body is greater. We tend to think of bone as rigid but that is not strictly true. Vertebrae are six times stiffer and three times thicker than the discs and only allow half the deformation, but they do have some elasticity. Micro-fractures may occur in the trabeculae and some authors suggest they may be a source of back pain, although there is no proof of this. Increased venous pressure in cancellous bone may occur

adjacent to osteoarthritis in peripheral joints, but we do not know if that is important in the vertebrae.

Disc

The disc forms the main articulation between the vertebral bodies. The mechanical properties of the disc depend on the tissues of the annulus and the nucleus. The annulus contains about 90 collagen lamellae, which are spiral and interdigitate like a modern car tire to give maximum strength. With age the collagen fibers and lamellae split and break. The young nucleus is about 90% water and is an incompressible gel. With age it dries out and loses much of its mechanical properties. The normal nucleus is under pressure even at rest and this increases to balance axial loads, which produces tension and slight bulging of the annulus. This disc bulge is *normal* and reflects the balance between the mechanical forces applied to the spine and the osmotic forces in the nucleus (Fig. 9.6). There is about 20% diurnal variation in disc height and volume. During the day, the load on the disc due to gravity and physical activity gradually overcomes the osmotic forces, and the disc is squashed. When we lie down at night, osmotic forces restore disc height. The pressure in the disc varies with posture and physical activity (see Fig. 9.4). Even distribution of stress within the disc depends on the intact nucleus and annulus, and becomes uneven with degeneration.

Discs are quite avascular and their nutrition depends on diffusion. The permeability of the vertebral end plates decreases with age. Movement is good for the disc, improving the transport of nutrients and disc metabolism. Continuous motion is more effective than intermittent motion, e.g. regular exercise once a day is better than once or twice a week.

Facet joints

The main functional posterior elements of the spine are the facet joints. The facets stabilize the spine and limit rotation and shift. The facet

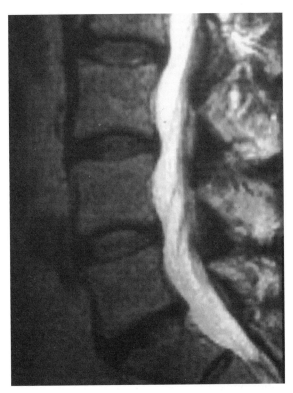

Figure 9.6 Disc bulging is normal. This is an incidental MRI finding in a healthy 55-year-old man. The more sensitive the investigation, the higher the false-positive rate in older patients. (From Dr N McMillan, with thanks.)

joint itself is subject to compression and shearing. The facets carry 20–25% of the axial load, although this may rise as high as 70% when the discs narrow with degenerative changes. They provide 40% of torsional and shear strength. The posterior elements may be more vulnerable to cyclic fatigue, as in spondylolysis.

Ligaments

Ligaments stabilize the spine and set the limits to movement. They are one of the main tensile elements acting as check reins to prevent excessive movement. They are relatively nonelastic, but they do give a little as they take up load. They are really visco-elastic: how much they stretch and how they fail depends on the rate of loading. However, the intervertebral ligaments are very strong. Trauma may rupture

collagen fibers, but complete rupture of the ligament probably only occurs with violent injury almost sufficient to dislocate the spine. Ligaments are subject to fatigue failure. Most importantly, ligaments can also heal, and we can see healed minor tears at autopsy.

In general, flexion puts tension on the posterior ligaments, and extension puts tension on the anterior ligaments. Muscles can act on ligaments and fascia to alter their tension. This may indirectly modify load bearing and help to control the range of movement.

Muscles

The spine depends on muscles for stability. The muscles control and position the spine and the trunk. They provide movement and power for voluntary activity. A spine held by ligaments alone, with all the muscle excised, buckles under loads of only 2 kg. Paralytic scoliosis provides a dramatic illustration of the role of the spinal muscles.

Of the flexor muscles, the psoas arises directly from the vertebral bodies while the more distant abdominal wall muscles act indirectly on the trunk. The extensor muscles run between the vertebral processes, both within each motion segment and over several segments. All the muscles work in synergy. When the anterior or posterior muscles contract symmetrically, they produce flexion or extension. When the left or right sides contract in various combinations, they produce lateral bending or rotation. Asymmetric positions cause very high muscle and joint loading.

Standing erect, there is little electrical activity in the extensor muscles. As we bend forward there is increasing muscle activity. Beyond about 35° of trunk flexion, this activity reduces. By full flexion the muscles are silent and the trunk is 'hanging on the ligaments'. Coming back up, movement begins with the hip extensors. Then, as we rise further, the spinal extensors take up the load. The trunk muscles can also raise the pressure in the abdomen and chest and convert the entire trunk into a semirigid cylinder.

These are all voluntary striated muscles. They are highly metabolic tissues, and they need a good and continuous supply of oxygen and nutrients. They fatigue: on sustained effort, EMG activity diminishes with time. They also take a finite time to react to sudden loads, and this time increases with fatigue.

Functional anatomy

Vleeming et al (1997) pointed out that the spine, pelvis and legs function as an integrated whole and that the pelvis has an essential role that we have often neglected. The human pelvis is unique because we are the only truly erect, bipedal animal. We walk by swivelling on each leg in turn, which places great loads across the pelvis and sacroiliac joints. The glutei have developed enormously compared with any other animal to become the largest muscle mass in the human body.

The thoracolumbar fascia plays an important role in load transfer between the trunk and legs. It is part of a 'corset' that surrounds the trunk. The erector spinae lies within its layers. Contractions of the latissimus dorsii, gluteus maximus and abdominal wall muscles tense the fascia, which effectively links the actions of these muscles. The biceps femoris tendon tenses the sacro-tuberous ligament below. This all acts as a muscle–tendon–fascia sling that provides a functional link between the trunk, the pelvis and the legs. This fascia also has a rich innervation for both proprioception and nociception.

There is long-standing dispute about the possible role of the sacroiliac joints in back pain. The closely matched shape of these joints and the very strong surrounding ligaments make it very unlikely that these joints are often damaged or 'displaced'. However, these ligaments contain mechanoreceptors. They permit a very small range of movement, but very little movement is required for them to act as strain gauges. Vleeming et al (1997) suggested that the sacroiliac joints may act as multi-directional force transducers, which could play a key role in the function of the lower back.

Biomechanics vs. clinical symptoms

The greatest problem lies in relating biomechanical knowledge to clinical symptoms of nonspecific low back pain.

DYSFUNCTION

Osteopathy, chiropractic, manual medicine and physical therapy all emphasize function. They each use different terms and stress different features, but they share many clinical observations and concepts. These ideas also agree with modern understanding of the neurophysiology of pain. The key concept is of a painful musculoskeletal dysfunction, which may occur in tissues that are structurally normal. It is a primary dysfunction arising in response to abnormal forces imposed on or generated within the musculoskeletal system. The normal functions of the locomotor system include:

- strength
- endurance
- flexibility
- coordination
- balance.

Dysfunction may involve disturbance of any or all of these functions. Abnormal muscle function, abnormal forces acting on musculoskeletal structures, abnormal posture or abnormal joint movement may all produce pain.

DiGiovanna & Schiowitz (1991) gave an osteopathic definition of *somatic dysfunction*: 'Somatic dysfunction is an impaired or altered function of related components of the somatic (body framework) system: Skeletal, arthrodial and myofascial structures, and related vascular, lymphatic, and neural elements.' The focus is on change in the normal functioning of a joint, or, in the case of the spine, a motion segment. It is implicit that it is a type of lesion suitable for manipulation.

DiGiovanna & Schiowitz (1991) based diagnosis on specific ART criteria:

- *Asymmetry or vertebral malposition.* The vertebrae may lie in an asymmetric position compared with normal and the neighboring vertebrae. This is still within the normal range.

- *Restriction of movement.* Movement may be painful, stiff, limited or abnormal. There may be 'barriers' to normal movement, in one or more planes. The physiologic barrier is the functional limit to the range of active movement. Further passive movement may be possible. The anatomic barrier is the limit of passive movement. This restriction is due to bone, ligament or tendon. Overcoming the anatomic barrier requires disruption of tissue.
- *Tissue changes.* There are palpable changes in the skin, fascia or muscle around the affected joint.

MacDonald (1988a,b) classified possible dysfunctions (Box 9.4).

Box 9.4 Musculoskeletal dysfunction. (After MacDonald 1988a,b, with permission)

- Abnormalities of posture
- Abnormalities of joint movement
  — limited movement
  — hypermobility
  — abnormal patterns of movement
  — acute joint locking (Droz-Georget 1980)
- Muscle
  — fatigue
  — weakness
  — tension: stress/anxiety
  — shortening, stretching
  — reflex muscle spasm
- Connective tissue (fascia, ligaments, joint capsule, muscle)
  — adhesions, scarring, contracture
  — 'trigger points'
  — 'fibrositis'
- Neuromuscular incoordination
  — muscle imbalance
  — abnormal patterns of movement
- Altered proprioceptor and nociceptor input and neurophysiologic processing

---

The locomotor system involves both musculoskeletal and neuromuscular functions. Many of the clinical findings listed in Box 9.4 fit a motion segment, or segmental dysfunction at one or more levels, e.g.:

- altered patterns of movement
- altered muscle function
- soft tissue changes due to changed autonomic function
- neurophysiologic changes
- psychophysiologic changes.

These are all integral elements of the one functional unit in normal function. Dysfunction also affects them all, perhaps to varying degrees, irrespective of where the problem starts.

Altered patterns of movement

Early concepts of vertebrae actually being out of place are now largely discredited. They placed too much emphasis on anatomy and structural pathology for which there is little evidence. Many manual therapists still focus on limitation of movement, but this also is now under question. Our study of physical impairment found that lumbar flexion is more or less normal in patients with chronic low back pain (Ch. 8). Burton et al (1989, 1990) questioned the role of simple limitation of movement in back pain, whether segmental or total. The range of movement is one of the crudest measures of spinal function, and may miss the point. We need to consider more complex, dynamic, *patterns* of movement (Marras et al 1993, Paquet et al 1994, Esola et al 1996, Steffen et al 1997). There may be a change in the balance of lumbar and pelvic movements, or between flexion and extension. There may be different mobility in the upper or lower lumbar spine. Spinal movement occurs in three dimensions and coupled movements may be disturbed. Velocity of movement is probably important. Perhaps most important of all is what happens during movement, and how the various components work and interact.

It may be possible to palpate altered patterns of movement at one or more segmental levels, either individually or in relation to each other. There may be postural disturbance with abnormal resting position of the vertebrae. There may be hyper- or hypo-mobility, or lack of joint play. The quality of joint movement may vary, with crepitus or altered 'end feel', or there may be 'locking'. Palpation of these abnormalities may produce tenderness or pain.

Altered muscle function

Palpable changes in segmental and limb muscles have been known for several centuries in 'rheumatic' conditions. These include hyper- or hypo-tonicity, fibrotic tissue, atrophy or hypertrophy. The muscle may contract or relax in response to movement. Focal areas of muscle spasm or contracture may be palpated. When these are tender and painful, they are sometimes described as 'trigger points'. In the limb muscles, these tender areas correspond to motor points (Fig. 9.7). There is little doubt about such clinical observations, although there is heated debate about their meaning. Some medical studies suggest they are unreliable, although that may simply reflect the lack of training and skill of physicians. Strender et al (1997) have shown that trained manual therapists can assess such segmental findings reliably, even if physicians cannot. Terms such as increased muscle tone, spasm or contracture are often used loosely and interchangeably. Few examiners attempt to differentiate connective

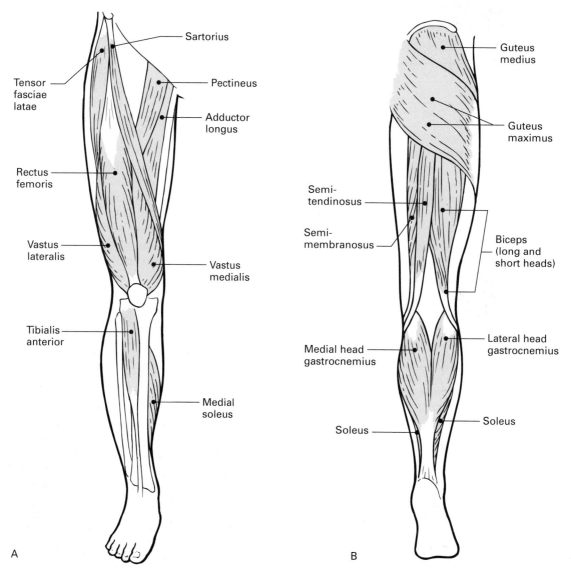

Figure 9.7 The site of tender motor points in the lower limb muscles. A: Anterior aspect. B: Posterior aspect. (From Gunn & Milbrandt 1976, with permission.)

tissue changes and neuromuscular effects. Pseudo-pathologic diagnoses include muscular rheumatism, fibrositis, or myofasciitis, to name but a few. Attempts to find an anatomic basis have failed, perhaps because these are expressions of disturbed physiology rather than structural pathology. This has all led to great confusion about the nature and meaning of these findings, but does not deny their existence or importance. Altered muscle tone and abnormalities of muscle function are key elements in movement disorders.

One of the most tender tissues, which is rich in nociceptors, is the junction of muscle, tendon, intermuscular septum, ligament or capsule with periosteum and bone. Increased muscle tension and contracture may stress these sensitive areas. Foci of hyper-irritable tissue may give myofascial, cutaneous, fascial, ligamentous or periosteal trigger points.

Environmental demands such as gravity, constrained positions, repetitive movements or inactivity alter the loads on the locomotor system. When muscles react to these loads, certain muscles show increased activity, while others are inhibited. Potential harm or pain may exaggerate that reaction. Grieve (1981) pointed out that different muscles contain varying proportions of slow and fast muscle fibers. Slow fibers maintain posture; they activate more easily, are capable of more sustained contraction, and tend to become shortened and tight. Fast or phasic fibers give dynamic, voluntary movement; they fatigue more rapidly and tend to weakness. Postural and phasic muscles are often antagonistic. Increased activity or contracture of the more postural muscle may not only mechanically limit the range of movement of its antagonist, but also inhibit that more phasic muscle. This produces an imbalance between the antagonists. Hypertrophy and atrophy occur at the same time in antagonistic muscles, which may lead to changes in resting length with contracture of the postural muscles and stretching of the phasic muscle. To exaggerate this, a sedentary lifestyle leads to overuse of postural muscles, while phasic muscles become weak with disuse. Muscle imbalance

gives typical patterns of postural disturbance. For example, there may be tightness of the erector spinae, iliopsoas and hamstrings, with weakness of abdominal muscles, glutei and anterior tibial muscles. This produces increased lumbar lordosis, and limitation of hip and knee extension. Muscle imbalance causes abnormal loads on joints and other structures, abnormal patterns of movement, muscle fatigue, and loss of coordination.

In patients with chronic low back pain, the paraspinal muscles are atrophied and contain an increased percentage of fat (Cooper et al 1992, Mooney et al 1997). They are weaker, and fatigue more easily. Hides et al (1994) have studied this closely, investigating 26 patients with a first episode of acute or subacute low back pain. They found local wasting in the multifidus muscle, which is the largest and most medial of the erector spinae (Fig. 9.8). Interestingly, the human lordosis is quite unique because of our upright posture, and this involves specific development of the multifidus muscle. The changes were segmental and unilateral, and corresponded to the level and side of symptoms. They found about 30% reduction in cross-sectional area. Because this wasting was so localized and developed so rapidly, they

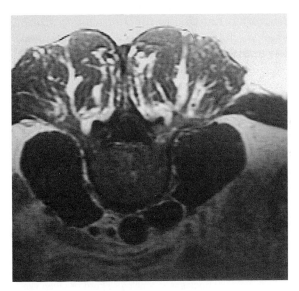

Figure 9.8 Multifidus muscle wasting in a patient with chronic low back pain. (From Dr V Mooney, with thanks.)

suggested that it was due to segmental inhibition rather than to a general effect of disuse. Acute low back pain usually resolves, but recurrent attacks are common. Even when symptoms settle, multifidus wasting may not recover spontaneously, and this may predispose to recurrence. Hides et al (1996) showed that specific, localized exercises for the multifidus may not make much difference to symptomatic recovery from the acute attack, but do produce better muscle recovery. Preliminary results suggest that they may reduce the recurrence rate (Richardson & Jull 1995).

The trunk muscles also play a key role in stabilizing the spine. Hodges & Richardson (1996) found that patients with back pain had delayed contraction of these muscles in anticipation of arm movements compared with normal controls. This may represent a loss of neuromuscular coordination. These changes were most marked and specific in the transversus abdominis.

Soft tissue changes

DiGiovanna & Schiowitz (1991) listed an extensive range of palpable changes in tissue texture, which form an important diagnostic tool. These vary between acute and chronic (Table 9.3). Disturbed autonomic function causes trophic changes in the skin and subcutaneous tissues of the spinal segment (Gunn & Milbrandt 1978). Vasomotor effects cause local change in the temperature of the skin – vasoconstriction usually makes the skin palpably colder. Sudomotor effects cause increased sweating. The pilomotor reflex is often hyperactive to produce visible 'goose bumps'. These changes may affect a dermatome or a local band of skin innervated by the posterior primary ramus. They may be transient, and appear only when the patient undresses to expose the skin to cold, or in response to painful stimuli.

These autonomic changes also lead to subcutaneous skin edema or trophedema. The skin is tight with loss of wrinkles, and the consistency of the subcutaneous tissues is firmer. Gently squeezing an area of skin and subcutaneous tissue produces a *peau d'orange* effect (Fig. 9.9).

Neurophysiology

We have already looked at how neurophysiologic changes may aggravate and perpetuate pain (Ch. 3). These changes directly affect neuromuscular activity and muscle function.

Some clinicians call this increased sensitivity 'neuropathic pain'. Unfortunately, this term may imply that the cause of pain is physical entrapment of a nerve root, which is not necessarily the case. The key concept is simply altered neuromuscular activity, what osteopaths called the 'facilitated segment'. There is hypersensitivity of joints and indeed the entire motion segment to mechanical strain and movement. Normal afferent input from mechano-receptors may become interpreted as pain. Musculoskeletal

Table 9.3 Tissue texture changes in acute and chronic somatic dysfunctions (from DiGiovanni & Schiowitz 1991, with permission)

Characteristic	Acute	Chronic
Temperature	Increased	Slight increase or decrease
Texture	Boggy, more rough	Thin, smooth
Moisture	Increased	Dry
Tension	Increased, rigid, board-like	Slight increase, ropy, stringy
Tenderness	Greatest	Present but less
Edema	Yes	No
Erythema test	Redness lasts	Redness fades quickly or blanching

Bogginess is a palpable sense of sponginess in the tissue, probably due to edema.
Ropiness is a palpable cord or string like feeling.
Stringiness is a palpable tissue texture characterized by fine or string-like myofascial structures.

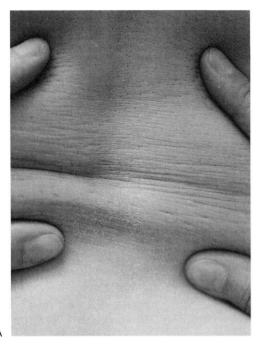 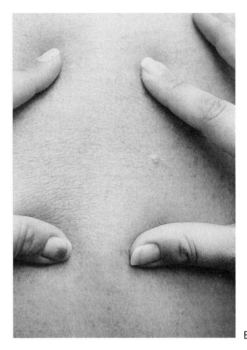

A   B

Figure 9.9 A: Trophedema due to disturbed autonomic function in a patient with acute low back pain. B: Normal. (From Dr C C Gunn, with thanks.)

structures may become tender to gentle pressure, and normal movements may become painful. These inputs may also lead to reflex response in muscle and autonomic activity.

This also leads to reprogramming of neuromuscular control. The CNS 'learns' new patterns of posture, locomotion and activities of daily living. These patterns of motor behavior become fixed and self-perpetuating.

These neurophysiologic changes imply that any of the segmental structures may become more sensitive. Experimental production of pain by stimulating one part of the segment does not identify the 'site' or the anatomic source of the pain, nor does it tell us anything about the original cause of the pain.

Psychophysiology

Psychologic states influence these neurophysiologic changes, and hence psychologic events can influence body physiology. Stress and anxiety lead to general autonomic arousal (Selye 1950). There may be lasting autonomic,

metabolic and endocrine changes, which might cause, exacerbate or maintain chronic pain. Experimentally, we can change physiologic responses to acute pain by conditioning. There is, however, very little evidence of such general arousal in patients with chronic back pain. Local and symptom specific mechanisms seem more likely (Flor & Turk 1989).

It is a common clinical observation that pain is associated with muscle spasm. Pain may produce reflex muscle spasm, and muscle spasm may produce pain, so there could be a pain–spasm–pain cycle. The traditional psychophysiologic model of muscle tension is a stress–spasm–pain cycle. The best known example is tension headache. Stress or anxiety causes increased tension in the temporal muscles which causes headache. Biofeedback works by teaching voluntary control of that muscle tension. It is possible that similar mechanisms could play a part in low back pain, although few workers would suggest they actually cause the pain. However, whatever the original cause of back pain, continued pain could be associated with increased muscle tension. This may initially be a normal physiologic response, but may become a learned, conditioned response.

Flor and her colleagues (Flor et al 1990, Flor & Birbaumer 1994) have reviewed the evidence on muscle tension. Experimental studies show that EMG activity in the erector spinae may be higher in patients with back pain in both standing and sitting. Increased muscle tension during physical or psychologic stress is probably more important than baseline activity. Increased muscle tension is local to patients' symptoms: in patients with back pain, raised muscle tension occurs in the paraspinal muscles but not in other parts of the body. It only occurs with pain or stress relevant to the individual. Muscle hyperactivity may continue after the stimulus stops, and only return slowly to baseline levels. Previous experience may lead to faster development and slower decay of the response. However, there are many limitations to this evidence. Any increase in static EMG activity in chronic low back pain is so small that it is of doubtful clinical significance. The concept of pain–spasm–pain is simple and attractive, but there is little evidence that static muscle tension plays a direct role in low back pain (Roland 1986, Orbach & McCall 1996).

This has led the latter authors to hypothesize about other possible indirect effects of muscle tension. Even slight increases in muscle tension could be enough to reduce resting muscle length. This may start as a mechanism to protect against painful movement. Attempts to move, and so stretch the muscle, could lead to increased muscle proprioception, and muscle contraction to guard against that movement.

The key may be that muscles are not static structures. Muscles *work*, and Watson et al (1998) stress the importance of dynamic testing. They used surface EMG of the paraspinal muscles to demonstrate changes in the flexion–relaxation phenomenon. As we have already noted, in normal people the extensor muscles go through a period of electrical silence during forward flexion from the erect position. In patients with back pain, this period of muscle relaxation is reduced or absent. This is one of the best documented muscle abnormalities in chronic low back pain, although it may develop at a much earlier stage. Main & Watson (1996) suggested that patients with low back pain may develop different patterns of dynamic muscle activity from normal, which may represent persisting physiologic dysfunction. These patterns improve with natural recovery (Haig et al 1993), rehabilitation (Ahern et al 1988) or a pain management program (Main & Watson 1995). This may correspond to clinical descriptions of 'muscle imbalance'; or we may best describe this as *guarded movement*.

The origin of dysfunction

From this point of view, the present state of dysfunction is more important than any original 'cause'. Dysfunction depends on the interaction over time, and imbalance between physical stresses and individual vulnerabilities (Fig. 9.10). This imbalance may be triggered by increased physical stress, such as a minor strain, or increased or unaccustomed use. But there does not have to be any such external cause. Any physiologic, neurophysiologic or psychophysiologic stress may increase vulnerability. Therefore, fatigue, lack of fitness, postural abnormalities, faulty movement patterns and activities may also cause imbalance and hence dysfunction. It may be only a question of degree when the normal bodily sensation of normal function becomes the discomfort or pain of dysfunction. Whatever the initial trigger, both psychologic and physiologic changes then take place, and dysfunction may become selfperpetuating.

If you still have difficulty accepting the concept of pain due to disturbed function

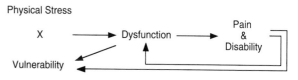

Figure 9.10 The origins of dysfunction. (From Manual Medicine, Osteopathic diagnosis of back pain, MacDonald R S, 3: 110–113, Fig. 2, 1988, with kind permission from Springer-Verlag.)

without any structural damage, try a few simple experiments for yourself:

- *Observation 1*. Lift a weight of a few pounds in your hand and stretch your arm out at shoulder height. Hold it there. After a few minutes it begins to hurt. The weight feels heavier. The pain spreads down the muscles of your shoulder and arm. You may try different ways of coping with the pain, but sooner or later it makes you lower your arm and put down the weight.
- *Observation 2*. Rest your left elbow on a table with your forearm upright. Extend your wrist and your fingers. Use your right hand to hyperextend your left middle finger as far as it will go. Hold it there. After a few minutes your finger becomes painful. Sooner or later the pain makes you release the finger and let it relax to a more normal position.
- *Observation 3*. We have all had muscle cramp. The acute pain persists until we manage to break the reflex arc.
- *Observation 4*. If we attempt prolonged strenuous exercise when we are unfit, our muscles and joints ache. If we measure them, we find the muscles are swollen. The ache may take several days to settle.

These are all examples of pain from normal muscles and joints. You do not need structural damage. It is pain from musculoskeletal dysfunction.

This concept of dysfunction also helps to deal with the vexed question of the duration of back pain. One of the common criticisms of the diagnosis of a soft tissue sprain or strain is that such an injury is normally followed by healing. Symptoms should settle over expected tissue healing time. If, however, the problem is dysfunction then symptoms can persist for as long as dysfunction continues. Dysfunction may be self-sustaining, so symptoms may persist indefinitely, but the other important implication is that dysfunction does not involve any permanent change, so it is always reversible. Even if dysfunction and symptoms may persist indefinitely, there is always still the potential for recovery by restoring normal function.

INTEGRATED FUNCTION

Most of the previous section dealt with segmental dysfunction, even if that might affect more than one level. However, functional anatomy, physical therapy, functional restoration and rehabilitation all stress that the body functions as a whole. The entire spinal column, its muscles and control system form a single, integrated system. The spine, pelvis and legs function together. Indeed, most normal daily activities and work depend on whole body function.

Health and fitness depend on continued use: 'use it or lose it'. Normal musculoskeletal function depends on movement, regular exercise and physical activity. These are essential for the development, maintenance and continuing function of the musculoskeletal system throughout life. They stimulate and maintain bone and muscle mass and strength, they aid nutrition, they help to maintain articular cartilage and joint range, and they improve endurance and coordination. They also stimulate neurophysiologic function and increase pain tolerance.

Prolonged immobilization leads to deterioration of the musculoskeletal, cardiovascular and central nervous systems. The ill effects of prolonged bed rest are a standard part of student teaching (Box 9.5). Bortz (1984) coined the term 'disuse syndrome'.

Most people with simple backache have less extreme degrees of inactivity, but the general principle is the same. Prolonged lack of use, of any degree, leads to loss of functional capacity. 'Use it or lose it' applies just the same. The more severe systemic effects do not seem to occur, although patients with chronic back pain do lose some cardiovascular fitness. The more common and important effect is loss of muscle strength and performance.

Mayer & Gatchel (1988) described this as a 'deconditioning syndrome'. Radiographs and clinical examination only give us a static snapshot of the musculoskeletal system. In the real world, musculoskeletal health shows in physiologic performance. Mayer believes that the deconditioning syndrome plays a major role in chronic low back pain and disability. He points to loss

---

Box 9.5   Effects of prolonged bed rest

- Catabolic, poor tissue nutrition, depressed metabolism
- Progressive loss of bone mineral and bone strength
- Stiffness due to loss of joint and soft tissue mobility, connective tissue contracture, fibrosis and adhesions
- Muscle wasting, 3% loss of muscle strength per day, decrease in time to fatigue, reduced endurance
- Loss of neuromuscular coordination and balance
- Ligaments lose strength
- Poorer healing, increased scar tissue formation
- Systemic effects
  — loss of cardiovascular fitness
  — anemia and thrombosis
  — respiratory and renal stagnation
  — endocrine changes
  — immune system, lowered resistance
- Loss of sensory and mental acuity
- Psychologic distress, depression
- Lower pain tolerance

---

of lumbar motion, trunk strength, cardiovascular fitness and lifting capacity. Patients with chronic back pain show lower muscle strength and performance on any form of dynamic testing. Mayer attributes much of this to disuse, and directs treatment to functional restoration.

AN EXPLANATION FOR PATIENTS

The reason that disc injuries are so popular is that the idea is easy to understand, plausible and acceptable to patients. It is amazing how many people with simple backache believe they have a 'disc out of place' or 'worn discs', with or without 'trapped nerves'. These ideas carry all the implications about permanent damage, fear of reinjury, and the need to rest or get fixed. We desperately need an equally simple, plausible and acceptable explanation that fits modern understanding of the physical basis of back pain. It must also support modern ideas of management. Let me try to use the ideas in this chapter to develop an alternative explanation suitable for patients.

First, back pain is a mechanical problem. It is a movement disorder or an activity-related disorder of the musculoskeletal system.

Second, back pain is only a symptom, not a disease. The most important message is that most back pain is not a signal of any serious disease or damage to the back.

Third, most back pain is simply a symptom of physical dysfunction. Pain and disability are intimately related to each other. The back is not working as it should. It is 'out of condition', like a car engine that is out of tune. This involves all the elements of dysfunction that we have discussed. Posture may be poor. The back is not moving as it should, but may be stiff or 'seized up'. This leads to fear and guarded movements. The muscles are not working as they should, but may be weak and wasted and tire easily. There may be loss of strength and endurance and of coordination. Loss of fitness makes it harder to rehabilitate. Changes in the nervous system lead to increased sensitivity, which together with stress and tension leads to a vicious circle. This whole pattern of painful dysfunction is the core of the problem and becomes self-perpetuating. It is much more important that any original, long gone, trigger for the pain.

Finally, this has obvious implications for management. The original cause or site of the pain really does not matter much any more. Whatever the original trigger, pain will continue as long as there is dysfunction. Recovery and relief of pain depend on getting the back working again and restoring normal function. The answer is to get moving. This leads to a sports medicine analogy, and sports medicine principles of rehabilitation. It also depends very much on the patient taking responsibility for what he or she does, rather than depending on the doctor or therapist.

An explanation for patients

- Back pain is a symptom, not a disease. Most back pain is not due to any serious disease or damage in your back
- Back pain is usually a symptom of *physical dysfunction*. Your back is simply not moving and working as it should. It is unfit or out of condition
- Recovery and relief of pain depend on getting your back moving and working again and restoring normal function

---

CONCLUSION

I am well aware that we have limited scientific evidence for many of these theories, which are based largely on clinical observation. However, I have argued already that we must seek the basic science that helps to explain our clinical findings, rather than trying to force patients to fit our basic science. I find it encouraging that so many health professionals from such different backgrounds have reached so much common ground – and that it fits modern neurophysiology. Dysfunction is a potentially rich but as yet untapped mine of knowledge. We still need much basic science and clinical research to develop and test these ideas. We should look more closely at the soft tissues and their physiology, at physical dysfunction and the effects of disuse. We should integrate clinical, psychophysiologic, biomechanical and functional knowledge. The traditional search for anatomic sites and structural causes of pain is simply inappropriate for nonspecific low back pain, and that is why it has failed. I believe that more physiologic concepts of dysfunction hold much greater promise.

REFERENCES

Adams M A, Dolan P 1995 Recent advances in lumbar spinal mechanics and their clinical significance. Clinical Biomechanics 10: 3–19

Ahern D K, Follick M J, Council J R, Laser-Wolston N, Litchman H 1988 Comparison of lumbar intervertebral EMG patterns in chronic low back pain patients and non-pain controls. Pain 34: 153–160

Bogduk N, Twomey L T 1991 Clinical anatomy of the lumbar spine. Churchill Livingstone, New York

Bortz W M 1984 The disuse syndrome. Western Journal of Medicine 141: 691–694

Buckwalter J A 1995 Spine update: aging and degeneration of the human intervertebral disc. Spine 20: 1307–1314

Burton A K, Tillotson K M, Edwards V A, Sykes D A 1990 Lumbar sagittal mobility and low back symptoms in patients treated with manipulation. Journal of Spinal Disorders 3: 262–268

Burton A K, Tillotson K M, Troup J D G 1989 Variation in lumbar sagittal mobility with low back trouble. Spine 14: 584–590

Cooper R G, Forbes W S T C, Jayson M I V 1992 Radiographic demonstration of paraspinal muscle wasting in patients with chronic low back pain. British Journal of Rheumatology 31: 389–394

DiGiovanna E L, Schiowitz S (eds) 1991 An osteopathic approach to diagnosis and treatment. Lippincott, Philadelphia

Droz-Georget J H 1980 High velocity thrust and pathophysiology of segmental dysfunction. British Osteopathic Journal 12: 2–17

Esola M A, McClure P W, Fitzgerald G K, Siegler S 1996 Analysis of lumbar spine and hip motion during forward bending in subjects with and without a history of low back pain. Spine 21: 71–78

Fiddler M 1980 Back pain without direct nerve root involvement. Unpublished report to ISSLS

Flor H, Birbaumer N 1994 Acquisition of chronic pain: psychophysiological mechanisms. American Pain Society Journal 3: 119–127

Flor H, Birbaumer N, Turk D C 1990 The psychobiology of chronic pain. Advances in Behavioural Research and Therapy 12: 47–84

Flor H, Turk D C 1989 Psychophysiology of chronic pain: do chronic pain patients exhibit symptom-specific psychophysiological responses? Psychological Bulletin 105: 215–259

Grieve G P 1981 Common vertebral joint problems. Churchill Livingstone, Edinburgh, p 112–121

Gunn C C, Milbrandt W E 1976 Tenderness at motor points. A diagnostic and prognostic aid for low back injury. Journal of Bone and Joint Surgery 58A: 815–825

Gunn C C, Milbrandt W E 1978 Early and subtle signs in low back sprain. Spine 3: 267–281

Haig A J, Weisman G, Haugh L D, Pope M, Grobler L 1993 Prospective evidence for change in paraspinal muscle activity after herniated nucleus pulposis. Spine 18: 926–930

Hides J A, Stokes M J, Saide M, Jull G A, Cooper D H 1994 Evidence of lumbar multifidus muscle wasting ipsilateral to symptoms in patients with acute/subacute low back pain. Spine 19: 165–172

Hides J A, Richardson C A, Jull G A 1996 Multifidus muscle recovery is not automatic after resolution of acute, first episode low back pain. Spine 21: 2763–2769

Hodges P W, Richardson C A 1996 Inefficient muscular stabilization of the lumbar spine associated with low back pain. A motor control evaluation of transversus abdominis. Spine 21: 2640–2650

Jackson R P, Jacobs R R, Montesano P X 1988 Facet joint injection in low-back pain. A prospective statistical study. Spine 13: 966–971

Kellgren J H 1938 Observations on referred pain arising from muscle. Clinical Science 3: 175–190

Kellgren J H 1939 On the distribution of pain arising from deep somatic structures with charts of segmental pain areas. Clinical Science 4: 35–46

Lilius G, Lassonen E M, Myllynen P, Harilainen A, Gronlund G 1989 Lumbar facet joint syndrome. A randomised clinical trial. Journal of Bone and Joint Surgery 71B: 681–684

MacDonald R S 1988a Primary dysfunction of the spine. Holistic Medicine 3: 27–33

MacDonald R S 1988b Osteopathic diagnosis of back pain. Manual Medicine 3: 110–113

Main C J, Watson P J 1995 Screening for patients at risk of developing chronic incapacity. Journal of Occupational Rehabilitation 5: 207–217

Main C J, Watson P J 1996 Guarded movements: development of chronicity. Journal of Musculoskeletal Pain 4: 163–170

Marras W S, Lavender S A, Leurgans S E et al 1993 The role of dynamic three-dimensional trunk motion in occupationally related low back disorders. Spine 18: 617–628

Mayer T G, Gatchel R J 1988 Functional restoration for spinal disorders: the sports medicine approach. Lea & Febiger, Philadelphia

Merskey H, Bogduk N (eds) 1994 Classification of chronic pain. Descriptions of chronic pain syndromes and definition of pain terms, 2nd edn. International Association of the Study of Pain (IASP) Press, Seattle

Mooney V, Gulick J, Perlman M et al 1997 Relationships between myoelectric activity, strength, and MRI of extensor muscles in back pain patients and normal subjects. Journal of Spinal Disorders 10: 348–356

Nachemson A 1975 Towards a better understanding of low back pain: a review of the mechanics of the lumbar disc. Rheumatology and Rehabilitation 14: 129–143

Nachemson A, Morris J M 1964 In vivo measurement of intradiscal pressure. Journal of Bone and Joint Surgery 46A: 1077–1092

Orbach R, McCall W D 1996 The stress-hyperactivity-pain theory of myogenic pain: proposal for a revised theory. Pain Forum 5: 51–66

Panjabi M M 1992 The stabilizing system of the spine. Part I. Function, dysfunction, adaptation and enhancement. Journal of Spinal Disorders 5: 383–389

Paquet N, Malouin F, Fichards C L 1994 Hip-spine movement and muscle activity patterns during sagittal trunk movements in low back pain patients. Spine 19: 596–603

Pope M H, Wilder D G, Krag M H 1991 Biomechanics of the lumbar spine: A. basic principles. In: Frymoyer J W (ed) The adult spine: principles and practice. Raven Press, New York, p 1487–1501

Richardson C A, Jull G A 1995 Muscle control – pain control. What exercises would you prescribe? Manual Therapy 1: 2–10

Roland M O 1986 A critical review of the evidence for a pain-spasm-pain cycle in spinal disorders. Clinical Biomechanics 1: 102–109

Selye H 1950 The physiology and pathology of exposure to stress. Acta Inc., Montreal

Steffen T, Rubin R K, Baramki H G, Antoniou J, Marchesi D, Aebi M 1997 A new technique of measuring lumbar segmental motion in vivo. Spine 22: 156–166

Strender L-E, Sjoblom A, Sundell K, Ludwig R, Taube A 1997 Inter-examiner reliability in physical examination of patients with low back pain. Spine 22: 814–820

van Tulder M W, Assendelft W J J, Koes B W, Bouter L M 1997 Spinal radiographic findings and non-specific low back pain. Spine 22: 427–434

Vleeming A, Mooney V, Dorman T, Snijders C, Stoeckart R (eds) 1997. Movement stability and low back pain: the essential role of the pelvis. Churchill Livingstone, New York

Watson P J, Booker C K, Main C J 1998 Evidence for the role of psychological factors in abnormal paraspinal activity in patients with chronic low back pain. Journal of Musculoskeletal Pain 37: 82–86

Wiltse L 1971 The effect of common anomalies of the lumbar spine upon disc degeneration and low back pain. Orthopedic Clinics of North America 2: 569–582

10

Illness behavior

Gordon Waddell   Chris J. Main

We looked briefly at pain behavior in Chapter 3 on pain and disability. We also found that we had to allow for the way in which patients behave in our assessment of physical impairment. Illness behavior is a key part of our story and it is now time to look at it more closely.

Illness behavior is what people say and do to express and communicate that they are ill. It depends very much on what and how they think about their symptoms and their illnesses.

We know that someone is ill, not by seeing disease or even by examining him or her, but by what he or she says and does. Consciously or unconsciously, we recognize that the way this person behaves is not well but ill.

If we drive past a traffic accident, we might see someone lying on the road in front of a car. From a distance we cannot see his broken leg. What draws our attention is the victim lying in the middle of the road. He is very still. A crowd of strangers stand around looking worried and trying to help. With little thought we interpret the scene as a road accident and an injured person waiting for help. We do not need to stop and ask what happened or look at his broken leg. We can tell by how he behaves – and how those about him behave.

You might think that his behavior is simply the physical effect of his broken leg, but that is not the whole story. Suppose he only had a sprained ankle. If you knew this, you might wonder why he was lying in the middle of the road waiting for an ambulance. However, he was knocked down and must have had a terrible fright. His ankle may feel broken and he might be afraid even to try to get up. People in the crowd may have told him that they had sent for the ambulance and that he should just lie there and wait. So his illness behavior may be out of proportion to his physical injury, but it is still easy to understand.

Now consider how two different patients cope with a sprained ankle. Let us suppose that each has a severe sprain with marked swelling and a lot of pain but no actual ligament instability. One patient will be completely unable to bear weight and will need crutches for a week or so, the other will laugh or be insulted at the very suggestion of crutches and will insist on having the ankle strapped up so that he can try to play an important game of football the next day. They both have a very similar physical injury but what they do about it is very different.

Now let us move on a year. Suppose we now find that the man with the sprained ankle is still using a cane and unable to work? His ligaments healed long ago, but his ankle is stiff and he has muscle wasting from lack of use. He is also very unfit. He may even have some disuse osteoporosis. It is not surprising that his ankle is still painful, but there is no clinical or radiologic evidence of any serious damage. Yet he still spends most of the day sitting or lying about the house. He keeps his ankle warm and supports it on a cushion. He does not go out of the house much, but when he does he uses his cane and makes no attempt to walk normally. His social life has suffered and his friends rarely visit him to talk about his injured ankle which is one of his main topics of conversation. He has really not considered going back to work. Indeed, when asked about it, he seems to be astonished by the question. He feels that it is obvious that he cannot even begin to think about work until his ankle fully recovers – though he cannot imagine how or when that magical event will ever occur. This whole pattern of illness behavior may have been reasonable for the first few days after the injury, but a year later it is now something more than just the physical effects of his original

minor injury or the current physical state of his ankle. His pattern of illness behavior and life-style of invalidity are now, in themselves, a major part of his disability.

This may seem an extreme and even ridiculous example. You might say that noone becomes permanently crippled by a sprained ankle. Now substitute 'back' for ankle, and 'strain' for sprain. Read that story again. You now have a clinical history that is all too common.

Examples of illness behavior in back pain

When we meet a friend who has back pain, we know if her back is troubling her again. We can tell by her awkward posture and guarded movements. She fidgets and grimaces and rubs her back. We get the message across the room before we exchange a word and without looking at her back. Not only do we know what is wrong, but the way she behaves gives us some idea of how bad her back is. This is normal. Most illness behavior simply reflects the physical problem. We must stress that *illness behavior is reasonable and normal.*

The fascination of back pain is how different patients react and behave so very differently. Several years ago, purely by chance, we had two patients with back pain in the same ward, shown in Fig. 10.1. The man standing up had undergone a small surgical biopsy of a thoracic vertebra earlier that day. The final histology showed a low-grade infection, but at that time we thought it was probably cancer. He had a serious disease in his spine, was in a lot of pain, and thought that it was something that would probably kill him. The healthy young man sitting down had a recurrent attack of nonspecific back pain. It was so severe that he had a morphine injection from his family doctor and was hospitalized in the middle of the night. On admission he was so agitated that we could hardly examine him. Within a few hours he settled and we could control his pain with nonsteroidal anti-inflammatory drugs (NSAID)s. There is no question that his back was in pain and that he had a lot of muscle

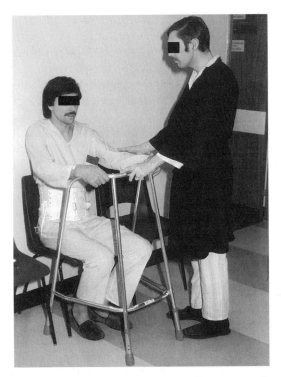

Figure 10.1 Different illness behaviors. The man standing up has just had a surgical biopsy of a spinal infection. The man sitting down was hospitalized as an emergency with simple backache.

spasm, but there was no evidence of any serious spinal disease or nerve root problem. Further tests were all normal. Over the next few days, the man with the spinal infection helped and encouraged the man with simple backache on to his feet. He used a walking frame and wore his lumbar support outside his clothes so that everyone could see how bad he was. A few days later, he was able to walk without any aids and went home, while the man with spinal infection waited for the result of his biopsy to learn whether he would live or die.

This does not mean it is a choice between either physical pathology or a psychologic problem. Both these men had a physical problem in their back. Our failure to make a precise diagnosis of back pain does not mean that the problem is psychologic. Nor does physical disease preclude a psychologic disturbance, any more than psychologic disturbance excludes a treatable physical disease.

Look at two other much rarer but instructive examples. The first was a 58-year-old lady with many years' history of chronic back pain, invalidity and depression. She had frequent medical and psychiatric hospitalization with multiple complaints. On this occasion she came in with an overdose of sleeping tablets and depression. Once again, she blamed this on her pain, but it was clear that her long-standing problems were mainly psychiatric rather than physical. When we listened carefully to her story, however, her recent attack of thoracic back pain was different from her usual chronic low back pain. Further investigation showed that she now had widespread breast metastases.

The second example was a 34-year-old man with a long history of psoriatic arthropathy (Fig. 10.2). He had been on systemic steroids for many years. He had severe arthritis of his hips, steroid-induced osteoporosis and vertebral collapse. He had a severe spinal deformity and a great deal of back pain. He also had considerable psychologic problems and depression. He was a very difficult patient who was very angry and uncooperative with treatment. He showed a great deal of illness behavior. He was almost completely house-bound. He was very demanding with his family and much of his family's life revolved around his illness.

- Illness behavior is normal
- Most patients have both a physical problem in their backs *and* varying degrees of illness behavior

CLINICAL OBSERVATION OF ILLNESS BEHAVIOR

We were all taught as students to use the clinical history and examination to diagnose disease, but we should also use them to learn about our patients. The great clinicians of the past established their reputations from their skill in differential diagnosis, but they also had an almost uncanny ability to assess patients. Much of their skill was subconscious and they could not explain or teach it. It seemed to come from natural aptitude and long experience. Nevertheless, we all should be able to dissect, teach, and learn this vital clinical skill. We would

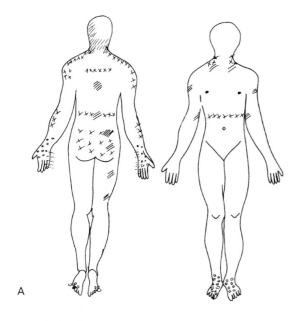

A

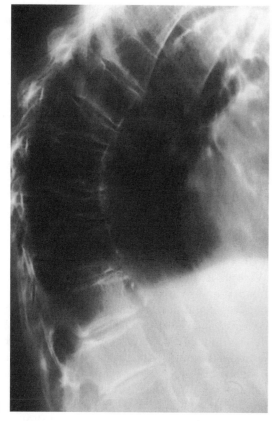

B

Figure 10.2 A man of 34 with marked distress and illness behavior (A) who also had severe steroid-induced osteoporosis (B).

suggest that these great clinicians were actually observing illness behavior – they just did not realize what they were doing. Modern professional training is all about the symptoms and signs of disease and we pay little attention to assessing the person. We leave that to 'clinical impression' and assume that we will learn somehow by osmosis and experience. Unfortunately, these impressions are unreliable, and we should instead learn how to assess illness behavior. There are a number of ways of doing this, which form an interrelated and homogeneous group of observations and which tell us a great deal about a patient's illness behavior.

The pain drawing

The pain drawing is the simplest example of illness behavior (Ransford et al 1976). Patients are quite willing to record their pain on an outline of the body. They regard it as a simple question about the physical pattern of their pain. However, the *way* in which they describe their pain also gives us information about how they are reacting and about how the pain is affecting them.

Figure 10.3 shows two pain drawings. Patient A is giving an anatomic description of her S1 pain and paresthesia due to a disc prolapse. Patient B is not paraplegic. He also has a disc prolapse, but he is trying to tell us how severe his pain is and how much he is suffering. This is a cry for help. The pain drawing describes the pain, but the way in which patients draw their pain can also tell us a lot about their psychologic state. The simplest signal is the sheer quantity of drawing – how large an area and how densely they fill it in (Ohlund et al 1996). Pain may be widespread or non-anatomic. It may expand to other areas of the body. It may even spread outside the body outline. Patients may put excessive detail into the drawing. They may add emphasis or comments on the severity of their pain. All these features reflect the patient's psychologic state. Thus, the simple pain drawing gives us both physical information about the pain and psychologic information about the patient. Once again, these are not alternatives. It is not a question of

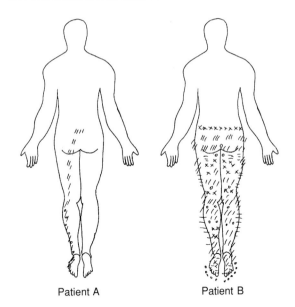

Patient A   Patient B

Figure 10.3 The pain drawing tells us about the physical and emotional characteristics of the pain. Patient A describes the anatomic pattern of S1 pain and paresthesia from a disc prolapse. Patient B is not paraplegic but also has a disc prolapse. This pain drawing is communicating distress. Many patients do both to varying degrees. (//, pain; 0, pins and needles; ×, ache; =, numbness.)

whether this is a physical drawing or a psychologic drawing. Remember that patients A and B both had a disc prolapse. Most pain drawings include both physical and psychologic information, although one aspect may dominate the picture. And sometimes, like here, illness behavior may obscure the underlying physical problem.

We may look at the McGill Pain Questionnaire (Fig. 3.5) in the same way. The physical drawing of pain is like the sensory adjectives: shooting, throbbing and burning. The drawing also shows the emotional characteristics of the pain experience, rather like the emotional adjectives: exhausting, terrifying or miserable. In both the questionnaire and the drawing, most patients describe their pain in some mixture of sensory and emotional ways.

We must not over-interpret the pain drawing. It is crude and cannot give a complete psychologic profile or diagnosis, and for this reason we have not described detailed ways to score the drawing. All that is important is to recognize that the patient's description of pain includes both sensory and emotional elements.

The pain drawing may be the first clue that you should assess this patient in more depth.

However, you cannot rely on the pain drawing alone. Most patients with an exaggerated pain drawing are distressed, but 50% of patients with distress will give a normal pain drawing (Parker et al 1995).

Behavioral symptoms

Clinical diagnosis depends on recognizing common patterns of symptoms and signs. Most patients with back pain describe their symptoms in a way that fits anatomy and mechanics. The symptoms often do not fit exactly, but they do make some kind of physical sense. However, patients occasionally describe their symptoms in a way that does not fit most clinical experience. These symptoms are vague and ill-localized. They lack the normal relationship with time and activity. Indeed, they seem to cross anatomic boundaries and contradict normal mechanics.

We tried to find those symptoms that seem to have more to do with illness behavior than physical disease (Waddell et al 1984). We found more than 30 possible symptoms from a literature review and pilot studies in our own Problem Back Clinic. We carried out a survey of 20 spinal surgeons who told us which symptoms they would regard as physically inappropriate. In the end, this told us more about the surgeons than about their patients, but it did give us ideas to explore. We tested these symptoms carefully. We did reliability studies. We looked at the symptoms in 180 patients with back pain and compared these with normal pain-free people. We had to discard many of the symptoms because they were unsatisfactory. Some were too rare for routine use, such as fainting with pain and written lists of symptoms. Some were common in normal people, such as their leg jumping. Some were not reproducible between different doctors, such as flattery or manipulative behavior. We then looked to see which symptoms correlated with psychologic factors. Our final result was a group of seven nonanatomic or behavioral descriptions of symptoms:

1. *Pain at the tip of the tailbone* (Fig. 10.4). Coccydynia can occur after direct injury. In a patient with nonspecific back pain it generally occurs together with other behavioral symptoms.

2. *Whole leg pain* (Fig. 10.5). The whole leg becomes painful in a stocking distribution. It usually affects a body image segment from the groin down or below the knee. You should distinguish this from the usual pattern of nerve root pain which at least approximates to a dermatome and does not affect the entire circumference of the leg. Whole leg pain is also quite different from the sclerotomal pattern of referred leg pain. Beware of multiple nerve root involvement, particularly in patients who have had spinal surgery.

3. *Whole leg numbness* (Fig. 10.6). This again affects the whole leg in a stocking distribution. It usually only occurs at times. Some patients describe this as the whole leg going dead.

4. *Whole leg giving way* (Fig. 10.7). The whole leg gives way or collapses, although few patients actually fall to the ground. Again, the key feature is that the whole leg gives way, although at other times it works quite normally. Like whole leg numbness, it is intermittent. It is quite different from local muscle weakness, such as going over on the ankle due to L5 weakness.

5. *Complete absence of any spells with very little pain in the past year*. Some patients insist that they have never been free of pain for a minute, for years on end. They often report that their pain is getting steadily worse on each consultation.

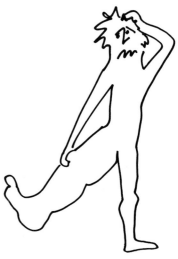

Figure 10.5 Whole leg pain. (Drawing by Mr J C Semple, with thanks.)

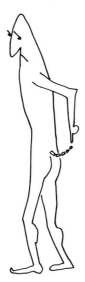

Figure 10.4 Pain at the tip of the tailbone. (Drawing by Mr J C Semple, with thanks.)

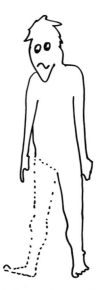

Figure 10.6 Whole leg numbness. (Drawing by Mr J C Semple, with thanks.)

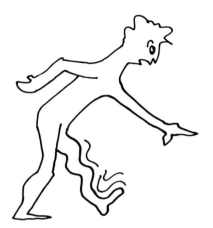

Figure 10.7 Whole leg giving way. (Drawing by Mr J C Semple, with thanks.)

6. *Intolerance of, or reactions to, many treatments.* Most of our treatments for back pain are quite ineffective, so we should never blame the patient if they do not help. Side-effects are also quite common although most are minor. A few patients, however, say that almost every treatment caused side-effects or complications or that they could not tolerate it for one reason or another: every tablet caused either dyspepsia or an allergy; the corset could not be worn because it made their asthma worse; and the therapist made the pain unbearable! This kind of patient is telling you more about their reaction to treatment than about their physical problem.

7. *Emergency admission to hospital with simple backache.* This does not refer to a road accident or a spinal fracture, but to emergency hospitalization because of the severity of simple backache. This may be inappropriate behavior on the part of those who sent the patient to the hospital, or those who admitted him, but it is a measure of what the patient is doing about the problem as well as of the pressure on those around him to do something. It is interesting to note that there are striking variations in the number of such admissions in different areas depending on admission attitudes.

You can also record these symptoms using a questionnaire:

- Specific questions
  — do you get pain at the tip of your tailbone?
  — does your *whole* leg ever become painful?
  — does your *whole* leg ever go numb?
  — does your *whole* leg ever give way?
  — in the past year have you had *any* spells with very little pain? (Score No = positive)

- Data gathered in routine history
  — intolerance of or reactions to treatments (plural)
  — emergency admission(s) to hospital with simple backache.

This group of behavioral symptoms is clearly separate from the common mechanical symptoms of back pain. We first developed these behavioral symptoms and signs in our Problem Back Clinic, where our aim was to clarify assessment of nerve root problems and decisions about surgery. This is still the simplest and clearest example. But the same principles apply to mechanical low back pain and referred leg pain (Table 10.1).

We can assess these behavioral symptoms simply and reliably as part of our routine clinical history. Patients offer these descriptions in response to the standard clinical questions. It is simply a matter of recognizing these patterns and realizing that they provide information about illness behavior.

Nonorganic or behavioral signs

In the same way, we have standardized a group of nonorganic signs or, more precisely, behavioral responses to examination (Waddell et al 1980).

We often assume that physical signs on clinical examination are objective. They *are* objective in the sense that they are assessed by an independent observer, but this does not necessarily mean that they are purely physical and independent of the patient. Some physical findings, like structural deformities, may remain the same even under general anesthesia. But with many 'signs' in the back, we deliberately

Table 10.1 The spectrum of clinical symptoms and signs

	Physical disease	Illness behavior
Pain		
Pain drawing	Localized Anatomic	Nonanatomic Regional Magnified
Pain adjectives	Sensory	Emotional
Symptoms		
Pain	Musculoskeletal or neurologic distribution	Whole leg pain Pain at the tip of the tailbone
Numbness	Dermatomal	Whole leg numbness
Weakness	Myotomal	Whole leg giving way
Time pattern	Varies with time and activity	Never free of pain
Response to treatment	Variable benefit	Intolerance of treatments Emergency hospitalization
Signs		
Tenderness	Musculoskeletal distribution	Superficial Nonanatomic
Axial loading	Neck pain	Low back pain
Simulated rotation	Nerve root pain	Low back pain
Straight leg raising	Limited on formal examination No improvement on distraction	Marked improvement with distraction
Motor	Myotomal	Regional, jerky, giving way
Sensory	Dermatomal	Regional

try to produce pain and see how the patient responds. In the assessment of impairment, we found that tenderness, lumbar movement and straight leg raising all depend to some extent on how the patient reacts. However, there are other signs that appear to depend much more on the patient's behavior during examination than on his or her physical disorder. These are the behavioral signs.

Once again we carried out a literature search and pilot studies to find nearly 30 possible signs. We tested them in the same way, and had to discard many of the signs because they were unreliable or prone to observer bias. Observer bias is a particular problem with these signs. Too many examiners fall into the trap of trying to make judgements rather than dispassionate

clinical observations. Our studies produced a final group of seven behavioral signs:

- tenderness
  - superficial
  - nonanatomic
- simulation
  - axial loading
  - simulated rotation
- distraction
  - straight leg raising
- regional
  - weakness
  - sensory disturbance

You can add or substitute many other signs but that makes little difference. This is a simple but comprehensive group of tests suitable for routine clinical use. It is easy to learn and quick to perform, and you can include it unobtrusively in your routine clinical examination. The tests work equally well in North America and in Britain.

Tenderness. You often cannot localize physical tenderness exactly but in most clinical practice you can usually find some kind of musculoskeletal pattern. Nonorganic tenderness is widespread, spreading far beyond any musculoskeletal anatomy. It may be superficial or nonanatomic (Fig. 10.8).

Superficial tenderness. The lumbar skin is tender to light pinch over a wide area. Nerve irritation can cause a local band of tenderness in the distribution of the posterior primary ramus which is physical.

Nonanatomic tenderness. This is deep tenderness over a wide area that crosses musculoskeletal boundaries. It may extend from the occiput to the coccyx and round to the midaxillary line on both sides.

Simulation tests. These give the impression that you are performing a test when you are not. It is usually simulation of a movement that causes pain. When you carry out a certain movement on formal examination, the patient reports pain. You then simulate the movement but it is not really taking place. If the patient still reports pain on the simulated test, this is due to expectation of pain rather than actual movement. The wording is important and you must minimize suggestion. You should ask, 'What do you feel when I do that?' and not 'Is that painful?'

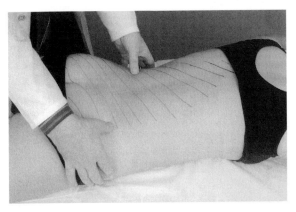

Figure 10.8 Superficial and nonanatomic tenderness.

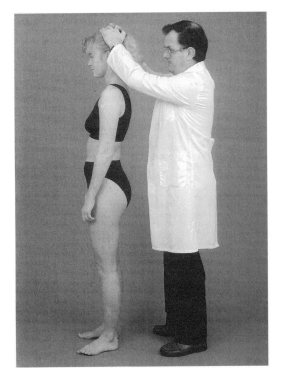

Figure 10.9 Axial loading.

Axial loading. Apply a few pounds of pressure to the top of the patient's skull with your hands (Fig. 10.9). This often produces neck pain that is physical, but to test the lower back you can then repeat the test on the shoulders. Low back pain on axial loading is surprisingly rare even in the presence of serious spinal pathology. If axial loading produces low back pain in a patient with simple backache or sciatica, it is behavioral.

Simulated rotation. Spinal rotation does often cause back pain. Now get the patient to stand relaxed with their hands at their sides. Hold the patient's hands against his or her pelvis and passively rotate his or her trunk. Move the shoulders and pelvis together so that they stay in the same plane (Fig. 10.10). There is no rotation taking place in the spine and any low back pain is behavioral. If the patient has nerve irritation, this test can produce nerve root pain, which is physical.

Distraction tests. Demonstrate a finding in the routine manner and then check the finding while the patient's attention is distracted.

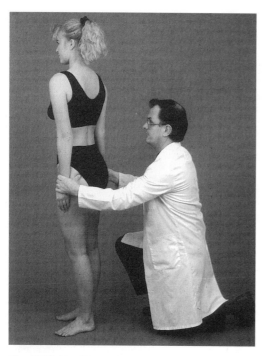

Figure 10.10 Simulated rotation.

Distraction must be nonpainful, nonemotional and non-surprising. In its simplest and most effective form, simply observe the patient all the time that they are in your presence, while they are not aware of being examined. This includes dressing and undressing, getting off the couch at the end of examination, and walking out of the office or clinic. When you are examining any one part, you should also observe what the patient is doing with the rest of his or her body. Any finding that is present at all times, during formal examination and when distracted, is likely to be physical. Findings that are present only on formal examination, but which disappear at other times, have a large behavioral element.

Straight leg raising. Straight leg raising (SLR) is the most useful distraction test (Fig. 10.11). SLR is part of the standard clinical examination, but if SLR is limited on formal examination you should always check it later while the patient is distracted. There are several ways to do this test. You may simply ask the patient to sit up on the couch, or you may sit the patient on the side of the couch with their legs hang-

ing over the edge. Test the knee and ankle reflexes and then lift their leg to examine the knee or test the plantar reflex. This is the 'flip test'. Let us sound a note of caution. There is 10–20° difference in SLR in the lying or sitting position due to a change in lordosis and the position of the pelvis, so only count this test positive if there is at least a 40° change between formal SLR and SLR on distraction. If SLR becomes normal when the patient is distracted then the apparent restriction on formal examination was not due to any physical limitation or nerve irritation. Distraction SLR is then positive and the original restriction was behavioral. This is also important to the physical examination and diagnostic triage. Distraction SLR may invalidate what you first thought was a sign of nerve irritation.

This is a suitable point to stress that improvement in SLR with distraction does not necessarily mean that the patient is faking or trying to deceive you. Many patients know the SLR

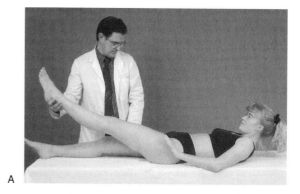

A

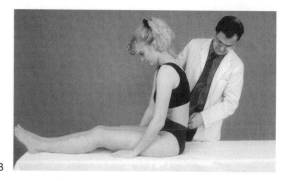

B

Figure 10.11 Straight leg raising apparently limited on formal examination (A), and improving with distraction (B).

test and have learned from past experience that it is painful. They anticipate pain and try to protect themselves by tensing and resisting SLR. They are in pain and your examination may already have made the pain worse. Remember that you are simply observing their pattern of response and behavior and must not over-interpret its cause.

Regional changes. Regional changes involve a widespread area. They often fit a body image or body segments such as the whole leg or from the knee down.

Regional weakness. Neurologic weakness approximates to a myotome. You may overcome a weak muscle with hand pressure, but resistance is steady and even. Nonorganic weakness is much more widespread. It involves many muscle groups that do not fit any neurology. Quite unlike physical weakness, nonorganic weakness is jerky 'giving way'. One minute there is more or less normal power but then there is sudden collapse of muscle resistance. If you test hip extension by lifting the patient's leg and telling him or her to keep it down on the couch, you may find almost no resistance. Instead, you may find that the patient is actually lifting the leg himself! Despite apparent severe weakness of many leg muscles on formal testing, the patient is then able to walk. However, test for regional weakness with caution. Patients may give way simply because of pain, and this often inhibits hip flexion or extension. If a patient has nerve irritation, you should ask him or her to flex their hips and knees to relieve the tension on the nerve before you test ankle and toe strength.

Regional sensory change. The best way to test for regional sensory change is with light touch. Classic hysterical anesthesia is now rare. There is usually only slight alteration in sensation so you can detect it best by comparison with the other leg. The key finding is the 'stocking' rather than dermatomal pattern (Fig. 10.12). Giving way and sensory changes often affect the same area. In patients with spinal surgery or spinal stenosis, you must take care not to mistake multiple nerve root damage for a regional disturbance.

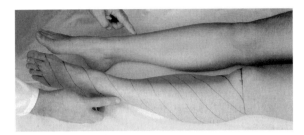

Figure 10.12   Regional sensory change.

It is important to look at the whole group of symptoms and signs, and at the whole pattern of behavior. In all our studies we found that most patients had either 0–1 behavioral signs or showed a constellation of three or more. Multiple behavioral symptoms and signs are reliable and consistent over time and correlate with other features of illness behavior. Isolated symptoms and signs are quite common in normal people with straightforward physical pathology and no other evidence of illness behavior. All clinical diagnosis depends on patterns of illness rather than isolated findings. You would not diagnose a disc prolapse from an isolated depressed ankle reflex without any other clinical features. In the same way you cannot assess illness behavior from one or two symptoms or signs. You must not over-interpret isolated behavioral symptoms or signs.

There are three situations where you cannot use the behavioral signs. You should ignore even multiple signs in these patients:

- Patients with possible serious spinal pathology or widespread neurology. You must carry out diagnostic triage and exclude these first. These behavioral symptoms and signs are only 'inappropriate' to mechanical low back pain and sciatica.
- Patients over about 60 years of age. These responses are common in elderly patients, who behave differently when they are ill. We do not know how to interpret these findings in elderly patients and it is better to ignore them.
- Patients from ethnic minorities. There are wide cultural variations in pain behavior. We have only standardized the behavioral symptoms and signs in white patients. If you

want to use these tests in other groups you need to standardize them for your patients. This merits further research.

Overt pain behavior

Our original description of the behavioral signs included over-reaction to examination. All experienced doctors and therapists recognize this. We see it in our physical examination or in minor procedures such as venepuncture. We are all aware of how patients react, but it is a very subjective judgement. It is unreliable and prone to considerable observer bias.

Keefe & Block (1982) have developed a much better way of looking at this. They looked at the expressions and body actions made by patients that communicate they are in pain. They called this 'overt pain behavior' (Box 10.1). They showed that these signs are reliable and free from observer bias. They found the same pain behaviors in other conditions such as cancer and rheumatoid arthritis. We have shown that doctors and therapists can assess overt pain behavior during a routine examination (Waddell & Richardson 1992). These findings are common during the examination of patients with back pain. They are much less common but even more significant if patients exhibit them spontaneously during interview. They do require careful training and standardized methods of observation. Of all the clinical tests that we use, these are the hardest to perform properly.

Box 10.1 Overt pain behavior (from Keefe & Block 1982, with permission)

- Guarding – abnormally stiff, interrupted or rigid movement while moving from one position to another
- Bracing – a stationary position in which a fully extended limb supports and maintains an abnormal distribution of weight
- Rubbing – any contact between hand and back, i.e. touching, rubbing or holding the painful area
- Grimacing – obvious facial expression of pain that may include furrowed brow, narrowed eyes, tightened lips, corners of mouth pulled back and clenched teeth
- Sighing – obvious exaggerated exhalation of air usually accompanied by the shoulders first rising and then falling. They may expand their cheeks first

---

History of illness behavior in daily life

These methods of assessing pain, behavioral symptoms and signs, and overt pain behavior are all measures of illness presentation in the context of a clinical history and examination. They provide useful information, but may be peculiar to the health care situation and may be colored by patient–professional communication. We now also have several powerful measures of illness behavior in daily life. These are all illness behaviors in *chronic* back pain and sciatica. They are of much less significance for a few days in an acute attack. They are obviously not a matter of illness behavior in patients with serious spinal pathology or widespread neurology.

Use of walking aids. This includes use of one or two canes, crutches or even a wheelchair because of chronic back pain (Fig. 10.13). These patients do not have any gross structural instability or major neurology. There is no physical reason why they are unable to walk. Indeed, when you examine them, they do usually walk more or less normally for a short distance. This is a behavioral response to pain.

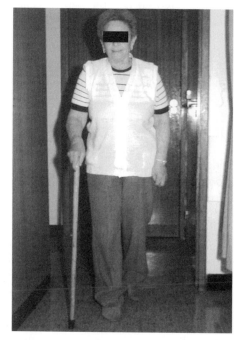

Figure 10.13 Illness behavior in daily life. Use of walking aids for chronic back pain.

Down-time: the amount of time spent lying down most days because of chronic pain (Fig. 10.14). You may take this as the average number of hours lying down between 7 a.m. and 11 p.m.

Help with personal care: frequent and wide-ranging help from a partner or family with bodily care, e.g. washing hair, dressing and putting on footwear. More extreme examples include helping to turn over in bed during the night. Again, there is no physical reason why these patients cannot do these personal tasks, although they may have to modify the way they do them. This is a behavioral response to pain.

Observations of illness behavior

- Pain drawing
- Pain adjectives and description
- Nonanatomic or behavioral descriptions of symptoms
- Nonorganic or behavioral signs
- Overt pain behavior
- Use of walking aids
- Down-time
- Help with personal care

UAB pain behavior scale

Richards et al (1982) developed the University of Alabama pain behavior scale independently (Box 10.2). It includes various aspects of illness behavior. They designed it for in-patients in a chronic pain clinic, but it is a simple method

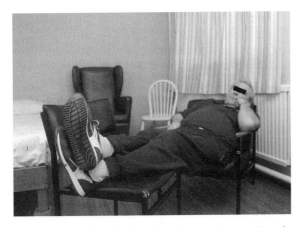

Figure 10.14 Chronic down-time: the average number of hours lying down between 7 a.m. and 11 p.m.

Box 10.2 UAB pain behavior scale. (From Richards et al 1982, with permission)

- Vocal complaints: verbal
- Vocal complaints: nonverbal (moans, groans, gasps, etc.)
- Down-time because of pain (none; 0–60 min; > 60 min/day)
- Facial grimaces
- Standing posture (normal; mildly impaired; distorted)
- Mobility: walking (normal; mild limp or impairment; marked limp or labored walking)
- Body language (clutching. rubbing site of pain)
- Use of visible physical supports (corset, stick, crutches, lean on furniture, TENS – none; occasional; dependent, constant use)
- Stationary movement (sit or stand still; occasional shift of position; constant movement or shifts of position)
- Medication (none; non-narcotic as prescribed; demands for increased dose or frequency, narcotics, analgesic abuse)

Score each item as follows: none, 0; occasional, 0.5; frequent, 1. This gives a total score of 0–10.

---

suitable for routine clinical use. Nurses or other staff can administer it in 5 minutes, and it gives reliable results and is sensitive enough to measure progress. Ohlund et al (1994) found that the UAB scale and some of our clinical methods of assessing illness behavior gave similar results.

Important caveats

These methods of observing illness behavior are powerful tools, but like most powerful tools they can be dangerous if you misuse them. You must use them with care and compassion, and must not over-interpret or misinterpret your clinical observations. This is equally true in both clinical practice and medicolegal assessment:

- Always carry out diagnostic triage first. Exclude serious spinal pathology or a widespread neurologic disorder before even thinking about illness behavior.
- Clinical observation of illness behavior depends on careful technique. It is important to avoid observer bias.
- Isolated behavioral symptoms and signs do not mean anything. Many normal patients

show a few such features. Only multiple findings, of several different kinds, are significant.

- Behavioral symptoms and signs do not tell us anything about the initial cause of the pain. They certainly do not mean that the patient does not have 'real' physical pain, and they do not mean that the pain is 'psychogenic' or 'hysteric'. Most back pain starts with a physical problem in the back. Illness behavior is only one aspect of the patient's current clinical presentation.
- It is not a differential diagnosis between physical disease and illness behavior. Most patients have *both* a physical problem in their backs and varying degrees of illness behavior. The fact that we cannot demonstrate the physical basis of the pain does not mean that the pain is psychogenic, any more than the presence of illness behavior excludes a treatable physical problem. Recognizing psychologic problems and illness behavior depends on positive psychologic and behavioral findings.
- Illness behavior is not a diagnosis. Clinical observations of illness behavior do not provide a complete psychologic assessment and do not give you a psychologic or psychiatric diagnosis. They are only a screening test to alert you to the need for a more thorough assessment of this patient, and of how he or she is reacting and behaving with back pain.
- Behavioral symptoms and signs are not medicolegal tests, but observations of normal human behavior in illness. They do not necessarily mean that the patient is acting, faking or malingering. Most illness behavior occurs in pain patients who are not in a compensation or adversarial legal situation.

THE DEFINITION OF ILLNESS BEHAVIOR

Up to now, we have looked at the clinical features of illness behavior. Let us now consider the theoretic concept. It originally came from medical sociology, for illness is a social event. Halliday (1937), one of the pioneers of modern social medicine, described illness as 'a mode of behavior of a person or community'. Mechanic (1968) defined illness behavior as 'the ways in which given symptoms may be differentially perceived, evaluated and acted (or not acted) upon by different kinds of persons and in different social situations'. Medical sociologists stress the role of mental events and of attitudes and beliefs in illness behavior. What people do depends very much on how and what they think about their symptoms and their illness.

Although beliefs about illness, psychologic events and actual illness behavior are all important and all interact, we should make a clear distinction between them. The dictionary defines behavior as acts, manners and conduct. Behavioral psychologists, after Fordyce (1976), emphasize that behavior relates to overt actions and conduct that we can observe. Illness behavior is what patients actually do and how they react to pain and clinical examination. This is not to deny the reality or importance of inner mental events. It simply recognizes that we cannot observe directly such purely subjective experiences but must rely on the patient's own report of them. We can only observe behavior. This is a pragmatic approach, and we must always remember that the behavior we observe is only the outward manifestation of these inner mental and emotional events. It is only one clinical perspective on the whole pattern of illness. Its particular value is that it is one of the few objective, external observations of pain. Against that background, we can define illness behavior as 'observable and potentially measurable actions and conduct that express and communicate the individual's own perception of disturbed health' (Waddell et al 1989).

Illness behavior is a normal part of human illness, and back pain is no different from any other illness. In most patients, illness behavior is in proportion to their physical problem. In some patients, however, illness behavior gets out of proportion and reflects these mental and psychologic events more than the underlying physical disorder. Illness behavior may then aggravate and perpetuate pain and suffering and disability. It becomes counter-productive and is then part of the continuing problem. However, this is not to say that there is 'normal' and 'abnormal' illness behavior. All illness behavior is part of human illness. It is a spectrum, and it does not help to label it normal or abnormal. It is more important to try to understand how each patient is reacting to and dealing with his or her illness.

The physical basis of illness behavior

The first and most important message is that illness behavior generally reflects the severity of the underlying physical problem. Some doctors seem to have the idea that if patients show illness behavior, then they do not have anything physically wrong with them. Or at least nothing much. In fact, that is the opposite of the truth. Illness behavior expresses and communicates the severity of pain and physical impairment. The more severe the physical problem, the more ill the patient behaves.

Regional and 'nonanatomic' symptoms and signs also reflect the neurophysiology of chronic pain. Remember that pain is always modulated at every level of the nervous system, and that response is plastic and may change in chronic pain. Animal experiments show that pain thresholds may rise or fall and receptive fields may enlarge. So a neurone may respond to stimuli from a wider area, or a localized stimulus may excite more neurones. Light touch or pressure may become pain or there may be reduction in sensation, and neurologic activity may persist after the stimulus stops.

We now have an animal model for neuropathic pain by ligating the lumbar nerve roots in the rat. This type of pain has multiple features:

- spontaneous pain
- persistent, intense, burning pain
- pain from innocuous stimuli such as light touch or pressure
- intense pain from normally painless stimuli.

These rats also show pain behavior. We can then reverse these changes by sympathectomy. Thus spinal cord mechanisms can produce hypersensitivity and 'nonanatomic' tenderness, regional pain and altered sensation, all from a local lesion.

We must therefore interpret our clinical findings with caution. We must recognize that clinical localization of symptoms and signs is never exact. They are often ill-localized and appear to spread. Poorly localized symptoms, nonanatomic tenderness and regional findings can all occur in isolation in patients with no other evidence of illness behavior.

However, we must not fall into the trap of trying to force every clinical symptom and sign into a physical or neurophysiologic explanation. Neither, must every clinical finding have *either* a neurophysiologic *or* a psychologic explanation. Every action depends on neurophysiology and muscle activity. That action depends on electrical activity in the nervous system, but also on mental events. Neurophysiology may help us to understand the *mechanisms* of pain, but we must also look at pain psychology and behavior if we want to understand these clinical presentations.

Psychologic factors in illness behavior

The weight of clinical evidence suggests that these clinical observations can also give us information about illness behavior. We can clearly separate the behavioral symptoms and signs, both clinically and statistically, from the symptoms and signs of physical disease or impairment. They often spread far beyond any likely neurophysiologic mechanism and tend to a body image distribution. They are closely related to other observations of illness behavior. Illness behavior is closely related to emotional arousal and psychologic distress. As a first over-simplification, we might regard illness behavior as the clinical equivalent or expression of distress.

Pilowsky (1978) integrated sociologic concepts of illness behavior with psychiatric observations of hypochondriasis. The key feature of hypochondriasis is a persistent preoccupation with health or disease. It is out of proportion to any physical pathology, and it persists despite investigation and reassurance. Illness behavior is closely related to disease conviction. Some patients are overwhelmed by pain and disability and become absolutely convinced that they have a serious physical illness, despite all the evidence to the contrary. They reject any suggestion that their mental or emotional reactions may play any part in their continuing pain problem. Their illness behavior is to some extent simply a magnified or more emphatic presentation of their problem. These patients are trying to get the message across that they really do have a physical problem. They are concerned about the problem, and feel that it is all getting out of control. They are distressed about its severity and persistence and the failure of treatment, and are trying to get help. From their experience up to now, these worries will not settle with simple reassurance. From this point of view, illness behavior is a powerful form of communication between patient and health professional. Up to a point, it may serve a useful purpose. Unfortunately, beyond a certain point it may become counter-productive, both for the patient and for communication with health professionals.

Illness behavior is closely linked to disability, loss of function or the limitation of normal activity. Illness behavior is what you do, or do not do, and how you behave. Depending on how you look at it, disability *is* illness behavior and illness behavior *is* disability.

Illness behavior is associated with chronic pain and disability, the amount of failed treatment, 'problem patient' status, and the duration of work loss. These all lead to increased illness behavior, but the cause and effect relationship is not entirely clear. Illness behavior is not only the consequence of chronic pain and disability. It occurs at an earlier stage than we previously believed, and it may be implicated in the process of developing chronic pain and disability. Patients who show marked illness behaviors have a lower success rate of any kind of treatment. Beliefs, distress and illness behavior all get better or worse with the success or failure of physical treatment. This may become a vicious circle,

which we will consider again from different perspectives in the following four chapters.

Illness behavior does not just happen: it is learned. It is not fixed, but is a dynamic process over time, and health care may play a key role in its development. The information and advice we give may color patients' beliefs about their illness and what they should do about it. In back pain, our 'treatment' often consists of direct advice to stop or restrict normal activities and to behave in a more ill manner. We may prescribe 'sick certification'. In more extreme cases, doctors or therapists may offer or support the use of walking aids, and the patient's partner or family may encourage and support illness behavior. Chronic pain patients often have repeated consultations and examinations and learn what to say and do for health professionals. They learn what to expect, and what is expected of them, and this modifies how they react and behave. Conflicting opinions and advice, failed treatment, disappointment and frustration all lead them to press their case more strongly. We teach, and they learn, illness behavior in their clinical presentation. All of this is unconscious, learned behavior. Unfortunately, traditional health care for back pain may do more to cause than to prevent illness behavior.

Clinical observation of illness behavior is clearly only one facet of a complex phenomenon. We must assess the whole clinical picture before we can begin to understand illness behavior:

- attitudes, fears and beliefs about illness
- distress
- a broad assessment of illness behavior in its clinical presentation and everyday life
- whether the patient has inappropriate beliefs about health that persist despite accurate information and reasonable reassurance
- disability and invalidity.

HOW ILLNESS BEHAVIOR AFFECTS CLINICAL MANAGEMENT

Before we consider psychologic issues in more detail (Ch. 11), we should note the value of observing illness behavior in routine practice.

If you recognize illness behavior, this helps to clarify your clinical assessment and removes a potential source of great confusion. Too often, in our Problem Back Clinic, we see patients with failed back surgery who have whole leg pain, apparent limitation of SLR that improves with distraction, and regional weakness. If we look carefully at their records, we find that they had these features before surgery. Unfortunately, their surgeon did not recognize that these were symptoms and signs of illness behavior and made a clinical diagnosis of a disc prolapse. The severity of pain and distress led to great pressure to do something and the MRI showed a bulge. So, surprise, surprise, they had a negative surgical exploration that made them worse. If the surgeon had recognized the illness behavior, he would have seen that these symptoms and signs were not of nerve root pain, nerve irritation, and combined L5 and S1 weakness, and that the patient had no specific symptoms or objective signs of a disc prolapse. There was never any clinical indication for surgery. The incidental findings on the MRI only completed the trap. Dr P Dudley White was President Eisenhower's personal physician, although it is not clear whether this political background led to his clinical insight! 'The doctor who cannot take a good history and the patient who cannot give one are in danger of giving and receiving bad treatment.'

In both assessment and management, it is not a question of *either* physical disease *or* illness behavior. Rather, we must recognize which symptoms and signs are behavioral in nature and which tell us about the physical problem and we must assess both. Recognizing illness behavior helps to clarify your physical assessment, but also alerts you to the need for further psychologic assessment. These patients may require both physical treatment of their physical disorder and more careful assessment and management of the psychosocial and behavioral aspects of their illness.

This is not only important for surgery. The concept of illness behavior is fundamental to understanding low back pain and disability and its clinical management. It is one of the keys to treating people rather than spines. Our aim is better understanding of the clinical presentation. It is not a question of credibility. We should believe both physical and behavioral observations, but each gives us different information about the patient and his or her illness. Illness behavior must not lead to moral judgements or to rejecting these patients. It is our job as health professionals to care for our patients, both their physical disorders and their illness behavior. The aim of recognizing illness behavior is to manage them more appropriately.

- Methods of assessing illness behavior are a powerful aid to understanding the clinical presentation of back pain. It is important to distinguish the symptoms and signs of illness behavior from those of physical disease
- This distinction clarifies the assessment of the physical problem
- These findings of illness behavior should also alert you to the need for more detailed psychosocial assessment. They do not, on their own, give a diagnosis of psychologic disturbance, or of exaggeration in a compensation or medicolegal context
- These patients may require *both* physical treatment of their physical problem *and* more careful management of the psychosocial and behavioral aspects of their illness
- Health care may have a profound influence on illness behavior

---

REFERENCES

Fordyce W E 1976 Behavioural methods for chronic pain and illness. Mosby, St Louis
Halliday J L 1937 Psychological factors in rheumatism: a preliminary study. British Medical Journal 1: 213–217, 264–269
Keefe F J, Block A R 1982 Development of an observation method for assessing pain behavior in chronic low back pain patients. Behavioral Therapy 13: 363–375
Mechanic D 1968 Medical sociology. Free Press, New York
Ohlund C, Lindstrom I, Areskoug B, Eeek C, Peterson L-E, Nachemson A 1994 Pain behavior in industrial subacute low back pain. Part I. Reliability: concurrent and predictive validity of pain behavior assessments. Pain 58: 201–209

Ohlund C, Palmblad S, Areskoug B, Nachemson A 1996 Quantified pain drawing in subacute low back pain: validation in a non-selected outpatient industrial sample. Spine 21: 1021–1031

Parker H, Wood P L R, Main C J 1995 The use of the pain drawing as a screening measure to predict psychological distress in chronic low back pain. Spine 20: 236–243

Pilowsky I 1978 A general classification of abnormal illness behaviours. British Journal of Medical Psychology 51: 131–137

Ransford A O, Cairns D, Mooney V 1976 The pain drawing as an aid to the psychological evaluation of patients with low back pain. Spine 1: 127–134

Richards J S, Nepomuceno C, Riles M, Suer Z 1982 Assessing pain behavior: the UAB pain behavior scale. Pain 14: 393–398

Waddell G, McCulloch J A, Kummel E, Venner R M 1980 Non-organic physical signs in low back pain. Spine 5: 117–125

Waddell G, Main C J, Morris E W, Di Paola M P, Gray I C M 1984 Chronic low back pain, psychologic distress, and illness behavior. Spine 9: 209–213

Waddell G, Pilowsky I, Bond M 1989 Clinical assessment and interpretation of abnormal illness behaviour in low back pain. Pain 39: 41–53

Waddell G, Richardson J 1992 Clinical assessment of overt pain behaviour by physicians during routine clinical examination. Journal of Psychosomatic Research 36: 77–87

11

Psychologic distress

Chris J. Main   Gordon Waddell

The fascination of back pain is the way in which different people react to it so very differently. Just compare the two patients shown in Figure 10.1. It should be clear by now that how people think and feel about back pain is central to what they do about it and how it affects them.

Pain is a 'passion of the soul'. Our modern definition of pain describes it as 'an unpleasant sensory and emotional experience'. Pain is highly personal and subjective, and always has an emotional and psychologic dimension, which we must allow in its clinical presentation and management. Hence:

- different patients react differently to the same physical pain
- placebos can give good pain relief
- anxiety and depression can make pain feel worse
- distraction can make pain feel better
- psychosocial factors play a major role in the development of chronic pain and disability.

Emotional changes with pain vary in different people and at different times. Acute pain raises natural fear and anxiety about its cause and possible future consequences. It leads to increased awareness and preoccupation with the cause of the pain and an urgent search for a remedy. People with acute pain are often more irritable and less tolerant than usual. It may distract them and cause poor concentration and faulty judgement. This may all lead to strained relations with family and fellow workers.

As pain becomes chronic, emotions change in nature and degree. Chronic pain almost inevitably implies failed treatment and this colors the emotions. Patients may still be afraid and anxious, but the focus changes to the prospect of chronic pain and disability. There is increasing conviction that the pain reflects a serious problem, and there is scepticism toward attempts at reassurance. The physical focus may lead to a desperate and unrealistic search for anyone who can offer a diagnosis or cure. Repeated failures to find an answer may lead to anger, distrust and hostility. There is pessimism about the future and the prospect of continued pain and disability. Many patients with chronic pain become depressed, helpless and hopeless. Drugs and surgery may produce side-effects and some chronic pain patients develop analgesic or alcohol dependence. Chronic pain and its associated emotions lead to progressive withdrawal from social activities. Pain and disability now have profound impact on family relationships and work. Many patients with back pain eventually lose their jobs, with all the economic, social and emotional consequences of unemployment.

Early clinical studies

Disc surgery has stood the test of time for more than half a century because 80–90% of carefully selected patients get good results. When the number of disc operations escalated after World War II, however, the failures were equally dramatic. By 1970, one of the pioneers of disc surgery was forced to admit the conundrum: 'No operation in any field of surgery leaves in its wake more human wreckage than surgery on the lumbar spine' (DePalma & Rothman 1970). Every study of failed back surgery has stressed the importance of psychologic factors which could also affect the patient's response to further surgery.

A classic study by Wiltse & Rocchio (1975) showed that psychologic tests could actually predict how patients with disc prolapse would respond to treatment. There was no question that these patients had physical pathology, yet

psychologic factors influenced the outcome of physical treatment. Other studies have now shown that psychologic factors influence how patients respond to every form of conservative or surgical treatment.

These studies stimulated further research into the role of psychologic factors. At first, the research was driven by an attempt to predict how patients might respond to surgery, so that selection for surgery might be improved. It was then realized that psychologic factors are of more fundamental importance in how patients react to back pain, the development of chronic pain and disability, and clinical management.

'Personality'

Most of the early psychologic studies on back pain focused on 'personality' and were thought to show that patients with chronic low back pain were 'neurotic'. The results of the early psychologic tests were interpreted as fixed characteristics of the person's psychologic make-up. These studies only looked at patients after they had developed chronic pain, but it was assumed that these were preexisting personality traits. Thus, people with certain types of personality would be more likely to develop chronic pain. The other, even more unfortunate, implication was that there was little they or anyone else could do about it.

Subsequent studies showed that these test findings are not fixed and immutable personality traits. When we look at people before they develop back pain and follow them through the acute stage and as they get better, we discover that these psychologic features develop and then get better with patients' clinical progress. We now realize that most of these findings reflect the patient's *present* emotional and psychologic state, and their current clinical situation. Noone has been able to identify any particular personality type that predisposes to back pain. People with back pain are no different from the rest of us, which is not surprising as we are all likely to get it at some time!

Personality, in the sense of our individual psychologic make-up due to our unique combination of nature and nurture, clearly does influence how we respond if we do develop back pain. It is the pond into which the stone of back pain drops to produce emotional and psychologic ripples. It sets our psychologic style, the defence mechanisms we use, and the ways in which we try to cope. Understanding patients' psychologic background may help us to understand their clinical presentation, their methods of communication and their responses to health care.

A number of recent reports from highly specialized pain clinics show that 30–50% of their chronic patients may have some type of 'personality disorder' (Polatin et al 1993, Weisberg & Keefe 1997). These clinics have a high proportion of patients with a history of physical or sexual abuse, alcohol and drug problems, and severe personality disorders. However, we must be careful not to over-interpret this. Only a very highly selected and atypical group of patients is referred to these clinics. There are still problems with the diagnosis of 'personality disorders', and the criteria used may give the same diagnosis in about 10% of normal people. It is doubtful if these studies tell us anything about the average patient with back pain.

Misconceptions

Before we go any further, we should clear away some misconceptions that seem to be common among some clinicians. We accept that some of our more knowledgeable readers may regard this as over-simplified and dogmatic, but we feel it is important to start with a clean slate.

First, back pain is usually not psychogenic. Emotional and psychologic disturbances and illness behavior do not tell us anything about the original cause of the pain. Most back pain starts with a physical problem in the back, even if it is only the simple backache that we all get at some time. Most emotional and psychologic changes occur secondarily to physical pain. Psychologic factors may make a person more aware of back pain or more likely to consult. They may also aggravate and perpetuate the pain, or even turn simple backache into chronic pain and disability. Physical treatment alone

may not then solve the problem, and by that stage we may also need to deal with the psychologic changes as well.

Second, we cannot divide pain into physical or psychologic, organic or nonorganic, real or imaginary. The IASP definition emphasizes that pain is an unpleasant sensory *and* emotional experience. Despite this, many doctors and therapists wrongly act as if pain is either physical or psychologic. If there are few physical findings to explain continued pain, then they assume the pain is psychologic. Clinical experience and many scientific studies show that this is not the case. Sensory and emotional dimensions are integral to pain itself. Physical pain and emotional changes are not alternatives: they are two sides of the same coin. Our failure to find the physical source of back pain does not mean that the pain is psychogenic, any more than the presence of emotional changes excludes a treatable physical problem. In clinical practice it is more realistic to accept that back pain has a physical cause. It is also safer and more helpful. Nothing destroys the doctor–patient relationship faster than trying to categorize pain in that way. Our inability to find the source of back pain is not the patient's fault, but rather reflects our limited knowledge. We should not diagnose psychologic events by exclusion, but must assess the patient's emotional state on positive psychologic and behavioral features.

Third, as we have already discussed, most ordinary patients with back pain have nothing wrong with their personality.

Fourth, patients with chronic back pain are not mentally ill. Most patients who present with a main complaint of low back pain do not have a primary psychiatric illness, and attempts at formal psychiatric diagnosis are inappropriate. This is why referral to a traditional psychiatrist is usually not much help. The psychiatrist simply replies, correctly, that the problem is in the patient's back and not his or her head. Clinicians should avoid pseudo-psychiatric diagnoses. The terms hysteria and hypochondriasis have been so variously used, misused and abused that we should discard them completely in the context of back pain.

Finally, few patients with back pain are malingering. Most of these emotional and psychologic changes and illness behavior occur in the absence of any claims for compensation. Patients cannot help how they react to pain. They do not want to have pain and they do not choose to be emotional or disabled. Emotions are generally outside our conscious control and most illness behavior is involuntary. Our professional role is not to sit in judgement, but to understand the problem with compassion and to provide the best possible management for each patient.

- Back pain arises from a physical problem in the back. It is usually not psychogenic
- We cannot divide back pain into physical or psychologic
- Most patients with back pain are no different from the rest of us:
  — they are not personality-deficient
  — they do not have a psychiatric disorder
  — they are not malingering

In summary, patients with back pain are not mad or bad or psychologically different from the rest of us. Most of them are normal people with pain in their back.

THE NATURE OF STRESS AND DISTRESS

Stress is a normal human emotion that is part of everyday living. It is how we become energized, and a certain level of stress is necessary for us to perform to our best. In situations requiring a high level of performance or concentration, the body releases chemicals and stress hormones. Biologically, we may think of this as a method of mustering our resources to cope with threat or danger. This 'fight or flight' reaction is well known in the animal kingdom, but even though humans now face similar challenges to a much lesser extent, we still react by the same biologic mechanisms. The first reaction to a stressful situation is to escape if possible. However, that is not always possible or it may have other unacceptable effects. When we face particularly severe or prolonged stress from which we cannot escape, we may become stressed. Too much stress can be unproductive.

Instead of raising our performance, it may make it worse. We become fatigued or 'burnt out'. We may worry and become distressed.

However, we need to distinguish *distress* from *stress* (see Box 11.1). We sometimes use the word stress to refer to the event that is stressful, such as a bereavement, a difficult situation at work, or financial worries. Strictly speaking, such an event is a *stressor*, and there are many of these in life. We also use the word stress to refer to the reaction to a stressor, such as irritability, difficulty sleeping or increased sweating. Strictly speaking, such reactions are *stress responses*. This kind of stress response can occur without the person being distressed. Thus, sometimes a person does not realize they are stressed, even though it may be obvious to family and friends. We should only use the term *distress* for excessive or abnormal stress responses. At its most severe, distress may require formal psychiatric treatment, but most pain patients do not require that. Simple reassurance will often be enough to defuse the patient.

People react to stress in different ways. The most common emotions are anxiety, depression and anger. These are not mutually exclusive, and some patients show features of all of these. Some patients wear their emotions on their

---

Box 11.1 Stress and distress

- *Stress is a normal human emotion in response to life*
- *Distress is an excessive or abnormal stress response*

The common underlying characteristic of stress is a feeling of being under pressure or overwhelmed. Other symptoms and signs of stress include:

- chronic fatigue
- loss of interest and enjoyment
- difficulty concentrating
- irritability and impatience
- anxiety
- withdrawal
- muscle tension
- aches and pains
- difficulty sleeping
- changed appetite
- trembling
- sweaty hands.

sleeve. They clearly state their anxiety, depression and frustration. It is important to spend time listening to such patients. If they feel they have had the opportunity to express their view, and that someone has been listening to their difficulties, a major step in their management will have been achieved.

However, not all patients find it easy to talk about their feelings. Some patients may instead present symptoms that appear to be physical but which actually indicate their underlying distress. In our research, we found that the most common indicators of distress in patients with back pain are increased awareness of bodily symptoms or depressive symptoms.

Finally, changes in established behavior patterns may also be indicative of distress. Changes in sleep; sexual interest or activity; food, alcohol and drug consumption; and personal relationships or social activities may also be indicators of distress.

Clinically, we can define psychologic distress as a disturbance of emotion and mood in which psychologic and physical symptoms occur. It is similar in nature, if not in scale, to the normal experience of exposure to stress. It is a normal human reaction to pain, a state of emotional arousal, disturbed emotions and suffering. Croft et al (1995) looked at psychologic distress associated with back pain in the general population, and found that 15–30% of people with back pain may have some degree of distress, sufficient to influence their pain and consulting.

Generalized vs. specific distress

Having determined that the patient is distressed, we should then try to evaluate the reason for his or her distress. This is not always as straightforward as it might appear. As a general rule, it is a good idea to take a *stress history* in the same way that you take a physical history. Be careful: you must be sensitive. Patients may be reluctant to disclose what they consider to be personal details that they feel are irrelevant to their back pain. Evaluate general life stress both historically and in the context of the present or recent past. Why should this very general history be so important? Simply put, experience may color the patient's view of his or her current difficulties. People's emotional reactions to stress in the past may cast light on their current reaction to their back pain and its effects. Some people may show a general tendency to become distressed or even depressed in the face of stress or unresolved conflict, while others may show a tendency to 'shrug things off'.

There is no doubt that back pain is a very powerful stressor. However, there may be other, unresolved difficulties that are confounding the current problem. These may need separate consideration and may need to be dealt with in their own right. Recent bereavement is an example. Sometimes a major marital problem has predated the onset of the back trouble. Ongoing litigation may be another 'obstacle' needing careful consideration. More extreme examples may need specific psychologic assessment and treatment. Any such life events may limit the range of therapeutic options or affect the outcome of treatment for back pain. They may even affect whether or not treatment for back pain should be offered at that time, or indeed at all.

Three specific examples of a 'stress history' merit special attention:

- First, a small but important group of chronic pain patients have a history of physical and sexual abuse, either in childhood or as part of their continuing problem. We generally think of such abuse being more common in females, but it is now clear that similar problems are not uncommon in men. If you elicit such a history, it is important to decide immediately whether the patient requires more specialized assessment and treatment. Such a patient should have the opportunity to talk to a skilled professional of the same sex, if he or she so wishes. Traumatizing physical or sexual abuse needs delicate handling.
- Secondly, if patients have been involved in a serious injury, you should always look for post-traumatic stress symptoms (see Box 11.2). You can carry out a rough screening as part

of the 'stress history', but if the symptoms have been more than transient they may need special investigation or treatment. Again, it is important to identify such symptoms and to evaluate their significance before deciding on the management of back pain.

Box 11.2 Post-traumatic stress disorder (Mendelson 1988)

- An event outside the usual range of experience that would markedly distress almost anyone
- Persistent re-experiencing of the traumatic event, e.g. distressing recollections, dreams, reliving
- Avoiding thoughts, activities or situations associated with the trauma
- Symptoms of physiologic arousal and psychologic distress
- Duration of symptoms for more than 1 month.

- Thirdly, some patients may have become distressed about seeing doctors or other health professionals. By the time you see them, they may already have received a whole range of opinions, which may be contradictory. They may have looked for a diagnosis and got no clear answer. They may not have understood what they were told, and they may feel they were not taken seriously. Other doctors may have implied that their pain is trivial or even imaginary, and may have seemed unsympathetic. Such experience colors and shapes the patient's attitude towards consultation. They may be angry. Before you blame the patient, listen carefully to the history. Remember, they may have very good reason to be angry and distressed. Part of your job is to put your patient at ease. In order to understand and help your patient, you need to establish rapport.

In summary, the stress history should assess the importance of other life stresses facing the patient, quite apart from those related to his or her back pain. It may at times be difficult to judge the relative importance of back pain among these other problems. You must set priorities, and make judgements about the place and value of treatment for the symptom of back pain.

CLINICAL PRESENTATIONS

Most studies of back pain agree that the main emotions associated with it are anxiety, increased bodily awareness, fear, anger and depression. Different patients present various combinations of these and there is no sharp divide between acute and chronic pain. These can all be part of the emotional impact of pain.

There is overlap and interaction between all these emotions. They share many symptoms in common, symptoms which are also common in pain. They are all part of the normal human response to pain and stress. Most patients with back pain show a complex but variable mixture of these emotions and the mix will vary according to their make-up and background. Apart from depression, individual emotions rarely reach the level of a specific psychiatric illness. Rather, these patients are emotionally aroused by their pain and disability and by failed treatment. In some patients, these emotional changes may be more severe and prolonged and appear to get out of control. This rich emotional broth may then aggravate and perpetuate pain and disability, and may itself become part of the problem (Sullivan & Katon 1993). It may reduce the success rate of treatment. At root, however, patients with back pain are quite simply distressed by their continued pain and disability and by our failure to solve their problem.

Anxiety

We all experience anxiety at some time, but it can become harmful if it is excessive or prolonged. We all respond differently to stress and vary in the extent to which we are prone to anxiety. We may tend to become anxious in response to a wide range of stresses, or we may only be anxious about a particular situation. Anxiety varies widely from a normal emotional reaction to a more exaggerated form of anxiety neurosis. Autonomic activity may produce physiologic and emotional changes and symptoms. The clinical presentation varies, with some patients openly expressing their emotional symptoms while others focus more on their physical symptoms. Some patients describe feelings of being 'tense', 'wound up' or 'on edge'. They may be anxious, nervous or suffer panic attacks. Others may be more aware of tachycardia, excessive sweating, dry mouth and tremor. They may describe their symptoms more dramatically as 'butterflies in the stomach', shortness of breath or choking. The anxious person is restless and unable to relax or settle for any length of time. They usually have difficulty getting to sleep and sudden waking during the night. They may have increased or reduced appetite.

The mental features of anxiety include:

- apprehension
- doubt about ability to cope or achieve
- loss of ability to take responsibility and increase in dependence on others
- feeling of tension
- difficulty with concentration.

Anxiety is one of the most basic emotions in illness, and has a major impact on consulting and health care (Leigh & Reiser 1980). However, in the context of back pain, anxiety is usually only one of several emotions and does not reach the stage of a frank anxiety neurosis.

Increased bodily awareness

There is a constant stream of bodily sensations from our somatic and autonomic nervous systems, but usually we are unaware of it. Most of us spend most of our lives blithely paying little conscious attention to our bodies. Again, this varies with the individual and some people are by nature and upbringing much more introspective. Usually, however, it is only when something goes wrong that we pay attention. It is then normal to become more aware of and concerned about bodily symptoms. Pain, anxiety and stress all lead to sympathetic activity and emotional arousal. This heightened emotional state produces 'sensitizing' to bodily sensations and physiologic events. We may then interpret them as discomfort or malaise and we are more likely to seek health care for them (Sullivan & Katon 1993).

Main (1983) assessed patients with back pain in an orthopedic outpatient clinic. These patients were clearly anxious and concerned about their pain. They described symptoms of increased sympathetic activity, which are closely allied to anxiety, but few met the criteria for anxiety neurosis. They did show an understandable concern about their physical problem, but very few met the criteria for hypochondriasis. The common theme seemed to be increased bodily awareness rather than anxiety or hypochondriasis. They simply seemed to be more aware of their bodily symptoms and function. Main (1983) developed a 'modified somatic perception questionnaire' (MSPQ) to measure this increased bodily awareness (Fig. 11.1).

Fears and uncertainty

Back pain can be frightening, especially if you do not know what is happening to you and no-one seems to have an answer. There are also overtones to do with back pain coming from behind us where we cannot see it and feel vulnerable. There is implied threat to our very backbone and physical capability. We all know that back pain now often leads to chronic disability and incapacity for work, so there can be a very real and realistic fear about the pain itself and its possible consequences.

Health professionals are not very good at allaying that fear. Frequently, we cannot give a diagnosis or a good explanation of the problem. Patients get a different story from every doctor and therapist they see, which undermines any reassurance. Most of our treatment has a low success rate and recurrences are common, which undermines faith and confidence.

Anger

Many patients with chronic low back pain also get angry and frustrated (Fernandez & Turk 1995). They are angry at the pain. Why should they have to suffer like this? They may blame the apparent cause of the pain, which may be their work or their employer. If treatment fails

Please describe how you have felt during the PAST WEEK by making a check mark (✓) in the appropriate box. Please answer all questions. Do not think too long before answering.

	Not at all	A little/slightly	A great deal/ quite a lot	Extremely/could not have been worse
Heart rate increasing				
Feeling hot all over*	0	1	2	3
Sweating all over*	0	1	2	3
Sweating in a particular part of the body				
Pulse in neck				
Pounding in head				
Dizziness*	0	1	2	3
Blurring of vision*	0	1	2	3
Feeling faint*	0	1	2	3
Everything appearing unreal				
Nausea*	0	1	2	3
Butterflies in stomach				
Pain or ache in stomach*	0	1	2	3
Stomach churning*	0	1	2	3
Desire to pass water				
Mouth becoming dry*	0	1	2	3
Difficulty swallowing				
Muscles in neck aching*	0	1	2	3
Legs feeling weak*	0	1	2	3
Muscles twitching or jumping*	0	1	2	3
Tense feeling across forehead*	0	1	2	3
Tense feeling in jaw muscles				

The questionnaire as given to patients does not include the scoring.
Only those items marked with an asterik (*) are scored and added to give a total score.

Figure 11.1 Modified somatic perception questionnaire (MSPQ). (From Main 1983, with permission.)

and back pain becomes chronic and disabling, they may blame the doctors and therapists who fail to find the cause or provide a cure. When each doctor and therapist gives them a different story, they get confused, suspicious and angry. Loss of their job and financial hardship make them angrier still at the injustice of it all. If they have a legal dispute, they get angry at 'the system', the lawyers or medical examiners.

Doctors and therapists also get angry at the patient with back pain. These patients fail to meet our disease stereotypes and fail to get better as they should with our treatment. They try our professional skills and expose our limitations. It is tempting and more comfortable to blame that on the patient rather than on ourselves, and we get angry at the patient for putting us in this predicament.

So patients, doctors and therapists may all get angry. Patients may express their anger openly as hostility, or it may be inhibited and result in non-cooperation with treatment. Doctors and therapists may lose sympathy and patience. There may be a complete breakdown in communication. All of these undermine the patient–doctor or patient–therapist relationship. All health care depends on mutual trust and cooperation, which may not survive anger and hostility. Anger may lead to failed treatment, which then makes the patient more angry, trapping them in a self-perpetuating rut of failure and frustration.

Depressive symptoms

Depression is the most common psychologic disturbance in chronic pain (Sullivan et al 1992). Various studies show that 30–80% of patients at a pain clinic have some depressive symptoms, and up to 20% meet the criteria for a major depressive disorder. These are selected groups of patients, but lesser degrees of depression are important in most patients with chronic pain (Romano & Turner 1985, Rudy et al 1988, von Korff et al 1993). Although some pain may be the result of depression, most research indicates that depression is secondary to pain (Averill et al 1996).

Depression involves negative beliefs, lowered mood and clinical symptoms. Patients may show different patterns. The key feature of depression is a negative view of oneself, the world and the future (see Box 11.3). There may be loss of interest and energy and slowing of mental function. Depressive symptoms include a sense of loss, sadness, hopelessness and pessimism about the future. Physical symptoms include disturbed appetite, sleep and sexual function. Aches and pains are also common and there may be an excessive and morbid concern with symptoms or with health. We can perhaps best describe this as learned helplessness. Depressive symptoms range from a normal emotional reaction to a depressive neurosis. It is a question of degree and clinical impact whether they meet the criteria of a depressive illness.

Box 11.3 Features of depression

- Hopelessness, pessimism
- Sense of failure, loss of self-esteem, loss of joy in life
- Indecision, apathetic, retarded, withdrawn
- Fatigue
- Guilt, shame, self-accusation
- Agitated, hostile, irritable
- Crying spells
- Thoughts of suicide
- Physical symptoms may include
  — early morning wakening
  — loss of libido
  — loss of appetite
  — constipation
- Clinical observation may reveal slowing of thought, speech and reactions

---

Psychologic questionnaires

Clinical psychologists often use questionnaires, which can collect information quickly and efficiently. They provide a simple screen for psychologic distress.

We have already seen that two of the most important emotional changes in low back pain are increased bodily awareness and depressive symptoms. So we would recommend the MSPQ (Fig. 11.1; Main 1983) and the Zung depressive inventory questionnaires (Fig. 11.2; Zung 1965,

Please indicate for each of these questions which answer best describes how you have been feeling recently.

	Rarely or none of the time (less than 1 day per week)	Some or little of the time (1–2 days per week)	A moderate amount of time (3–4 days per week)	Most of the time (5–7 days per week)
1. I feel downhearted and sad	0	1	2	3
2. Morning is when I feel best	3	2	1	0
3. I have crying spells or feel like it	0	1	2	3
4. I have trouble getting to sleep at night	0	1	2	3
5. I feel that nobody cares	0	1	2	3
6. I eat as much as I used to	3	2	1	0
7. I still enjoy sex	3	2	1	0
8. I notice I am losing weight	0	1	2	3
9. I have trouble with constipation	0	1	2	3
10. My heart beats faster than usual	0	1	2	3
11. I get tired for no reason	0	1	2	3
12. My mind is as clear as it used to be	3	2	1	0
13. I tend to wake up too early	0	1	2	3
14. I find it easy to do the things I used to do	3	2	1	0
15. I am restless and can't keep still	0	1	2	3
16. I feel hopeful about the future	3	2	1	0
17. I am more irritable than usual	0	1	2	3
18. I find it easy to make a decision	3	2	1	0
19. I feel quite guilty	0	1	2	3
20. I feel that I am useful and needed	3	2	1	0
21. My life is pretty full	3	2	1	0
22. I feel that others would be better off if I were dead	0	1	2	3
23. I am still able to enjoy the things I used to	3	2	1	0

The questionnaire as given to patients does not include the scoring.
All items are scored as marked and added to give a total score.

Figure 11.2 The modified Zung depression questionnaire. (From Zung 1965, Main & Waddell 1984, with permission from Macmillan Press Ltd.)

Main & Waddell 1984). There are many alternatives, but these have the advantage of being widely used in back pain and we have found them most useful. Main et al (1992) used the MSPQ and Zung as the basis for the 'distress and risk assessment method' (DRAM). The DRAM is a simple and straightforward method of screening patients. It classifies them into those showing no psychologic distress, those at risk, and those who are clearly distressed (Table 11.1).

The DRAM may assist selection for referral for more formal psychologic assessment. Those showing no distress can have routine clinical management, without particular concern for psychologic issues. Those who are 'at risk' can also be managed routinely, but with awareness and monitoring of the possible development of distress, and the risk of chronic pain and disability. Management of those who are 'clearly distressed' must address both physical and psychologic issues. These patients need more than just physical treatment. They need more comprehensive psychologic assessment to decide if they also require formal pain management. Burton et al (1995) showed that the DRAM predicted 1 year outcomes in primary care patients (Table 11.2), and we have found that it also predicts response to a pain management program.

You should be aware of the strengths and limitations of psychologic tests (Table 11.3). Most are questionnaires that the patient fills in alone without assistance (see Figs 11.1 and 11.2). Answers are then scored and groups of related questions summed to obtain several measures or scales of different psychologic traits. Questionnaires have a number of advantages over clinical interview. They are very carefully designed and tested. They eliminate observer variation and bias. They can give a very precise and detailed assessment of a particular psychologic feature, allowing it to be measured in numbers. They are reproducible, so they can observe change over time or with treatment. They also have some weaknesses. They usually focus on particular psychologic features that we know are important in most patients. They will miss less common features that may be important in the individual patient. The patient must be fluent in the language, have sufficient mental ability, and be able to read and write. They must be cooperative and honest, or the questionnaires may be liable to bias.

You must also interpret the results with care. Numbers sometimes give an illusion of accuracy. You cannot diagnose psychiatric illness from psychologic questionnaires alone. Nor can they turn an untrained clinician into an amateur psychologist. If you do decide to use these questionnaires, you should get advice, and probably work closely with a clinical psychologist. Background reading is essential. Even then, questionnaires are only a first stage screening test, either to support clinical impression or to alert you to the need for more thorough psychologic assessment.

Questionnaires, then, may supplement, but cannot replace, the clinical interview. Questionnaires may be most useful in particular situations, such as for patients with chronic pain and disability, before surgery, or when planning a rehabilitation or pain management program.

MANAGEMENT OF PSYCHOLOGIC DISTRESS

We should be clear about our aims. All health professionals should have sufficient understanding of psychologic issues to provide understanding, reassurance and support for the

Table 11.1 The DRAM method of assessing psychologic distress (Main et al 1992)

Classification	Zung and MSPQ scores
Normal	Modified Zung <17
At risk	Modified Zung 17–33 and MSPQ, <13
Distressed, somatic	Modified Zung 17–33 and MSPQ, >12
Distressed, depressive	Modified Zung >33

Table 11.2 DRAM prediction of 1 year outcome in primary care patients (based on data from Burton et al 1995)

DRAM at presentation	DRAM at 1 year		
	Normal	At risk	Distressed
Normal (79)	87% (69)	9% (7)	4% (3)
At risk (59)	46% (27)	44% (26)	10% (6)
Distressed (34)	18% (6)	35% (12)	47% (16)

Numbers in brackets refer to the numbers of patients in each group.

Table 11.3 The advantages and disadvantages of clinical interview and questionnaires

	Clinical interview	Questionnaires
Advantages	Can be adapted to individual patient Incorporates clinical experience and judgement Link to goals for treatment	Quick, easy to administer Standardized Easy to score
Disadvantages	May be time-consuming Potential observer bias May be misleading unless skilled	Require reading and language skills Limited perspective May be too sensitive and susceptible to patient bias

patient with back pain. We should also be able to recognize those few patients who require referral for more thorough psychologic assessment and possibly treatment. It is also important to recognize our limitations: most health professionals do not have the background and experience to provide specialized help. Fortunately, very few patients with back pain, even chronic pain and disability, need formal psychologic or psychiatric treatment. But emotional changes are so common that every doctor and therapist should be aware of them and must deal with them. This is also fundamental to a good patient–doctor relationship (Balint 1964).

Understanding

Most doctors and therapists rely on their 'clinical impression' of the patient's emotional state. With all our experience in this field, both of us have learned to distrust our own gut reactions – they are usually misleading. A typical medical history and examination do not provide an adequate basis for psychologic

diagnosis or management. There is much room for improvement.

It is perhaps most important simply to be aware of emotions and psychologic distress. They should form part of the routine clinical assessment. Start with the patient's description of pain. Listen to the adjectives used. How strong are the emotions? Next, listen to the patient's symptoms and the impact on his or her life. Obviously the patient will describe the physical problem, but is he or she also describing emotional reactions? Ask how he or she feels about the pain. What are his or her hopes, fears and anxieties? Encourage him or her to talk and ensure you listen. Too often, especially in a short clinical consultation, we focus on physical symptoms and disease and do not give our patients the chance or the time to talk about *their* problem. With most patients, it only takes a moment to get a more balanced picture that will help better management and save time in the long run. In a few patients, it may open an unexpected can of worms that you cannot possibly deal with in a few minutes.

These patients may then need another longer consultation at a more convenient time, and they may need further help. However, these are the very patients who are most in need of early recognition of their psychologic problems so that better management can be provided. Your clinical assessment should also include illness behavior (Ch. 10), which may alert you to the need for more thorough assessment.

Remember also that these emotional changes may occur much earlier than we used to believe. Understanding these emotional changes provides the basis for dealing with them. Listening and understanding lead to empathy, which is a therapy in itself, and should also make us think more carefully about the information and advice that we offer to patients with back pain. The psychologic impact of our advice may be much more profound and important than any physical effect.

Reassurance

We must address our patients' fears and anxieties with firm, consistent and if necessary repeated reassurance. This is one of the major roles of the doctor in dealing with back pain – to provide reassurance that there is no serious disease. It depends on confident assessment of the problem. We must provide accurate and reasonable information and advice. We should be able to give a simple factual explanation of the illness, a plan of management, and a long-term outlook. This must be honest and realistic, but also optimistic. Indeed, that is what a large part of this book is about.

We must also avoid creating unnecessary worry. Too often, doctors and therapists encourage fear and anxiety about back pain by what we say and do, blithely unaware of how our patients think and feel about it.

Support

Psychologic support is every bit as important as physical treatment. This is one of the primary social roles of the health care professions, even if we cannot always cure all back pain.

We provide professional help to share the patient's burden: 'a problem shared is a problem halved' (see Box 11.4). The opportunity to talk about emotional problems to an understanding listener is sufficient support for many patients. Bringing emotional problems into the open may help to defuse them and enable the patient to handle them.

Box 11.4 The doctor–patient relationship (Balint 1964)

- Listening and taking time to listen are important
- Warmth: demonstrate an unconditional positive regard for the patient as a human being; not judgement or like/dislike.
- Accurate empathy: convey to the patient that you have an accurate understanding of their problem and experience
- Genuineness: 'be yourself'; do not hide behind a professional facade. This does not mean disclosing personal details about yourself
- Provide continuity of support over time
- Draw the line between support and counseling and do not try to be an amateur psychiatrist

---

Time to listen and talk to patients provides simple psychotherapy, although the quality of communication may be more important than what is actually said or the length of the consultation. Effective communication establishes a good relationship and provides reassurance, support and encouragement. It builds on the more basic human virtues of faith, hope and caring. For many patients with back pain, physical treatment alone is enough. Many others need physical treatment and better management of the whole illness. But for some, the more ancient role of adviser and comforter may meet the most important need of all.

Drugs

Sometimes, it may be appropriate to consider the use of psychotropic drugs such as antidepressants or hypnotics. Low-dose amitriptyline at night is often used in chronic pain patients to help reestablish a more normal sleep pattern. However, you should only prescribe such drugs if you have the necessary professional knowledge and experience.

REFERENCES

Averill P M, Novy D M, Nelson D V, Berry L A 1996 Correlates of depression in chronic pain patients: a comprehensive examination. Pain 65: 93–100

Balint M 1964 The doctor, his patient, and the illness. International Universities Press, New York

Burton A K, Tillotson K M, Main C J, Hollis S 1995 Psychosocial predictors of outcome in acute and subacute low-back trouble. Spine 20: 722–728

Croft P R, Papageorgiou A C, Ferry S, Thomas E, Jayson M I V, Silman A J 1995 Psychologic distress and low back pain: evidence from a prospective study in the general population. Spine 20: 2731–2737

De Palma A F, Rothman R H 1970 The intervertebral disc. WB Saunders, Philadelphia, p 347

Fernandez E, Turk D C 1995 Clinical review: the scope and significance of anger in the experience of chronic pain. Pain 61: 165–175

Leigh H, Reiser M F 1980 The patient: biological, psychological and social dimensions of medical practice. Plenum, New York, p 39–69

Main C J 1983 The modified somatic perception questionnaire. Journal of Psychosomatic Research 27: 503–514

Main C J, Waddell G 1984 The detection of psychological abnormality in chronic low back pain using four simple scales. Current Concepts in Pain 2: 10–15

Main C J, Wood P L R, Hollis S, Spanswick C C, Waddell G 1992 The distress and risk assessment method: a simple patient classification to identify distress and evaluate the risk of poor outcome. Spine 17: 42–52

Mendelson G 1988 Psychiatric aspects of personal injury claims. CC Thomas, Springfield, IL, p 122–123

Polatin P G, Kinney R K, Gatchel R J, Lillo E, Mayer T G 1993 Psychiatric illness and low back pain. Spine 18: 66–71

Romano J, Turner J A 1985 Chronic pain and depression: does the evidence support a relationship? Psychological Bulletin 97: 18–34

Rudy T E, Kerns R D, Turk D C 1988 Chronic pain and depression: toward a cognitive-behavioral mediation model. Pain 35: 129–140

Sullivan M J L, Reesor K, Mikail S, Fisher R 1992 The treatment of depression in chronic low back pain: review and recommendations. Pain 50: 5–13

Sullivan M, Katon W 1993 Somatization: the path between distress and somatic symptoms. American Pain Society Journal 2: 141–149

von Korff M, Resche L L, Dworkin S F 1993 First onset of common pain symptoms: a prospective study of depression as a risk factor. Pain 55: 251–258

Weisberg J N, Keefe F J 1997 Personality disorders in the chronic pain population. Pain Forum 6: 1–9

Wiltse L L, Rocchio P D 1975 Pre-operative psychological tests as predictions of success of chemonucleolysis in the treatment of the low back syndrome. Journal of Bone and Joint Surgery 57A: 478–483

Zung W W K 1965 A self-rated depression scale. Archives of General Psychiatry 32: 63–70

12

Beliefs about back pain

Gordon Waddell   Chris J. Main

THE NATURE OF BELIEFS

Man, above all else, is the thinking animal. The power of human thought can move mountains and transform our lives. It is our strength and our weakness, which sets us apart from all the other beasts. Beliefs are the mental engine that drives human behavior, and may raise us to the skies or cast us down to the depths of hell.

Beliefs are basic and relatively fixed ideas about the nature of reality. Beliefs are ideas written in stone. They become fixed and the only way to change them may be to break the mould.

Beliefs are shaped from childhood onwards and are influenced by parents, education and culture. We each develop our individual beliefs, but share them to a greater or lesser extent with our families, peer groups and fellow workers. Some beliefs are very general, but others are highly specific to our particular situation. Personal experience moulds our beliefs, but once they become established they may then persist despite contrary experience. Beliefs mould our perceptions of ourselves and our worries, and shape the meaning of our lives.

Pain beliefs are the patient's own ideas about what pain is and what it means for them. Psychologic studies suggest four general components to patients' beliefs about illness (DeGood & Shutty 1992):

- the nature of the illness – beliefs about the nature of the illness and the symptoms the person regards as part of the illness

- future course of the illness – beliefs about the future course and duration of the illness
- consequences – expected effects of the illness and its impact on the individual's life
- cure or control – beliefs about how to deal with the illness including personal responsibilities and expectations of health care.

These beliefs provide a framework for us to make sense of our experience and to decide what to do about it, including decisions about health care and taking sick leave. Every patient brings a set of beliefs to the consulting room. Indeed, the fact that they consult at all shows certain beliefs about health care. Earlier psychologic studies focused on general beliefs and we have only recently begun to appreciate the importance of specific beliefs about back pain.

Pain beliefs range from the very general to the highly specific. They range from broad philosophic perspectives about the meaning of life to very specific beliefs about the nature of back pain and treatment. The most general beliefs are basic philosophic assumptions about pain and disability and work. Such beliefs are highly personal but at the same time strongly rooted in a particular culture. They are often inconsistent and contradictory, and are very difficult to change. More specific beliefs include basic personal characteristics such as introspection about health, self-confidence and ability to cope. We must recognize and allow for each patient's personal characteristics, but we cannot change them. Finally, there are specific beliefs about pain and how patients think it should be managed, both by themselves and by others. These are the 'nut and bolts' that directly affect what we do about the pain, our illness behavior and disability. They are specific to the particular pain context. Patient's beliefs about their own particular pain may be quite distinct from their knowledge and ideas of pain in general. These specific beliefs are also more open to positive or negative influence by health care.

Patients often have a simplistic view of the nature of pain. They do not understand why pain persists and may express a desire to 'have the bit which hurts cut out'. They may have received different diagnoses from different doctors, so that by the time you see them, they may be confused and distressed. It is too easy simply to blame the patient for this state of affairs. If a patient has more than a trivial problem, in terms of either impact or duration, you should look carefully at their beliefs about their pain and disability. It is important to appreciate the power of folklore and 'old wives' tales'. Popular magazines are full of advice about back pain. Hardly a month passes without another miracle cure. It is essential to find out just what your patient thinks. Mistaken beliefs may prevent them from participating in treatment and it is essential to identify any such obstacles to treatment.

Box 12.1 shows some common beliefs about chronic pain.

Box 12.1 Common beliefs about chronic pain (From DeGood & Shutty 1992, with permission)

- Etiology of pain
  - somatic only vs. interaction of multiple factors
  - external vs. internal, e.g. accident vs. aging
  - someone is to blame vs. unfortunate chance
  - pain as symptom vs. benign
- Diagnostic expectations regarding
  - medical history
  - clinical examination
  - laboratory tests, especially radiologic
  - psychosocial assessment
- Treatment expectations
  - patient passive vs. active, e.g. surgery or medications vs. exercise or pain counseling
  - invasive vs. noninvasive
  - fix or repair vs. rehabilitation
  - somatic and medical vs. psychologic and behavioral
- Outcome goals
  - cure vs. control
  - rapid vs. gradual change
  - complete vs. partial freedom from pain
  - sensory change only vs. quality of life

Beliefs about damage or disease

Pain is the most universal physical and emotional stress that human beings experience. Thirty-five per cent of patients regard pain as the most stressful event in their lives. The amount of any stress depends not only on the severity of the threat but also on the extent to which we feel we can deal with it or that it may tax and exceed our resources.

Clinical studies show that patients' main fears and concerns about back pain are:

- that it may be due to serious disease
- the cause of the pain
- the likelihood of persistent pain.

This includes both concern about damage that has already occurred and the possibility of future damage. Humans are probably the only animals who can imagine and worry about the future. Fear of what may happen to us in the future can be even more important than present pain.

Tarasuk & Eakin (1994) interviewed people who applied for workers' compensation for back injuries. They focused on the workers' own perceptions and experience of what their back injury meant to them. How did their experience of back pain influence how they viewed their bodies, their work and their future?

A central feature was that many of these workers felt that their back problems were permanent. This belief sometimes arose from their current experience of chronic and persisting pain, combined with other aspects of their current life situation. For most of them, however, it was linked to a belief that their back was permanently vulnerable to reinjury. Even some who had only injured their backs a few weeks previously were convinced they would have back problems for life. Others feared their condition would get worse and lead eventually to permanent disability. Even if their back pain settled completely, they still had this fear of reinjury or recurrent back pain. Many of them had a sense of fragility. These beliefs had a strong influence on return to work.

Symonds et al (1995, 1996) looked more closely at beliefs about the future course and inevitability of back pain, and developed a new 'back beliefs questionnaire' (BBQ) for their studies (Fig. 12.1). It is short, simple and suitable for patients with back pain and also for workers with or without back pain. They found that workers with a previous history of low back pain were more likely to believe that their

backs would give continuing problems. They were also more negative about their ability to control the pain and to take personal responsibility. The greater the number of previous spells and the longer the amount of time off work with back pain, the more negative were their beliefs. Those who had low back pain at the time of the study also had more negative beliefs. People who believe they will inevitably have continuing back trouble are more negative in their approach to rehabilitation and return to work.

Szpalski et al (1995) also found that patients who believed that low back pain is a lifetime problem sought more health care, took more bed rest and used more medication. Carosella et al (1994) found that patients' own expectations about return to work were the best predictor of whether they were likely to drop out of an intensive rehabilitation program. It was more powerful than severity of pain, the patient's perception of their work environment or time off work. Sandstrom & Esbjornsson (1986) found that patients' beliefs were the best predictor of return to work after rehabilitation. They questioned patients before a rehabilitation program, and those who believed they would not be able to return to work were much less likely to do so. In other words, patients who are convinced they will continue to have back pain and remain disabled are likely to fulfill their own prophecy, quite apart from their physical condition.

Fear of hurting/harming

Fear is a basic instinct throughout the animal kingdom. Some fears, such as fear of the dark or fear of snakes, may be biologic rather than based on personal experience. Pain is aversive and frightening, as it is commonly a warning signal of actual or impending tissue damage. This fear has an important and useful purpose. If a child touches something hot, it will burn itself. The sudden pain leads the child instinctively to withdraw its hand, thus minimizing tissue damage. The child does not think about withdrawing its hand. There is no time. In

We are trying to find out what people think about low back trouble. Please indicate your general views towards back trouble, *even if you have never had any.*

Please answer *ALL* statements and indicate whether you *agree* or *disagree* with each statement by circling the appropriate number on the scale.

1 = COMPLETELY DISAGREE, 5 = COMPLETELY AGREE

1	2	3	4	5
Completely disagree				Completely agree

		Disagree			Agree	
1	There is no real treatment for back trouble	1	2	3	4	5
2	Back trouble will eventually stop you from working	1	2	3	4	5
3	Back trouble means periods of pain for the rest of one's life	1	2	3	4	5
4	Doctors cannot do anything for back trouble	1	2	3	4	5
5	A bad back should be exercised	1	2	3	4	5
6	Back trouble makes everything in life worse	1	2	3	4	5
7	Surgery is the most effective way to treat back trouble	1	2	3	4	5
8	Back trouble may mean you end up in a wheelchair	1	2	3	4	5
9	Alternative treatments are the answer to back trouble	1	2	3	4	5
10	Back trouble means long periods of time off work	1	2	3	4	5
11	Medication is the *only* way of relieving back trouble	1	2	3	4	5
12	Once you have had back trouble there is *always* a weakness	1	2	3	4	5
13	Back trouble *must* be rested	1	2	3	4	5
14	Later in life back trouble gets progressively worse	1	2	3	4	5

The inevitability scale uses nine of these statements: items 1, 2, 3, 6, 8, 10, 12, 13, 14.
Calculate the scale by reversing the scores (i.e. 5, 4, 3, 2, 1) and adding the nine scores.
© 1993 University of Huddersfield, UK

Figure 12.1   The back beliefs questionnaire (BBQ). (From Symonds et al 1996, with permission.)

many such situations, pain is biologically useful, but because it is unpleasant and linked to such experiences, we become afraid of it.

Recent research has shown that fear of pain, and fear of hurting and harming, is a frequent and powerful influence in back pain. In the first instance, most people's reaction to back pain is instinctive and automatic: they attempt to avoid what seemed to be the cause of the pain. However, fear may subsequently lead to continued attempts to avoid the situation. Up to a point this is reasonable. Unfortunately, depending on circumstances, all sorts of misunderstandings about back pain may develop. The intensity of the fear will depend on the context of the pain, and particular situations will be more likely to cause strong painful memories associated with fear (Turk et al 1996). Fear may become associated not only with recurrent injury, but also with pain itself. Such fears may develop into fixed beliefs about hurt and harm, and become a barrier to treatment or rehabilitation. If patients wrongly believe that pain from unfit muscles means continuing damage, it may seem natural and indeed logical that they should not exercise. And if they believe that pain *always* means that further damage is taking place, they may not only 'avoid' any treatment that involves pain, e.g. when trying to mobilize, but give up treatment or rehabilitation altogether. Inappropriate fears about back pain, based on misunderstandings or on painful emotional memories, are an important barrier to treatment and rehabilitation (Dehlin et al 1981, Sandstrom & Esbjornsson 1986, Feuerstein 1991).

However, pain does not always produce fear or anxiety. For example, sportsmen accept pain as a normal part of training, especially when unfit or when recovering from injury. This is a useful analogy for patients with back pain.

Fear avoidance beliefs

With experimental pain in the laboratory, fore-warning of pain may relieve its impact, particularly if subjects feel they have some control over what is happening. Anticipation of uncontrollable pain makes the pain more intense. In clinical pain also, expectations and fear of pain affect the pain and what we do.

Fear is a powerful negative drive in humans and in animals, closely allied to pain. Fear is to some extent an innate, inborn instinct, but to a greater extent it is learned. We learn from experience to fear situations or stimuli that have caused us stress or pain, and we then try to avoid them. If we avoid the situation and do not have pain, this may reinforce our belief and fear about the cause of the pain, and reward our efforts to avoid it. Philips (1987) stressed the importance of such beliefs and 'avoidance learning' in chronic pain.

Patients who believe that physical activity may aggravate their pain, whether from their past experience or because of their understanding of the pain, will expect and fear more pain if they are active. Note that this is all a matter of fears and expectations about what *may*

happen. Schmidt (1985) showed that patients with chronic low back pain do not do as much on a treadmill task and have lower pain tolerance when they immerse their forearm in ice water. However, it is not simply a question of the severity of pain during the task. Treadmill performance depends more on previous reports of pain than on current pain. Cold tolerance depends more on beliefs about how well one can cope.

Lethem et al (1983) and Troup et al (1987) used these ideas to develop a 'fear avoidance model of exaggerated pain perception' in chronic low back pain (Fig. 12.2). Their main focus was on patients' beliefs as the driving force for behavior. They drew attention to the central role of fear of pain leading directly to pain avoidance behavior.

Measuring fear avoidance beliefs

We later used Lethem et al's and Troup et al's ideas to develop the *Fear Avoidance Beliefs Questionnaire* (FABQ), which measures beliefs about physical activity and work (Fig. 12.3;

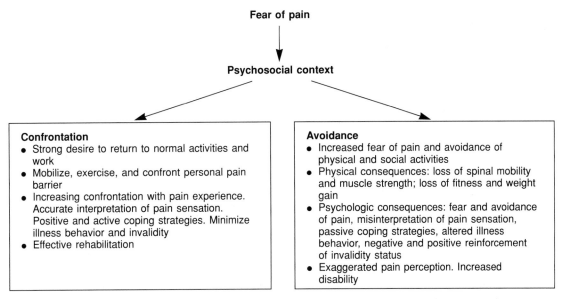

Figure 12.2   Fear avoidance: confronters and avoiders. In reality, of course, many people fall between these two extremes. (Adapted from Lethem et al 1983.)

Waddell et al 1993). People with back pain may believe that physical activity or work could increase their pain, injure their back or damage their back. These beliefs are closely allied to their conviction that they should not or cannot do these activities. We showed that these fear avoidance beliefs help to explain self-reported disability in activities of daily living and loss of time from work. The analysis in Table 12.1 shows how much fear avoidance beliefs *add* to disability, over and above the effects of pain itself. Indeed, we found that low back disability depends more on fear avoidance than on pain or physical pathology. Fear of pain may be more disabling than pain itself.

In our study (Waddell et al 1993), fear avoidance beliefs about work were more powerful than fear avoidance beliefs about physical activity in general. We have already looked at Sandstrom & Esbjornsson's (1986) study of how patients predicted their return to work after rehabilitation. One of the most important statements was: 'I am afraid to start working again, because I don't think I will be able to manage.' Changing an attitude such as this is fundamental to successful rehabilitation.

The development of fear avoidance beliefs

It may at first seem that fear avoidance beliefs are a natural and accurate interpretation of pain as a signal of injury, but that is only part of the story. In fact, certainly by the time pain becomes chronic, there is very little relation between fear avoidance beliefs and pain itself. In our study, fear avoidance beliefs about physical activity were only weakly related to the severity of pain. Fear avoidance beliefs about work bore no relation at all to any measure of pain. None of the fear avoidance beliefs was related to duration of pain. Fear avoidance beliefs seemed to relate more to the uncertainty of diagnosis than to the severity of the physical problem.

Fear avoidance beliefs may start from experience that physical activity or work aggravates back pain, although even this may have more to do with the patient's understanding or expectation than with reality. Only 36% of patients with low back pain say that physical activity such as walking makes their pain worse. When you question them carefully, 45% say it makes no difference and 16% say it makes their pain better. Even if physical activity does aggravate pain, that is quite different from being the cause of the pain. Temporary aggravation may also be quite different from any long-term effect. To use the sports analogy again, training may cause temporary musculoskeletal aches but lead to long-term benefit. Moreover, patients' perception of physical activity and its relation to pain is often inaccurate. Several studies have shown that patients with back pain over-estimate the physical demands of their job compared with healthy fellow workers. Patients tend to over-predict the pain they will get on exercise. Treadmill endurance of patients with chronic low back pain is only 75% that of normal controls (Schmidt 1985). However, this form of exercise does not increase their pain. Both groups rate their exertion similarly, but the patients with back pain actually show lower levels of physiologic demand. They stop because they over-estimate their exertion rather than because of increased pain. Exercise to the limit of pain tolerance is very dependent on feedback. In the absence of feedback, chronic pain patients increase their performance on an incremented exercise program at the same rate as normal, pain-free subjects. Fear avoidance beliefs may start from the experience of pain and physical activity, but all the evidence suggests that those fear avoidance beliefs then develop a life of their own which may diverge greatly from reality.

The crucial point is that fear of pain is more about expectancy of future pain than about current reality. Avoidance behavior may reduce nociception at the acute stage. Later, these avoidance behaviors may persist in anticipation of pain rather than as a response to it. If we do not attempt the activity and do not have increased pain, then we may be given a false reinforcement. There is no need for any external reinforcement to maintain the behavior.

Here are some of the things which other patients have told us about their pain. For each statement please circle any number from 0 to 6 to say how much physical activities such as bending, lifting, walking or driving affect or would affect *your* back pain.

		COMPLETELY DISAGREE		UNSURE			COMPLETELY AGREE	
1	My pain was caused by physical activity	0	1	2	3	4	5	6
2	Physical activity makes my pain worse	0	1	2	3	4	5	6
3	Physical activity might harm my back	0	1	2	3	4	5	6
4	I should not do physical activities which (might) make my pain worse	0	1	2	3	4	5	6
5	I cannot do physical activities which (might) make my pain worse	0	1	2	3	4	5	6

The following statements are about how your normal work affects or would affect your back pain.

		COMPLETELY DISAGREE		UNSURE			COMPLETELY AGREE	
6	My pain was caused by my work or by an accident at work	0	1	2	3	4	5	6
7	My work aggravated my pain	0	1	2	3	4	5	6
8	I have a claim for compensation for my pain	0	1	2	3	4	5	6
9	My work is too heavy for me	0	1	2	3	4	5	6
10	My work makes or would make my pain worse	0	1	2	3	4	5	6
11	My work might harm my back	0	1	2	3	4	5	6
12	I should not do my normal work with my present pain	0	1	2	3	4	5	6
13	I cannot do my normal work with my present pain	0	1	2	3	4	5	6
14	I cannot do my normal work until my pain is treated	0	1	2	3	4	5	6
15	I do not think that I will be back to my normal work within 3 months	0	1	2	3	4	5	6
16	I do not think that I will ever be able to go back to that work	0	1	2	3	4	5	6

Figure 12.3 The Fear Avoidance Beliefs Questionnaire (Waddell et al 1993).

Avoidance behavior itself reinforces fear avoidance beliefs in a vicious circle. It is like the dog that barks every time the postman appears. The postman never has and never will break into the house, but the dog believes that is because it has chased him away. The very fact that the threat never materializes encourages the dog to go on barking.

Table 12.1 The influence of pain and fear avoidance beliefs on disability (based on data from Waddell et al 1993)

	Disability in activities of daily living	Work loss
Pain		
Anatomic pattern ⎫		
Time pattern ⎬	14%	5%
Severity ⎭		
Fear avoidance beliefs	+ 32%	+ 26%
Total identified	56%	31%

These are the additive effects, after allowing for severity of pain. It is usually only possible to identify a modest proportion of any biologic relationship.

The fear may not be only of pain itself but more specifically of reinjury (Vlaeyen et al 1995). The patient wrongly assumes that movement, physical activity and work may cause (re)injury. It is always difficult to restart physical activity or work after a lay-off. The longer the lay-off, the greater the loss of physical fitness and the worse the disuse syndrome, the harder it will be. Return to work may then lead to some temporary increase in low back pain. Unfortunately, this reinforces fear avoidance beliefs. If the patient stops work again, this failure will strongly reinforce fear avoidance beliefs. Fear avoidance beliefs about work are most important in patients with work-related back pain and compensation claims.

The effect of fear avoidance beliefs

From the fear avoidance model (Fig. 12.2), Lethem et al (1983) described patients as 'confronters' or 'avoiders'. Confronters may have severe pain, but they have little fear of pain. They remain positive and confident and able to confront their pain. They gradually increase their activities even if they have some temporary aggravation of pain. They gain confidence in their ability to cope with the pain and to maintain daily activities despite some pain. Success reinforces their beliefs and ability to cope. Avoiders have similar pain, but they also have a strong fear of pain. This leads them to avoid activities that are painful, or which they think may be painful. Indeed, they do everything possible to avoid the experience of pain, fearing

reinjury and fearing that pain means further damage. They rest a lot and wait for the pain to get better. Avoidance behavior, however, maintains and exacerbates fear, which may even become a phobia.

Vlaeyen et al (1995) found that patients who were afraid of reinjury showed more fear and avoidance behavior when they were asked to do a simple movement. Fear of movement and reinjury was more closely linked to depressive symptoms and catastrophizing than to pain itself. Klenerman et al (1995) studied 300 patients attending their family doctor with acute low back pain, and found that fear avoidance beliefs at the acute stage predicted outcome at 2 and 12 months. Some patients ignored their pain, carried on and took physical exercise, while others took analgesics and rested. Those who used the more active coping strategies had less pain and disability and sick leave at 2 and 12 months. Klenerman et al showed that fear avoidance beliefs are important at the acute stage, and not just in chronic pain and disability.

Fear avoidance of physical activity and exercise is one of the major barriers to physical therapy and rehabilitation.

There are many aspects to fear:

- Beliefs about injury and damage
- Pain and fear; expectations and fear of future pain and reinjury
- The assumption that hurt means harm
- Fear avoidance: 'confronters' and 'avoiders'
- Increased pain behavior and disability
- Barriers to rehabilitation

Personal responsibility and control

Psychologists have shown that from early childhood, one of the main goals of the infant is to try to gain some control over his or her environment. The attempt to reduce uncertainty and establish control seems to be one of the most fundamental human drives. One of the key aspects of personality is the strength of this drive and the balance between our personal needs for control and the needs of others. These beliefs are probably not innate, but more likely a product of learning and social conditioning. The human arena is one of potential conflict. In rearing children, every parent has to find the right balance between affection and nurturing on the one hand, and the imposition of control on the other. If our needs are frustrated we become angry and unsettled, and try to impose control. Our self-confidence is related in part to the extent to which we have established sufficient control over our environment to meet our needs. We also differ in our tolerance of lack of control. Sometimes the socialization process goes drastically wrong. At one end of the scale are people so ruthless in their attempts to impose control that they disregard totally the needs of others. Many such people end up in prison. At the other end of the scale are people who are desperately shy and withdrawn, with no confidence in trying to assert any control over their environment.

As a result of this life experience, we all form beliefs about the extent to which we are able to get control of our lives. At one extreme are those who are totally fatalistic and who believe that they are powerless to affect their own future. They are passive and wait for life or other people, including health professionals, to take control for them. They believe that their lives and the affairs of men are determined by fate or the position of the planets and that all their actions are predetermined – it does not matter what they do, the die is already cast. At the other extreme are those who believe that they can and indeed must exercise control over every aspect of their lives. They are hell-bent on establishing control. Not only do they have

confidence that they can establish control, but they try at every opportunity to do it, and become various sorts of 'power freaks'. If they transgress the norms of society, they will be locked up. If they manage to stay within the law and manipulate the system satisfactorily, they become powerful and successful. Some of them become doctors! We might describe these extremes as being either *externally* or *internally* controlled.

Of course, it is easy to caricature such personality types. Most people fall somewhere in between. But this concept of control has an important influence on how people react to adversity and illness (Williams & Keefe 1991, Jensen et al 1994). In particular, it influences how people seek and respond to treatment. *Internals* seek less health care, and respond well to management approaches in which they can play an active part, whereas *externals* seek more health care, and are more likely to rely on health professionals to make them better.

Clinical impression and psychologic studies suggest that patients who accept personal responsibility for their pain do better than those who leave it to 'others'. Those who feel it is entirely up to doctors or therapists or someone else to cure them do worse. Accepting personal responsibility is closely allied to feelings of control. People who feel in control of their own destiny are more able to take responsibility for their own health and do better than those who feel that they cannot do much about it.

Gaining control over back pain means actually mastering the pain and associated disability. The ability to do this is largely dependent upon the individual's own judgement of their capabilities as shown in Sandstrom & Esbjornsson's (1986) study. Psychologists call this a lack of 'self-efficacy', where self-efficacy is the belief that you can *successfully* gain control and mastery. People are more likely to attempt and complete activities that they believe they are able to do. We do not attempt the daily tasks that constitute low back disability without thinking about it first. We evaluate the task, our own ability and our fear of possible pain or harm. This inner debate largely predetermines our performance, when we decide to stop, or whether we decide even to try. Lackner et al (1996) showed that patients with chronic low back pain predicted quite accurately their performance at a set of lifting, carrying, pushing and pulling tasks. Indeed, patients' own rating of their expected ability was more closely related to their performance than pain, fear of pain or fear of reinjury. Estlander et al (1994) found that back patients' beliefs in their ability to endure physical activity were the best predictor of isokinetic performance. Anthropometric measures, pain and disability levels were all less important. Hildebrandt et al (1997) found the same in a multidisciplinary treatment program. They asked patients before the program if they believed that it would enable them to return to work after discharge. Poor expectations were one of the strongest predictors of failure to return to work (Table 12.2).

People who regard themselves as capable have more confidence in their own ability. They try harder, they persevere despite their symptoms, and they show fewer signs of anxiety. People who regard themselves as less able do not try as hard, are less persistent, get frustrated, and give up more easily. They show more distress and they do not cooperate as well with treatment and advice. Patients with strong beliefs in their own abilities commit themselves more firmly to their tasks and are more highly motivated to complete them despite temporary setbacks. They also function better psychologically and show less distress.

Many of the beliefs described in previous sections may influence patients' estimates of what they can do, but the research described here suggests that patients' own expectations of what they can do may be one of the most powerful and direct psychologic mechanisms to influence performance. People with high self-efficacy are more confident in their ability to achieve control of their pain, and live up to their own expectations.

Beliefs about treatment

Beliefs about health care and the outcome of treatment are also extremely important (DeGood & Shutty 1992, Main & Benjamin 1995). Patients vary widely in their expectations. One patient may arrive with a straightforward and realistic expectation, while another may believe that their spine is crumbling, that they will end up in a wheelchair, and that noone can do anything to prevent it. You should always try to find out what the patient expects in terms of treatment and its likely outcome. These beliefs about treatment obviously depend also on what the patient believes about the nature and cause of his or her pain. You must correct misunderstandings, if the patient is to accept and benefit from treatment. You must also give a clear and honest account of the range of possible treatment options. Do not be tempted into offering second-rate treatment simply because the patient is distressed and you feel sorry for him or her. Patients must have realistic expectations of treatment if they are to make sensible choices and not be disappointed. Patients and health professionals must share the same beliefs and expectations concerning treatment if they are to work in harmony to a common goal. This is also one of the keys to satisfaction with care.

Table 12.2 The impact of patients' beliefs about return to work on the outcome of a multidisciplinary treatment program (based on data from Hildebrandt et al 1997)

	Outcome of program	
	Did return to work	Did not return to work
Beliefs before treatment:		
Will return to work	31 (81%)	7
Will not return to work	12 (46%)	14

THE NATURE OF COPING

Coping refers to the way in which we deal with problems. More precisely, coping strategies are the purposeful mental efforts we make to manage or reduce the impact of stress (Lazarus & Folkman 1984). We try to prevent problems from taxing or exceeding our resources and endangering our mental well-being. People cope with stress or adversity, or pain, in many different ways. Broadly speaking, coping strategies are used either to confront (in an attempt to deal with) the stress, or to try to escape from or avoid the situation. *Problem-focused* coping aims to control the pain, e.g. by avoiding situations or activities that cause or increase the pain, or by doing things that reduce it. *Emotion-focused* coping aims to reduce its emotional impact, e.g. by avoiding thinking about the pain or trying to distract one's attention from it. This does not mean that we only use one or other kind of coping strategy exclusively. We all use varying combinations of problem-focused and emotion-focused strategies to cope.

In theory, the most effective coping strategy is to avoid a stressful situation entirely. For example, it may be possible to avoid certain activities that cause or aggravate back pain. Such 'accommodation' can be thought of as a set of successful coping strategies, based essentially on avoidance. Unfortunately, avoidance is not always possible or may have a cost, and sometimes the cost is high. You may try to reduce aggravations of back pain by avoiding lifting, but that may cost you your job. If sitting is painful, you may avoid travel and a wide range of social situations, but that will significantly impair your quality of life. Avoiding sex lest it increase back pain may put strain on a valued relationship. The balance of costs and benefits of avoidance is a matter for the individual. It depends on the person's circumstances and needs. If avoidance causes too much disruption to family life or work, other coping strategies will be required. In fact, back patients employ a wide range of behaviors and coping strategies to limit the effects of pain. Much coping may be 'trial and error', based on advice from friends, relatives or health professionals. The choice of strategy will be based on the patient's understanding of the problem. As we discussed previously, the strategies people choose depend on their beliefs about the pain, its cause, and its likely outcome. This choice also depends on their confidence in being able to influence events, and their repertoire of coping skills and behaviors.

Coping with back pain

Most people with back pain, even chronic pain, cope with the pain, adjust and continue to lead more or less normal lives. Chronic pain is not synonymous with disability and depression. So how is it that some people cope with the pain successfully while others become disabled? What are the different mental strategies they use to cope with the stress (Jensen et al 1991)?

Coping strategies may be active or passive (Snow-Turek et al 1996). Active coping strategies are positive attempts to manage the pain, e.g. exercising, staying active and ignoring the pain. Passive strategies succumb to the pain, e.g. withdrawal, giving up control, rest and analgesics. Active coping strategies help to reduce pain, depression and disability, whereas passive strategies are associated with increased pain, depression and disability. Passive coping strategies also predict poorer outcomes over time.

The most widely used measure of coping is the *Coping Strategies Questionnaire* (Fig. 12.4; Rosensteil & Keefe 1983). This shows that the most harmful coping strategy in patients with back pain is catastrophizing, which is negative and distorted thinking and worrying about the pain and one's inability to cope — 'fearing the worst.' This may be clearer in some examples from the *Coping Strategies Questionnaire*:

'It is terrible and I feel it is never going to get any better.'
'It is awful and it overwhelms me.'
'I worry all the time about whether it will end.'
'I feel I can't stand it any more.'
'I feel like I can't go on.'

There are complex links between beliefs, coping strategies and pain behavior (Williams

---

Cognitive coping strategies

1. *Diverting attention*: thinking of things that serve to distract one away from the pain.
   Sample item: I count in my head or run a song through my head.

2. *Reinterpreting pain sensations*: imagining something which, if real, would be inconsistent with the experience of pain.
   Sample item: I just think of it as some other sensation, such as numbness.

3. *Coping self-statements*: telling oneself that one can cope with pain, no matter how bad it gets.
   Sample item: I tell myself to be brave and carry on despite the pain.

4. *Ignoring pain sensation*: denying that pain hurts or affects one in any way.
   Sample item: I tell myself it doesn't hurt.

5. *Praying or hoping*: telling myself to hope and pray that the pain will get better someday.
   Sample item: I pray to God that it won't last.

6. *Catastrophizing*: negative self-statements, catastrophizing thoughts and ideation.
   Sample item: I worry all the time about whether it will end.

Behavioral coping strategies

1. *Increasing activity level*: engaging in active behaviors which divert one's attention away from pain.
   Sample item: I do something active, like household chores or projects.

2. *Increasing pain behavior*: overt pain behaviors that reduce pain sensations.
   Sample item: I take my medication.

Effectiveness ratings

1. Control over pain

2. Ability to decrease pain

Figure 12.4 The Coping Strategies Questionnaire. (From Rosenstiel & Keefe 1983, with permission.)

& Keefe 1991, Jensen et al 1994). Beliefs frame our mental image of the pain problem; they have a direct effect on mood and may lead to depression. They also affect how we try to cope. Coping strategies are the mental and psychologic links between beliefs and behavior. A sense of personal control and self-efficacy are associated with positive and active coping strategies and better mental adjustment. Negative thoughts and coping strategies lead to maladaptive behavior. They impair psychologic and physical adjustment to pain and increase chronic pain and illness behavior. Lack of personal control and feelings of helplessness are associated with passive coping strategies and catastrophizing. Catastrophizing is closely related to depressive symptoms and is maladaptive: it is irrational and harmful and leads to psychologic and physical dysfunction.

Widely differing beliefs and coping strategies help to explain the very different outcomes of back pain. People tend to cope either quite well or quite badly. People who catastrophize do particularly badly. This fits with clinical experience that most people cope well with low back pain and get on with their lives more or less normally despite the pain. A few become chronic back cripples from simple backache.

Conclusions about beliefs and coping

There is currently a huge amount of research into the relationship between beliefs and coping styles, and adjustment to pain and disability. Much of this psychologic research is quite technical and there is a lot of overlap between, and confusion about, different questionnaires. Despite this, there is emerging agreement on a number of key themes:

- Beliefs about pain and coping strategies can influence not only the perception of pain but adjustment to it.

- Such beliefs derive from a wide variety of sources.
- Patients often get 'mixed messages' from health care providers.
- Patients may develop mistaken beliefs about back pain and treatment.
- Such beliefs can be thought of as 'obstacles to treatment'.
- Some coping strategies are more useful or effective than others.
- Individuals differ in their adoption of coping strategies.
- Much disability is psychologically mediated and therefore preventable.
- Cognitive therapy focuses specifically on mistaken beliefs and for some patients is the best way to help them manage their back pain.
- A combination of cognitive and behavioral coping strategies may offer a powerful therapeutic alternative to the traditional medical approach.

HOW BELIEFS AFFECT HEALTH CARE

Beliefs about back pain determine what we do about it, including whether we seek health care and how we respond to treatment (DeGood & Shutty 1992).

There are some common threads to most of these beliefs and coping strategies for dealing with back pain. At one end of the spectrum are people with back pain who are not unduly concerned about it. Although they have pain, which may be persistent or recurring, they do not believe it is a serious problem. They have little fear and are not worried about its long-term consequences. They believe it is up to them to deal with the problem, they take control, and they get on with their lives despite the pain. They seek relatively little health care. If they do decide to see a doctor to make sure there is nothing seriously wrong, we can reassure them relatively easily. They then only seek health care occasionally for help to control more acute episodes or for short-term sick certification. At the other end of the spectrum are patients

whose back pain is a serious problem that takes over their attention and their lives. They are convinced it is due to some serious disease which noone has yet been able to identify. They are dominated by fear. They are pessimistic about the future, believing they will continue to have back pain indefinitely and that it will inevitably disable them. They feel that it is all out of their control, there is nothing they can do about it, and it is up to health professionals to find out what is wrong and to cure them. They catastrophize. They show avoidance behavior. Their beliefs and coping strategies are closely linked to depression, and depression in turn distorts their beliefs and makes them even more pessimistic and helpless.

Modern patients, like most doctors and therapists, generally start from the belief that pain is a warning signal that something is wrong with their bodies. If it is severe or if it does not settle, we believe we should seek health care to diagnose and treat the underlying problem. That is an appropriate response to trauma or acute illness. However, if our expectations of diagnosis and cure are not met, fear soon appears. It then turns to anger and depression as we begin to feel a loss of control over the course of our lives. These beliefs are not simply a product of the chronic pain experience which will disappear once we get the correct diagnosis or treatment. Rather, beliefs about the pain, its course, its likely impact on our lives, and the prospects for getting adequate help lie at the heart of the chronic pain problem.

One of the most striking features of some patients with chronic pain is their maladaptive beliefs about the diagnosis and treatment of their pain. Despite repeated negative investigations, they still demand more tests in their desperate search for a 'cause' for their pain. Despite multiple failed treatments, they are still pathetically ready to undergo more of the same, even if there is little realistic hope that it will help. Indeed, their own experience may show that it is more likely to make them worse. Such wishful thinking may be an understandable result of their desperation, but such beliefs and behavior are maladaptive. They are unrealistic and harmful, and they trap these patients into a hopeless cycle of treatment, preventing them from seeking a more realistic and effective approach.

HOW HEALTH CARE INFLUENCES BELIEFS ABOUT BACK PAIN

The information and advice we give to our patients can have a profound effect on their beliefs. Too often, this effect is negative. The harmful effect of medical 'labeling' was first shown in hypertension. A population survey detected people with asymptomatic hypertension. Before the survey they were unaware of their condition, had no symptoms and were not ill. After the survey told them they had hypertension, they developed symptoms and became ill. There was no change in their blood pressure, but labeling them sick made them ill and turned them into patients.

There is now some evidence that is equally true in back pain. Tarasuk & Eakin (1994) explored how workers' sense of permanent vulnerability in their back was related to their health care. Many of these patients' beliefs seemed to come from, or at least be reinforced by, health care professionals. This was partly due to the information and advice they received: 'Your back is injured, it is damaged, and it could be reinjured. You should avoid those activities that might cause reinjury.' Unfortunately, these activities often included daily activities and work. Some of the messages were more subtle. Medical uncertainty and the absence of a definite diagnosis or prognosis cast doubt on the possibility of full recovery. Conflicting opinions and treatments implied that noone would be able to find the answer. Advice to change your lifestyle and even your job means that your back will permanently change your life. Rose et al (1998, unpublished data) found that medical advice and information, and disagreement between health professionals, seemed to contribute to fear avoidance beliefs and pessimism about future recovery.

Deyo & Diehl (1986) found that patients' most frequent reason for dissatisfaction with medical care was failure to receive an adequate explanation for their back pain. Fifteen per cent of patients did not believe that the doctors and nurses understood their pain problem. Patients who felt that their explanation was inadequate wanted more diagnostic tests, did not cooperate as well with treatment and had poorer outcomes at 3 weeks.

Think about what we tell patients with simple backache, for example, if the lumbar spine X-rays show normal age-related changes: 'You have wear and tear in your spine or degenerate disc disease.' To the patient, this means serious deterioration; it is irreversible, and will continue to deteriorate as they get older. If I am like this now what will I be like in 10 years? Will I end up in a wheelchair? It is no use then saying, 'But it is nothing to worry about.' The damage is done. We have labeled them with a disease that may make them ill.

Our advice on management is just as bad. Too often, the implicit message we give is: 'Pain is a signal that you are damaging your back and that you should stop whatever you are doing. The treatment is rest. Rest until it gets better.' This kind of advice leads directly to fear of reinjury, fear avoidance and avoidance behavior. And then we are surprised at our patients' beliefs? It is too late then to tell them to stop worrying and that it is time to get active again.

Health professionals are also guilty of taking over. Patients bring their problems to us and we take responsibility for diagnosis and treatment. Unfortunately we have no magic cure for backache, but we take over anyway. Instead of advising patients on how they themselves can best deal with their problem, we prescribe our treatment. If the patient gets better, there is no problem, but if he or she does not get better quite quickly he or she is trapped. Instead of patients taking responsibility and coping with their own situation, they have handed over responsibility, lost control and now wait helplessly to be 'fixed', with all the negative effects on disability and outcomes.

All doctors and therapists should be much more conscious of how what we say may affect our patients' beliefs and their ability to cope with back pain. This may be more important than any direct effect of our advice on their physical condition.

There are several good examples of how information and advice about back pain can have more positive and helpful effects on patients' beliefs. Symonds et al (1995) gave a simple pamphlet to workers in an industrial setting. They designed the pamphlet to shift beliefs by simple messages: 'Back pain is not usually a serious problem. Continued back pain is not inevitable. Most people can take care of it themselves.' This pamphlet produced a large and positive shift in beliefs about the inevitability of back pain and ability to control their pain. It was most effective in workers with no previous history of low back pain. People with previous experience of low back trouble may require more powerful persuasion to shift their beliefs. These changed beliefs led to a 60% reduction in extended sickness due to back pain.

Dolce et al (1986a,b) showed that exercise quotas increase exercise performance and expectancies of exercise capability while reducing anxiety about exercise. Newton et al (1993) found that an isokinetic exercise program reduced patients' fears and improved their confidence in their own abilities. These changes in beliefs occurred faster and may be more important than any physiologic effect.

Many studies in the United States and Europe have shown that pain management programs can improve beliefs about pain control and self-efficacy, and reduce distress and disability in patients with chronic pain (Flor et al 1992).

All this clinical evidence suggests that patients' beliefs and ability to cope play a very important role in low back pain and disability, and may form a major barrier to recovery (Fig. 12.5). Tackling and overcoming harmful beliefs and improving a patient's own ability to cope are key elements in management. We should perhaps target our information and advice to patients more at these goals, rather than thinking that it is all about physical management. We should have more faith in the power of human thought and in our patients' own capabilities. Beliefs *can* move mountains.

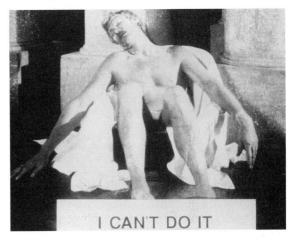

Figure 12.5 'I can't do it.'

REFERENCES

Carosella A-M, Lackner J M, Feuerstein M 1994 Factors associated with early discharge from a multidisciplinary work rehabilitation program for chronic low back pain. Pain 57: 69–76

DeGood D E, Shutty M S 1992 Assessment of pain beliefs, coping and self-efficacy. In: Turk D C, Melzack R (eds) Handbook of pain assessment. Guilford Press, New York, ch 13, p 214–234

Dehlin O, Berg S, Andersson G B J, Grimby G 1981 Effect of physical training and ergonomic counselling on the psychological perception of work and on the subjective assessment of low back insufficiency. Scandinavian Journal of Rehabilitation Medicine 13: 1–9

Deyo R A, Diehl A K 1986 Patient satisfaction with medical care for low back pain. Spine 11: 28–30

Dolce J J, Crocker M F, Moletteire C, Doleys D M 1986a

Exercise quotas, anticipatory concern and self-efficacy expectancies in chronic pain: a preliminary report. Pain 24: 365–372

Dolce J J, Doleys D M, Raczynski J M, Lossie J, Poole L, Smith M 1986b The role of self-efficacy expectancies in the prediction of pain tolerance. Pain 27: 261–272

Estlander A-M, Vanharanta H, Moneta G B, Kaivanto K 1994 Anthropetric variables, self-efficacy beliefs, and pain and disabilty ratings on the isometric performance of low back pain patients. Spine 19: 941–947

Feuerstein M 1991 A multidisciplinary approach to the prevention, evaluation and management of work disability. Journal of Occupational Rehabilitation 1: 5–12

Flor H, Fydrich T, Turk D C 1992 Efficacy of multidisciplinary pain treatment centers: a meta-analytic review. Pain 49: 221–230

Hildebrandt J, Pfingsten M, Saur P, Jansen J 1997 Prediction of success from a multidisciplinary treatment program for chronic low back pain. Spine 22: 990–1001

Jensen M P, Turner J A, Romano J M, Karoly P 1991 Coping with chronic pain: a critical review of the literature. Pain 47: 249–283

Jensen M P, Turner J A, Romano J M, Lawler B K 1994 Relationship of pain-specific beliefs to chronic pain adjustment. Pain 57: 301–309

Klenerman L, Slade P D, Stenley I M et al 1995 The prediction of chronicity in patients with an acute attack of low back pain in a general practice setting. Spine 20: 478–484

Lackner J M, Carosella A M, Feuerstein M 1996 Pain expectancies, pain, and functional self-efficacy expectancies as determinants of disability in patients with chronic low back disorders. Journal of Consulting Clinical Psychology 64: 212–220

Lazarus R A, Folkman S 1984 Stress, appraisal & coping. Springer, New York

Lethem J, Slade P D, Troup J D G, Bentley G 1983 Outline of a fear avoidance model of exaggerated pain perception. Behavioral Research and Therapy 21: 401–408

Main C J, Benjamin S 1995 Psychological treatment and the health care system; the chaotic case of back pain. Is there a need for a paradigm shift? In: Mayou R, Bass C Sharpe (eds) Treatment of functional somatic symptoms. Oxford University Press, Oxford, ch 12, p 214–230

Newton M, Thow M, Somerville D, Henderson I, Waddell G 1993 Trunk strength testing with iso-machines. Part II. Experimental evaluation of the Cybex II Back Testing System in normal subjects and patients with chronic low back pain. Spine 18: 812–824

Philips H C 1987 Avoidance learning and its role in sustaining chronic pain. Behavioral Research and Therapy 25: 273–279

Rosenstiel A K, Keefe F J 1983 The use of coping strategies in chronic low back pain patients: relationship to patient characteristics and current adjustment. Pain 17: 33–44

Sandstrom J, Esbjornsson E 1986 Return to work after rehabilitation. The significance of the patient's own prediction. Scandinavian Journal of Rehabilitation Medicine 18: 29–33

Schmidt A J 1985 Cognitive factors in the performance level of chronic low back pain patients. Journal of Psychosomatic Research 29: 183–189

Snow-Turek A L, Norris M P, Tan G 1996 Active and passive coping strategies in chronic pain patients. Pain 64: 455–462

Symonds T L, Burton A K, Tillotson K M, Main C J 1996 Do attitudes and beliefs influence work loss due to low back pain? Occupational Medicine 48: 3–10

Symonds T L, Burton A K, Tillotson K M, Main C J 1995 Absence resulting from low back trouble can be reduced by psychosocial intervention at the work place. Spine 20: 2738–2745

Szpalski M, Nordin M, Skovron M L, Melot C, Cukier D 1995 Health care utilization for low back pain in Belgium. Influence of sociocultural factors and health beliefs. Spine 20: 431–442

Tarasuk V, Eakin J M 1994 Back problems are for life: perceived vulnerability and its implications for chronic disability. Journal of Occupational Rehabilitation 4: 55–64

Troup J D G, Foreman T K, Baxter C E, Brown D 1987 The perception of back pain and the role of psychophysical tests of lifting capacity. Spine 12: 645–657

Turk D C, Okifuji A, Starz T W, Sinclair J D 1996 Effects of type of symptom onset on psychological distress and disability in fibromyalgia syndrome patients. Pain 68: 423–430

Vlaeyen J W S, Kole-Snijders A M J, Boeren R G B, van Eek H 1995 Fear of movement/(re)injury in chronic low back pain and its relation to behavioral performance. Pain 62: 363–372

Waddell G, Somerville D, Henderson I, Newton M, Main C J 1993 A fear avoidance beliefs questionnaire (FABQ) and the role of fear avoidance beliefs in chronic low back pain and disability. Pain 52: 157–168

Williams D A, Keefe F J 1991 Pain beliefs and the use of cognitive-behavioral coping strategies. Pain 46: 185–190

13

Social interactions

Aristotle, in the 4th century BC, recognized that 'man is by nature a social animal', and laid out the principles of social influence and persuasion. We live and act, and fall ill and die, in concert with our fellow man – and woman. Our whole lives take place in the context of human society. Social interactions are the stuff of drama and tragedy. The poet John Donne put it simply: 'No man is an island'.

It is not possible to be truly human except as an integrated member of society. A human child raised in isolation is not truly human. He will look human, and will have the same mental abilities, but he will simply not have learned to *be* human. He will not be able to talk or communicate with his own kind, and literally will not know how to act or behave like a human being. We start with a clean slate, with great potential abilities but few innate skills or instinctive knowledge. It is our capacity to learn through an extended childhood that lets us acquire the knowledge and experience of past generations to take our place in human society. This social and cultural heritage has let the human race evolve over the last 10 000 years far faster than any possible biologic change. The need to learn means that our social and cultural milieu has a powerful influence on how we think, what we believe and how we behave (see Box 13.1).

This is also true with illness and pain and back pain. Social influences apply as in every other human activity (Skevington 1995). The biologic imperatives of diseases such as cancer may set the physical limits of health and death,

---

Box 13.1   Social influences

- Culture
- Family
- Nurture
- Learning
- Social context
- Social support

---

but even then there is much scope for how we behave when we are ill and even for the manner of our dying. With a much more subjective experience such as back pain, there is even greater scope for what we do about it. The less clear and more frightening the experience, the greater the social influences on how we think and behave: 'When reality is unclear, other people become a major source of information' (Aronson 1984).

SOCIAL INFLUENCES

Culture

Zborowski (1952) made the classic observation of how ethnic background affects the expression of pain. He studied 103 patients – all men – in a US veterans hospital; 87 had chronic pain, mainly spinal. He compared 31 men of Jewish background, 24 Italians, 11 Irish and 26 'old Americans', who might best be described as WASPs (white Anglo-Saxon protestants). Pain threshold is more or less the same irrespective of nationality, sex or age, but Zborowski observed that these different groups expressed their pain in very different ways. Italians and Jews showed a more 'emotional' response. They gave free expression to their feelings in words, sounds and gestures, and were not ashamed of this, wanting support and company. However, their underlying concerns varied. The Italians' main concern was about their present pain and its immediate impact. They wanted analgesics and had faith in doctors. The Jews' main concern was about the meaning of the pain and its effect on their future. They refused analgesics, were sceptical of doctors, and pessimistic about the future. The old Americans simply 'reported' their pain and did not express their emotions.

They were concerned with the meaning of the pain. They were very health conscious, though in a mechanistic sense, and optimistic about a 'fix'. They behaved well as patients and cooperated with the treatment team but tended to withdraw from intimate contact.

These patterns of behavior varied with the degree of Americanization, socioeconomic background, education, religion and occupation. Zborowski thought that culture had more effect on attitudes and beliefs about pain, but that individual background and peer pressure had more effect on actual behavior.

Looking at very different cultures shows the importance of this kind of social and cultural learning on pain and illness behavior even more dramatically. Honeyman & Jacobs (1996) studied back pain in Australian aboriginals (Fig. 13.1). On close questioning, nearly one-third of the men and half the women admitted to long-term back pain, although it was difficult to assess. They kept their pain 'private', not communicating it to others or seeking health care. In that society, there are strong cultural pressures about tolerating and not displaying pain. This is reflected in painful and mutilating initiation rights.

Volinn (1997) recently reviewed surveys of back pain in different countries. In most high-income countries, such as the United States and Europe, the annual prevalence of back pain is about 20–40%. In low-income countries, urban populations have a comparable level of 23–35%, but rural populations only report 7–18%. This is despite the much harder and more physically demanding life of rural workers. However, selected groups of workers in 'enclosed workshops' in low- and middle-income countries report a prevalence of 38–68%. There are a lot of problems with such studies across different languages and cultures. It is difficult to know if the questions are exactly the same or how different cultures choose to answer. These surveys tell us more about how different groups *report* their pain than about the physical condition of their backs or the neurophysiology of their pain. Even so, urbanization and rapid industrialization seem to be associated with increased reports of back pain.

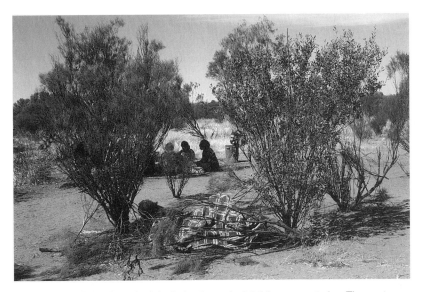

Figure 13.1 Australian aboriginals lead very 'public' lives even today. They get back pain but it is 'private' and they do not express or communicate their pain.

In summary, back pain is common to all societies, but different cultural groups do not perceive or respond to this pain in the same way. There is cultural variation in attitudes, expectations, and the meanings we attach to pain. Distress levels vary. Culture influences how we express pain and emotions, our pain behavior, and whether and how we communicate our pain to others, including health professionals. It affects how we seek and respond to treatment. However, there is a risk to this kind of ethnic stereotyping. Cultural patterns are not fixed but fluid. Zborowski (1952) found that as his different groups became Americanized, they changed their attitudes and behavioral patterns to conform to their new society. Stereotyping also ignores the great individual variation in learning and experience about pain and illness within each cultural group.

Social context

Beecher (1959) first pointed out how the context of pain influences its meaning. He observed that battle casualties on the Anzio beachhead in World War II seemed to need very little analgesia for serious injuries compared with civilian casualties. He suggested that their injuries represented an honorable escape from danger and stress, and so caused less pain and distress than a civilian 'accident'. I must confess to some doubt about this classic observation. In my experience, most road traffic accident victims with serious injuries do not require much analgesia at the acute stage either. However, once again, this may simply reflect my particular clinical situation and expectations.

Torstensen (1996) looked at back pain in top Norwegian athletes, comparing them with chronic low back pain patients in the general population. About 10% of all athletic injuries involve the

Table 13.1 A comparison between top athletes with back pain and chronic back pain patients in the general population (from Vikne 1996 and Torstensen 1996, with permission)

	Top athletes	Chronic LBP patients in the general population
Age	15–30 years	Peak 40 years
Higher education	52%	13%
Smokers	12%	54%
Physical activity	100% enjoy physical activity and feel physically healthy	9% physically active; 90% unsatisfied with their physical health

spine, but 25–40% of these are serious problems such as fractures or spondylolysis. Chronic disability due to a simple back strain is rare in athletes. Even among elite soccer players who get frequent musculoskeletal injuries, low back disability is almost unknown.

Patients with chronic low back pain and disability in the general population present a very different picture (Table 13.1):

- 74% do strenuous physical work
- 59% are unsatisfied with their work
- 30% want to change their work
- 55% are dissatisfied with their leisure activities
- 38% are generally dissatisfied with their lives.

Athletes, on the other hand, love their sport and are highly motivated to get back to it as fast as possible. They seem to have very different expectations about back pain and what they should do about it. They also receive very different health care (Table 13.2).

The outcomes and impact of back pain in these two groups are very different. Many factors play a part: what people think and do about it; their whole social situation; and their health care. However, we should not over-interpret this example. This was a very selected group of elite athletes and also a very selected group of workers with chronic pain and disability. Most workers with back pain also recover quite rapidly. Suffice it to say that even in a homogeneous ethnic and cultural group, the social setting can affect attitudes to back pain and the development of chronic disability.

We all know the importance of the social context of pain and illness from our own experience. We have all had a bad cold or flu. If your partner asks you to do a household chore you have been putting off for a while, your symptoms feel worse and you do not feel up to it. When you are watching an exciting ball game on television, however, your symptoms make a magic, if temporary, recovery. Even my dog responds the same way. She recently had a sore paw. When the family were all concerned, examining her leg and patting her, she limped around the room on three legs. Real pathetic. However, when I offered the command 'walk' she rushed to the door without a trace of a limp. On the walk the limp gradually reappeared as she tired, but never so dramatically as in the family setting. It is perfectly normal for pain and illness behavior to vary with social context.

Social learning

Obviously, we must learn this kind of social behavior. It is part of socialization and growing up. We probably learn it mostly in childhood, both consciously and unconsciously. As in most social learning, the family is the first and most powerful learning situation. Balague et al (1995) looked at how school children report pain. There is little evidence that family background actually affects the occurrence of back pain, but it does seem to influence children's attitudes,

Table 13.2 Organization of health care for top athletes and the general population with back pain in Norway (after Torstensen 1996, with permission)

General population	Top athletes
Weak organization, 15 minute GP assessment	Good organization, medical team
Waiting lists for treatment	Immediate access
Poor communication between health professionals	Good communication within team
Health professionals focus on symptomatic treatment. Little interest or focus on rehabilitation or return to work?	Health professionals highly motivated to rehabilitate and retrain
Common goal – return to work??	Athlete and professionals share common goal of return to sport as rapidly as possible

reporting of symptoms and behavior. As we grow up, our social peer groups may become equally or even more influential.

There are three interrelated processes to learning or changing social behavior (Aronson 1984):

- communication
- feedback
- conforming.

All social intercourse depends on communication and humans have the richest means of communication of any animal. The most sophisticated is language, and linguistic studies cast light on each culture's views of pain and its expression. Sayings such as 'the backbone of ...' or 'a pain in the neck' reflect cultural beliefs about the spine and spinal pain. Nonverbal communication is equally important, the human face being particularly expressive. We all subconsciously pay as much attention to facial expression and to the way in which the message is delivered as to the spoken word. Indeed, when the nonverbal message conflicts with the verbal message, serious doubt is cast on what is said. We have already seen in Chapter 10 that overt pain behavior is a powerful form of communication. We use it with little conscious thought. We recognize it and interpret it with ease. More complex illness behaviors such as failing to meet social duties or staying off work, and resting or lying down, make an even stronger social statement.

Because of the nature of human society, feedback is unavoidable. Social communication is always a two-way interaction. Conversation, by definition, is an exchange of ideas, thoughts and feelings. Talk of pain, pain behavior and illness behavior are almost impossible to ignore and we have to make some kind of response. Even if we deliberately ignore them, this in itself gives a powerful message. All that we say to the person in pain, whether directly or not, and whether or not we consider it carefully, contributes to the background of his or her thinking about the pain. Attitudes and feelings are probably more important than actual information or advice.

Several factors may affect the strength of this feedback. The more entrenched the patient's own ideas and attitudes, the harder he or she will be to change. The more important the person who provides the feedback, in the sense of social importance to the patient, the greater the influence. Hence the spouse or partner and immediate family are likely to have the most influence. They also provide some of the earliest feedback before ideas become entrenched. The influence of health professionals will depend on what the patient thinks of them. The more immediate, relevant and personal the feedback, the stronger it will be. Fordyce (1976) first applied behavioral principles to pain. He suggested that there is always powerful positive or negative social reinforcement of pain behavior and that this determines whether or not that behavior will continue. Attention, sympathy and social support encourage the patient to express his or her pain and his or her feelings about it, and continue his or her pain behavior. Ignoring pain expressions and behavior, rejecting emotions, withholding social support, and expecting the person to fulfill social duties all discourage the communication of pain.

Underlying this is a strong social pressure to conform. Human society can only survive if we all share a large measure of common attitudes, beliefs and behavior. This effect is most powerful in small, intimate social groups such as the family or peer groups. Our opinions and behavior are strongly influenced by real or imagined pressure from other members of the group. This will depend on the strength and importance of these common ideas, the unanimity of opinion, and on who holds these opinions. But if we identify with our group, we must in large measure identify with these ideas and adopt them as our own.

This all leads to a social role – a set of expectations in the sense that it is how we *should* behave. These expectations are our own, other people's and society's. We each fill several roles, and these roles may change over time. Of particular interest in this context is the change from the social role of a healthy, active member of society, a productive worker, and the breadwinner of a family, to the role of a patient with chronic low back pain and disability. This involves a radical shift in your attitudes, beliefs and expectations about yourself. It changes your needs and duties in relation to your family, work and society. It also means that your partner and family, your fellow workers and employers, your friends and society at large take a very different view of you and your place in society.

Low back pain and disability are truly psychosomatic in the sense that they depend as much on psychologic and behavioral factors as on the underlying physical problem. What we do about it depends very much on our attitudes and beliefs and emotions about the pain. Shorter (1992) pointed out that cultural and social pressures are even more important in this situation. Patients always tend to present symptoms that are acceptable to their society, and so they conform to current ideas of legitimate, (organic) disease. As medical and social ideas about disease change, so the pattern of psychosomatic symptoms changes to match: 'The history of psychosomatic disease is one of ever-changing steps in a *pas-de-deux* between doctor and patient.' Perhaps at this point it may be illuminating to reconsider the history of back pain and our current epidemic (Ch. 4).

Social support

One of the major strengths of human society is the social support that it provides, particularly in times of difficulty. In general, social support helps us to cope with crisis and adapt to change, and provides protection against stress. It reduces psychologic impact and levels of distress, and increases compliance with treatment, aids recovery and improves general health.

The most important source of social support is a partner or confidante – someone with whom you can share your problems. Is there someone you can talk to about problems like illness, money or personal relationships? Does he or she live close at hand and can you see and speak to him or her easily? Can you discuss your most intimate problems with him or her,

and does he or she trust you equally with his or her problems? We also get support from a wider network of family, friends and fellow workers. How many people do you feel that you know and can share your life with among your family, neighbors, friends and fellow workers?

Note that this is all about how you feel. It is not a question of material support or services. It is more the feedback you get from others that leads you to believe that you are cared for, esteemed and loved. It is a common and shared network of communication and mutual obligation. More than anything else, it is about emotional support.

There is a good theoretic framework and considerable empiric evidence that this kind of social support helps us to cope with life's problems and stresses, and reduces ill health. There is very little evidence about its effect in back pain. Most people cope with back pain, recover rapidly from acute attacks, and get on with their lives. Social support probably helps them to do so. But for those who become chronic back cripples, social support may become a double-edged sword. Chronic disability is simply not possible without social support, and that support may also reinforce and perpetuate disability.

Engel (1959) and Szasz (1968) pointed out that most chronic pain patients have a 'partner in pain' (Fig. 13.2). The more extreme forms of chronic low back pain and disability are probably not possible without such support, usually from a spouse, partner, parent or child. There is almost always one main partner, although other members of the family or friends may assist. In 20 years of clinical practice, I think I have seen a chronic pain patient in whom I could not identify a partner only once. For the partner is intimately involved in the 'pain game'. Chronic pain patients and their partners play active, mutually supporting roles, and the pain may become a major focus in their whole relationship. Their whole social milieu may become pervaded by pain and disability, medical values and health care. Chronic pain and caring may become almost full-time careers, with both partners equally committed.

In extreme cases, this may actually provide a more satisfying emotional relationship for both of them.

Leaving aside these extreme examples, the partner of a chronic pain patient is always involved to some extent (Block & Boyer 1984). They usually share many of the patient's attitudes and beliefs and expectations about the pain. Spouses show intense emotional responses to the patient's expression of pain, particularly if they have a close and satisfactory relationship. If the patient is very distressed, the spouse is also likely to be distressed. If the marital relationship is poor, the spouse is also more likely to be emotionally disturbed and the pain may increase marital distress. Schwartz et al (1996) found that if there was marital conflict, the patient showed more pain behavior. This led to a more negative response and more punitive behavior from the spouse, which in turn was associated with greater disability and distress in the patient. On the other hand, good marital adjustment may lead to other problems (Block & Boyer 1984). The spouse will adjust better emotionally and be more optimistic. However, such a spouse is also more likely to view the patient as being severely disabled, focus more on the physical problem, and be more solicitous. Such an approach may be better for the emotional state of the spouse, but is more likely to reinforce the patient's pain behavior and disability. Romano et al (1995) videotaped chronic pain patients and their spouses while they did common household tasks together. More solicitous responses from the spouse led to the pain patient showing more nonverbal pain behavior and increased disability.

Social impact on family

All back pain and disability that last more than a few weeks impact on the patient's spouse and family. Whatever the emotional impact, chronic pain and disability always have a major social and financial impact. Halmosh & Israeli (1982) gave a graphic description of the wife of an injured worker, whom they described as the 'associate victim'.

During the first acute stage, when the patient is under active treatment, family and friends rally round and there is little or no immediate financial impact. Everyone is optimistic about rapid recovery. After a few weeks or months, however, the support of family and friends begins to fade. The wife is put under growing strain to maintain the family and home. She has to take on more of the patient's normal duties. Sooner or later, financial problems begin to arise. At this stage, the patient may at first still feel he is doing fine. He is freed of his normal duties. His wife, on the other hand, becomes tense and tired, and inside she also feels angry and guilty. As time passes, the patient becomes aware of these changes in his wife, but may misinterpret them as concern that he is more severely injured than he has been told. Both may find it difficult to communicate.

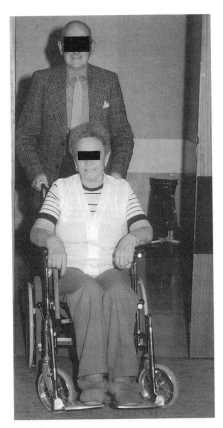

Figure 13.2 The 'partner in pain'.

Gradually, everything seems to grind to a halt and both patient and spouse sooner or later come face to face with hard reality. This happens simultaneously on several levels of consciousness and with very different perspectives for husband and wife. Active treatment comes to an end or is clearly not getting anywhere. He becomes worried and concerned about his lack of progress and pessimistic about his future recovery. They are both thrown back on their resources, and these resources are often diminishing as income drops and family and friends reduce their support to get on with their own lives. If the patient is unable – or feels unable – to return to his previous work, that raises serious questions about his whole existence. Not only how they will cope financially, but also who is he really and what is he worth? He may express this anxiety in several ways. He may increase his physical complaints, which means that as long as he still has pain he can postpone these difficult questions. Continued pain also legitimizes his situation. His wife shares these doubts and worries, and is under increasing strain. She begins to question herself, more or less consciously. Is this the life I am going to lead from here on? What is going to become of *me*? What is going to become of *us*? There may be further breakdown of communication, increase in marital stress and mutual recriminations.

The duration of the marriage, the strength of the relationship, and past experience all help to determine the outcome. Tragically, some marriages fail and each partner is then forced to make a fresh start in their lives. Most couples join forces, face up to the difficult questions of rehabilitation, retraining or reemployment, and survive a very traumatic phase of their lives. At the other extreme, some couples put the blame on outside forces such as the accident, slow healing and unsuccessful health care. They focus their anger and frustration on a common enemy in their fight for a cure or compensation.

THE SICK ROLE

The onset of illness always triggers a social process that in turn shapes the person's response to the ailment. The sick role is not a medical condition or diagnosis, but a status accorded to the individual by other members of society. The individual must also accept and assume the sick role. Often, particularly for chronic illness or financial support, the individual must also receive medical certification to legitimize it.

Parsons (1951) looked at illness as a social phenomenon and tried to define the social rights and duties of the person in the sick role. He started from the assumption that sickness is something unfortunate that occurs outside our control and involves some degree of helplessness.

- Rights
  — exempt from responsibility for incapacity
  — relieved from normal social duties and responsibilities
  — entitled to special attention and support.

On the other hand anyone who claims these rights when he or she is not 'really' sick will be judged to be malingering.

- Duties
  — accept that to be sick is undesirable and that there is an obligation to try to get well
  — obligation to seek professional help and to cooperate in the process of getting well.

So health professionals and society will disapprove of those who do not try to get well.

The concept of the sick role immediately takes illness beyond mere disease. It treats illness as part of the much broader relationship between the individual and society. Health professionals should not regard themselves as somehow being above or outside this system. If anything, we interpret the sick role conditions and what we expect of patients more rigidly than any other members of society.

Parsons (1951) based these ideas on acute physical illness. We must modify his analysis for chronic pain and disability, which we cannot understand purely in terms of physical disease and treatment. With chronic illness we must modify our expectations of health care and 'getting well'. Nor does this analysis fit well with chronic disability, where the person's beliefs and behavior may be part of the problem. Waddell et al (1989) gave a modified analysis of the sick role for chronic pain and disability:

- Rights
  — the sick person is not responsible for the original physical problem
  — the sick person may modify normal social obligations to a degree that is proportionate to the illness.

- Duties
  — recognize that to be ill is undesirable and that there is an obligation to reduce illness behavior and disability as much as possible
  — the sick person must share responsibility for his or her own health and disability.

This analysis recognizes that the sick role is not static but dynamic. It may change with time and the stage of the illness. It allows scope for adapting and coping. What is a normal sick role in acute illness, as in Parsons' original model, may even become maladaptive in chronic illness. It means some shift in responsibility from health professionals to the individual. It raises questions about the relative rights and duties of the sick role, and society's views and obligations to the chronically sick person.

Many of these questions are now in flux. New understanding of low back pain and disability and their management undermines the old Parsonian sick role of a simple social perspective on physical disease. Society will need to rethink what it does about this. Also, alas, much of this is only theory. It sounds reasonable, but there have been very few empiric studies of this social framework in back pain or disability, or indeed in other illness. Despite that, society and politicians on its behalf must make hard decisions on health care and social support for chronic low back disability. Life, and politics, is the art of drawing sufficient conclusions from insufficient information.

WORK

In current Western society, work, in the form of gainful employment, occupies a major place in our lives. It provides our financial status and security, and it defines who we are and our role in society (Box 13.2). If we are asked to describe ourselves, it is one of the first things that most of us say: 'I'm Dr Waddell' immediately puts me in a particular social position and evokes a particular set of social responses.

Box 13.2 The value of work

- Income (Should this come first or last?)
- Activity
- Occupies and structures our time
- Creativity/mastery
- Social interaction
- Sense of identity
- Sense of purpose

All workers get these to varying degrees, although their relative importance varies with the individual and the job.

The physical demands of work may make little difference to the chances of getting back pain (Ch. 6) but they certainly affect its impact. When you do have back pain, it is more difficult to continue a heavy physical job where there is little help or freedom to modify the nature or speed of your work. It is also more difficult to restart work, and the longer you are off, the harder it will be.

Nonphysical characteristics of work may be even more important. Bongers et al (1993) reviewed the way in which psychosocial factors affect musculoskeletal disorders (Box 13.3). High work demands, lack of clear direction and conflict at work all lead to more work stress and less job satisfaction. Low control over work, poor career development and poor social support at work may make it harder to cope with this stress. These all lead to increased absenteeism. There is some evidence that monotonous work may be associated with more reports of back pain, but there is contradictory evidence about working under time pressure. There is little clear evidence about the effect of job demands such as concentration, responsibility, career prospects and personal control. Bongers et al (1993) found one longitudinal study that showed that poor social support at work was associated with more reports of back trouble, but several cross-sectional studies were contradictory. In summary, monotonous work, perceived workload and work under time pressure seem to lead to more general musculoskeletal complaints. These are more consistently related to a combination of greater job demands and lack of support.

Box 13.3 Psychosocial factors that may be associated with musculoskeletal symptoms (summarized from Bongers et al 1993)

- Monotonous work
- Time pressure
- High concentration
- High responsibility
- High workload
- Few opportunities to take breaks
- Lack of clarity
- Low control and little autonomy
- Poor social support from colleagues
- Poor social support from superiors

Work involves a whole set of educational and social characteristics and attitudes that we share to a greater or lesser extent with our fellow workers. The prevailing work culture and how closely we identify with these common ideas will affect whether or not we stay off work and how rapidly we return. When workers were off work with back pain, Wood (1987) got their supervisor to phone up and say: 'How are you? We are thinking about you. You are a vital part of the team. Your work is important and your job is waiting for you.' This simple act of communication cut the number who stayed off long-term from 7.1% to 1.7%.

Hunt & Habeck (1993) reviewed different managerial approaches to reducing back injury claims and disability. They found that ergonomic approaches and wellness orientation were not effective. Disability case monitoring could actually be counterproductive, probably because it is adversarial. Safety training, active safety leadership, and pro-active return to work programs were most effective, probably because they all improve relationships between workers

and employers and supervisors. Green (1996) also stressed the importance of good relations between workers and employers, supervisors and fellow workers. There should be mutual respect and trust, and there should be regular communication, reinforcing the worker's importance and value. There should be cooperation and support. Good industrial relations make successful rehabilitation and return to work more likely.

Over the last decade, several Scandinavian studies have suggested that low job satisfaction may make workers more likely to take time off work with back pain. The *Boeing Study* (Bigos et al 1991) found that workers saying they 'hardly ever' enjoyed their job was one of the best predictors of reporting a back injury over the next 4 years. However, it was actually a very weak predictor. Again, the only reason it got so much attention was because so many of the findings of the *Boeing Study* were negative.

The *South Manchester Study* carried out a more careful longitudinal investigation of this relationship in the general UK population (Papageorgiou et al 1997). The initial cross-sectional study showed a very slight increase in reported back pain in workers with low job satisfaction. The longitudinal study over the next year showed that those who were markedly or severely dissatisfied with their work were at higher risk of getting back pain. Job satisfaction did not, however, make any difference to consulting their doctor about back pain.

Job satisfaction has received a lot of attention in recent years. The evidence suggests that it does have some effect on work loss due to back pain, but the effect is actually quite weak. However, it may simply be that it is too crude a measure and fails to tap more important attitudes about work.

There have been a few attempts to measure general socioeconomic influences on back pain. Volinn et al (1991) showed that age less than 40 years, low wages and lack of family support (widowed or divorced with no children) all produced a modest increase in chronic work loss due to back pain. The *South Manchester*

Study also looked at these kinds of general socioeconomic influences. In the initial cross-sectional study, perceived inadequacy of income, poor work satisfaction and problems getting on with fellow workers were all associated with a very slight increase in back pain. Income was more important in men, while problems getting on with fellow workers were more important in women. In the longitudinal study, only marked or severe work dissatisfaction was a modest predictor of back pain over the next year. However, lower social status (social classes IV and V) and perceived inadequacy of income were strong predictors of seeking health care for back pain. Unfortunately, that study did not record work loss. However, in view of the close link between consulting and sick certification in the UK, that is probably also related. These social influences remained important even after they allowed for psychologic distress. Again, these social factors only seemed to account for about 5% of back pain. Remember that these social measures are quite crude, and complex social factors may be much more important in individual cases.

Incapacity for work

Capacity and incapacity for work depend on complex interactions between the worker's medical condition and physical capabilities, ergonomic demands of the job and psychosocial factors (Feuerstein 1991). The factors that influence stopping work may be different from those that influence staying off and going back to work.

The relations between sickness, incapacity for work, employment and social benefits are complex (CSAG 1994). Look at three possible scenarios. First, back pain may be the direct cause of time off work, job loss, and unemployment, leading to sick certification and sickness benefits. Second, the physical, psychologic and social ill effects of unemployment may interact with and aggravate back pain and disability. Third, people with back pain who lose their job (for whatever reason) may be more likely to receive sick certification and benefits. These

correspond broadly to three routes of entry to invalidity benefits identified in a Department of Social Security (DSS) study in the UK (Ritchie & Snape 1993):

- *Condition-led entry*. The nature and severity of the illness and disability lead to long-term or permanent incapacity. Coming off benefits depends on the nature of the incapacity and treatment received and the availability of employment.
- *Employment-led entry*. Restricted employment opportunities combined with illness/disability (and often also age) cause loss of employment or inability to gain work and hence the start of benefits. The main barriers to coming off benefits are employment opportunities, availability of rehabilitation or retraining, and age.
- *Self-directed entry*. Some interaction between the person's condition, employment opportunities and motivation to continue or gain employment results in sickness benefits being seen as a possible option. This could be either with the support of the family doctor or negotiated with the family doctor. The main barriers to coming off benefits are age, low motivation and restricted employment opportunities, often related to their condition. Coming off benefits largely depends on external triggers, usually an independent medical review by the DSS or the family doctor's decision to stop sick certification.

Ritchie et al (1993) found that many complex factors influenced family doctors' judgements of their patient's capacity for work when giving sick certificates. The patient's medical condition and its impact on employment potential were always high on the list, but they were almost immediately linked to a whole range of non-medical factors. These included the patient's prospects of finding work, their age, their motivation to find work, the financial and psychologic consequences of returning to unemployment or job search, and the potential for rehabilitation or training.

The social process of becoming disabled and starting sickness benefits may occur insidiously and unconsciously rather than as a conscious decision. Once the person is assigned to benefit status, however, that may be almost irreversible in the current economic climate. This is especially the case if the person is approaching retirement age anyway.

Unemployment

As work is such an important part of our social fabric, it is not surprising that loss of work and unemployment are catastrophic. Unemployment causes the loss of all of the social and emotional advantages of work. It undermines our whole social position and status and is one of the greatest personal failures in a material society. Benefit status involves loss of social value, loss of respect and isolation. It is not surprising that unemployment causes pessimism, depression and fatalism. Unemployment, poverty and social deprivation lead to poor physical and mental health, with increased suicide and mortality rates. Lack of work causes loss of physical fitness and increased weight, psychologic distress and depression, and loss of work-related attitudes and habits, all of which are associated with low back disability. Volinn et al (1988) carried out a small area analysis in Washington state, which confirmed that disabling back pain was related to the unemployment rate, the percentage receiving food stamps, and income.

Enterline (1966) showed that the general sickness rate is inversely proportional to the unemployment rate. At that time, he found that on an average day about 7% of US workers were not at work, being either unemployed or sick. As unemployment rates rise, so sickness rates fall, and vice versa. Stopping work because of back pain is ultimately a decision made by the worker, with or without the advice or agreement of a health professional. Enterline (1966) suggested that when a worker falls ill, he or she is more likely to stay off work if there is:

- little risk of losing the job (because of low unemployment and labor shortage)
- little or no economic loss (because of continued pay or good wage replacement rates)
- little or no disapproval from fellow workers

and supervisors – which is closely linked to little or no disruption of their work.

The decision to stay off work depends on the relative attractiveness and price of the alternatives.

Over the past decade or two, there has been a change in attitudes to disability, which has become much more socially acceptable. This has been supported by policy attempts to improve the social facilities and status of disabled people. For the disabled, it has clearly been helpful. It means, however, that entry to disability status has also become more socially acceptable. Indeed, sickness and disability may now appear to be more socially acceptable than unemployment. Over the same period, pain *per se* has also become acceptable as a basis for chronic disability and benefits (Fordyce 1995). Enterline (1966) commented that in the 1950s and 1960s 'the right not to go to work when feeling ill appears to be part of a social movement that has swept across Europe'.

Higher unemployment rates produce greater competition for available work and higher selection criteria by employers. More jobs are also now shorter term with greater turnover of labor, which increases the frequency with which workers must seek and gain jobs. Any degree of mental or physical impairment, whether due to age, illness, or a poor sickness record, may make it harder to get or hold work than in better economic times when work was more readily available. A mild degree of incapacity may then lead a person to adopt the sick role who would otherwise have been able to continue to work without their symptoms being a health problem.

Once again, however, these social relationships are complex. There is actually very little difference in the prevalence of back pain between the employed and the unemployed (Table 13.3). The unemployed do seek more health care for back pain, but the most dramatic increase is in sick certification. DSS statistics from the UK show that nearly half the benefits paid for back pain now go to people who were not employed when they started benefits (Table 13.4). Sickness benefits are generally better than unemployment benefits and have less social stigma. There is a strong suspicion that many doctors try to help their patients by giving sick certificates for social rather than medical reasons.

Table 13.3 Relationship of back pain to lack of employment (based on data from Mason 1994 and DSS data)

	Employed	Not employed
Prevalence of back pain		
Point prevalence	11%	9%
1 year prevalence	37%	42%
Lifetime prevalence	65%	62%
Medical care for back pain in the past year	13%	20%
Sick certification for the last 4 weeks because of LBP	1%	20%

Chew & May (1997) looked at the dilemma faced by the family doctor in such a situation. They suggested that back pain may be a social resource for some patients, which has major implications for how patient and doctor approach the consultation. They pointed out that:

- chronic low back pain permits withdrawal from normal social obligations
- patients recognize that their doctor is not able to help, but view the doctor as a resource through which their social and economic inactivity can be legitimized
- patients do recognize the relation between psychosocial factors and pain
- chronic low back pain involves both the patient and the doctor negotiating conflicting roles.

Table 13.4 UK sickness and incapacity benefits for back pain (million days benefits per annum, 1990–91; based on DSS data)

	Start of benefit	
Employment status at start of benefit	Present year	Continued from previous year
Employed	4.3	26.6
Self-employed	1.9	2.6
Not employed	6.7	23.7

It appears that lack of employment may have different effects in different situations. When unemployment rates are high and job security is low, there may be more pressure on workers to stay at work when they feel unwell. This may reduce absenteeism due to back pain. However, once someone has lost their job, there may be social and financial advantages to sickness benefit, which may increase sick certification for back pain among those who are not employed.

Early retirement

Incapacity for work and sickness benefits related to low back pain are a particular problem in people over the age of about 50 years, in whom they are associated with early retirement.

Over the last few decades, there have been falling levels of employment within 10 years of retirement age. There has been a great increase in the number of workers who retire early, at some time in their 50s. In the Netherlands between 1971 and 1985, the number of men aged 55–59 in employment fell from 90 to 70%. In the UK, this trend has accelerated since that time. Some commentators suggest that some countries have encouraged early retirement as a more politically acceptable alternative to unemployment.

There is a dramatic change in the social acceptability and expectations of early retirement. A recent Australian survey found that a *majority* of workers now hope to retire before the present official retirement age. Some workers who retire early get various pension packages or redundancy payments as part of industrial reorganization. Despite slow general improvements in health, rising numbers of workers take early retirement on medical grounds, which may be the only mechanism available to many of them. In the UK between 1971 and 1981, the number of men aged 50–54 classified as 'permanently sick' rose from 1.3 to 11%.

In the UK, about 50% of all men and 40% of all women on long-term sickness benefits are now within 10 years of retirement age. Sick certification for back pain also rises rapidly in this age group, despite little change in prevalence, and a more modest rise in disability and consulting (Table 13.5).

Table 13.5 Age distribution of sick certification for back pain (based on data from Mason 1994, with permission from the Office of National Statistics)

Age	% with sick certification in last 4 weeks	% with sick certification throughout last 4 weeks
16–24	1.1	0
25–44	1.4	1.0
45–54	3.0	2.7
55–64	3.0	3.0

We have already seen the dramatic rise in early retirement with back pain in Sweden between 1971 and 1993 (Fig. 5.9). Erens & Ghate (1993) studied 1545 new recipients of long-term sickness benefits in the UK.

Among recipients aged 50+, their health condition appeared to be only one of several considerations in determining their attitudes towards returning to work. Attitudes to work appear to change quite dramatically around age 50. It would appear that personal considerations and labor market conditions play a prominent role in shaping the attitudes of recipients aged 50+.

Although low back pain is one of the most common health reasons given for early retirement, it is part of a more general problem and is not unique to back pain. Sickness benefits appear to be a transitional mechanism by which people within about 10 years of retirement age move from regular employment to early retirement.

Once again, the changes seem to be more social than biologic. Older people may have more difficulty coping with back pain, with heavy physical work, or especially with a combination of the two. However, any biologic change in the back with age seems to be only part of the story. Early retirement due to back pain is not restricted to workers with heavy jobs. Over the last two decades, during which there has been a marked increase in sickness benefits for back pain, there has been no change in back pain, and the number of people in heavy manual jobs has fallen.

On the present data, we cannot determine the relative importance of these various mechanisms linking employment status, low back disability and early retirement. It is probable that each is important in some people. More than one mechanism may operate simultaneously. Back pain and disability may contribute to job loss. The physical, mental and social ill-effects of loss of employment may interact with and aggravate low back pain and disability, and there may then be social and financial advantages to sick certification and sickness benefits.

COMPENSATION

Secondary gain

Few issues concerning back pain have given rise to more controversy than the question of compensation and secondary gain. *Secondary gain* is a vague term that suggests the person is somehow rewarded economically, physically or emotionally as a result of their injury or illness (Fishbain 1994, Fishbain et al 1995).

All illness involves some secondary gains. Illness may provide an excuse for avoiding all kinds of activities and lead to increased social support. For some people, it may provide an emotional crutch to deal with life's problems. Some people simply do not have the emotional and social resources to deal with life, particularly in times of adversity. Some people are passive and dependent, and health professionals offer a ready source of support. There is another group of people who have always coped remarkably well, but when illness does strike they never manage to return to their previous hyperactive state. They then have difficulty adjusting and 'never seem to get over it'. That does not mean that any of these people consciously contrive their situation. They are not malingering. They have genuine symptoms. It is just that they are not able to cope with them well and may continue to varying degrees in the sick role.

Too often, however, secondary gain focuses on money and implies malingering. Any benefit

---

I am indebted to Dr R Teasell (personal communication) for much of the material in this section.

such as disability payments or a concerned family member then casts suspicion on the legitimacy of the patient's symptoms. If treatment fails, secondary gain makes a good excuse. This is all a very circular argument, which may say more about the bias of the observer than the motivation of the patient. Noone raises questions of secondary gain about the patient with a stroke.

The courts and the media have drawn attention to videos of workers doing strenuous physical activities while they are claiming sickness benefit. That is clearly fraudulent, but it is rare. Boden (1996) estimated that, at most, 3% of injured workers in the United States fall into this category. Most workers have entirely 'genuine' physical pain and disability, although reasonable people may reasonably disagree about the degree of recovery and the appropriate duration of time off work.

Despite these philosophic comments, financial gain is a major motivating force in a material society. We all respond to financial incentives and disincentives. Indeed, before we cast any stones, we should recognize that all health professionals make much greater secondary gains from back pain than any patient ever did.

Miller (1976) was one of the first to calculate that benefits of much over 50% of wages led to an increase in the days of disability claimed by insured persons. His report to the US House of Representatives, Committee on Ways and Means, is still frequently quoted. There have been many such studies, recently reviewed by Loeser et al (1995). The evidence is not fully consistent, and not all studies show any effect. However, the best available literature suggests that a 10% increase in workers' compensation benefits produces a 1–11% increase in the number of claims, and a 2–11% increase in the average duration of claims. That is an average increase of 2–5 days off work with back pain. It is important to stress that these effects are similar for 'verifiable' injuries like fractures, as well as more subjective, soft tissue injuries. Loeser et al (1995) also pointed out that these figures may not accurately reflect other benefit systems.

These discussions usually neglect the fact that secondary gains are balanced by secondary losses (Fishbain 1994). Money is only one part of the secondary gains and losses of stopping work and going sick, and it is probably not the most important. Loss of all the other social benefits of working, loss of financial and social status, and the major change from a working role to a sick role are probably all more important. For most patients, they greatly outweigh any emotional gains. Even if we confine the argument to money, we should not overestimate the value of compensation. Nagi & Hadley (1972) showed that 82% of disabled people in the US were financially worse off than when they were working; 17% had little change, and only 1.5% were better off (Table 13.6). This has not changed. Despite anecdotal comments about the UK welfare state, few people on benefits are better off than when they were working. Half receive less than 50% of their previous net earnings, and only one in eight receive more than 80% of previous net earnings (Erens & Ghate 1993). We found that only 5% of our patients with back pain were financially better off sick than working. These few were generally part-time or very poorly paid workers whose wages were so low that they gave little financial incentive to work at all. Looking at their whole social situation, the vast majority of people off work with back pain are much worse off in many ways. Workers' compensation or other sickness benefits are a very inadequate replacement.

Economists often play down the role of health care and psychosocial factors in their studies, just as health care providers often overlook economic and administrative issues. Disability, health care and compensation are closely linked. We have no hard data on the

Table 13.6 Monthly income level before and after injury in 1961–1964 US dollars (based on data from Nagi & Hadley 1972)

	Before	After
< $200	9%	52%
> $500	41%	9%

influence of health care and its providers on the submission and duration of claims, although clinical experience suggests it may be considerable. Taylor et al (1996) suggested that compensation may even influence the decisions taken by patients and professionals about back surgery. Conversely, these clinical decisions have a major impact on health care costs, and on the duration and costs of compensation. Before we pass moral judgements on how compensation incentives influence workers, we should also consider how they influence employers, health professionals and lawyers.

Financial incentives certainly modify people's behavior in a particular situation. So, once back injuries occur, better benefits will increase the number and duration of claims. But there is no evidence to suggest that compensation increases the amount of back pain or changes the condition of anyone's back. The level of compensation is probably a very small factor in the decision to stop work, and only one factor in maintaining the sick role (Box 13.4). As we have already noted, there have been great changes in attitudes to work and disability and compensation over recent decades. There is rapid change in conditions of employment, with much more unemployment, job insecurity and job turnover. The average job tenure in the US is now less than 3 years. This has inevitably changed attitudes to work, employers and unemployment. These changed attitudes are all probably much more important than the actual level of compensation.

Box 13.4 Socioeconomic issues affecting workers' compensation

- Work demands
- Work environment
- Availability of modified work
- Income
- Job security
- Advancement/career potential
- Pension
- Natural job attrition
- Job availability
- Compensation

Clinical studies

Let us turn now to clinical studies of compensation, where there seems to me to be a striking dichotomy in the literature. At one extreme, some pain clinic studies and experts say that there is no clinical difference between compensation and noncompensation patients. At the other extreme, some medicolegal experts, who are mainly orthopedic surgeons, imply that many of the claimants they see are little short of frank malingerers. The difference seems to be a combination of case selection and observer bias, in both directions.

Rohling et al (1995) have made the most careful review, although they caution that most studies are in pain clinic settings and the results may not apply to more routine compensation patients. They found 32 studies that gave usable data on 3802 compensated and 3849 noncompensated patients. Compensation patients consistently reported more pain, although the difference was quite small, about 6%. Rohling et al and another review by Walsh & Dumitru (1988) concluded that the outcomes of conservative treatment, back surgery and chronic pain rehabilitation programs are consistently poorer in compensation patients. Compensation does seem to delay clinical recovery. There is conflicting evidence on the magnitude of this effect, with estimates ranging from 0 to 30%. Many studies show that there is very little difference in the physical findings and levels of distress in compensation patients, but some suggest that compensation patients are more depressed. To put this in context, we should also remember that 75–90% of compensation patients do respond well to health care, and do recover and return to work rapidly.

It is too easy to assume that this is all a direct effect of compensation, but that does not allow for other differences in these patients. Leavitt (1992) pointed out that compensation patients usually have heavier physical jobs. They are generally younger, male, less educated and from a lower social class. They form a very different occupational, social and economic group. Their selection and referral patterns are also quite different. These differences may have a more direct and much greater impact on their clinical progress and return to work than compensation itself. There is conflicting evidence on this. Dworkin et al (1985) found that employment status had most effect on the outcome of pain management, and compensation or litigation did not add anything. Sanderson et al (1995) found that both unemployment and compensation affected disability, but employment status was most important. Leavitt (1992) showed the importance of job demands. Nevertheless, he found that work-related injury and compensation led to more prolonged disability, even after allowing for job demands. Nagi & Hadley (1972) suggested that in patients with more severe physical injuries, social factors are less important. In those with less severe injuries, higher education, higher income, greater loss of income and more dependants seemed to produce higher motivation to return to work.

Box 13.5 Effects of compensation

Effect of compensation level on claims
- There is no evidence that it changes the actual injury rate
- 10% increase in compensation level produces 1–11% increase in claims rate
- 10% increase in compensation level produces 2–11% increase in duration of disability
- This affects 'verifiable' injuries like fractures as much as more subjective, soft tissue injuries

Effect of compensation on surgical outcome
- Compensation patients are less likely to have a good result of back surgery
- These findings have been criticized:
  — these men often have heavier physical jobs
  — they may get over-aggressive surgical intervention
- Despite this, more than 75% do return to their previous work

Effect of compensation on rehabilitation outcome
- Compensation patients respond less well to pain management and rehabilitation
- These findings have been criticized:
  — there are methodologic flaws in many of these studies. They are often small samples of highly selected patients with poor diagnostic criteria. Follow-up is poor. There is failure to allow for other factors such as job demands
  — differences are small
- Despite this, many compensation patients do benefit

There is little doubt that compensation affects what people do when they have back pain. It affects their response to treatment and their return to work. But it does not cause the pain or create the situation in which these patients find themselves. It is only one of the (probably less powerful) social influences on what they do to get out of that situation. Secondary losses usually greatly outweigh secondary gains.

Despite all this, most patients do respond to treatment, recover and return to work.

Box 13.5 summarizes the effects of compensation.

HEALTH CARE

Health care has reappeared throughout this chapter. The World Health Organization defines health as a state of complete physical, mental and social well-being and not simply the absence of disease or infirmity. The ultimate social role of health care is to make patients healthy and enable them to take their place in society.

We must consider our own role as health professionals in this process (Bennet 1979). Patients and health professionals have an intimate social relationship, because we are equally involved, in our very different ways, in the illness. We each have very different needs and demands and duties. Patients face illness as a personal and threatening experience. At a clinical level, health professionals may take a more detached view, but illness also provides us with our livelihood and identity. Society takes a much broader view of the social and economic impact of illness, and of health care. These views are very different, but they are simply different perspectives on a common problem. How these views blend or collide affects the quality and success of health care.

Doctors and other health professionals also play a key social role in disability and the provision of social support. We certify and legitimize the process, often with little insight into the consequences for the patient, their family, their work and society.

It is naive to think that all we do is treat disease to make our patients better. It should be clear by now that, quite apart from the

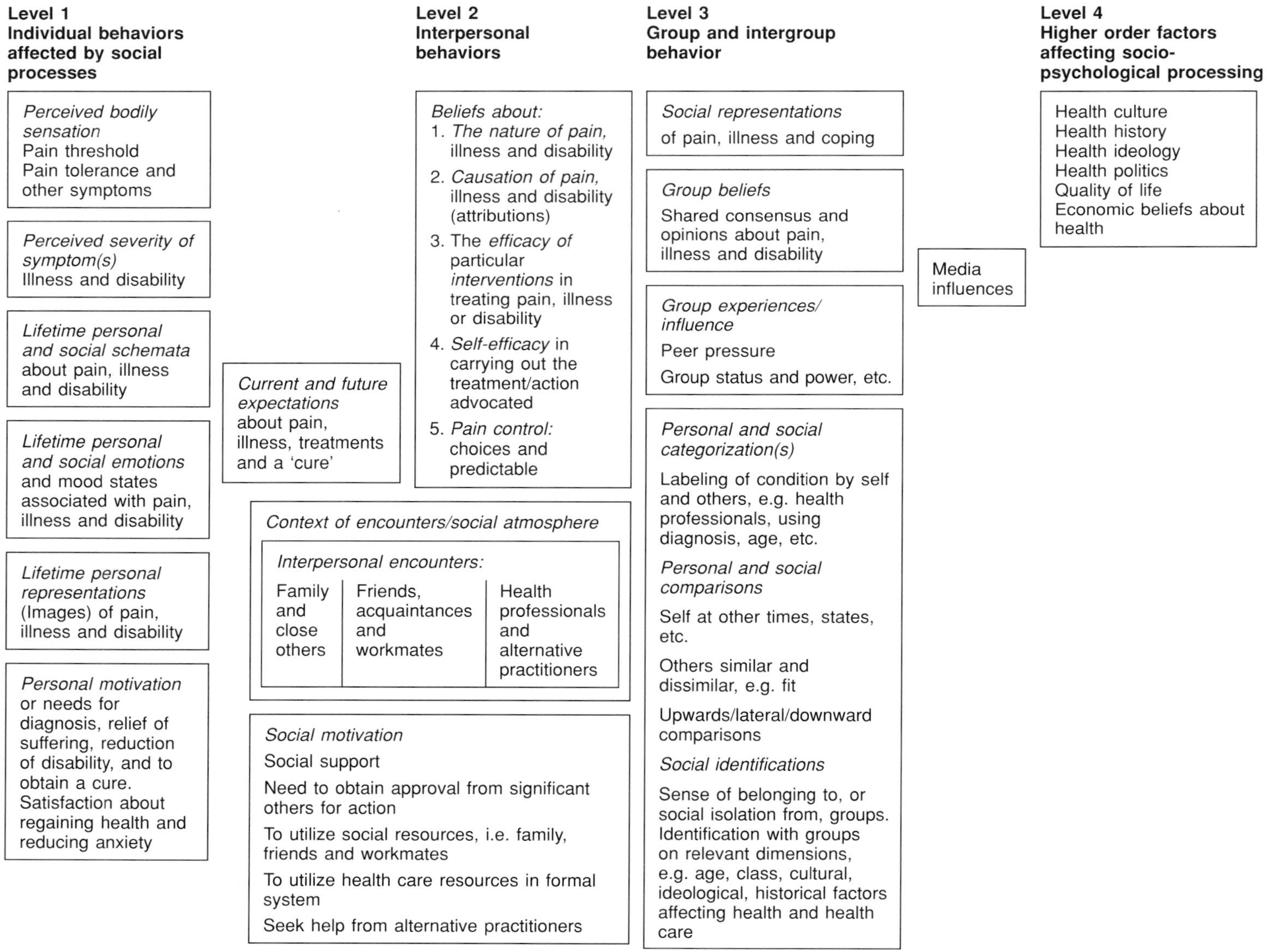

**Level 1
Individual behaviors affected by social processes**

Perceived bodily sensation
Pain threshold
Pain tolerance and other symptoms

Perceived severity of symptom(s)
Illness and disability

Lifetime personal and social schemata about pain, illness and disability

Lifetime personal and social emotions and mood states associated with pain, illness and disability

Lifetime personal representations (Images) of pain, illness and disability

Personal motivation or needs for diagnosis, relief of suffering, reduction of disability, and to obtain a cure. Satisfaction about regaining health and reducing anxiety

**Level 2
Interpersonal behaviors**

Beliefs about:
1. *The nature of pain,* illness and disability
2. *Causation of pain,* illness and disability (attributions)
3. *The efficacy of particular interventions* in treating pain, illness or disability
4. *Self-efficacy* in carrying out the treatment/action advocated
5. *Pain control:* choices and predictable

Current and future expectations about pain, illness, treatments and a 'cure'

Context of encounters/social atmosphere

Interpersonal encounters:

Family and close others	Friends, acquaintances and workmates	Health professionals and alternative practitioners

Social motivation
Social support
Need to obtain approval from significant others for action
To utilize social resources, i.e. family, friends and workmates
To utilize health care resources in formal system
Seek help from alternative practitioners

**Level 3
Group and intergroup behavior**

Social representations
of pain, illness and coping

Group beliefs
Shared consensus and opinions about pain, illness and disability

Group experiences/influence
Peer pressure
Group status and power, etc.

Personal and social categorization(s)
Labeling of condition by self and others, e.g. health professionals, using diagnosis, age, etc.

Personal and social comparisons
Self at other times, states, etc.
Others similar and dissimilar, e.g. fit
Upwards/lateral/downward comparisons

Social identifications
Sense of belonging to, or social isolation from, groups. Identification with groups on relevant dimensions, e.g. age, class, cultural, ideological, historical factors affecting health and health care

Media influences

**Level 4
Higher order factors affecting socio-psychological processing**

Health culture
Health history
Health ideology
Health politics
Quality of life
Economic beliefs about health

Figure 13.3 Psychosocial processes and social factors implicated in chronic pain and disability. (Reproduced with permission from Skevington 1995.)

'treatment' we offer, we are a powerful *social change agent* (Phillips 1994). We must consider and allow for all these social factors and consequences in our management of the patient with back pain. We must be sure that our contribution is to the patient's overall benefit. From a social perspective, that is what this whole book is about.

CONCLUSION

We must end this chapter with a strong note of caution. I have no doubt that these kinds of social influences and interactions are very important in chronic low back pain and disability. There is no evidence of any biologic change in low back pain and it is very unlikely that human psychology has changed in the last 20 years. The speed with which our current epidemic of chronic low back disability has developed makes it much more likely to be a result of change in social attitudes and behavior. Understanding these social factors may be the key to controlling the epidemic.

However, these social factors are complex (Fig. 13.3) and our understanding is limited. We have very little good evidence as to which social factors are important in back pain or how important they are. We have great difficulty identifying and defining them; and much more measuring them and their effects; never mind understanding how they work. We must be very careful not to make moral judgements, which often reflect our own social views and values more than anything about our patient's situation. I believe this is one of the most promising but unexplored fields for back pain research.

REFERENCES

Aronson E 1984 The social animal, 4th edn. Freeman, New York

Balague F, Skovron M-L, Nordin M, Dutoit G, Waldburger M 1995 Low back pain in school children. A study of familial and psychological factors. Spine 20: 1265–1270

Beecher H K 1959 Measurement of subjective responses: quantitative effect of drugs. Oxford University Press, New York

Bennet G 1979 Patients and their doctors. Baillière Tindall, London

Bigos S J, Battie M C, Spengler D M et al 1991 A prospective study of work perceptions and psychological factors affecting the report of back injury. Spine 16: 1–6

Block A R, Boyer S L 1984 The spouse's adjustment to chronic pain: cognitive and emotional factors. Social Science and Medicine 19: 1313–1317

Boden L I 1996 Work disability in an economic context. In: Moon S, Sauter S L (eds) Psychosocial aspects of musculoskeletal disorders in office work. Taylor & Francis, London, p 287–294

Bongers P M, de Winter C R, Kompier M A J, Hildebrandt V H 1993 Psychosocial factors at work and musculoskeletal disease. Scandinavian Journal of Work and Environmental Health 19: 297–312

Chew C A, May C 1997 The expert patient and the benefits of back pain. Presented to back pain management meeting, Chester, England

Clinical Standards Advisory Group (CSAG) 1994 Epidemiology review, the epidemiology and cost of back pain. Annex to the CSAG report on back pain. HMSO, London

Dworkin R H, Handlin D S, Richlin D M, Brand L, Vannucci C 1985 Unraveling the effects of compensation, litigation and employment on treatment response in chronic pain. Pain 23: 49–59

Engel G L 1959 Psychogenic pain and the pain prone patient. American Journal of Medicine 26: 899–918

Enterline P E 1966 Social causes of sick absence. Archives of Environmental Health 12: 467–473

Erens B, Ghate D 1993 Invalidity benefit: a longitudinal study of new recipients. Department of Social Security Research Report no. 20. HMSO, London.

Feuerstein M 1991 A multidisciplinary approach to the prevention, evaluation and management of work disability. Journal of Occupational Rehabilitation 1: 5–12

Fishbain D A 1994 Secondary gain concept: definition, problems and its abuse in medical practice. American Pain Society Journal 3: 264–273

Fishbain D A, Rosomoff H L, Cutler R B, Rosomoff R S 1995 Secondary gain concept: a review of the scientific evidence. Clinical Journal of Pain 11: 6–21

Fordyce W E 1976 Behavioral methods for chronic pain and illness. Mosby, St Louis

Fordyce W E 1995 Back pain in the workplace. Report of an International Association for the Study of Pain Task Force. IASP Press, Seattle, p 1–75

Green J F 1996 Management of debilitating injuries in a large industrial setting. Journal of Back and Musculoskeletal Rehabilitation 7: 167–174

Halmosh A F, Israeli R 1982 Family interactions as modulator in the post-traumatic process. Medicine and Law 1: 125–134

Honeyman P T, Jacobs E A 1996 Effects of culture on back pain in Australian aboriginals. Spine 21: 841–843

Hunt H A, Habeck R V 1993 The Michigan disability prevention study. WE Upjohn Institute for Employment Research, Kalamazoo MI

Leavitt F 1992 The physical exertion factor in compensable work injuries. A hidden flaw in previous research. Spine 17: 307–310

Loeser J D, Henderlite S E, Conrad D A 1995 Incentive effects of workers' compensation benefits: a literature synthesis. Medical Care Research and Review 52: 34–59

Mason V 1994 The prevalence of back pain in Great Britain. Office of Population Censuses and Surveys, Social Survey Division (now office of National Statistics), HMSO, London, p 1-24

Miller J H 1976 Preliminary report on disability insurance. Public Hearings before the Subcommittee on Social Security of the Committee on Ways and Means of the US House of Representatives. US Government Printing Office, Washington, DC, p 115–153

Nagi S Z, Hadley L W 1972 Disability behavior, income change and motivation to work. Industrial and Labor Relations Review 25: 223–233

Papageorgiou A C, Macfarlane G F, Thomas E, Croft P R, Jayson M I V, Silman A J 1997 Psychosocial factors in the workplace – do they predict new episodes of low back pain? Spine 22: 1137–1142

Parsons T 1951 The Social System. Free Press, New York

Phillips R B 1994 Social theory of chiropractic, 3rd edn. In: Leach R A (ed) The chiropractic theories: principles and clinical applications. Williams & Wilkins, Baltimore, p 365–371

Ritchie J, Ward K, Duldig W 1993 A qualitative study of the role of GPs in the award of invalidity benefit. Department of Social Security Research Report no. 18. HMSO, London

Ritchie J, Snape D 1993 Invalidity benefit; a preliminary qualitative study of the factors affecting its growth. Social & Community Planning Research SCPR, London

Rohling M L, Binder L M, Langhinrichsen-Rohling J 1995 Money matters: a metaanalytic review of the association between financial compensation and the experience and treatment of chronic pain. Health Psychology 14: 537–547

Romano J M, Turner J A, Jensen M P et al 1995 Chronic pain patient – spouse behavioral interactions predict patient disability. Pain 63: 353–360

Sanderson P L, Todd B D, Holt G R, Getty C J M 1995 Compensation, work status, and disability in low back pain patients. Spine 20: 554–556

Schwartz L, Slater M A, Birchler G R 1996 The role of pain behaviors in the modulation of marital conflict in chronic pain couples. Pain 65: 227–233

Shorter E 1992 From paralysis to fatigue, a history of psychosomatic illness in the modern era. Free Press, New York

Skevington S M 1995 Psychology of pain. Wiley, Chichester

Szasz T S 1968 The painful person. The Journal – Lancet 88: 18–22

Taylor V M, Deyo R A, Ciol M, Kreuter W 1996 Surgical treatment of patients with back problems covered by workers' compensation versus those with other sources of payment. Spine 21: 2255–2259

Torstensen T A 1996 Comparing likes and unlikes of non-athletes with low back pain versus elite athletes. Presented to Sports Medicine Symposium, Telemark Norway

Vikne J 1996 What are the characteristics of top elite athletes? MSc thesis, Norwegian University of Sport and Physical Education

Volinn E, Lai D, McKinney S, Loeser J D 1988 When back pain becomes disabling: a regional analysis. Pain 33: 33–39

Volinn E, Koevering D V, Loeser J D 1991 Back sprain in industry: the role of socioeconomic factors in chronicity. Spine 16: 542–548

Volinn E 1997 The epidemiology of low back pain in the rest of the world, a review of surveys in low and middle income countries. Spine 22: 1747–1754

Waddell G, Pilowsky I, Bond M 1989 Clinical assessment and interpretation of abnormal illness behaviour in low back pain. Pain 39: 41–53

Walsh N E, Dumitru D 1988 The influence of compensation on recovery from low back pain. Occupational Medicine 3: 109–121

Wood D J 1987 Design and evaluation of a back injury prevention program within a geriatric hospital. Spine 12: 77–82

Zborowski M 1952 Cultural components in responses to pain. Journal of Social Issues 8: 16–30

14

A new clinical model of low back pain and disability

Gordon Waddell   Chris J. Main

We have looked at many facets of low back pain and disability. It is now time to try and look at the whole picture, to seek a better understanding of the clinical and social problem.

We will start with the disease model, and compare it with modern neurophysiologic concepts of pain. We will then build up a biopsychosocial model in three stages. First, we will consider the elements that are important, and how they present clinically at one point in time. Secondly, we will consider how they interact over time in the process of developing and maintaining chronic pain and disability. Thirdly, we will consider decision points that may lead to some people becoming chronic back cripples, while most manage to cope with back pain most of the time and lead more or less normal lives. Finally, we will offer a brief introduction to the implications of this model for health care, which is really the theme of the rest of this book.

We must emphasize from the very start that this is not a causal model. We are not talking about the original cause of back pain. Of course, pain arises from musculoskeletal and neurophysiologic processes, but what we are trying to understand is how some patients then go on to develop chronic pain and disability.

THE DISEASE MODEL

For more than a century, Western health care has been based on the disease model. All our health professions share common philosophic

223

ideals, which we try to adhere to in our professional conduct. But if you look at our practice, it is all about a disease model of illness (Box 14.1; Virchow 1858).

Box 14.1 The disease model

• Recognize patterns of illness (behavior)	Symptoms and signs
• Infer underlying pathology	Diagnosis
• Apply physical therapy to underlying pathology	Treatment
• Expect illness (behavior) to improve	Cure

This disease model uses a Cartesian model of pain, with pain as a signal of tissue damage. Actually, that is rather unfair to Descartes (1664). This approach developed after the Renaissance under his influence, but it was really his followers who created such a strict mind-body dichotomy in which the body was nothing but a machine. Descartes himself took a more philosophic view, and considered feelings of pain a prime example of 'confused perceptions' or 'passions'. He felt they could not be referred to either the body alone or the mind alone, but rather arose from 'the close and intimate union of the mind with the body'. We should not decry Descartes' understanding!

An historic perspective (Ch. 4)

- Human beings have had back pain all through history, and it is no more common or severe than it has always been
- What has changed is how we understand and manage the symptom of pain in the back
- Three key ideas in the 19th century laid the foundation for traditional 20th century management:
  — back pain comes from the spine and involves the nervous system
  — it is due to injury
  — the back is irritable and should be treated by rest
- The epidemiology shows an epidemic of chronic disability attributed to simple backache, in all Western countries
- Traditional health care has not solved the problem, and may even have contributed to it

---

Nevertheless, medicine used this more mechanistic view of pain as a simple reflex response to physical injury. This concept of pain as a signal of injury, tissue damage and nociception is deeply entrenched in the way patients, doctors and therapists think. Despite all the recent advances in our knowledge of pain, it still dominates routine clinical practice.

From the disease model, we assume that:
- pain = tissue injury
- tissue injury → physical impairment → disability and handicap
- if we cure the pain, then disability will also get better.

This approach has worked well for clear-cut pathology such as a spinal fracture or a disc prolapse, but not for simple backache. We believe that is because some of the basic assumptions of the disease model do not apply to a symptom like nonspecific low back pain:

- We cannot identify any structural lesion in most patients.
- Pain is not the same as tissue injury. The Cartesian model fails to explain many clinical observations of pain (compare it with modern ideas about the neurophysiology of pain).
- Having back pain is not the same as being disabled by it. Most of us get back pain at some time in our lives but few of us become disabled.
- Different people respond very differently to the same physical injury or disease. Many patients who become disabled by back pain have no more objective abnormality in their backs than other people who manage to function quite normally.
- Individual beliefs, psychologic distress and illness behavior have a powerful influence on pain and disability and on how we respond to treatment.
- Cultural and socioeconomic factors have a profound influence on the epidemiology of low back disability.

Treatment of back pain according to the disease model has failed because there is a fundamental flaw to the approach. The disease model views low back pain and disability only in terms of spines and physical disease. It does not allow for complex human responses to pain and disability.

The neurophysiology of pain

Pain is 'an unpleasant sensory and emotional experience associated with actual or potential tissue damage, or described in terms of such damage' (Merskey 1979).

The gate control theory (Melzack & Wall 1965) and modern neurophysiology have made major contributions to our understanding of pain (Fig. 14.1). They suggest mechanisms by which other neurophysiologic and psychologic activity can modulate pain, and help to explain the complexity of clinical pain. They bridge the mind–body dichotomy. The danger comes when we fall into the trap of thinking that all pain is just a matter of neurophysiology, and that further knowledge will let us force pain back into an expanded neurophysiologic version of the disease model. That is a false path. We cannot solve all the problems of pain by moving the same physical approach to treatment one or two neurones up the CNS. We must also recognize and deal with psychologic and social issues.

A BIOPSYCHOSOCIAL MODEL

Let us briefly review the elements we need to build this model:

- physical dysfunction ⎫
- beliefs and coping   ⎪
- distress   ⎬ • pain and disability
- illness behavior   ⎪
- social interactions ⎭

Pain and disability (see Ch. 3)

- Pain and disability are not the same. We must make a clear distinction between them, both conceptually and in clinical practice
- Pain is a complex, sensory and emotional experience. It is much more than just a signal of tissue damage
  — pain signals do not pass unaltered to the cerebral cortex; they are always and constantly modulated within the CNS before they reach consciousness
  — pain, emotions and pain behavior are all integral parts of the pain experience
  — the CNS is plastic in nature, and there may be neurophysiologic changes over time with the development of chronic pain
- Clinical assessment depends on the patient's *report* of pain and disability, which depends on how the patient thinks and feels, and how he or she communicates the experience

---

Low back pain and disability often go together, but the relationship between them is much weaker than most patients and clinicians assume (Fig. 14.2). Many other authors have shown similar results (Linton 1985, Riley et al 1988, Cooper et al 1996). We cannot explain low back disability purely in terms of physical disease and pain. We need a more comprehensive, biopsychosocial model that allows for all these physical, psychologic and social aspects and for their interaction.

Physical dysfunction. The symptom of back pain usually arises, at least initially, from nociception in the back. However, we have argued that nonspecific low back pain is mainly a

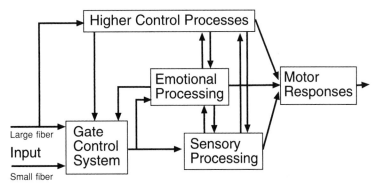

Figure 14.1 How the gate control system might link psychologic and neurophysiologic aspects of pain. (After Melzack & Casey 1968, with permission.)

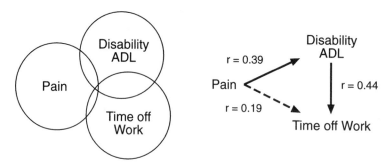

Figure 14.2 The relation between low back pain, disability in activities of daily living and work loss. *r* is the correlation coefficient, where 0 is no relation at all and 1 is complete identity. *r* = 0.30 is about 10% overlap in common, and *r* = 0.50 is about 25%.

matter of *dysfunction* or physiologic impairment. Dysfunction depends on the level of demand or stress, the capacity of the musculoskeletal system to cope with these, and the imbalance between them. It *may* start from increased load or injury. Equally, it may be due to reduced capacity to cope, whether due to personal state, loss of fitness, fatigue or other reasons that cannot be identified. There is always a background of subconscious and conscious sensation from normal musculoskeletal function, and any symptoms depend on how we perceive them against this background. Further, if back pain is due to disturbed function then it always has the potential to recover. As the epidemiology shows, most back pain should be benign and self-limiting, even if recurrent pain is common.

Painful musculoskeletal dysfunction (see Ch. 9)

- May occur in structurally normal tissues
- A primary dysfunction arising in response to abnormal forces imposed on or generated within the musculoskeletal system
- Abnormal patterns of muscle function, abnormal forces acting on musculoskeletal structures, abnormal posture or abnormal joint movement may all produce pain
- Segmental soft tissue changes; neurophysiologic and psychophysiologic changes

---

Disability depends on anatomic and physiologic abilities, but also on psychologic and social resources. Performance depends on effort. We cannot separate body and mind. Physical defects affect the person's beliefs and expectations about their situation. On the other hand, beliefs and expectations help to shape the impact of physical defects on function. We must not underestimate the extent to which psychologic and social processes influence physical function, and vice versa. Disability is not only a question of functional capacity. It is a question of performance. We must consider all the possible influences on that person's performance. Remember:

- capacity is determined by physiologic limits.
- performance is determined by psychologic factors.

Beliefs and coping. Human thought has a major influence on pain. How people think and feel about back pain is central to what they do about it and how it affects them. Anticipation of pain, anxiety and attention, the meaning and context of the pain, suggestion and placebos, past experience, prior conditioning and health care. These beliefs partly reflect the physical condition of the back, but they have more to do with our perceptions of the pain. Once they are established they may become fixed and difficult to change.

Distress. Pain, emotional arousal and psychologic distress are closely linked. Distress may raise awareness of bodily sensations, increase the severity of pain, and lower pain tolerance. It makes us more concerned about the pain and more likely to seek health care.

Beliefs about back pain (Ch. 12)
Beliefs   • Beliefs about damage and disease   • Fear of hurt and harming   • Fear avoidance beliefs   • Personal responsibility, control and self-efficacy   • Beliefs and expectations about treatment   *Coping*   • Active or passive   • Catastrophizing   • Beliefs affect health care: health care affects beliefs   *Fear of pain and what we do about pain may be more disabling than back pain itself.*

Psychologic distress (Ch. 11)
• Anxiety   • Increased bodily awareness   • Fear and uncertainty   • Anger   • Depressive symptoms

Illness behavior. Beliefs about the pain, coping strategies and psychologic distress all affect what we do – our illness behavior. Illness behavior reflects the severity of the physical problem, but in its final expression it may depend more on these psychologic events than on the underlying physical problem.

There is now a great deal of evidence that beliefs, distress and illness behavior are powerful influences on low back disability (see Tables 14.1 and 14.2).

Social interactions. Low back pain and disability occur in a particular social setting. Family, work and wider social networks influence how beliefs, coping strategies and illness behavior develop. Chronic low back disability can only develop with family and financial support. The availability, nature and strength of these social influences may either reinforce or discourage illness behavior and disability. In

Table 14.1 Fear of pain may be more disabling than pain itself (based on data from Waddell et al 1993)

Main elements of illness	Extent to which these account for chronic low back disability	
	In activities of daily living %	In loss of time from work %
Severity of pain	14	5
Fear avoidance beliefs	+32	+26
Total identified	46	31

These are the additive effects, after allowing for severity of pain.
It is unusual to be able to identify such a high proportion of any biologic relationship.

Table 14.2 Psychologic distress and illness behavior may be as disabling as physical impairment (based on data from Waddell et al 1984)

Main elements of illness	Extent to which these account for chronic low back disability	
	In activities of daily living %	In loss of time from work %
Physical impairment	40	22
Psychologic distress Illness behavior }	+31	+7
Social interactions	?	?
Total identified	71	29

These are the additive effects of distress and illness behavior, after allowing for physical impairment.

turn, pain and pain behaviors are powerful means of communication to other people, including health professionals.

A biopsychosocial model. We tried to put these elements together in a biopsychosocial model of chronic low back pain and disability (Fig. 14.3; Waddell et al 1984). Turk et al (1988) took a similar 'multi-axial view of impairment due primarily to pain'. They stressed the need to integrate physical findings, behavioral manifestations and loss of function.

The model in Figure 14.3 illustrates a number of important features. It is a model of human illness, rather than pain alone. Back pain may arise from nociception in the back, but its clinical expression involves all of these other aspects. Patients and health professionals alike see that physical symptom as if through a series of filters. When we observe its final clinical presentation, we can only look directly at behavior, which we must analyze more carefully to infer underlying events.

Some people have criticized this model because it seems to suggest that low back pain *starts* as a physical problem and all the psychosocial changes develop secondarily (Reilly 1993). There is indeed considerable evidence

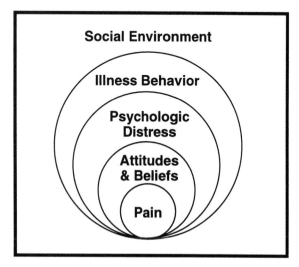

Figure 14.3 A biopsychosocial model of the clinical presentation and assessment of low back pain and disability at one point in time. (After Waddell et al 1984, with permission from the BMJ Publishing Group.)

that most of these psychologic and behavioral changes are secondary to pain, and get better or worse with clinical progress. However, we should recognize that distress may both precede and follow the physical problem. The patient's personality and preexisting psychologic state may modify the whole process. This is not a causal model, but only a static cross-section of the clinical presentation at one point in time. The model explores the psychologic and behavioral factors that may help to explain current levels of pain and disability. It does not allow for how these various aspects develop and interact. This is also a model of illness rather than wellness. It does not consider how most people manage to cope with back pain and get on with their lives more or less normally, while others become severely and even permanently disabled.

The development of chronic low back pain and disability

Pain and disability, even chronic pain and disability, are not static. They do not just occur suddenly, but develop over time. It is a dynamic process. So the real question is: how do chronic pain and disability develop? Here, the disease model is of little help, and biomedical factors are poor predictors of which patients will develop chronic, intractable problems. Back pain may arise from a physical problem in the back, but all the evidence shows that psychosocial factors have more influence on the development of chronic pain and disability.

Philips & Grant (1991a,b) made one of the earliest longitudinal studies of acute back pain, and questioned the traditional distinction between acute and chronic pain. By the end of the first week, 44% of patients were already improving and 31% were getting worse. Most patients still expected to recover gradually over a period of 3 or 4 weeks. They were mildly frustrated and anxious about their pain, but they did not have clinical anxiety or depression. The main effect of acute pain was reduced exercise tolerance, and there was less impact on their housework, social activities and family relationships. Most chronic pain patients were broadly similar. The main differences were that they reported much greater impact of pain on their lives and lower expectations of recovery.

At 6 months, 40% of patients reported continuing pain. If we define chronic pain purely by duration, then they had chronic pain. Half of them described their pain as moderate or severe. However, most of them gradually adjusted and returned to their usual activities despite continuing pain. Very few went on to chronic intractable pain and disability. Philips & Grant found that most of the emotional changes developed within the first 3 months and then remained quite stable. In contrast, the impact of their pain and their level of disability reduced, and they continued to improve up to 6 months.

Philips & Grant's study included few real 'chronic pain patients'. It probably tells us more about how most normal people deal with continuing pain than about the few who become 'problem pain patients'. Hadjistavropoulos & Craig (1994) compared patients with acute back pain and a group of chronic back pain sufferers. They also found that most acute and chronic patients are actually quite similar. It is a small subgroup of patients who develop emotional and behavioral problems out of proportion to their physical problem; and some of these patients develop these changes at an early stage. It is this subgroup of patients who are different, rather than there being any difference between acute and chronic pain.

It is now clear that many of the psychologic and behavioral changes that we used to associate with chronic pain can appear much earlier. Burton et al (1995) found that 18% of patients had significant distress when they first presented in primary care. Roberts (1991) found distress at 3 weeks in an acute attack. Ohlund et al (1994) found pain behavior by 6 weeks. It is clear, then, that these emotional and behavioral changes can develop within 3–6 weeks.

All of these studies raise doubts about the traditional division between acute and chronic pain. Acute pain merges into chronic pain, but although many people with back trouble continue to have pain, most of them adjust to it, and manage to return to most activities and a reasonably normal lifestyle. Chronic pain may not be something new or different that develops with time. Rather, we may understand chronic pain better as a failure of acute pain to resolve as it should. Chronic pain patients continue to present as if they still had an acute problem, rather than developing new reactions and behavior. Many of the changes may depend more on the severity and impact of pain and disability than on the duration of symptoms. Failure to restore normal function appears to be worse than chronic pain alone. The rate of development and severity of these changes also vary from patient to patient. Acute and chronic pain are not different in kind, but rather in effect. The major difference may be in the established nature of chronic pain, its impact on the patient's life and its intractable nature – and this may develop surprisingly early. If this is correct, we should look for factors that delay or prevent recovery, rather than factors that cause chronicity. We should also look at the influence of health care. It may be not just that chronic pain patients continue to present as if they had acute pain. It may be also that doctors and therapists treat them as if they still had acute pain.

In Chapter 7 we reviewed the evidence that psychosocial factors are better predictors of clinical progress and outcome than any biomedical data. They play an important part in the *process* of developing chronic pain and disability. They not only develop earlier than we previously thought, but also influence this process at an early stage.

Coste et al (1994) studied primary care patients with acute low back pain within 3 days of onset. Roland et al (1983), Lehmann et al (1993), Burton et al (1995), Gatchel et al (1995) and Klenerman et al (1995) all studied patients within the first 2–8 weeks. Within the first few days, severity of symptoms is probably the best predictor of symptomatic recovery. It is much more difficult at that stage to predict return to work, or which patients are at risk of chronic disability. Probably within the first 3 weeks, and certainly within 6–8 weeks, psychologic factors become more important. They are then much better predictors of clinical progress, pain and disability at 1 year, and return to work than any biomedical measures.

Social interactions also have an important influence on clinical progress. It is very difficult to become a chronic pain patient without family support or a 'partner in pain'. Return to work depends more on work-related factors than on the physical state of the patient's back. Patients who are unemployed or who lose their jobs have much greater difficulty returning to work. Most clinical studies show that patients on compensation or in an adversarial legal situation have slower and poorer outcomes, especially for return to work.

Let us emphasize again that we are not saying that these patients have psychogenic pain. We believe that their pain arises from a physical source in their back, although we have debated the nature of their continuing nociception. However, even in patients with clear physical pathology in their back, psychosocial factors can have a profound influence on whether it leads to chronic pain and disability.

The development of chronic pain and disability

- The symptom of back pain arises from a physical process in the back and nociception
- The key to chronic pain and disability may be failure to recover as it should, rather than the development of a different syndrome
- As pain becomes chronic (and this process may start within 3–8 weeks), attitudes and beliefs, distress and illness behavior play an increasing role in the development of chronicity and disability
- This all occurs within a social context, and leads to social interactions with others, including in particular family, work and health care

---

The link between psychologic and physiologic events

How do these physical and psychologic events interact? Chronic low back pain and disability does not depend on *either* physical *or* psychologic mechanisms. Rather, it is a question of how psychologic events influence physiologic processes, and the interactions between them over time.

There are close links between physiologic and psychologic events:

- Nonspecific low back pain seems to be mainly a matter of disturbed function or painful musculoskeletal dysfunction.
- Disability is reduced function. It is a matter of what we do (or do not do) and of altered performance.
- Pain behavior or illness behavior is also a matter of what we do (or do not do).
- Disability involves both physical dysfunction and illness behavior, which in a sense are simply two sides of the same coin. Behavior always involves motor and physiologic activity; and physiologic processes always have behavioral expressions. Behavior changes at both subjective and physiologic levels.

This combination of dysfunction and behavior is the crux of the problem (Fig. 14.4). It is not a question of whether physical dysfunction or altered behavior comes first or which is more important, but rather how they interact and reinforce each other (Ahern et al 1990). What is the effect of pain and disability on mental and psychologic events, which in turn influence behavior? How do these psychologic processes and altered behavior aggravate and perpetuate musculoskeletal dysfunction?

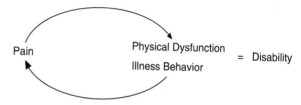

Figure 14.4 Physical dysfunction and illness behavior are intimately linked to each other. They lie at the heart of the process of developing chronic low back pain and disability. Low back pain leads to physical dysfunction and altered behavior, which in turn aggravate and perpetuate the pain. Physical dysfunction and illness behavior lead to low back disability or, in another sense, *are* disability.

Psychologic events may affect physiologic processes by several mechanisms:

- increased muscle tension
- guarded movements
- disuse syndrome.

These are not mutually exclusive, but may all play a role.

As we saw in Chapter 9, there is little evidence that static muscle tension plays an important role in low back pain (Flor & Birbaumer 1994). Our backs and our muscles are for working, and dynamic processes are much more important. Guarded movements appear to be particularly important, and could be closely linked to psychologic processes (Main & Watson 1996, Watson et al 1998). Guarded movements bear little relationship to current pain, but are strongly related to fear avoidance. Fear of pain or reinjury, and the patient's own perception of their ability – or lack of ability – to perform movements and activities despite pain may all lead to guarded movements. Exacerbations of back pain are common and may further reinforce this conditioning. These patterns may start as a physiologic response to injury or primary dysfunction, but persist due to psychophysiologic rather than physiologic processes alone (Box 14.2). They may become unconscious and relatively independent of current back pain. They may produce physical changes such as disturbed posture and gait, reduced range of movement, loss of strength and fatigue.

Box 14.2 Psychophysiologic links

- Withdrawal, catastrophizing and depression
- Passive coping strategies
- Avoidance learning
  — anticipation of pain
  — avoidance of physical activity
  — avoidance of social activities and situations
  — non-occurrence of pain is a powerful negative reinforcer for reduced activity
- Increased muscle tension, muscle imbalance, guarded movements, gait disturbance

---

Studies in gait biomechanics suggest that limping may be another form of guarded movements. Keefe & Hill (1985) showed that patients with chronic low back pain walk more slowly, with shorter steps and asymmetric gait patterns. Limping again bears little relation to the severity of pain, but more to anticipation of pain and pain behavior.

Guarded movements and lack of normal use lead in turn to physical and psychologic deconditioning. This 'disuse syndrome' is the direct consequence of reduced activity and illness behavior (Bortz 1984). Disuse has a profound effect on the physical condition of the back which aggravates and maintains physical dysfunction, and leads directly to more severe disability. As well as this physical or physiologic loop, there is feedback and reinforcement of behavior. What we do, our activity level and illness behavior, reinforce our beliefs about the pain and the coping strategies we use to deal with it. Illness behavior, disability and work loss reinforce distress and depression, which increase illness behavior and disability. These are all interlocking, vicious circles.

Deconditioning may be the end result of altered behavior

- Circulatory, tissue nutrition and metabolic changes
- Muscle wasting, loss of strength and endurance
- Loss of neuromuscular coordination
- Muscle imbalance
- Guarded movements
- Reduced range and patterns of movement
- Disturbed posture and gait
- Physical dysfunction and illness behavior

A dynamic model of low back pain and disability

Low back pain and disability are part of a dynamic process over time. Low back pain arises from a physical problem in the back, but physical dysfunction and altered behavior then aggravate and perpetuate pain and disability. The factors that influence clinical progress, their relative importance, and the interactions between them vary over time as the process evolves. Time itself – the duration of pain and, particularly, time off work – also plays a major role (Frank et al 1996).

The core of this process is how physical dysfunction and illness behavior develop and interact over time. We can look at this process on several levels: neuromuscular, neurophysiologic and psychophysiologic. Figures 14.5–14.7 offer a series of possible links and feedback loops between fear avoidance, guarded movements and physical dysfunction. Figure 14.5 shows more of the possible musculoskeletal mechanisms, Figure 14.6 is a more neurophysiologic perspective, and Figure 14.7 shows more of the possible psychologic processes. We suggest that all these levels are interlinked and develop simultaneously. These are not alternative models, but rather different levels or perspectives of the one process. We have a good theoretic basis for this kind of dynamic model, but little direct evidence on the exact links. We simply offer these figures as hypotheses for further testing and experiment.

Flor et al (1990) stressed the role of learning in the development and maintenance of chronic pain and disability. Chronic pain and inactivity lead to preoccupation with physical symptoms. Withdrawal, distress and depression increase bodily awareness and aggravate the pain. Pain patients often misinterpret their sensations. They

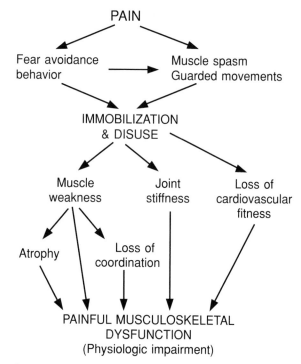

Figure 14.5 A more physical perspective of the relationship between altered behavior and dysfunction: the relation between fear avoidance and painful musculoskeletal dysfunction. (Based on ideas from Liebenson 1996.)

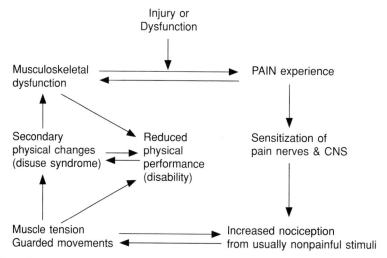

Figure 14.6 A more neurophysiologic perspective of the relationship between altered behavior and dysfunction: possible neurophysiologic mechanisms of guarded movements. (With contributions from Dr C Spanswick, with thanks.)

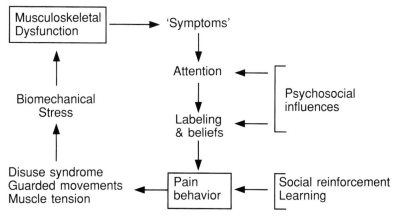

Figure 14.7 A more psychologic perspective of the relationship between altered behavior and dysfunction: possible mechanisms linking psychologic and behavioral processes with guarded movements. (With contributions from P Watson, with thanks.)

develop maladaptive beliefs about the cause and meaning of their pain, and what they should do about it. Once these beliefs become fixed, they are very resistant to change, even when they are clearly inaccurate and unhelpful. Avoidance learning and passive coping strategies may be particularly important and difficult to reverse, particularly if they lead to physiologic changes:

$$\text{Learning} \rightleftarrows \text{changed behavior} \rightleftarrows \text{physiologic changes}$$

Vlaeyen et al (1995a,b) looked at more specific fears of movement/(re)injury. There is a strong association between such fears and physical activity or behavior, independent of the severity of pain (McCracken et al 1993, Crombez 1994, Menard et al 1994, Vlaeyen et al 1995a,b). Crombez (1994) and Vlaeyen et al (1995a,b) showed that chronic low back pain patients with high fear levels and avoidance behavior perform less well at motor tasks. Reduced activity and avoidance behavior lead to disuse, depression and increased disability (Philips 1987, Council et al 1988). Cross-sectional studies by Rose et al (1992) and Waddell et al (1993) supported this analysis. Longitudinal studies by Klenerman et al (1995) and Burton et al (1995) showed that these fears act at an early

stage and contribute to the development, not just to the maintenance, of chronic pain and disability.

These psychophysiologic and behavioral mechanisms may all combine in the following way:

- fear of movement/(re)injury
- reduced activity level and avoidance behavior
- guarded movements
- deconditioning
- chronic pain and disability.

Why do some people recover and others become disabled?

The models described above show the process by which chronic low back pain and disability can develop. They do not explain how some people develop chronic pain and disability, while others recover. Clearly, quite different mechanisms must operate in different people. There must be 'decision points' and different paths that lead to widely divergent outcomes. (Of course, that does not mean that these are necessarily conscious decisions.)

Clinical progress is not smooth and uninterrupted, but involves crises. Frank et al (1996) looked at concepts of equilibrium and thresholds. Back pain is often a persistent or recurrent problem over time. Most people cope with this up to a certain point, but then an exacerbation of pain, increased demand or reduced ability to cope may disturb their equilibrium. They reach a crisis or breakpoint, at which they may slide or fall uncontrollably into a different situation (Fig. 14.8). It may then be much more difficult to return to their previous state. The most dramatic example is when they stop work. They then face a very different set of influences and obstacles to return to work, which requires recrossing the threshold in the opposite direction.

Beliefs, coping strategies and behavior may play a major role in these crises and decision points. People have different beliefs about their pain, and they try to learn different strategies to cope. Each strategy has its costs and benefits, and gives different expectations of success. The most powerful negative drive is fear. Fear may lead to avoidance of the activity or situation that caused the fear or pain, in an attempt to reduce it. Personal experience, catastrophizing, depression and social context may increase fear avoidance. Avoiders do not have significantly different demographics, pain or medical history from other back pain sufferers, but they do have a greater fear of pain and reinjury. Confronting and avoiding are very different strategies with different short- and long-term costs and benefits (Lethem et al 1983). Vlaeyen et al (1995a,b) sug-

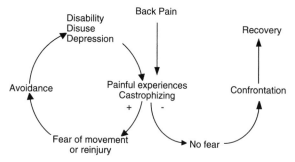

Figure 14.9 Confrontation or avoidance of pain can lead to very different outcomes: fear of movement and reinjury can determine how some people recover from back pain while others go on to chronic pain and disability. (Adapted from Vlaeyen et al 1995b, with permission.)

gested that confrontation or avoidance can lead to very different outcomes (Fig. 14.9). This fits clinical observations of the dramatic contrast between most people who cope successfully with low back pain and the few who become chronic pain patients. The unanswered questions are what determines whether we confront or avoid pain, and how we may change this.

Krause & Ragland (1994) proposed a phase model that offers a social perspective on how work disability develops over time (Fig. 14.10). Phase 1 is the onset of symptoms before any health care or work loss. This has little social impact, although it may interfere with work performance to some extent. Phase 2 is the formal reporting of an injury or medical certification of the condition, which is the official, public registering of sickness. Phase 3 covers most acute episodes of low back pain. The worker may rely on self-treatment, or seek medical care or alternative health care. Most acute attacks settle rapidly, sufficient to permit return to work with minor social, work and economic impact.

Phase 4 is work disability for 1–7 weeks. Virtually all patients are receiving health care by this time. This is commonly regarded as the 'normal healing time' or, perhaps more accurately, the normal recovery time. Treatment is most likely to be effective. Most Western countries require medical certification, and some form of sick pay or sickness benefit begins. Krause & Ragland regard this phase as the

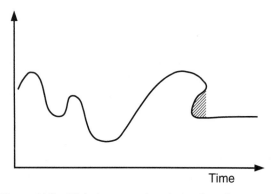

Figure 14.8 Clinical progress is not smooth and uninterrupted but involves crises and sudden shifts from one state to another. (Based on Catastrophe Theory.)

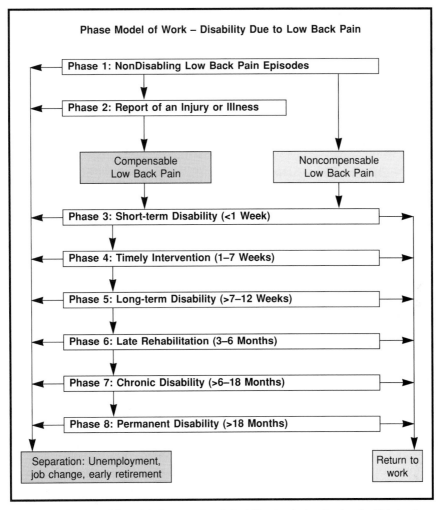

Figure 14.10 A social model of occupational disability due to low back pain. This implies break-points and shifts from one social state to another. (From Krause & Ragland 1994, with permission.)

opportunity for 'timely' health care and ergonomic or administrative action.

In phase 5, the worker is beginning to enter the chronic stage, with all its medical and social implications. Prognosis and expectations deteriorate. By phase 6, the chance of successful medical treatment falls and there is now a major rehabilitation challenge. Through phases 6–8 there is increasing social and economic impact on the worker and his family, loss of employability, need for retraining or placement, and major social adaptation. Society must meet

escalating health care costs and financial support, and there may be adversarial legal proceedings. The perspective changes. Instead of a medical condition with social implications, chronic back pain becomes a disability problem with medical implications.

Once again, we would stress that disability is not static but dynamic. The disabling process evolves through distinct phases over time, and each phase involves a different set of social interactions. Capacity for work deteriorates, and the difficulties of rehabilitation and returning to work increase. Patients have to revise their expectations about getting well and being able to return to work. Their social status changes through each of these phases, at some points quite dramatically. The outcome of any intervention may be quite different in different phases, so the timing of health care is critical.

HEALTH CARE FOR BACK PAIN FROM A BIOPSYCHOSOCIAL PERSPECTIVE

The successes and failures of treatment for spinal disorders reflect the value and limitations of the disease model, and the need for a biopsychosocial approach. The success of physical treatment depends on accurate diagnosis of a treatable lesion, as Spangfort (1972) showed in surgery for disc prolapse (Table 14.3).

However, the classic study by Wiltse & Rocchio (1975) showed that psychologic factors also affect how patients respond to surgery (Table 14.4). Many other studies have now shown this to be equally true of all conservative therapies, surgery, pain management programs and rehabilitation. Psychologic distress and illness behavior lead to poorer relief of pain, more disability and more work loss (Table 14.5). This is true whether or not the patient has a verifiable pathology such as a disc prolapse, or an 'unverifiable' soft tissue problem.

We investigated the interaction of physical and psychologic factors in a prospective study of 195 surgical patients (Waddell et al 1986), and found that the physical outcome of surgery depended on physical factors: accurate diagnosis

Table 14.4 Psychologic distress predicting symptomatic outcome from chemonucleolysis for disc prolapse (based on data from Wiltse & Rocchio 1975)

Preoperative Hs and Hy scores on the MMPI*	Excellent or good symptomatic relief
5+	10
75–84	16
65–74	39
55–64	72
54–	90

*The mean score for normal people is 50.

of a surgically treatable lesion, good surgery and avoiding complications. If surgery was successful, then the patient's emotions and illness behavior also got better; but if surgery failed, it could make the patient psychologically worse. Psychologic factors could affect outcome in two ways. They could affect pain and disability directly and so affect the patient's and surgeon's judgement of outcome. They could also influence surgical decisions and hence affect outcomes indirectly. Most often, psychologic factors aggravated pain and disability and led to more pressure to 'do something'. Most dangerous of all, illness behavior could lead to inappropriate surgery. The patient was desperate, conservative treatment had failed and the surgeon wanted to help. Surgery carried out for the wrong reasons led to predictably poor results. It not only failed to provide relief, but could also make the patient's pain and distress worse, which in turn would lead to more illness behavior and disability.

Hasenbring et al (1994) found the same in Germany. The 111 patients in their study all had proven disc prolapse, and two-thirds of them underwent surgery. Hasenbring et al

Table 14.3 Relief of sciatica and back pain according to the degree of herniation found at surgery (based on data from Spangfort 1972)

Operative findings	Relief of sciatica		Relief of back pain (%)
	Complete (%)	Partial (%)	
Complete herniation	90	9	75
Incomplete herniation	82	16	74
Bulging disc	63	26	54
No herniation	37	38	43

Table 14.5 Outcome of treatment related to the amount of illness behavior (based on collected data from various sources)

Treatment	Success rate of treatment (%) in patients with:	
	No behavioral signs	Multiple behavioral signs
First lumbar surgery	80–90	30–50
Chemonucleolysis	60	10
Repeat lumbar surgery	50–60	20–40
Rehabilitation	50–60	10
Behavioral modification	60–80	40–50

studied preoperative findings and long-term outcomes. Persistent pain at 6 months was predicted by a combination of physical, psychologic and social measures. The physical measures included the degree of disc displacement and the presence of scoliosis due to severe muscle spasm. The clinical outcome at 6 months, however, depended much more on how patients reacted to and coped with the pain. Nineteen of these patients applied for early retirement and the best predictors were depression and stress at work.

The moral is clear. We must distinguish the underlying physical problem from the patient's reaction and illness behavior. We should direct physical treatment, especially potentially dangerous treatment such as surgery, to the physical problem. At the same time we must also recognize and deal with these important psychosocial issues. If this is true of a clear-cut physical pathology like a disc prolapse which fits the disease model, it is even more important in a nonspecific symptom like back pain.

From a biopsychosocial point of view, it is not surprising that traditional treatment of back pain as a purely biomedical problem has failed. Back pain is a symptom, not a disease. If it is a symptom of dysfunction, that would explain why the traditional medical search for a structural lesion has been futile. By focusing on physical pathology, the disease model neglects important psychosocial issues. If low back pain and disability are much more than just a physical problem, we cannot expect physical treatment alone to provide the answer. By focusing on pain, it neglects disability. Although we think

Table 14.6 The influence of different elements of illness on the amount of conservative treatment that patients receive for low back pain (from Waddell et al 1984, with permission from the BMJ Publishing Group)

Identifiable influences	Extent to which these account for the amount of treatment received (%)
Duration of symptoms	14
Physical severity	+11
Psychologic distress	+9
Illness behavior	+15
Total identified	**50%**

These are additive.

that we direct physical treatment rationally to physical disease, this is not entirely true. In practice, treatment for a poorly understood condition such as back pain depends more than we realize, or like to admit, on nonphysical factors (Table 14.6).

The problem is that we give the wrong treatment for the wrong reasons. Treatment may not only be ineffective for the physical disorder, but may also make the psychosocial aspects worse and cause iatrogenic disability (Fig. 14.11). Health care can have a profound effect on all of these processes. Formal information and advice may have some influence on patients' beliefs about back pain. Our whole management strategy may have much greater impact on their beliefs, coping strategies, illness behavior and disability. Advice to stop work and sick certification are direct adjuncts to work loss and even loss of employment and early retirement. Health care also affects patients' families and workplaces, as well as their attitudes and what they do.

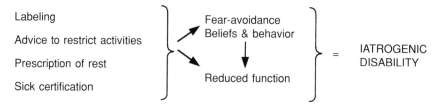

Figure 14.11 Health care for back pain can have a profound effect at all levels in a biopsychosocial model. Unfortunately, it may lead to iatrogenic disability.

Chronic disability due to nonspecific low back pain is never simply a matter of physical pathology. A 'medical condition' and sick certification are prerequisites for long-term social support, but disability for work is essentially a social phenomenon. This is why medical diagnosis and treatment alone cannot solve the problem. But health professionals also play a vital role in the interactions among the individual, employment, society and legal systems.

The biopsychosocial model of low back pain and disability leads to a very different approach to management. It lets us consider low back disability as a human illness rather than low back pain as a spinal disease, and shifts our focus from structural damage to disturbed function and neurophysiology. We must consider all the physical, psychologic and social aspects of the illness. Of course, we must exclude serious spinal disease, and provide simple, safe, symptomatic measures to control pain. We must also recognize psychologic distress and distinguish the symptoms and signs of illness behavior from those of physical disease. This model changes our focus from pain alone to pain and disability; from relief of symptoms to an equal goal of restoring function. It stresses the social impact of back pain and the need to get patients back to work.

This all helps us to put into practice our common ideal of treating our patients as individual human beings. Instead of thinking only about how to treat their physical condition, we must also consider how our management affects their beliefs and behavior. We should recognize, and try to change, mistaken beliefs and fears at an early stage to prevent chronicity. The key to successful rehabilitation may be to overcome these fears and change behavior, as much as any physical reconditioning. We must always keep in mind that the ultimate goal and outcome of health care is not only to relieve, or at least control, pain, but also to help our patients to get on with their normal lives.

All of this is not to deny that these patients have a physical problem in their backs and real pain. They do, and this analysis may help us to understand the nature and depth of their suffering. It is not our intention to deny them health care, but they need a different kind of health care. They need physical treatment for their physical problem, but, more importantly, they may also need support and help to cope with the pain and to restore normal activity and behavior.

The biopsychosocial model is simply a set of tools to better understand low back pain and disability, and to treat patients rather than their spines.

Pain — dysfunction

- Epidemiologically and clinically, the main problem is not back pain alone but the combination of pain and disability
- NOT treatment of pain as a signal of tissue damage
- NOR symptomatic treatment of pain as an end in itself
- INSTEAD treatment of pain as a symptom of dysfunction
- The logical treatment for the pain is to restore normal function:
  — physiologic
  — behavioral
  — work

REFERENCES

Ahern D K, Hannon D J, Goreczny A J, Follick M J, Parziale J R 1990 Correlation of chronic low back pain behavior and muscle function examination of the flexion-relaxation response. Spine 15: 92–95

Bortz W M 1984 The disuse syndrome. Western Journal of Medicine 141: 691–694

Burton A K, Tillotson M, Main C J, Hollis S 1995 Psychosocial predictors of outcome in acute and sub-chronic low back trouble. Spine 20: 722–728

Cooper J E, Tate R B, Yassi A, Khokhar J 1996 Effect of an early intervention program on the relationship between subjective pain and disability measures in nurses with low back injury. Spine 21: 12 329–12 336

Coste J, Delecoeuillerie G, Lara A C, Le Parc J M, Paolaggi J B 1994 Clinical course and prognostic factors in acute low back pain: an inception cohort study in primary care practice. British Medical Journal 308: 577–580

Council J R, Ahern D K, Follick M J, Kline C L 1988 Expectancies and functional impairments in chronic low back pain. Pain 33: 323–331

Crombez G 1994 Pain modulation through anticipation. PhD thesis, University of Leuven, Belgium

Descartes R 1664 Traite de l'homme. Angot, Paris

Flor H, Birbaumer N, Turk D C 1990 The psychobiology of chronic pain. Advances in Behavioural Research and Therapy 12: 47–84

Flor H, Birbaumer N 1994 Acquisition of chronic pain: psychophysiological mechanisms. American Pain Society Journal 3: 119–127

Frank J W, Kerr M S, Brooker A-S et al 1996 Disability resulting from occupational low back pain. Spine 21: 2908–2929

Gatchel R J, Polatin P B, Mayer T G 1995 The dominant role of psychosocial risk factors in the development of chronic low back disability. Spine 20: 2702–2709

Hadjistavropoulos H D, Craig K D 1994 Acute and chronic low back pain: cognitive, affective, and behavioral dimensions. Journal of Consulting and Clinical Psychology 62: 341–349

Hasenbring M, Marienfeld G, Kuhlendahl D, Soyka D 1994 Risk factors for chronicity in lumbar disc patients. Spine 19: 2759–2765

Keefe F, Hill W 1985 An objective approach to quantifying pain behavior and gait patterns in low back pain patients. Pain 21: 153–161

Klenerman L, Slade P D, Stanley I M et al 1995 The prediction of chronicity in patients with an acute attack of low back pain in a general practice setting. Spine 20: 478–484

Krause N, Ragland D R 1994 Occupational disability due to low back pain: a new interdisciplinary classification based on a phase model of disability. Spine 19: 1011–1020

Lehmann T R, Spratt K F, Lehmann K K 1993 Predicting long-term disability in low back injured workers presenting to a spine consultant. Spine 18: 1103–1112

Lethem J, Slade P D, Troup J D G, Bentley G 1983 Outline of a fear-avoidance model of exaggerated pain perception. Behavioural Research and Therapy 21: 401–408

Liebenson C 1996 Rehabilitation of the spine. Williams & Wilkins, Baltimore, p 13–31

Linton S J 1985 The relationship between activity and chronic pain. Pain 21: 289–294

Main C J, Watson P J 1996 Guarded movements: development of chronicity. Journal of Musculoskeletal Pain 4: 163–170

McCracken L M, Gross R T, Sorg P J, Edmands T A 1993 Prediction of pain in patients with chronic low back pain: effects of inaccurate prediction and pain-related anxiety. Behavioural Research and Therapy 31: 647–652

Melzack R, Casey K L 1968 Sensory, motivational and central control determinants of pain: a new conceptual model. In: Kenshalo D (ed) The skin senses. C C Thomas, Springfield, IL, p 423–443

Melzack R, Wall P D 1965 Pain mechanisms: a new theory. Science 150: 971–979

Menard M R, Cooke C, Locke S R, Beach G N, Butler T B 1994 Pattern of performance in workers with low back pain during a comprehensive motor performance evaluation. Spine 19: 1359–1366

Merskey H 1979 Pain terms: a list with definitions and notes on usage. Recommended by the IASP Subcomittee on Taxonomy. Pain 6: 249–252

Ohlund C, Lindstrom I, Areskoug B, Eeek C, Peterson L-E, Nachemson A 1994 Pain behavior in industrial subacute low back pain. Part I. Reliability: concurrent and predictive validity of pain behavior assessments. Pain 58: 201–209

Philips H C 1987 Avoidance learning and its role in sustaining chronic pain. Behavioural Research and Therapy 25: 273–279

Philips H C, Grant L 1991a Acute back pain: a psychological analysis. Behavioural Research and Therapy 29: 429–434

Philips H C, Grant L 1991b The evolution of chronic back pain problems: a longitudinal study. Behavioural Research and Therapy 29: 435–441

Reilly J P 1993 The efficacy of a pain management programme for people with chronic low back pain. PhD thesis, University of Liverpool

Riley J F, Ahern D K, Follick M J 1988 Chronic pain and functional impairment: assessing beliefs about their relationship. Archives of Physical Medicine and Rehabilitation 69: 579–582

Roberts A 1991 The conservative treatment of low back pain. MD thesis, University of Nottingham

Roland M O, Morrell D C, Morris R W 1983 Can general practitioners predict the outcome of episodes of back pain? British Medical Journal 286: 523–525

Rose M, Klenerman L, Atchinson L, Slade P D 1992 An application of the fear-avoidance model to three chronic pain problems. Behavioural Research and Therapy 30: 359–365

Spangfort E V 1972 The lumbar disc herniation. A computer aided analysis of 2504 operations. Acta Orthopaedica Scandinavica (Supplement) 142: 1–95

Symonds T L 1995 Attitudes, beliefs and associated absence: impact of a psychosocial back pain pamphlet in an industrial setting. PhD thesis, University of Huddersfield

Turk D C, Rudy T E, Stieg R L 1988 The disability determination dilemma: toward a mutiaxial solution. Pain 34: 217–229

Virchow R 1858 Die Cellular pathologie in Ihrer Begrundurg auf physiologische und pathologische. A Hirschwald, Berlin

Vlaeyen J W S, Kole-Snijders A M J, Boeren R G B, van Eek H 1995a Fear of movement/(re)injury in chronic low back pain and its relation to behavioral performance. Pain 62: 363–372

Vlaeyen J W S, Kole-Snijders A M J, Rottevel A, Ruesink R, Heuts P H T G 1995b The role of fear of movement/(re)injury in pain disability. Journal of Occupational Rehabilitation 5: 235–252

Waddell G 1987 A new clinical model for the treatment of low back pain. Spine 12: 632–644

Waddell G, Bircher M, Finlayson D, Main C J 1984 Symptoms and signs: physical disease or illness behaviour? British Medical Journal 289: 739–741

Waddell G, Main CJ, Morris EW, DiPaola M, Gray ICM 1984 Chronic low back pain, psychologic distress and illness behaviour. Spine 9: 209–213

Waddell G, Morris E W, Di Paola M P, Bircher M, Finlayson D 1986 A concept of illness tested as an improved basis for surgical decisions in low back disorders. Spine 11: 712–719

Waddell G, Somerville D, Henderson I, Newton M, Main C J 1993 A fear-avoidance beliefs questionnaire (FABQ) and the role of fear-avoidance beliefs in chronic low back pain and disability. Pain 52: 157–168

Watson P J, Booker C K, Main C J 1998 Evidence for the role of psychological factors in abnormal paraspinal activity in patients with chronic low back pain. Journal of Musculoskeletal Pain 5: 82–86

Wiltse L L, Rocchio P D 1975 Pre-operative psychological tests as predictions of success of chemonucleolysis in the treatment of the low back syndrome. Journal of Bone and Joint Surgery 57A: 478–483

15

Rest or stay active?

This new model of illness raises fundamental questions about our whole strategy of management for back pain. What should we advise patients with back pain to do: rest or stay active? The biopsychosocial model and the disease model give radically different answers.

THE HISTORY OF REST FOR BACK PAIN

Restriction of activity, rest and even bed rest are the traditional medical treatment for back pain and sciatica. At least through the early 1990s, rest was the most common treatment advised by physicians apart from analgesics (Table 15.1). Bed rest is the first line of treatment for 'acute attacks'.

Historically, rest is relatively new. Seriously ill people had always gone to the 'sick bed', but that was a consequence of disease and not a treatment. Sydenham (1734) had always kept arthritic or rheumatic patients mobile: 'For keeping bed constantly promotes and augments the disease.'

John Hunter (1794) first proposed rest as a treatment, in a treatise on wounds and inflammation. The concept of therapeutic rest seems to have arisen about that time, based on new pathologic ideas of inflammation:

The first and great requisite for the restoration of injured parts is rest, as it allows that action, which is necessary for repairing injured parts, to go on without interruption, and as the injuries excite more action than is required, rest becomes still more necessary.

Table 15.1 Treatment for low back pain reported by 500 patients attending an orthopedic clinic

Treatment advised at some time	One course	Repeated courses	Total
Analgesics	18%	69%	87%
Bed rest	21%	27%	48%
Lumbosacral support	14%	17%	31%
Physical therapy	10%	14%	24%
Manipulation	5%	5%	10%

Hunter dealt with this principle in two pages, but the theme is implicit in his whole book.

Hilton popularized this in *Rest and Pain*, a course of lectures to the Royal College of Surgeons in 1860–1862 (Hilton 1887). In his introduction, he considered the influence of mechanical and physiologic rest in the treatment of accidents and surgical diseases, and the diagnostic value of pain. He proposed rest as a curative agent or natural therapeutics in surgical practice. His argument was intriguing. He ranged from biblical quotations to contemporary ideas about cardiac, liver, renal, pulmonary and brain disease. The divine gift or solace for mankind is rest from his labors. Night-time sleep has a restorative function and is essential for the growth of plants and children. He linked psychiatric disease to physical and mental exhaustion. More prosaically, after Hunter, he said that rest is the natural treatment for the inflammation of injury and wounds. Hilton's contribution was to link rest to pain. Pain is the prime agent 'suggesting the necessity and indeed compelling to seek rest'. Hilton laid out this thesis in 14 introductory pages. The remainder of his book contains 17 lectures on a wide range of surgical conditions.

Both Hunter and Hilton were surgeons, dealing with surgical disease, yet their ideas had an impact across the whole of medicine. Once back pain came to be regarded as an injury, these principles applied. The links were injury → pain → rest → healing, and pain → inflammation (irritability) → rest. These were powerful and influential ideas, even if there was never much actual evidence. I do not think it is unkind to suggest that the most influential part of Hilton's book was its seductive title

Rest and Pain. Over the next century, physicians used rest as treatment for a wide range of conditions, from myocardial infarction to normal childbirth.

Hugh Owen Thomas (1874), the father of English orthopedics, applied the concept of rest to the newly emerging specialty of orthopedics. Therapeutic rest must be 'enforced, uninterrupted and prolonged'. Orthopedics achieved this by bracing, by bed rest and later by surgical fusion. This was a rational treatment for serious diseases such as fractures, tuberculosis and joint infection, before antibiotics and modern surgery. But even today, student textbooks still describe rest as a basic principle of orthopedic treatment.

As sciatica and later back pain came under the care of orthopedic doctors, so they prescribed orthopedic treatment. Like all professionals, when we do not know what to do, we do what we are trained to do. So, when these doctors did not know how to treat back pain and sciatica, they prescribed treatment according to the orthopedic principle of rest. So began 'modern' treatment for back pain. Orthopedics proposed rest for back pain in the latter part of the 19th century, and by 1900 a standard orthopedic text recommended 2–6 weeks' bed rest for acute lumbosacral pain.

The discovery of the ruptured disc in 1934 was the key marketing idea that allowed orthopedics to dominate back problems. World War II diverted society's and the profession's attention for a time, but also led to a great expansion in the specialty of orthopedic surgery. After the war, orthopedic surgeons had to find alternative civilian work. This coincided with improved health care and surgery, better resources and access, and rising public expectations. Within a generation, between the late 1940s and the 1970s, orthopedics became the leading specialty dealing not only with spinal disorders but also with nonspecific low back pain.

As late as 1966, family doctors in Britain felt that there was little discussion of back pain in their training, but that soon changed. From the 1960s to the mid-1990s, standard student textbooks of orthopedics trumpeted the message. They still give a strong impression that back pain is all about prolapsed intervertebral discs, and continue to advise rest. Through 1995, one British textbook actually stated unequivocally: 'The principle is to provide rest for the lumbar spine … (either) by a plaster jacket or bed rest …. Rest for the spine must be continued for six to twelve weeks according to progress.' This was finally updated in a new edition in 1995. Another blithely continues at the time of writing in October 1997 'REST: With an acute attack the patient should be kept in bed, with hips and knees slightly flexed and 10 kg traction to the pelvis … for two weeks.' By implication this is in hospital (Fig. 15.1).

With that kind of teaching, it is not surprising that there is still widespread professional and public perception that the appropriate treatment for back problems is rest. A postgraduate questionnaire in the UK in 1992

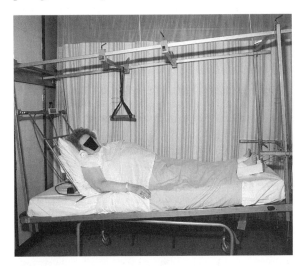

Figure 15.1 Strict hospital bed rest on traction: a stranded whale. Once you get the whale beached, it is very difficult to get her back into the water.

described a 38-year-old man with a 2 week history of nonspecific low back pain: 67% of family doctors selected bed rest as the 'correct' treatment. Coste et al (1994) looked at practice in France in 1991, and found that 49% of patients who attended their family doctor with acute nonspecific low back pain for less than 72 hours were prescribed bed rest. There has certainly been some change in thinking over the last 2 or 3 years, but speaking to patients in 1997 it is clear that this is slow to percolate into practice. Many doctors still routinely advise reduced activity and staying off work with back pain. They also continue to prescribe bed rest for 'acute attacks'.

However, that traditional orthopedic teaching did not go unchallenged. The French school of orthopedics, from Nicholas Andre in the early 18th century, continued to promote mobilization. One of the earliest English orthopedic texts on back pain was a lecture by Johnson (1881), who advised against bed rest. Indeed, he thought bed rest was a cause of back pain!

When the nutrition of the muscles has been impaired by long inaction, the results of confining to bed by illness or mechanical injury … pains in the back and limbs often follow the first attempts at exercise during convalescence. And these pains usually continue with more or less severity until by degrees the muscles regain their normal state of nutrition and vigour.

By 1923, one major orthopedic textbook qualified their prescription of bed rest for back pain: 'As soon as possible movement must be encouraged and bed forbidden.' Asher (1947) waxed lyrical:

It is my intention to justify placing beds and graves in the same category and to increase the amount of dread with which beds are usually regarded …. There is hardly any part of the body which is immune to its dangers.

Cyriax (1969) was his usual forthright self: 'Recumbency admits failure and should be the doctor's last thought, not his first.' But these were voices in the orthodox orthopedic wilderness. The principle of therapeutic rest became the traditional medical treatment for back pain.

Table 15.2 Proportion of different health professionals who advise bed rest for back problems (based on data from Cherkin et al 1988, Battie et al 1994)

Percentage who advise bed rest	Patient vignettes		
	Acute sciatica	Acute back pain	Chronic back pain
Medical specialists	87%	70%	31%
Family physicians	86%	52%	18%
Chiropractors	51%	30%	8%
Physical therapists	38%	0	0

There are still fascinating professional differences in recommendations about bed rest. Cherkin et al (1988) and Battie et al (1994) gave patient vignettes to various professional groups in the US (Table 15.2).

There is also considerable individual variation. von Korff et al (1994) found that physicians' advice about bed rest depended on their educational background and practice style. Patients also vary. Those who are better educated are less likely to use bed rest and more likely to stay active (Svensson & Andersson 1989). Those who are less well educated are more likely to heed medical advice!

However, this orthodox medical approach to back pain never gained universal public acceptance. Bone setters, like their descendants, the osteopaths and chiropractors, continued to treat the everyday aches and strains for which orthodox medicine had no good answer. They continued, and still continue, to follow the competing principle of mobilization.

The rationale of rest

The rationale of rest for back pain was a mixture of ideas based on the disease model. The orthopedic principle of rest started from the belief that back pain and sciatica were due to injury and traumatic inflammation. As Hunter and Hilton suggested, rest was essential for healing, so chronic pain would develop unless they treated the initial injury with rest. This was closely linked to the lingering idea that the spine and the nervous system were 'irritable'. Movement and physical activity may increase pain, and so must be harmful. Above all, the patient must avoid repeated injuries, for these would aggravate inflammation, prevent healing and lead to chronic pain.

This thinking was then updated in terms of the disc. The ruptured disc is clearly an injury – the disc comes 'out'. Disc pressure is lowest when lying down, so perhaps recumbency somehow let the disc 'go back'.

Unfortunately, none of these ideas has much pathologic validity. Orthopedics has also greatly confused the understanding and management of disc prolapse and nonspecific low back pain. Most of these ideas probably have nothing to do with simple backache. The reasoning is also illogical. Rest is, at best, an ineffective method of symptomatic relief (Table 15.3), and even if it does produce temporary relief, it does not necessarily have a corresponding effect on the natural history or clinical outcome.

It should come as no surprise that there was never any scientific evidence to support the dogma of bed rest for back pain.

The harmful effects of rest

The ill-effects of prolonged immobilization are a standard part of basic medical and nursing teaching (see Box 9.5, p. 152). Prolonged bed rest

Table 15.3 Effect of physical activities on back pain in 200 osteopathic patients (from Dr K Burton, with thanks)

	Aggravates	Relieves
Sitting	30%	23%
Walking	22%	12%
Movement	17%	16%
Lying	9%	35%

is the most effective method known of producing a severe disuse syndrome (Bortz 1984).

Lesser degrees of deconditioning probably play a part in most cases of chronic low back pain (Mayer & Gatchel 1988, Hides et al 1994) and, as every sportsman knows, this begins within a week or two of inactivity. Deconditioning leads to loss of:

- strength
- endurance
- flexibility
- coordination
- fitness.

Treatment by rest also ignores its psychosocial impact. Physical deterioration, psychologic withdrawal and social inactivity reinforce each other. Rest is a completely passive approach that leads to fear avoidance, catastrophizing and depression. It actually prescribes iatrogenic disability and illness behavior (see Fig. 14.11, p. 238).

THE SCIENTIFIC EVIDENCE

By the mid-1980s, research workers began to question the *duration* of bed rest for acute back pain. There were two key randomized controlled trials (RCTs). Deyo et al (1986) showed that patients who were advised to take 2 days' bed rest returned to work faster than those who were advised to take 7 days. Gilbert et al (1985) showed that those who had no bed rest reported less restriction of daily activities and returned to normal activities faster than those who had 4 days' bed rest. These two studies had a major impact. The scientific world of back pain accepted that short periods of 2–4 days bed rest were better than longer periods. This formed the basis for recommendations in the US and UK clinical guidelines for acute back pain (AHCPR 1994, CSAG 1994). However, most experts still accepted the basic principle of rest or modified activity, and recommended short periods of bed rest for acute attacks.

That was soon to change. We can actually interpret these two trials in two ways. The general view was that they showed that short periods of a few days' bed rest were better than longer periods. Equally, however, they could mean that 7 days' bed rest was proportionately more harmful than 2–3 days! I had already made an impassioned theoretic argument against bed rest for back pain (Waddell 1987, 1993):

There is no evidence that rest has any beneficial effect on the natural history of low back pain. On the contrary, there is strongly suggestive evidence that rest, particularly prolonged bed rest, may be the most harmful treatment ever devised and a potent cause of iatrogenic disability.

Two influential Scandinavian RCTs put this to the test. Was there any evidence for even short periods of bed rest?

In Finland, Malmivaara et al (1995) studied patients with acute nonspecific low back pain, with an average duration of 5 days. They randomly assigned them to one of three treatments: 2 days' bed rest; back mobilizing exercises; or ordinary activities to be continued as tolerated. In the original experimental design, they used ordinary activities as the control group. At 3 and 12 weeks, the control group did best. They had significantly less duration and severity of pain, less disability and fewer days off work. Recovery was slowest in those who had bed rest. Malmivaara et al concluded that continuing ordinary activities within the limits permitted by the pain leads to more rapid recovery.

In Norway, Indahl et al (1995) looked at the effect of regarding low back pain as a benign, self-limiting condition and treating it by light normal activity. They studied nearly 1000 patients who had been off work for more than 8 weeks. Patients in the study group were carefully assessed and reassured that there was no serious disorder in their backs. Indahl et al tried to correct common misunderstandings about back pain, and explained about pain and tension, muscle spasm and guarding. They reassured patients that light activity and mobilization would not cause further damage, but would more likely help recovery. They put considerable effort into overcoming fears about back pain and illness behavior. Their main practical advice was for patients to walk normally and to be as flexible as possible, and a therapist demonstrated how to implement these principles. Indahl himself is a most charismatic speaker, and I have no doubt that he delivered the message forcibly and convincingly.

Patients in the control group were not examined, but received standard treatment in the Norwegian health care system.

Indahl et al's management produced a highly significant, 50% reduction in the number of patients still on chronic sick leave after 6 months. They have now maintained this up to 2 years. They concluded that information and advice designed to reduce fear and to encourage patients to continue light normal activity with an emphasis on keeping flexible were better than standard medical treatment for back pain.

A review of the evidence

We have recently reviewed the evidence on bed rest and advice to stay active (Waddell et al 1997). We made a systematic literature search for all RCTs published up to April 1996. The main symptom had to be acute back pain of up to 3 months' duration. We included all the trials we could find of bed rest, regardless of setting. Trials of advice and activity had to be in a primary care setting, including general family practice, osteopathy, chiropractic or occupational health. Advice and activity are not indexed in the standard literature databases, so we checked all published RCTs of low back pain to find these treatments. The main intervention had to be advice about maintaining activity levels, given to the individual patient by a practitioner. We excluded trials of specific back exercises, back education classes and educational booklets. We looked at patient-centered outcomes including rate of recovery from the acute attack, relief of pain, restoration of function, satisfaction of treatment, days off work and return to work, development of chronic pain and disability, recurrent attacks and future health care. We also rated the quality of the trials.

We found 10 trials of bed rest and eight trials of advice to stay active. Table 15.4 presents the trials of bed rest with information on the patients, settings, interventions, main outcomes and results. Table 15.5 presents the review of advice to stay active. Two trials directly compared bed rest and advice to stay active, and we included them in both tables (Malmivaara et al 1995, Wilkinson 1995).

Two of the trials of bed rest stand out from the others, and we need to consider them separately. Pal et al (1986) showed that bed rest with continuous traction gave no benefit over bed rest with sham traction. However, their trial did not provide any information on the effect of bed rest itself. The trial by Wiesel et al (1980) involved young male army recruits under army discipline. The subjects, setting, interventions and outcomes were all atypical and we cannot generalize them to the general back pain population in primary care. This probably explains why its results are completely different from all the other trials.

All the other trials showed that bed rest was not effective. Two trials showed that longer periods of 7 days' bed rest are no different from shorter periods of 2–3 days. Five trials showed that short periods of 2–4 days are no different from or worse than no bed rest at all. Bed rest is not significantly different from placebo or no treatment. It is either no different from or less effective than the alternative treatments with which it was compared for rate of recovery, relief of pain, return to daily activities and days lost from work. It has no effect on recovery of objective clinical measures. There are no direct comparisons of bed rest in hospital and at home, but the hospital trials of bed rest also failed to demonstrate any value.

Despite widespread practice, there is little evidence available on bed rest for patients with sciatica. What evidence there is questions its value (Coomes 1961, Pal et al 1986, Postachinni et al 1988). However, we still need further, well-designed trials of bed rest for patients with clear evidence of nerve root pain and disc prolapse.

All eight trials of medical advice to stay active, encourage physical activity and continue

Table 15.4 Evidence table of randomized controlled trials of bed rest for acute back pain or sciatica in order of methodologic score (from Waddell et al 1997, with permission)

Study	n	Patients	Setting	Intervention	Control(s)	Follow-up	Outcome measures	Results
Malmivaara et al (1995)	186	Acute back pain (average 5 days)	Occupational health clinics	2 days bed rest	c1 – back mobilizing exercises c2 – ordinary activity	3 and 12 weeks	Rate of recovery Pain Disability Satisfaction Days off work Flexion and SLR	Worse Worse Worse NS Worse NS
Gilbert et al (1985) Evans et al (1987)	252	Acute back pain (average 35 days)	Family practice	4 days bed rest	c1 – physio + education c2 – no treatment (factorial	10 days 6 and 12 weeks	Rate of recovery Pain Disability Flexion and SLR	NS NS Worse NS
Deyo et al (1986)	203	Acute back pain (78% <30 days)	Hospital walk-in patients	7 days bed rest (actual average 3.9 days)	2 days bed rest (actual average 2.3 days)	3 weeks 3 months	Disability Satisfaction Days off work Flexion and SLR	NS Worse NS NS
Wilkinson (1995)	42	Acute back pain (<7 days)	Family practice	48 hours bed rest (actual average daytime rest 12.6 hours)	Stay mobile daytime rest (actual average daytime rest 6.1 hours)	7 and 28 days	Rate of recovery Disability Flexion and SLR	Slower (NS) Worse (NS) Worse (NS)
Pal et al (1986)	41	Back pain and sciatica	Admitted to hospital	Bed rest + continuous traction	Bed rest + sham traction	1 and 2 weeks	Pain Return to work SLR and neurology	NS NS NS
Wiesel et al (1980)	80	Acute back pain	Army medical service	Bed rest until ready for full duties	Kept ambulatory Restricted duties	15 days	Rate of recovery Pain Days off work	Faster Better
Postachini et al (1988)	398	Acute back pain ± radiating pain (male)	Hospital outpatient	20–24 hours/day bed rest for 4–6 days; 15–20 hours/day for next 2 days	1. Manipulation 2. NSAIDs 3. Physical Therapy 4. Placebo	3 weeks 2 and 6 months	Combined score pain, disability and spinal movement	Worse than c1 Equal to c2 and c3 Better than c4 at 3 weeks only
Szpalski & Hayez (1992)	51	Acute back pain	Hospital outpatient	7 days bed rest	3 days bed rest	1, 5 and 9 days	Pain Isostation B200	NS NS
Coomes (1961)*	40	Sciatica (average 34 days)	Hospital outpatient	Bed rest at home*	Epidural anes No advice re. bed rest	Weekly, 10 weeks	Rate of recovery Pain	Slower Worse
Rupert et al (1985)*	145	Separate data on acute (<30 days)	Hospital	Bed rest c\o orthopedic specialist*	1. Manipulation 2. Sham manipulation	2 weeks	Pain	Worse than c1 NS c2

NS, no significant difference.
Outcomes are significant (*P* <0.05), unless otherwise stated.
*Originally control group.

Table 15.5 Evidence table of randomized controlled trials of advice on activity for acute and subacute back pain in order of methodologic score (from Waddell et al 1997, with permission)

Study	n	Patients	Setting	Intervention	Control(s)	Follow-up	Outcome measures	Results
Malmivaara et al (1995)	186	Acute back pain (average 5 days)	Occupational health clinics, Finland	'Ordinary activity' Avoid bed rest Continue routine activity as normally as possible	c1 – back mobilizing exercises c2 – 2 days bed rest	3 and 12 weeks	Rate of recovery Pain Disability Satisfaction Days off work	Better Better Better NS Better
Lindequist et at (1984)	56	Acute back pain ± referred leg pain	Family practice, Sweden	Back school, physical therapy training programme, encourage physical activity despite back pain	Analgesics PRN Advice not to stain back	Initial recovery, 1 year	Rate of recovery Days off work Satisfaction Recurrences 1 year sick leave Chronic disability	NS NS Better Fewer and shorter Less (NS) NS
Wilkinson (1995)	42	Acute back pain (<7 days)	Family practice, UK	Stay mobile and no daytime rest	48 hours strict bed rest	7 and 28 days	Rate of recovery Disability Flexion and SLR	Faster (NS) Better (NS) Better (NS)
Indahl et at (1995)	975	Back pain, off work 8–12 weeks	Population-based (NI claims), Norway	Intense personal advice, reduce fear, activity, normal walking, reduce sick behavior, set goals	'Conventional medical' system	1–2 years	Days off work Return to work Chronic disability	Less More Less
Fordyce et at (1986)	17	Acute back pain (1–10 days)	Family practice, emergency room orthopedic OP, US	Time-contingent analgesics and programed restoration of activity	Traditional analgesics as required, 'let pain be your guide'	6 weeks 1 year	6 week assessment Disability Chronic sickness Further health care use	NS NS Less Less
Lindstrom et al (1992a,b)	13	Subacute back pain 8–12 weeks	Industrial blue collar workers Sweden	Graded activity program, workplace behavioral principles	Traditional medical care by own physician	1 year	Days off work 1 year sick leave Chronic disability	Less Less Less (NS)
Linton et al (1993)	198	Acute back or neck pain	Primary care and occupational health, Sweden	'Early activation' Reinforce healthy behavior, maintain daily activities, training	'Treatment as usual' Analgesics, rest and sick leave	1 year	Pain Disability Satisfaction 1 year sick leave Chronic disability	NS NS Better Less Less
Philips et at (1991)	117	Acute back pain, first episode <15 days	Family practice or emergency room, Canada	Graded reactivation ± behavioral counseling	'Let pain guide' return to normal, (factorial design)	6 months	Pain Rate of recovery (return to activities) Chronic pain	NS Faster Less (NS)

NS, no significant difference.
Outcomes are significant ($P < 0.05$), unless otherwise stated.

ordinary activities as normally as possible showed consistent findings (Table 15.5). This advice made little, if any, difference to the pain or to initial recovery, but despite that, patients were more satisfied with their treatment. Three trials showed that advice to stay active led to faster return to work, while one found no significant difference. All the trials which considered chronic disability and health care use for back pain in the following year showed that these outcomes were reduced. There was no evidence that early activity had any harmful effects or led to more recurrences. Three trials showed that patients advised to stay active had fewer recurrences and less time off work in the following year (Lindequist et al 1984, Lindstrom et al 1992a,b, Linton et al 1993).

The two, high-quality trials that compared advice to stay active directly against bed rest both showed that ordinary activity produced faster recovery.

These reviews provide strong empiric evidence against bed rest and in favor of advice to stay active. Almost all the trials show that bed rest is not an effective treatment for acute back pain, but may delay recovery. Acute back pain may force patients to modify their activities, and some patients may be confined to bed for a few days. However, we should regard that as an undesirable consequence of their pain rather than a treatment. There is no justification for actually prescribing bed rest for back pain. Advice to stay active and to continue ordinary activities as normally as possible is likely to result in faster recovery, faster return to work and less chronic disability. Most important, despite common fears about reinjury, it does not cause more recurrent problems. It actually leads to fewer recurrent problems and less sick leave over the next 1–2 years.

These conclusions are supported by other evidence. Careful assessment, adequate explanation and reassurance can produce positive shifts in patients' beliefs about back pain and improve their satisfaction with health care (Deyo & Diehl 1986, Haig et al 1990, Bush et al 1993). Conversely, 'labeling' can do powerful harm (Hall et al 1994, Abenhaim et al 1995).

Systematic reviews show the benefits of back schools and that active exercise therapy is effective for chronic low back pain (van Tulder et al 1996). Physical training can increase patients' perception of their own ability (Dehlin et al 1981). People who are active and physically fit get fewer and shorter recurrent attacks (Cady et al 1979). Three RCTs showed that active exercise programs may reduce recurrences in people with a previous history of back pain (Linton et al 1989, Kellett et al 1991, Gundewall et al 1993).

There are no RCTs of medical advice about work for patients with back pain. However, there is other evidence that advice to return to work as early as possible may reduce work loss both initially and over the following year (Catchlove & Cohen 1982). There is conflicting evidence as to whether advice to return to temporary modified work is associated with an earlier return to work (Skovron et al 1994), makes little difference (Skovron et al 1998) or actually acts as a barrier to return to work (Hall et al 1994). Most important, all the evidence in this review shows that early return to work does not increase the chance of recurrence of back pain.

Based on this evidence, the latest British clinical guidelines on the management of acute low back pain (RCGP 1996) are much more positive (Box 15.1).

RESTORATION OF NORMAL ACTIVITY

From the disease model, many doctors and therapists traditionally assume that pain is the initial and main problem and disability is secondary. So, if they just treat the pain, disability will automatically go away:

Pain → Disability

That does not work. It often *appears* to work, because while we give symptomatic treatment the usual natural history of back pain is for acute exacerbations to recover by themselves: *'Je le pensai, Dieu le guerit'* (Ambrose Pare). But it does not always work, partly because

---

Box 15.1 RCGP (1996) guidelines

Conclusions
- For acute or recurrent LBP with or without referred leg pain, bed rest for 2–7 days is worse than placebo or ordinary activity. It is not as effective as the alternative treatments to which it has been compared for relief of pain, rate of recovery, return to daily activities and days lost from work
- Prolonged bed rest may lead to debilitation, chronic disability and increasing difficulty in rehabilitation
- Advice to continue ordinary activity can give equivalent or faster symptomatic recovery from the acute attack, and lead to less chronic disability and less time off work than 'traditional' medical treatment with analgesics as required, advice to rest and 'let pain be your guide' for return to normal activity
- Graded reactivation over a short period of days or a few weeks, combined with behavioral management of pain, makes little difference to the rate of initial recovery of pain and disability, but leads to less chronic disability and work loss
- Advice to return to normal work within a planned short time may lead to shorter periods of work loss and less time off work

Recommendations
- Do not recommend or use bed rest as a treatment for simple back pain
- Some patients may be confined to bed for a few days as a consequence of their pain but this should not be considered a treatment
- Advise patients to stay as active as possible and to continue normal daily activities
- Advise patients to increase their physical activities progressively over a few days or weeks
- If a patient is working, then advice to stay at work or return to work as soon as possible is probably beneficial

---

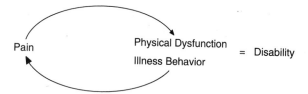

Figure 15.2 Physical dysfunction and altered behavior lie at the heart of chronic low back pain and disability.

patient. At a more holistic level we must restore normal healthy behavior and social function.

The rationale of treatment

- Back pain should be a benign, self-limiting symptom, even if it is often persistent or recurrent
- Its major impact is when it leads to physical dysfunction and illness behavior, which aggravates and perpetuates pain and disability
- The basic strategy of treatment is to restore normal function and behavior
- To do this we must overcome barriers to recovery

Pathologic view of disease vs. physiologic view of health

Rest. *Restore. Restoration* of function. This is a very pathologic review of human disease.
Contrast this with a physiologic view of health:

- continued use is essential to maintaining health: 'use it or lose it'
- function stimulates and maintains structure
- use leads to improved functional capacity, fitness and performance
- movement promotes healing

Reactivation

The goal is clear; the best methods of achieving it are not. There is considerable theory and clinical experience of rehabilitation. There is not nearly enough scientific knowledge. Few of these methods would stand up to systematic review of proven effectiveness. Let us simply try to identify a few tentative principles from these trials and related work.

Consistency of information

We must have a consistent strategy of management and give consistent information and advice to patients. One of the most common complaints

---

symptomatic treatment has little effect on the natural history of back pain, but also because disability is a key part of the problem, rather than just a secondary effect (Fig. 15.2).

My whole argument is that back pain *should* settle unless physical dysfunction and illness behavior block recovery. The basic management strategy should be to overcome dysfunction and illness behavior, to restore normal function and behavior, and so permit the pain to settle. We must do this at several levels simultaneously. At a musculoskeletal level we must provide adequate pain control, restore normal movement and gait patterns, and recondition the from patients with back pain, and the most common cause of dissatisfaction, is to do with conflicting messages from different health professionals (Deyo & Diehl 1986). The strategy must be consistent over time. It is no use telling patients to rest, and then, when that has failed and they are already chronic, telling them to reverse the strategy and to become active. If you do that, the pattern is already fixed and difficult to change. The basic strategy must be set and clear from the very beginning. All health professionals involved with the patient should give consistent information and advice. There is some evidence that patients are then more likely to accept and to adhere to that advice (Cherkin et al 1996).

Analgesia

Patients need adequate pain control to increase their activity level. Pain is the main reason that most back patients seek health care. I have argued strongly that dysfunction is the underlying problem, and that overcoming dysfunction is the best means of preventing chronic pain and disability, and obtaining long-term pain relief. But the problem is back *pain*, not just 'activity intolerance'. It is quite illogical to ignore the pain and focus *solely* on function. Patients rightly do not accept that.

Patients with back pain need adequate analgesia. This is particularly important at the acute stage, for the first few weeks, which should be the stage when they are increasing their activity level. Adequate pain control is also important during the initial stages of an active exercise and rehabilitation program. Analgesia should be in fixed doses at fixed times, based on the duration of drug action, to give continuing pain control. Drugs should *not* be on a p.r.n. basis, waiting until the pain gets out of control and then rewarding pain complaints and behavior with further analgesics. Analgesia should be time-dependent, not pain-dependent (Berntzen & Gotestam 1987).

Strong analgesia should also be time-limited. We must make clear from the start that pain control by drugs is not an answer in itself or a long-term solution. It is a temporary measure, for a fixed period of days or up to a few weeks, the aim of which is to control the pain and so enable the patient to become active. The long-term answer is the restoration of activity. We need further experiments on the timing and speed of reducing and withdrawing analgesics. It may also may be possible to progressively reduce the strength of analgesia in a drug cocktail, either with or without forewarning the patient.

Oral analgesics do not provide adequate pain control for some patients, either during the acute attack or when starting exercise. Various local anesthetic injections are in common use for acute attacks, particularly for nerve root pain. They appear clinically to give reasonable, short-term, pain relief, even if there is little scientific evidence of any effect on clinical outcomes for back pain. We could perhaps consider such trigger point, nerve block or epidural injections to give better pain control in order to start exercise and rehabilitation programs. They sometimes give longer relief than we would expect from the duration of drug action. The only justification for such invasive procedures is if they do enable increased exercise and activity levels. They should not be used, especially repeatedly, purely for symptomatic relief, and they should be strictly limited in number and time. I know of a number of discussions and early experiments in this field, but not of any published scientific work. This has considerable potential, but we need much more careful experiment.

Increasing activity levels

Activity levels should increase by planned, fixed increments over time. It may be reasonable to set the starting point according to the patient's present symptoms and capacity. From this point on, there should be steadily increasing increments of activity level and exercise quotas. These are time-dependent, not symptom-dependent (Fordyce et al 1986): do what you plan, not what you feel. However, the rate of increase must be realistic. It is no use trying to do too much, too fast, provoking a pain crisis and abandoning the effort (Fig. 15.3).

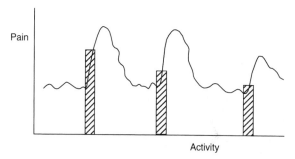

Figure 15.3 The problem of over-enthusiastic bursts of activity and the need for pacing. (After Hazard, personal communication.)

Many patients need to pace themselves, particularly at first. The rate and size of the increments will depend on the severity and duration of the patient's symptoms. It is a question of judgement and experiment to find a balance between what is realistically possible and achieving the goal within a reasonable time-scale. For most acute patients, this may be a matter of days or a few weeks. Even for chronic patients, it should usually be over a period of weeks or a few months at most if it is to have any chance of success.

The most important message is that, contrary to common belief, progressive, incremented exercise levels lead to progressive decrease in pain (Fig. 15.4). But we must accept, and warn our patients, that there may be some temporary exacerbations of pain along the way. That is normal, and must be accepted and overcome.

The value of early motion is now generally accepted in fractures and after joint replacement. It reduces swelling and inflammation, and promotes tissue nutrition and healing. In some situations, we now use machines immediately postoperatively, to move joints through a modest range of 'continuous passive motion'. This appears to benefit postoperative recovery and rehabilitation. It may be worth experimenting with a similar approach in back pain rehabilitation.

Active rehabilitation

Active rehabilitation is not the same as exercise. The aim is to increase activity levels and restore normal function. Exercise is only a means to this end, not a cure in itself. Specific back exercises may aim to strengthen muscle groups, and improve movement or posture, but the evidence is that these have little effect on clinical outcomes. The benefit seems to lie in increasing ordinary activities and returning to work.

Active rehabilitation uses exercise, but concentrates also on functional activities such as walking. It uses exercise as a means to achieve its goals of restoring full function and regaining physical fitness. Rehabilitation is also more intensive and structured. It is the difference between prescribing quadriceps exercises for an elderly lady with a fractured femur or teaching her to walk again (Fig. 15.5).

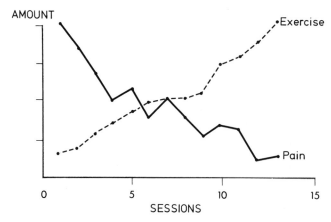

Figure 15.4 The importance of incremented increases in activity levels. Contrary to common belief, increased exercise does not cause increased pain, but actually leads to progressive reduction in pain levels. (From Fordyce et al 1981, with permission.)

Physical therapy is the rehabilitation specialty *par excellence*. This is what therapy is all about in most other musculoskeletal disorders. The 84-year-old lady in Figure 15.5 fractured the neck of her femur 36 hours before that photograph was taken, and had a major life-threatening operation. That morning, two bright young therapists came to her bedside: 'Right, Granny, we're here to get you walking again.' She looked at them in astonishment: 'But I can't walk, I've broken my hip.' 'We know,' they replied, 'but you've had your operation, and you've got a pin to hold the bone in place.' 'But I can't walk,' she repeated. 'We know, but we're here to help you.' 'But it's still painful,' the lady protested once more. 'Of course it is, you'd expect that at this stage. But your pain killers should be working soon, and that won't stop you walking.' The therapists do not pay much attention to the pain, but instead

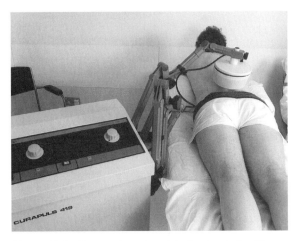

Figure 15.6 Too much treatment for back pain is still passive symptomatic modalities. Compare this with Figure 15.5!

concentrate on getting her walking again. And, if she survives, this gives her the best chance of getting mobile, independent, and back to her own home. What a contrast with back pain! In back pain, we often seem to be more concerned with ineffective symptomatic treatments, and are afraid to start active rehabilitation until the pain settles (Fig. 15.6). If this analysis is correct, rehabilitation is doomed to failure. My argument is simply that therapists should apply the same rehabilitation principles and professional skills to back pain that they use in every other musculoskeletal condition (Fig. 15.7).

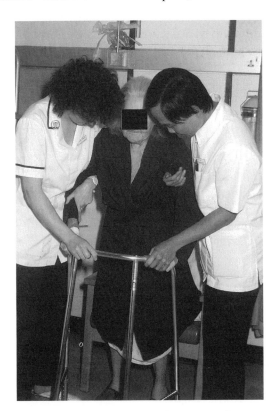

Figure 15.5 An elderly patient making her first attempt to walk, 24 hours after major surgery for a fractured neck of femur.

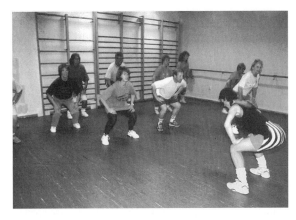

Figure 15.7 A back training class in Norway. (From H B Finckenhagen, with thanks.)

Changing beliefs

We generally think of rehabilitation as restoring physical and physiologic function. However, reactivation and rehabilitation may be as much a matter of changing patient's beliefs and behavior as any physiologic change.

We found a totally unexpected effect of exercise on fear avoidance beliefs (Newton et al 1993). We were doing reliability studies on isokinetic assessment and got 20 patients to repeat the test four times over 7–10 days. Before we tested them we carried out a complete clinical assessment, including self-report of disability, and they told us all the things they could not do. We then put them on the isokinetic equipment. From the outside this equipment looks rather frightening, but it actually gives patients a feeling of support and security. We put them through a test protocol and at the end of it, several patients turned to us in amazement: 'I never thought I could do that!' So we tested their fear avoidance beliefs over the series of four assessments (Table 15.6).

Remember, this was only a test protocol. These patients did not do enough physical exercise to have any physiologic effect. We had also explained the study honestly. The patients knew it was only an assessment, and we did not pretend it was treatment. Yet their experience of what they could do in a single assessment session produced a significant shift in their fear avoidance beliefs about physical activity. The series of four tests over 7–10 days gave a further shift in fear avoidance beliefs, which in turn led to improvement in their pain and disability. The amount of exercise was too small, and the change too rapid, for any possible physiologic effect.

Providing information and advice is a very weak method of changing behavior. (This is equally true of patients and health professionals!) Actions speak louder than words. Personal experience that challenges existing misconceptions and forces the patient to rethink their whole approach to the problem is a much more powerful agent for change. Perhaps we need to redesign our therapy and rehabilitation for back pain specifically to meet these goals, rather than thinking it is all a question of muscle physiology.

Overcoming negative beliefs

Overcoming negative beliefs and maladaptive behavior may be the most important aspect of treatment. Jensen (1997) recently reported preliminary results from a pain management program in Seattle. This produced a marked improvement in self-reported disability and depressive symptoms, with a slight increase in satisfaction with life, and marked reduction in health care visits for pain. These effects were maintained over 12 months. The main focus of the study, however, was to investigate how this worked. They found that improvement in emotional state and disability was linked to increased feelings of control and reduced fear of harm. The patients began to use more positive (active) coping strategies and less negative (passive) coping strategies. The researchers then looked at the interactions between these beliefs and behaviors. Clinical improvement depended most on reducing guarding, rest and catastrophizing (Table 15.7).

Overcoming these negative *obstacles to clinical progress* or *barriers to recovery* seems to be tremendously important. Jensen suggested that exercise may be a powerful method of changing patients'

Table 15.6 Change in fear avoidance beliefs (FABs) with isokinetic assessment (unpublished data from Dr M Newton, with thanks)

	Baseline	After one assessment	After four assessments
FAB activity beliefs	17.2	14.0*	10.3***
Pain	48.7	45.9	36.5***
Disability	9.4	8.9	7.1*

*$P < 0.05$; ***, $P < 0.001$

Table 15.7 Changes in beliefs and coping strategies that relate to improvement in disability (from Jensen 1987 with permission)

Change	Partial correlation coefficient
Reduce guarding	0.52
Reduce use of rest for pain	0.41
Reduce catastrophizing	0.36
Increased feelings of control	0.31

beliefs in his or her own ability, which can lead in turn to changes in behavior. Theoretically, from a psychologic perspective, exercise may function best as *antiguarding treatment*. This fits with some of the successful trials quoted in Table 15.5.

Taking responsibility

Patients must take personal responsibility for their own clinical progress and health. Restoring function depends entirely on patients' active participation. No therapist can do that for them. In this more active approach the doctor's and therapist's role is to guide and support the patient's own efforts. The patient must accept, and health professionals must relinquish, the main responsibility for rehabilitation. This is closely linked to beliefs about personal responsibility and control (see Ch. 12).

Context of rehabilitation

Any gains in activity level and function must be transferred from a health care setting to normal life. Performing exercise in a physical therapy department, ordinary activities of daily living, and working for a living, are three quite different scenarios. The demands, physical capacity required and performance are all different. Unfortunately, many beliefs, behaviors and performance are quite specific to their setting, so transfer does not always happen automatically. Management must devote as much attention and effort to restoring activity levels in normal life as to performance in a health care setting.

Capacity for work depends to some extent on physical capacity and performance, but it also depends on how these match work demands. To return to work the patient must surmount a whole different set of social barriers (Chs 13 and 14). Rehabilitation must take account of and deal with these issues. It is striking that some of the most successful back schools and early activation programs (Table 15.5) take place in an occupational setting.

Planning for relapse

Most health care and rehabilitation takes a short-term perspective, to help the patient to recover from the acute attack and to return to work. But back pain is often a persistent or recurrent problem, and so maintaining gains and preventing relapse are equally important. Some of these trials show that improvement continues for 6–24 months, while others show that initial improvements regress after a few months. Even when health care is effective, there is little evidence that it has any effect on recurrence rates and the long-term natural history.

It is essential for health professionals and patients to recognize and plan for recurrences and relapses. The first and most vital step is to face up to the fact that they are almost inevitable. They are normal, and do not mean that treatment has failed. Therefore, they are not a reason for abandoning the strategy and going back to square one to seek a different medical cure. If this management strategy worked before, this is a good reason for continuing the same approach. Hopefully, continuing experience should lead to faster recovery, and to less frequent and less severe relapses.

There is an ongoing debate about the role of health care in dealing with recurrences. Many orthodox practitioners provide health care for each attack, almost ignoring the previous history and likely future course. Some therapists and alternate practitioners argue for long-term 'maintenance therapy', although I do not know of any scientific evidence to suggest that is effective. The problem is that it may create dependency, and discourage the patient from taking personal responsibility and control. A few pain specialists raise the question of 'booster sessions' or support groups to maintain initial gains.

Perhaps the most important support of all is the family, and some pain management programs argue that changing family attitudes and behavior is just as important as dealing with the patient.

We need much more research into how to maintain any improvements we achieve and how to reduce recurrences and relapses.

Principles of reactivation

- Consistent strategy of management
- Adequate pain control, particularly when starting to get active and exercising
- Incremented, time-depended increase in activity/exercise levels
- Increased activity level > specific exercises
- Changing behavior may be equally, or more, important than physical changes
- Overcoming negative beliefs and coping may be most important of all
- Personal experience is a much more powerful influence than information or advice
- The patient must take personal responsibility
- These changes must be transferred into normal life and everyday activities
- Rehabilitation must be linked to return to work
- Maintenance of gains is important, in view of the probability of persistent or recurrent symptoms

---

EARLY INTERVENTION

There are strong theoretic arguments for early intervention. Workers who are still off sick after 3–6 weeks begin to show physical deconditioning, and the risks of chronic pain and disability rise rapidly. Treatment at this stage is likely to be more effective, and it is clearly preferable to prevent chronic pain and disability.

The rationale and scientific evidence for this approach are clear (Table 15.5). Implementing it in practice is more difficult. The evidence on early intervention in practice shows conflicting results as to whether it is effective and cost-effective.

Wiesel et al (1984) first showed the value of monitoring case management to see how it meets an agreed protocol of diagnosis and management. This can improve the quality and efficiency of health care delivery, and at the same time reduce work loss and both health care and compensation costs. Miller et al (1995)

reported the 10-year results in a public utility company with a stable work force of 5000 workers. Patients chose their own physicians, but each patient was also assessed by an independent orthopedic consultant, who saw them within 1 week of injury and compared their treatment with the algorithm. When care diverged from the algorithm, the consultant discussed this on a peer basis with the treating physician. If there was no adequate explanation, he ordered an independent examination. This approach usually led to a change in management, closer to the algorithm. The 10-year results of this program are impressive (Box 15.2).

Box 15.2 Results of monitoring case management against an agreed algorithm (from Miller et al 1995, with permission)

- Quality control was ensured with adherence to the established algorithms by unbiased physicians who could not take part in the patients' ongoing care
- The number of days lost from work fell by 55%
- The number of new injuries reported fell by 51%
- The average time lost per injury dropped by 40%
- The number of surgical procedures performed decreased by almost 70%, and the operative success rate increased dramatically
- There was a 60% reduction in expenditures for lost time and replacement wages
- Overall, the program resulted in a 10-year saving of more than $4.1 million

---

Haig et al (1990) studied aggressive early management by a specialist in physical medicine and rehabilitation. He saw patients without delay, but gave standard treatment. Simply delivering care earlier and more efficiently reduced the average number of days off to 6.7, compared with 11.8 days for historic controls. However, this was largely due to a dramatic improvement in a few patients with neck pain. For the much more common problem of back pain, the reduction was from a mean of 8.8 to 7.5 days.

Greenwood et al (1990) looked at an early intervention, case management approach in West Virginian coal miners. This was an RCT within 2 weeks of injury. Patients with psychosocial risk factors saw a nurse and counselor who offered guidance; coordinated their primary care, specialist care and physical therapy; and, if necessary, arranged psychologic services. This intervention did not change the time off work, but medical costs rose. The intervention was neither effective nor cost-effective. A recent report from the Ontario Workers' Compensation Board (Sinclair et al 1997) also suggested that providing intensive rehabilitation at an earlier stage may actually be counterproductive. It made little difference to the rate of recovery of pain or disability, but *increased* time off work while workers were attending the program!

Cooper et al (1996) tested an early intervention program for nurses with low back injuries. They gave physical assessment and treatment under the direction of a rehabilitation physician. If patients were off work for 4 days, they had an occupational therapy assessment. Modified work was available for up to 7 weeks. This produced some improvement in pain and disability but the change was not significant.

Ryan et al (1995) tested an early intervention program for back pain in a new mine in central Queensland, Australia. They included work-force education, early injury reporting, acute back care at the mine by a trained first aid officer, early referral to a general practitioner and support for early return to work. They stressed the importance of changing work place perceptions:

- early intervention
- allay fears about permanent damage to the back
- treatment by encouraging activity and return to work.

This intervention led to fewer back injury claims and lower costs per claim, compared with a neighboring mine. The median time off was 10 days, and no worker was off for more than 60 days with a back injury. This program was easy to introduce and inexpensive.

van Doorn (1995) tested an early intervention program in a mutual insurance company in the Netherlands for doctors, physical therapists, dentists and vets. These groups have a much lower sickness rate for back pain, but those who do stop work may then be off much longer, presumably because they only go off work when they have more serious problems. This program cut the mean time off work from 136 to 98 days. It reduced the number of people off work for a year or more by 56%.

Ehrmann-Feldman et al (1996) studied compensation records of 2147 workers in Quebec with back injuries. They found that those who were referred to physical therapy within 1 month of injury were much more likely to return to work within 2 months. This appears to support the value of early physical therapy. However, this was not a prospective or randomized controlled trial. There was probably selection of cases, and those who were referred earlier may not have been the same as those who were referred later. This evidence is suggestive, but does not *prove* that it was the early physical therapy that led to early recovery and return to work.

These varying results suggest that it is not simply a matter of early intervention. It also depends very much on what that intervention is. Simply providing routine care faster does not make any difference; it may not be cost-effective and may even be counter-productive. Perhaps that is not surprising if routine care is ineffective. Wiesel et al's results suggest that monitoring and peer pressure to improve the quality and efficiency of health care delivery according to an algorithm or guideline may be more effective. Referral for physical therapy at the subacute stage of 1 month may be more effective than leaving it for many months. However, the most effective early interventions seem to be those that try to implement the scientific evidence (Ryan et al 1995, van Doorn 1995).

van Doorn lists the principles of early intervention:

- a time-dependent approach, in which non-specific low back pain is distinguished from specific low back pain
- an evaluation of medical, psychosocial and ergonomics factors, at the first consultation

- active rehabilitation including early, gradual return to work
- mutual trust between the physician and the claimant to create a win-win situation
- good communication between the insurance physician and the attending physician.

Most of these studies of early intervention are explorations of practice rather than scientific investigations. This is quite acceptable. We have the scientific evidence. Now we need to see how we can put it into routine practice on a large scale. Nevertheless, we must be very cautious about the results of these trials. We still need a great deal of research into the nature and timing of the most effective interventions, and into what settings and under what conditions they are likely to be effective and cost-effective.

CONCLUSION

Patients need clear and unambiguous advice. Professional advice to rest or to stay active is potentially one of the most potent influences on what patients do about their back pain. How patients deal with their pain has a major impact on clinical outcomes and on the development of chronic disability. Traditional management of back pain by rest is now discredited. The biopsychosocial model provides a powerful theoretic argument for an active strategy of management

for back pain (Nachemson 1983, Mayer et al 1985, Waddell 1987). The goal and the means should be to maintain or return to ordinary activities as rapidly as possible (Table 15.8).

We no longer use bed rest to treat any other musculoskeletal condition. The whole emphasis of trauma treatment is now on early mobilization and ambulation. We subject elderly, unfit patients with fractures to major surgery and aggressive physiotherapy to avoid the risks of prolonged immobilization. We have stopped bed rest for myocardial infarction and childbirth. Yet we continue to treat patients with simple backache as if they were more seriously ill than patients with myocardial infarction who now routinely get early ambulation.

If you are still not fully convinced, let me suggest a final, brutal test. How do you deal with your own back pain? Would you let anyone treat you the way you treat your patients? At one recent meeting, 60% of 230 doctors said they had back pain. About 20% said they had had an acute attack. Most had never taken any bed rest. Only two out of 230 had ever stayed in bed for 2 weeks, and none had ever had any longer period. Yet doctors continue to treat patients with simple backache in a way they would never treat themselves. I suspect that most of us already follow many of these principles. All I am pleading is that you should treat your patients the same way that you treat

Table 15.8 Disease model vs. biopsychosocial approach

Traditional assumptions based on a disease model	A biopsychosocial approach + empiric evidence
Etiology	
Low back pain is an injury	Physical dysfunction (not really an injury)
Often work related	Not really 'caused' by work
Pain = disability	Pain and disability are not the same thing
Activity/work causes	
Increased pain	Reduced pain in the long run
Reinjury	(It isn't really an injury)
Recurrences and risk of chronicity	Fewer recurrences and less risk of chronicity
Treatment	
Rest	Stay active
Activity limitation	Temporary activity modification
Routine sick certification	Stay at work if at all possible

yourself. I don't believe the excuses about doctors neglecting themselves. When it comes to something as important as this, doctors treat themselves in the best way they know. If it is good enough for us, perhaps it is also best for our patients.

The goal and the strategy seem clear (Box 15.3), even if there are still many practical questions about how best to achieve this. The value is not in exercise *per se*, but in restoring normal function in ordinary activities. So, what is the most effective way of getting patients to increase their activity level, particularly if they still have pain? What is the role of exercise, and what exercises? How do we coordinate pain control and increasing activity? To what extent is it a question of correcting physical dysfunction, or correcting fear avoidance behaviors? What are the main barriers to recovery, and how do we overcome them? How do we get patients (and health professionals) to change their behavior? How do we get them to maintain these changes?

All the available evidence suggests that changing from a passive strategy of rest to a more positive, active strategy could improve clinical outcomes and reduce the personal and social impact of back pain. There is a very simple choice: rest or stay active? rest or restoration of function? rest or recovery? The challenge is to develop simple but effective methods of achieving this in practice.

Box 15.3 Principles of management

Acute
- Simple symptomatic measures
- Advise to continue ordinary activities as normally as possible
- Aim: avoid developing physical dysfunction and illness behavior

Subacute
These patients are at risk, and beginning to develop physical dysfunction and illness behavior. Aims and principles of treatment are:
- Overcome guarded movements and improve flexibility
- Reduce negative beliefs and coping strategies, and illness behavior
- Increase activity levels and return to work

Chronic
- Established physical dysfunction and illness behavior
- Much more difficult to reverse

Prevention is better than cure. Early intervention is important. *Avoid iatrogenic disability.*

REFERENCES

Abenhaim L, Rossignol M, Gobielle D, Bonvalot Y, Fines P, Scott S 1995 The prognostic consequences in the making of the initial medical diagnosis of work-related injuries. Spine 20: 791–795

AHCPR 1994 Clinical Practice Guideline Number 14. Acute low back problems in adults. Agency for Health Care Policy and Research, US Department of Health and Human Services, Rockville MD

Asher R A J 1947 The dangers of going to bed. British Medical Journal 967–968

Battie M C, Cherkin D C, Dunn R, Clol M A, Wheeler K J 1994 Managing low back pain: attitudes and treatment preferences of physical therapists. Physical Therapy 74: 219–226

Berntzen D, Gotestam K G 1987 Effects of on-demand versus fixed-interval schedules in the treatment of chronic pain with analgesic compounds. Journal of Consulting and Clinical Psychology 55: 213–217

Bortz W M 1984 The disuse syndrome. Western Journal of Medicine 141: 691–694

Bush T, Cherkin D, Barlow W 1993 The impact of physician attitudes on patient satisfaction with care for low back pain. Archives of Family Medicine 2: 301–305

Cady L, Bischoff D, O'Connel E 1979 Strength and fitness and subsequent back injuries in firefighters. Journal of Occupational Medicine 21: 269–272

Catchlove R, Cohen K 1982 Effects of a directive return to work approach in the treatment of workmen's compensation patients with chronic pain. Pain 14: 181–191

Cherkin D C, MacCornack F A, Berg A O 1988 Managing low back pain – a comparison of the beliefs and behaviors of family physicians and chiropractors. Western Journal of Medicine 149: 475–480

Cherkin D C, Deyo R A, Street J H, Hunt M, Barlow W 1996 Pitfalls of patient education. Limited success of a program for back pain in primary care. Spine 21: 345–355

Coomes E N 1961 A comparison between epidural anaesthesia and bed rest in sciatica. British Medical Journal 1: 20–24

Cooper J E, Tate R B, Yassi A, Khokhar J 1996 Effect of an early intervention program on the relationship between subjective pain and disability measures in nurses with low back injury. Spine 21: 2329–2336

Coste J, Delecoeuillerie G, Lara A C, Le Parc J M, Paolaggi J

B 1994 Clinical course and prognostic factors in acute low back pain: an inception cohort study in primary care practice. British Medical Journal 308: 577–580

CSAG 1994 Back pain Clinical Standards Advisory Group report. HMSO, London

Cyriax J 1969 Textbook of orthopaedic medicine. Williams & Wilkins, Baltimore

Dehlin O, Berg S, Andersson G B J, Grimby G 1981 Effect of physical training and ergonomic counselling on the psychological perception of work and on the subjective assessment of low back insufficiency. Scandinavian Journal of Rehabilitation Medicine 13: 1–9

Deyo R A, Diehl A K 1986 Patient satisfaction with medical care for low back pain. Spine 11: 28–30

Deyo R A, Diehl A K, Rosenthal M 1986 How many days of bed rest for acute low back pain? New England Journal of Medicine 315: 1064–1070

Ehrmann-Feldman D, Rossignol M, Abenhaim L, Gobielle D 1996 Physician referral to physical therapy in a cohort of workers compensated for low back pain. Physical Therapy 76: 150–157

Evans C, Gilbert J R, Taylor W, Hildebrand A 1987 A randomized controlled trial of flexion exercises, education and bed rest for patients with acute low back pain. Physiotherapy Canada 39: 96–101

Fordyce W E, McMahon R, Rainwater G et al 1981 Pain complaint-exercise performance relationship in chronic pain. Pain 10: 311–321

Fordyce W E, Brockway J A, Bergman J A, Spengler D 1986 Acute back pain: a control group comparison of behavioural -vs- traditional management methods. Journal of Behavioral Medicine 9: 127–140

Gilbert J R, Taylor D W, Hildebrand A 1985 Clinical trial of common treatments for low back pain in family practice. British Medical Journal 291: 791–794

Greenwood J G, Harvey H J, Pearson J C, Woon C L, Posey P, Main C F 1990 Early intervention in low back disability among coal miners in West Virginia: negative findings. Journal of Occupational Medicine 32: 1047–1052

Gundewall B, Liljeqvist M, Hansson T 1993 Primary prevention of back symptoms and absence of work. A prospective randomized study among hospital employees. Spine 18: 587–594

Haig A J, Linton P, McIntosh M, Moneta L, Mead P B 1990 Aggressive early medical management by a specialist in physical medicine and rehabilitation; effect on lost time due to injuries in hospital employees. Journal of Occupational Medicine 32: 241–244

Hall H, McIntosh G, Melles T, Holowachuk B, Wai E 1994 Effect of discharge recommendations on outcome. Spine 19: 2033–2037

Hides J A, Stokes M J, Saide M, Jull G A, Cooper D H 1994 Evidence of lumbar multifidus muscle wasting ipsilateral to symptoms in patients with acute/subacute low back pain. Spine 19: 165–172

Hilton J 1887 Rest and pain, 4th edn. In: Jacobson W H A (ed) A course of lectures at the Royal College of Surgeons of England. Bell & Sons, London

Hunter J 1794 A treatise on the blood, inflammation and gun-shot wounds. Nicol, London

Indahl A, Velund L, Reikeraas O 1995 Good prognosis for low back pain when left untampered. A randomized clinical trial. Spine 20: 473–477

Jensen M 1997 Changing pain beliefs, coping and function

through pain management. Presented to the 6th national Conference on Pain Management Programmes, Manchester, September 18–19

Johnson G 1881 A lecture on backache and the diagnosis of its various causes with hints on treatment. British Medical Journal 1: 221–224

Kellett K M, Kellett D A, Nordholm L A 1991 Effects of an exercise program on sick leave due to back pain. Physical Therapy 71: 283–293

Lindequist S, Lundberg B, Wikmark R, Bergstad B, Loof G, Ottermark A-C 1984 Information and regime at low back pain. Scandinavian Journal of Rehabilitation Medicine 16: 113–116

Lindstrom I, Ohlund C, Eek C et al 1992a The effect of graded activity on patient with subacute low back pain: a randomized prospective clinical study with an operant-conditioning behavioral approach. Physical Therapy 72: 279–291

Lindstrom I, Ohlund C, Eek C, Wallin L, Peterson L-E, Nachemson A 1992b Mobility, strength and fitness after a graded activity program for patients with subacute low back pain. Spine 17: 641–652

Linton S J, Bradley L A, Jensen I, Spangfort E, Sundell L 1989 The secondary prevention of low back pain: a controlled study with follow-up. Pain 36: 197–207

Linton S J, Hellsing A-L, Andersson D 1993 A controlled study of the effects of an early intervention on acute musculoskeletal pain problems. Pain 54: 353–359

Malmivaara A, Hakkinen U, Aro T et al 1995 The treatment of acute low back pain – bed rest, exercises or ordinary activity? New England Journal of Medicine 332: 351–355

Mayer T G, Gatchel R J, Kitchino N et al 1985 Objective assessment of lumbar function following industrial injury. Spine 10: 482–493

Mayer T G, Gatchel R J 1988 Functional restoration for spinal disorders: the sports medicine approach. Lea & Febiger, Philadelphia

Miller M W, McAndrews B G, Wiesel S W, Feffer H L 1995 Health care for the injured worker. A management challenge. Orthopedic Physical Therapy Clinics of North America 4: 367–373

Nachemson A 1983 Work for all: for those with low back pain as well. Clinical Orthopaedics and Related Research 179: 77–85

Newton M, Thow M, Somerville D, Henderson I, Waddell G 1993. Trunk strength testing with iso-machines. Part II. Experimental evaluation of the Cybex II Back Testing System in normal subjects and patients with chronic low back pain. Spine: 18–812

Pal P, Mangion P, Hossian M A, Diffey L 1986 A controlled trial of continuous lumbar traction in the treatment of back pain and sciatica. British Journal of Rheumatology 25: 1181–1183

Philips H C, Grant L, Berkowitz J 1991 The prevention of chronic pain and disability: a preliminary investigation. Behavioral Research and Therapy 29: 443–450

Postacchini F, Facchini M, Palieri P 1988 Efficacy of various forms of conservative treatment in low back pain: a comparative study. Neuro-Orthopedics 6: 28–35

RCGP 1996 Clinical guidelines for the management of acute low back pain. Royal College of General Practice, London

Rupert R L, Wagnon R, Thompson P, Ezzeldin T 1985 Chiropractic adjustments: results of a controlled trial in Egypt. ICA International Review of Chiropractic: 58–60

Ryan W E, Krishna M K, Swanson C E 1995 A prospective study evaluating early rehabilitation in preventing back pain chronicity in mine workers. Spine 20: 489–491

Sinclair S, Hogg-Johnson S, Mondloch M V, Shields S A 1997 Evaluation of effectiveness of an early, active intervention program for workers with soft tissue injuries. Spine 22: 2919–2931

Skovron M L, Hiebert R, Nordin M, Brisson P M, Crane M 1998 Work restrictions and outcome of non-specific low back pain, in press.

Skovron M L, Szpalski M, Nordin M, Melot C, Cukier D 1994 Sociocultural factors and back pain: a population-based study in Belgian adults. Spine 19: 129–137

Svensson H, Andersson G 1989 The relationship of low-back pain, work history, work environment and stress. A retrospective cross-sectional study of 38- to 64-year-old women. Spine 14: 517–522

Sydenham T 1734 The whole works of that excellent physician Dr Thomas Sydenham, 10th edn (transl. John Pechey). W Feales, London

Szpalski M, Hayez J P 1992 How many days of bed rest for acute low back pain? Objective assessment of trunk function. European Spine Journal 1: 29–31

Thomas H O 1874 Contributions to medicine and surgery. Lewis, London

van Doorn J W 1995 Low back disability among self-employed dentists, veterinarians, physicians and physical therapists in the Netherlands. Acta Orthopaedica Scandinavica 66 (supplement 263): 1–64

van Tulder M W, Koes B W, Bouter L M (eds) 1996 Low back pain in primary care: effectiveness of diagnostic and therapeutic interventions. Institute for Research in Extramural Medicine, Amsterdam

von Korff M, Barlow W, Cherkin D, Deyo R A 1994 Effects of practice style in managing back pain. Annals of Internal Medicine 121: 187–195

Waddell G 1987 A new clinical model for the treatment of low back pain. Spine 12: 632–644

Waddell G 1993 Simple low back pain: rest or active exercise? (Editorial) Annals of Rheumatic Diseases 52: 317–319

Waddell G, Feder G, Lewis M 1997 Systematic reviews of bedrest and advice to stay active for acute low back pain. British Journal of General Practice 47: 647–652

Wiesel S W, Cuckler J M, Deluca F, Jones F, Zeide M S, Rothman R H 1980 Acute low back pain. An objective analysis of conservative therapy. Spine 5: 324–330

Wiesel S W, Feffer H L, Rothman R H 1984 Industrial low back pain: a prospective evaluation of a standardized diagnostic and treatment protocol. Spine 9: 199–203

Wilkinson M J B 1995 Does 48 hours bed rest influence the outcome of acute low back pain? British Journal of General Practice 45: 481–484

16

Treatment: the scientific evidence

The earlier chapters are based on careful clinical and epidemiologic observation and on solid scientific theory. Now, it is time to get down to the nuts and bolts. What are the best treatments for back pain? What works? The scientific gold standard for any therapy is the randomized controlled trial (RCT): what do the various RCTs show to be effective treatment for back pain?

Background

The first attempt to answer these questions was the Quebec Task Force (Spitzer et al 1987). This was an independent and comprehensive review of the many treatments for low back pain. It gave two main messages. Most important and most disappointing, there was very little scientific evidence available at that time. What evidence there was failed to show that most treatment for back pain was much better than a combination of time and natural history; or no treatment at all. They highlighted the need for more good RCTs. Alf Nachemson has waged a one man crusade for RCTs over the past decade, and we should give him much of the credit for stimulating and encouraging the studies that are now available.

The US clinical guidelines (AHCPR 1994) provided the most comprehensive review of the evidence ever undertaken. The Agency for Health Care Policy and Research spent more than 2 years and nearly $1 million reviewing and evaluating more than 10 000 articles. However, although the guidelines were published in December 1994, they only included the evidence published up to 1992. Since 1992 there have been many more RCTs and a number of systematic reviews in key areas.

The review presented in this chapter was prepared for the Royal College of General Practitioners, as the evidence base for the second British guidelines in September 1996 (RCGP 1996). Like every review and national guideline since 1994, we built on the AHCPR review and updated it with further evidence published from January 1993 through April 1996. We carried out systematic reviews of four key areas

of management: bed rest, advice on staying active, manipulation and exercise. Our reviews of bed rest and advice on staying active (Waddell et al 1997) form the basis of Chapter 15. We cross-checked the latter two reviews against independent reviews of manipulation by Shekelle (1995) and Koes et al (1996a), and of exercise by Faas (1996). A number of reviews published since 1992 cover other areas of management (Table 16.1). Much of this evidence was presented and discussed at the first International Forum for Primary Care Research on low back pain in Seattle (Cherkin 1996). We also drew on two recent major reviews of this complete field by van Tulder et al (1996a) and Evans & Richards (1996).

Table 16.1 Systematic reviews of treatment for back pain since AHCPR (1994)

Authors	Subject	Number of RCTs	Comment	Change from AHCPR
van den Hoogen et al (1995)	Accuracy of history, physical examination and ESR	36 (cohort studies)	Meta-analysis of sensitivity and specificity	No
Koes et al (1996b)	NSAIDs	26		No
Turner & Denny (1993)	Antidepressants	6	For chronic low back pain	No
Koes & van den Hoogen (1994)	Bed rest	5		No
Waddell et al (1997)	Bed rest	10	RCGP review	Stronger against
Waddell et al (1997)	Advice on activity	8	RCGP review	New
Koes et al (1994)	Back schools	16	6 in acute or recurrent LBP	No
Cohen et al (1994)	Back schools	13	3 in acute LBP	No
Koes et al (1996a)	Manipulation	36	Presented First Primary Care Research Forum 1995	No
Faas (1996)	Back exercises	11 (since 1990)	Presented First Primary Care Research Forum 1995	Weaker but see Activity
Koes et al (1995)	Epidural steroids	12	9 RCTs on acute or subacute LBP and sciatica	No
Gam & Johannsen (1995)	Ultrasound	2	22 RCTs on various musculoskeletal disorders 2 RCTs in LBP	No
van der Heijden et al (1995)	Traction	14	+ 3 RCTs on neck pain	No
Koes & van den Hoogen (1994)	Orthoses	5		No

This is our assessment of the current evidence on the primary care management of acute low back pain in adults. In future, the Cochrane Collaboration should provide a complete and constantly updated systematic review of the evidence, but it may take several years for that to be fully on-stream.

Evidence ratings

We rated the evidence on a three-star system (see Box 16.1). We judged therapies on RCTs and, wherever possible, gave references to systematic reviews or to key RCTs. However, RCTs are simply not applicable to some important areas such as assessment, epidemiology and natural history, and complications of treatment. There the evidence comes mainly from prospective cohort studies of acute low back pain in primary care.

Box 16.1 Evidence rating and sources

*** Generally consistent finding in a majority of multiple acceptable studies

** Either based on a single acceptable study, or a weak or inconsistent finding in some of multiple acceptable studies

* Limited scientific evidence, which does not meet all the criteria of acceptable studies

- 'Acceptable' studies of therapy
  — randomized controlled trial
  — acute (<3/12) or recurrent LBP
  — relevant to primary care
  — at least 10 patients in each group
  — patient-centered outcome(s)
- 'Acceptable' studies of assessment and natural history
  — prospective cohort study
  — acute or recurrent LBP
  — relevant to primary care
  — at least 100 patients
  — at least 1 year follow-up

Most of the present conclusions and the three-star ratings are based on our review.

Where we have not changed the conclusions from AHCPR the text is printed like this, in smaller type.

We then also show the original AHCPR ratings in brackets for comparison. The original AHCPR (1994) ratings are:

- A – strong research-based evidence (multiple relevant and high-quality scientific studies)
- B – moderate research-based evidence (one relevant high-quality scientific study or multiple adequate scientific studies)
- C – limited research-based evidence (at least one adequate scientific study in patients with low back pain)
- D – panel interpretation of information that did not meet inclusion criteria as research-based evidence.

AHCPR applied this grading very strictly and did not rate any evidence on acute back pain better than B.

ASSESSMENT
Diagnostic triage

Both AHCPR (1994) and the Clinical Standards Advisory Group (CSAG) (1994a) considered diagnostic triage to be fundamental to clinical management and the organization of services for back pain. Although there is general agreement on the importance and basic principles of differential diagnosis, there is little empiric evidence on triage in primary care. Individual clinical features may have low sensitivity and specificity.

The statements presented are originally from AHCPR and modified by CSAG.

* Diagnostic triage forms the basis for decisions about referral, investigation and management.

* Diagnostic triage of acute low back problems should be based on the clinical history and examination:
  — simple backache (nonspecific low back pain)
  — nerve root pain
  — possible serious spinal pathology (tumor, infection, inflammatory disorders, cauda equina syndrome, etc.)

(Waddell 1982, Deyo et al 1992, van den Hoogen et al 1995)

Initial assessment methods (adapted from AHCPR 1994)

** The patient's age, the duration and description of symptoms, the impact of symptoms on activity and work, and the response to previous therapy are important in the care of back problems. (B)

** The initial clinical history can identify 'red flags' of possible serious spinal pathology. Such inquiries are especially important in patients over the age of 55. (B)

* Symptoms and signs of cauda equina syndrome, widespread neurologic involvement and severe or progressive motor weakness are 'red flags' for severe neurologic risk. (C)

* A history of significant trauma relative to age (e.g. a fall from a height or a motor vehicle accident in a young adult, or a minor fall or heavy lifting in a potentially osteoporotic or older patient) raises the question of possible fracture. (C)

** Initial assessment should include psychologic and socioeconomic problems in the individual's life, since such nonphysical factors can complicate both assessment and treatment. (B)

** Straight leg raising (SLR) should be assessed and recorded in young adults with sciatica. In older patients with spinal stenosis, SLR may be normal. (B)

** Examination for neurologic deficits should emphasize ankle and knee reflexes, ankle and great toe dorsiflexion strength, and distribution of sensory complaints. (B)

(Waddell et al 1982, Deyo et al 1992, van den Hoogen et al 1995)

X-rays

The American recommendations on x-rays from the AHCPR guidelines are presented in their original form. No further review of evidence was undertaken.

Plain X-rays are not recommended for routine evaluation of patients with acute low back problems within the first month of symptoms unless a red flag is noted on clinical examination. (B)

Plain X-rays of the lumbar spine are recommended for ruling out fractures in patients with acute low back problems when any of the following red flags are present: recent significant trauma (any age), recent mild trauma (patient over age 50), history

of prolonged steroid use, osteoporosis, patient over age 70. (C)

Plain X-rays in combination with a complete blood count (CBC) and erythrocyte sedimentation rate (ESR) may be useful for ruling out tumor or infection in patients with acute low back problems when any of the following red flags are present: prior cancer or recent infection, fever over 100°F, IV drug abuse, prolonged steroid use, low back pain worse with rest, unexplained weight loss. (C)

In the presence of red flags, especially for tumor or infection, the use of other imaging studies such as bone scan, CT, or MRI may be clinically indicated even if plain X-rays are negative. (C)

A bone scan is recommended to evaluate acute low back problems when spinal tumor, infection, or occult fracture is suspected from red flags on medical history, physical examination, corroborative lab test or plain X-ray findings. Bone scans are contraindicated during pregnancy. (C)

The routine use of oblique views on plain lumbar X-rays is not recommended for adults in light of the increased radiation exposure. (B)

(Deyo & Diehl 1988)

Table 16.2 gives the British recommendations on X-rays from the Royal College of Radiologists (RCR).

Psychosocial factors

There is now a great deal of evidence on psychosocial factors in chronic low back pain. Several recent prospective cohort studies show that psychosocial factors are important at a much earlier stage than previously believed.

*** Psychologic, social and economic factors play an important role in chronic low back pain and disability (Waddell 1992, Waddell & Turk 1992).

** Psychosocial factors are important at a much earlier stage than previously believed (Deyo & Diehl 1988, Burton et al 1995, Gatchel et al 1995, Klenerman et al 1995).

*** Psychosocial factors influence a patient's response to treatment and rehabilitation (Waddell 1992, Waddell & Turk 1992).

Table 16.2 British recommendations on X-ray of the lumbar spine

RCR (1993, 2nd ed)

Circumstance	Guidelines	Exceptions
Back pain	Not recommended routinely Acute back pain is usually due to conditions which cannot be diagnosed by plain film radiography. Pain correlates poorly with the severity of degenerative change found on radiology	Symptoms getting worse or not resolving Neurological signs History of trauma
Asymptomatic patients, e.g. pre-employment screening	Not recommended There is no correlation between radiological findings and likelihood of future disability	

RCR (1995, 3rd ed)

Clinical problem	X-ray	Guideline	Comment
Chronic back pain with no pointers to infection or tumor	Plain	Not routinely indicated	Degenerative changes are common and nonspecific Main value in younger patients (spondylolisthesis) ankylosing spondylitis, etc) or in older patients with possible vertebral collapse
Back pain with adverse features: sphincter or gait disturbance, saddle anaesthesia, severe or progressive motor loss, widespread neurological deficit, previous carcinoma, systemically unwell, HIV	Imaging	Indicated	Together with URGENT SPECIALIST REFERRAL MRI is usually the best examination. Imaging should not delay specialist referral. Bone scan is also widely used for possible bone destruction. 'Normal' X-rays may be falsely reassuring
Acute back pain ? disc herniation Sciatica with no adverse features (see above)	Plain	Not routinely indicated	Acute back pain is usually due to conditions which cannot be diagnosed on plain X-ray (osteoporotic collapse an exception) 'Normal' X-rays may be falsely reassuring. Demonstration of disc herniation
	MRI/CT	6 week suggestion	requires MRI or CT and should be considered immediately after failed conservative management MRI generally preferred (wider field of view, conus, postoperative changes, etc.) and avoids irradiation MRI better than CT for postoperative problems

Risk factors for chronicity

There are now a number of prospective cohort studies in primary care which identify risk factors for chronicity: (Roland & Morris 1983 and Roland et al 1983 (same study); Troup et al 1981 and Lloyd & Troup 1983 (same study); Biering-Sorensen 1984; Biering-Sorensen & Thomsen 1986; Deyo & Diehl 1988; Burton & Tillotson 1991; Burton et al 1995; Klenerman et al 1995; Gatchel et al 1995).

** A number of clinical features are risk factors for developing chronic pain and disability (Roland et al 1983, Lloyd & Troup 1983, Biering-Sorensen 1984, Biering-Sorensen & Thomsen 1986, Burton & Tillotson 1991).

** Psychosocial features are more important risk factors for chronicity than biomedical symptoms and signs (Deyo & Diehl 1988, Burton & Tillotson 1991, Burton et al 1995, Klenerman et al 1995, Gatchel et al 1995).

Note. There are not at present any RCTs that demonstrate whether psychosocial assessment or interventions in acute low back pain affect clinical outcomes.

MANAGEMENT

** Medical management can have a major impact on patients' clinical progress and outcomes.

* Initial management should include:

— a thorough clinical history and brief physical examination
— reassurance that there are no red flags of any serious spinal pathology (avoid 'labeling')
— reassurance that there is no need for special investigations in the absence of red flags
— accurate information on the good prognosis for rapid recovery
— reassurance that light physical activity is not harmful
— practical advice on:
  — maintaining daily activities
  — return to work.

(AHCPR 1994)

Information to patients

** Appropriate information and advice can reduce anxiety and improve patient satisfaction with care (Deyo & Diehl 1986, Jones et al 1988, Roland & Dixon 1989, AHCPR 1994).

There is evidence to support the following statements:

*** Most severe back pain and severe activity limitation improves considerably in a few days or at most a few weeks, but milder symptoms may persist longer, often for a few months.

*** Most patients will have some recurrences of back pain from time to time. Recurrences are normal and do not mean that you have reinjured your back or that your condition is getting worse.

** About 10% of patients will have some persisting symptoms 1 year later, but most of them can manage to continue with most normal activities. Patients who return to normal activities feel healthier, use less analgesics and are less distressed than those who limit their activities.

(Pedersen 1981, Troup et al 1981 and Lloyd & Troup 1983 (same study), Roland & Morris 1983 and Roland et al 1983 (same study), Chavannes et al 1986, Coste et al 1994, Von Korff et al 1993, von Korff & Saunders 1995, Croft et al 1997)

*** The longer someone is off work with back pain, the lower their chance of returning to work (McGill 1968, Abenhaim et al 1995, Waddell 1987).

** Back pain does not usually increase with age, but becomes (slightly) less common after age 50–60. However, older patients who do continue to have back pain may have more persistent symptoms and more activity limitation (CSAG 1994b).

TREATMENT: SYMPTOMATIC MEASURES

Drug therapy

Paracetamol, paracetamol-weak opioid compounds, NSAIDs

** Paracetamol and paracetamol-weak opioid compounds prescribed at regular intervals effectively reduce acute low back pain. Comparisons of effectiveness to NSAIDs are inconsistent.

*** NSAIDs prescribed at regular intervals effectively reduce simple backache.

*** Different NSAIDs are equally effective for the reduction of simple backache.

*** NSAIDs can have serious adverse effects particularly at high doses and in the elderly. Ibuprofen followed by diclofenac have the lowest risk of gastrointestinal complications.

** NSAIDs are less effective for the reduction of nerve root pain.

** Clinicians find that paracetamol-weak opioid compounds may be effective alternatives when paracetamol or NSAIDs alone do not give adequate pain control. Adverse effects include constipation and drowsiness.

(de Craen et al 1996, Henry et al 1996, Koes et al 1996b, van Tulder et al 1996b)

Muscle relaxants

Trials of muscle relaxant treatment for patients with acute back pain have used a wide range of agents including diazepam, baclofen and dantrolene.

*** Muscle relaxants effectively reduce acute back pain.

** Comparisons of effectiveness between muscle relaxants and NSAIDs are inconsistent. There are no comparisons to paracetamol.

** Muscle relaxants have significant adverse effects, including drowsiness and potential physical dependence even after relatively short courses (i.e. 1 week).

(Henry et al 1996, Koes et al 1996b, van Tulder et al 1996b)

Strong opioids

Strong opioids appear to be no more effective in relieving low back symptoms than safer analgesics such as paracetamol, aspirin or other NSAIDs. (C)

Strong opioids have significant adverse effects such as decreased reaction time, clouded judgement, drowsiness and potential physical dependence. (C)

Antidepressant medications

* Antidepressant medications have been widely used for the treatment of chronic low back pain, though there is little scientific evidence on their effectiveness. There is no evidence available on the use of antidepressants in acute low back pain. (C) (Turner & Denny 1993)

Bed rest

There are now 10 RCTs of bed rest for acute or recurrent LBP with or without referred leg pain. These show consistently that bed rest is not effective. The only trial showing positive results for bed rest was very atypical and the results can not be applied to primary care. (Wiesel et al 1980). Despite widespread practice, there is little evidence on the efficacy of bed rest for disc prolapse or nerve root pain. The only RCT is a very early trial of poor methodologic quality, which showed that bed rest is not as effective as epidural anesthesia (Coomes 1961). There is no evidence that bed rest in hospital is any more effective.

*** For acute or recurrent LBP with or without referred leg pain, bed rest for 2–7 days is worse than placebo or ordinary activity. It is not as effective as the alternative treatments to which it has been compared for relief of pain, rate of recovery, return to daily activities and days lost from work.

** Prolonged bed rest may lead to debilitation, chronic disability and increasing difficulty in rehabilitation.

(Koes & van den Hoogen 1994, Waddell et al 1997; see Ch. 15)

Advice on staying active

There are now eight RCTs of advice to stay active with consistent findings.

*** Advice to continue ordinary activity can give equivalent or faster symptomatic recovery from the acute attack, and lead to less chronic disability and less time off work than 'traditional' medical treatment with analgesics as required, advice to rest and 'let pain be your guide' for return to normal activity.

*** Graded reactivation over a short period of days or a few weeks, combined with behavioral management of pain, makes little difference to the rate of initial recovery of pain and disability, but leads to less chronic disability and work loss.

* Advice to return to normal work within a planned short time may lead to shorter periods of work loss and less time off work.

(Waddell et al 1997; see Ch. 15)

Physical therapies

Manipulation

There are now 36 RCTs of manipulation for low back pain, although many are of poor quality. Overall, 19 report 'positive' results and a further five report 'positive' results in one or more subgroups. There are also even more systematic reviews of these trials, but the reviews sometimes reach conflicting conclusions. There is very little evidence available on manipulation in patients with nerve root pain.

*** Within the first 6 weeks of onset of acute or recurrent low back pain, manipulation provides better short-term improvement in pain and activity levels and higher patient satisfaction than the treatments to which it has been compared. However, there is no firm evidence that it is possible to select which patients will respond or what kind of manipulation is most effective.

** The evidence is inconclusive as to whether manipulation for low back pain of more than 6 weeks' duration provides clinically significant improvement in outcomes compared with other treatments. There is conflicting evidence from RCTs and systematic reviews on the effectiveness of manipulation in chronic low back pain.

(Shekelle 1995, Koes et al 1996a)

** The risks of manipulation for low back pain are very low, provided patients are selected and assessed properly and it is carried out by a trained therapist or practitioner. Manipulation should not be used in patients with severe or progressive neurologic deficit in view of the rare but serious risk of neurologic complication (Haldeman & Rubinstein 1992).

Back exercises

There are now 28 RCTs of specific back exercises for low back pain, but many are of poor quality.

*** On the evidence available at present, it is doubtful that specific back exercises produce clinically significant improvement in acute low back pain, or that it is possible to select which patients will respond to which exercises.

** McKenzie exercises may produce some short-term symptomatic improvement in acute low back pain. (Koes et al 1991, Faas 1996)

** There is some evidence that exercise programs and physical reconditioning can improve pain and functional levels in patients with chronic low back pain (Evans & Richards 1996, van Tulder et al 1996a).

* There are strong theoretic arguments for commencing exercise programs and physical reconditioning by 6 weeks rather than later (AHCPR 1994, CSAG 1994a).

Physical agents and modalities

This includes ice, heat, short-wave diathermy, massage and ultrasound.

** Although commonly used for symptomatic relief, these passive modalities do not appear to have any effect on clinical outcomes (Gam & Johansson 1995).

Traction

There are now 24 RCTs of various forms of traction in neck and back pain but they are generally of poor quality.

*** Traction does not appear to be effective for low back pain or radiculopathy (van der Heijden et al 1995).

Transcutaneous electrical nerve stimulation (TENS)

** There is inconclusive evidence on the efficacy of TENS in patients with acute low back problems. (C)

Shoe insoles and shoe lifts

* Limited evidence suggests that shoe insoles may reduce back pain in some individuals with mild back complaints. There is no evidence that they provide any long-term benefit. (C)

* Leg length differences of less than 2 cm are unlikely to be significant. (D)

Lumbar corsets and supports

* There is no evidence that lumbar corsets or support belts are effective for treating patients with acute low back problems (D) (Koes & van den Hoogen 1994).

Trigger point and ligamentous injections

* Limited evidence, in studies that included chronic patients, suggests that the efficacy of trigger point or ligamentous injections is equivocal. There is little evidence specifically for acute low back problems. (C)

* Ligamentous and sclerosant injections are invasive and can expose patients to serious potential complications. (C)

Acupuncture

* Weak and equivocal evidence suggests that acupuncture may reduce pain and permit increased activity in patients with chronic low back pain. There is no evidence on the efficacy of acupuncture for acute low back problems. (D)

Epidural steroid injections

There are now 12 RCTs of epidural steroid injections, many of which are of reasonable quality.

** Epidural injections of steroids with or without local anesthetic appear to produce better short-term relief of acute low back pain with sciatica than the treatments to which they have been compared (Koes et al 1995).

* Limited evidence suggests that epidural injections of steroids, local anesthetics, and/or opioids lack proven efficacy for acute low back pain without radiculopathy. (D)

** Epidural injections are invasive and pose rare but serious potential risks. (B)

Facet joint injections

* Studies in chronic low back pain show that facet joint injections do not produce pain relief or global improvement. Neither the type of agent injected nor the site of injection makes a significant difference to outcomes. There is no evidence on the efficacy of facet injections in acute low back problems. (C)

** Facet injections are invasive but the potential serious complications are rare.

Biofeedback

* There is conflicting evidence on the effectiveness of biofeedback for chronic low back problems. There is no evidence available on the effectiveness of biofeedback in acute low back problems. (C)

Group education: back school

There is wide variation in the format and content of 'back schools'. There are two good Swedish RCTs which show positive results, but reviews of all the other available studies are inconclusive.

** Group education in (modifications of) the 'Swedish back school' may be effective in occupational settings (Bergquist-Ullman & Larsson 1977, Hurri 1989).
* The efficacy of back schools in non-occupational settings has yet to be demonstrated (Cohen et al 1994, Koes et al 1994b).

Treatments that are contraindicated

There is no evidence that these treatments are of any benefit for low back pain or sciatica. In every case there are simpler and safer alternatives. They are all associated with potential hazards or complications.

Narcotics for more than 2 weeks (CSAG 1994a)

* Pain of such severity requires further investigation and assistance with management.

Benzodiazepines (diazepam) for more than 2 weeks (CSAG 1994a)

** Benzodiazepines carry a significant risk of habituation and dependency (Owen & Tyrer 1983, Edwards et al 1990).

Colchicine (AHCPR 1994)

* There is limited and conflicting evidence that oral or intravenous colchicine is an effective treatment for acute low back problems. Serious potential side-effects have been reported. (B)

Systemic steroids (AHCPR 1994)

** The limited available evidence suggests that oral steroids are not effective for acute low back problems. (C)

* Serious potential complications are associated with long-term use, but potential complications appear minimal with short-term use. (D)

Bed rest with traction (CSAG 1994a)

** The evidence shows that bed rest with traction is not effective. It adds the complications of immobilization to the deleterious effects of bed rest: in particular, joint stiffness, muscle wasting, loss of bone mineral, pressure sores and thromboembolism (see also bed rest, p. 269) (Pal et al 1986).

Manipulation under general anesthesia (CSAG 1994a)

* There is no evidence that manipulation under general anesthesia is effective. It is associated with an increased risk of serious neurologic damage (Haldeman & Rubinstein 1992).

Plaster jacket (CSAG 1994a)

* There is no evidence that a plaster jacket is an effective treatment for acute low back pain or sciatica. It may cause spinal stiffness, muscle wasting, plaster sores and respiratory complications. It has major psychosocial impacts.

REFERENCES

Abenhaim L, Rossignol M, Gobielle D, Bonvalot Y, Fines P, Scott S 1995 The prognostic consequences in the making of the initial medical diagnosis of work-related injuries. Spine 20: 791–795 (cohort study)
AHCPR 1994 Clinical Practice Guideline Number 14. Acute low back problems in adults. Agency for Health Care Policy and Research, US Department of Health and Human Services. Rockville MD
Bergquist-Ullman M, Larsson U 1977 Acute low back pain in industry. Acta Orthopaedica Scandinavica (supplement) 170: 1–117 (RCT)
Biering-Sorensen F 1984 Physical measurements as risk indicators for low-back trouble over a one-year period. Spine 9: 106–119 (cohort study)
Biering-Sorensen F, Thomsen C 1986 Medical, social and occupational history as risk indicators for low-back trouble in a general population. Spine 11: 720–725 (cohort study)
Burton A K, Tillotson K M 1991 Prediction of the clinical course of low-back trouble using multivariable models. Spine 16: 7–14 (cohort study)
Burton A K, Tillotson M, Main C J, Hollis S 1995 Psychosocial predictors of outcome in acute and subchronic low back trouble. Spine 20: 722–728 (cohort study)
Chavannes A W, Gubbels J, Post D, Rutten G, Thomas S 1986 Acute low back pain: patients' perceptions of pain four weeks after initial diagnosis and treatment in general practice. Journal of the Royal College of General Practitioners 36: 271–293 (cohort study)
Cherkin D 1996 Proceedings of the First International Forum for Primary Care Research on low back pain, Seattle, October 1995. Spine 21(4): 2819–2929
Cohen J E, Goel V, Frank J W, Bombardier C, Peloso P, Guillemin F 1994 Group interventions for people with low back pain: an overview of the literature. Spine 19: 1214–1222 (systematic review)
Coomes E N 1961 A comparison between epidural anaesthesia and bed rest in sciatica. British Medical Journal 264: 20–24 (RCT)
Coste J, Delecoeuillerie G, Cohen de Lara A, Le Parc J M, Paolaggi J B 1994 Clinical course and prognostic factors in acute low back pain: an inception cohort study in primary care. British Medical Journal 308: 577–580 (cohort study)
Croft P, Papageorgiou A, Mcnally R 1997 Low back pain. In: Stevens A, Raferty J (eds) Health care needs assessment, 2nd series. Radcliffe Medical Press, Abingdon, p 129–181 (epidemiologic review)
CSAG 1994a Back pain. Clinical Standards Advisory Group Report. HMSO, London
CSAG 1994b Epidemiology review: the epidemiology and cost of back pain. Annex to the CSAG Report on Back Pain. Clinical Standards Advisory Group Report. HMSO, London
de Craen A J M, Di Giulio G, Lampe-Schoenmaeckers A J E M, Kessels A G H, Kleijnen J 1996 Analgesic efficacy and safety of paracetamol-codeine combinations versus paracetamol alone: a systematic review. British Medical Journal 313: 321–325 (systematic review)

Deyo R A, Diehl A K 1986 Patient satisfaction with medical care for low back pain. Spine 11: 28–30 (*cohort study*)

Deyo R A, Diehl A K 1988 Psychosocial predictors of disability in patients with low back pain. Journal of Rheumatology 15: 1557–1564 (*review*)

Deyo R A, Rainville J, Kent D L 1992 What can the history and physical examination tell us about low back pain? Journal of the American Medical Association 268: 760–765 (*review*)

Edwards J G, Cantopher T, Olivieri S 1990 Benzodiazepine dependence and the problems of withdrawal. Postgraduate Medical Journal 66 (supplement 2): S27–S35

Evans G, Richards S 1996 Low back pain: an evaluation of therapeutic interventions. Health Care Evaluation Unit, University of Bristol, Bristol (*mega-analysis*)

Faas A 1996 Exercises: which ones are worth trying, for which patients and when? Spine 21: 2874–2879 (*systematic review*)

Gam A N, Johannsen F 1995 Ultrasound therapy in musculoskeletal disorders: a meta-analysis. Pain 63: 85–91 (*systematic review*)

Gatchel R J, Polatin P B, Mayer T G 1995 The dominant role of psychosocial risk factors in the development of chronic low back disability. Spine 20: 2702–2709 (*cohort study*)

Haldeman S, Rubinstein S M 1992 Cauda equina syndrome in patients undergoing manipulation of the lumbar spine. Spine 17: 1469–1473 (*review*)

Henry D, Lim L L Y, Rodriguez L A G et al 1996 Variability in risk of gastrointestinal complications with individual non-steroidal anti-inflammatory drugs: results of a collaborative meta-analysis. British Medical Journal 312: 1563–1566 (*systematic review*)

Hurri H 1989 The Swedish back school in chronic low back pain. Part I. Benefits. Scandinavian Journal of Rehabilitation Medicine 21: 33–40 (*RCT*)

Jones S L, Jones P K, Katz J 1988 Compliance for low-back pain patients in the emergency department: a randomized trial. Spine 13: 553–556 (*RCT*)

Klenerman L, Slade P D, Stanley I M et al 1995 The prediction of chronicity in patients with an acute attack of low back pain in a general practice setting. Spine 20: 478–484 (*cohort study*)

Koes B W, Assendelft W J J, Van der Heijden G J M G, Bouter L M 1996a Spinal manipulation for low back pain: an updated systematic review of randomized clinical trials. Spine 21: 2860–2873 (*systematic review*)

Koes B W, Bouter L M, Beckerman H, van der Heijden C J M G, Knipschild P G 1991 Physiotherapy exercises and back pain: a blinded review. British Medical Journal 302: 1572–1576 (*systematic review*)

Koes B W, Scholten R J P M, Mens J M A, Bouter M 1995 Efficacy of epidural steroid injections for low-back pain and sciatica: a systematic review of randomized clinical trials. Pain 63: 279–288 (*systematic review*)

Koes B W, Scholten R J P M, Mens J M A, Bouter L M 1996b Efficacy of NSAIDs for low back pain: a systematic review of randomised controlled trials of 11 interventions. In: van Tulder M W, Koes B W, Bouter L M (eds) Low back pain in primary care: effectiveness of diagnostic and therapeutic interventions. Institute for Research in Extramural Medicine; Amsterdam, p 171–190 (*systematic review*)

Koes B W, van den Hoogen H M M 1994 Efficacy of bed rest and orthoses of low back pain. A review of randomized clinical trials. European Journal of Physical Medicine and Rehabilitation 4: 86–93 (*systematic review*)

Koes B W, van Tulder M W, van der Windt D A W M, Bouter L M 1994 The efficacy of back schools: a review of randomized clinical trials. Journal of Clinical Epidemiology 47: 851–862 (*systematic review*)

Lloyd D C E F, Troup J D G 1983 Recurrent back pain and its prediction. Journal of Social and Occupational Medicine 33: 66–74 (*cohort study*)

McGill C M 1968 Industrial back problems: a control program. Journal of Occupational Medicine 10: 174–178 (*cohort study*)

Owen R T, Tyrer P 1983 Benzodiazepine dependence: a review of the evidence. Drugs 25: 385–398 (*review*)

Pal P, Mangion P, Hossian M A, Diffey L 1986 A controlled trial of continuous lumbar traction in the treatment of back pain and sciatica. British Journal of Rheumatology 25: 1181–1183 (*RCT*)

Pedersen P A 1981 Prognostic indicators in low back pain. Journal of the Royal College of General Practitioners 31: 209–216 (*cohort study*)

RCGP 1996 Clinical guidelines for the management of acute low back pain. Royal College of General Practitioners, London

RCR 1993 Making the best use of a department of radiology: guidelines for doctors, 2nd edn. Royal College of Radiologists, London

RCR 1995 Making the best use of a department of clinical radiology. Guidelines for doctors, 3rd edn. Royal College of Radiologists, London

Roland M, Dixon M 1989 The role of an educational booklet in managing patients presenting with back pain in primary care. In: Roland M, Jenner J (eds) Back pain: new approaches to education and rehabilitation. Manchester University, Manchester (*RCT*)

Roland M O, Morrell D C, Morris R W 1983 Can general practitioners predict the outcome of episodes of back pain? British Medical Journal 286: 523–525 (*cohort study*)

Roland M, Morris R 1983 A study of the natural history of low-back pain. Part II: development of guidelines for trials of treatment in primary care. Spine 8: 145–150 (*cohort study*)

Shekelle P 1995 Spinal manipulation and mobilization for low back pain. Paper presented to the International Forum for Primary Care Research on Low Back Pain, Seattle, October 1995 (*review*)

Spitzer W O, LeBlanc F E, Dupuis M et al 1987 Scientific approach to the assessment and management of activity-related spinal disorders. (Report of the Quebec Task Force on Spinal Disorders.) Spine 12 (suppl 7S): 1–59 (*review*)

Troup J D G, Martin J W, Lloyd D C E F 1981 Back pain in industry: a prospective survey. Spine 6: 61–69 (*cohort study*)

Turner J A, Denny M C 1993 Do antidepressant medications relieve chronic low back pain? Journal of Family Practice 37: 545–553 (*systematic review*)

van den Hoogen H M M, Koes B W, van Eijk J T H M, Bouter L M 1995 On the accuracy of history, physical examination and erythrocyte sedimentation rate in diagnosing low-back pain in general practice. A criteria-based review of the literature. Spine 20: 318–327 (*systematic review*) van der Heijden G J M G, Beurskens A J H M, Koes B W, de Vet H C W, Bouter L M 1995 The efficacy of traction for back and neck pain: a systematic, blinded review of randomized clinical trial methods. Physical Therapy 75: 93–103 (*systematic review*)

van Tulder M W, Koes B W, Bouter L M (eds) 1996a Low back pain in primary care: effectiveness of diagnostic and therapeutic interventions. Institute for Research in Extramural Medicine Amsterdam, p 1–285 (*mega-analysis*)

van Tulder M W, Koes B W, Bouter L M 1996b Conservative treatment of acute low back pain: a systematic mega-review of 81 randomised controlled trials of 11 interventions. In: van Tulder M W, Koes B W, Bouter L M (eds) Low back pain in primary care: effectiveness of diagnostic and therapeutic interventions. Institute for Research in Extramural Medicine, Amsterdam (*systematic review*)

von Korff M, Deyo R A, Cherkin D, Barlow W 1993 Back pain in primary care: outcomes at one year. Spine 18: 855–862 (*cohort study*)

von Korff M, Saunders K 1996 The course of back pain in primary care. Spine 21: 2833–2839

Waddell G 1982 An approach to backache. British Journal of Hospital Medicine 28: 187–219 (*cohort study*)

Waddell G 1987 A new clinical model for the treatment of low back pain. Spine 12: 632–644 (*review*)

Waddell G 1992 Biopsychosocial analysis of low back pain. Clinical Rheumatology 6: 523–557 (*review*)

Waddell G, Turk D C 1992 Clinical assessment of low back pain. In: Turk D C, Melzack R (eds) Handbook of pain assessment. Guilford Press, New York, ch 2, p 15–36 (*review*)

Waddell G, Feder G, Lewis M 1997 Systematic reviews of bedrest and advice to stay active for acute low back pain. British Journal of General Practice 47: 647–652 (*systematic review*)

Wiesel S W, Cuckler J M, Deluca F, Jones F, Zeide M S, Rothman R H 1980 Acute low back pain. An objective analysis of conservative therapy. Spine 5: 324–330 (*RCT*)

17

Clinical guidelines

In the last 5 years there has been growing interest in clinical guidelines. Practice guidelines are 'systematically developed statements to assist practitioner and patient decisions about appropriate health care for specific clinical circumstances' (Institute of Medicine 1992). They describe good practice for the typical patient with a common clinical problem. Their aim is to improve standards of care and clinical effectiveness. All health professionals have always tried to apply the best and most up-to-date knowledge to clinical practice. Guidelines are simply a way of presenting this knowledge in a form that is accessible and easy to use (see Box 17.1)

Guidelines are based on two main principles:

- the best scientific evidence that is currently available
- the widest possible professional and patient consultation and consensus.

Box 17.1 The qualities of good guidelines (Institute of Medicine 1992, NHS Executive 1994)

- State clearly the population they apply to, and exceptions
- Be scientifically valid and robust
- State the strength of evidence for each recommendation
- Be user-friendly and suitable for use by all grades of staff
- Note areas where patients should be involved in decisions about their health care
- Point out the implications for health care process and provision
- Be suitable for clinical audit
- State the review date so that the guideline stays up to date
- Have documented support
- Have plans to distribute and implement the guidelines

There is a heated debate surrounding evidence-based medicine and clinical guidelines (Farmer 1993, Feder 1994, Meeker 1995, Sackett et al 1996). Some regard it as the most fundamental advance in medicine during the last quarter of a century, and the road to improved health care in the next millenium. To others, it is the greatest threat to clinical freedom and the road to bureaucratic control of professional practice. This is not the place for that debate. Whether we like them or not, guidelines are here to stay. They are only a tool, but a powerful tool. The argument is, perhaps, not about guidelines but about how we use them. It is up to all of us to use them wisely and to make sure that they are not abused. I will simply offer the available guidelines for acute back pain and leave it to you to decide if and how you want to use them.

Box 17.2 The more specific clinical aims of guidelines for acute low back pain (Feder 1994)

- Improve clinical assessment of patients who present with low back symptoms
- Promote appropriate investigations
- Promote appropriate prescribing
- Promote appropriate referral for physical therapy or specialist investigation and treatment
- If possible, prevent chronic low back pain and disability

CLINICAL GUIDELINES FOR ACUTE LOW BACK PAIN

I have included the national guidelines for the US, the UK and New Zealand. Most of the main messages are the same, with subtle shifts over time which reflect new evidence and current thinking. Each guideline offers very different presentations and you can take your pick.

The American guideline was developed by the Agency for Health Care Policy and Research (AHCPR) and published in December 1994. AHCPR put a great deal of effort and resources into this project. They carried out the most thorough review ever performed of the scientific evidence on back pain up to 1992. Indeed, the American guideline is the father of all other national guidelines for acute back pain. The

complete AHCPR guideline is 160 pages long. It gives a complete evidence review, rates the strength of the evidence, and links the evidence to the recommendations. Here, I have included the abstract and the 'Quick Reference Guide for Clinicians'.

The first UK guidelines were developed by the Clinical Standards Advisory Group (CSAG) and were also published in December 1994. The CSAG group worked closely with the American panel and based the UK guidelines on the AHCPR evidence. However, rightly or wrongly, we decided to present the UK guideline in a much simpler, user-friendly form. We did not attempt to include all the scientific evidence, but simply referred to the background detail in the American guideline and the full CSAG report.

It may help to put things into perspective if we look at the brief for the CSAG guidelines:

- Purpose – to review the scientific evidence on effective treatment for acute low back problems
- Subjects – adult males and females over 18 years of age
- Clinical condition – acute low back pain lasting up to 3 months, with or without related leg symptoms
- Definition of effective treatments – that relieve pain and improve physical function
- Outcomes – low back symptoms, level of physical function, patient satisfaction and complications
- Users of guideline – practitioners and therapists in primary care.

All guidelines stress the need for regular update as more evidence and knowledge become available. The UK is the only country in the world that has actually done this for back pain. The second edition of the UK guidelines was developed by the Royal College of General Practitioners (RCGP) and published in September 1996. This was a truly primary care group of family doctors, physical therapists, osteopaths, chiropractors and the national patients' organization. There has been much new scientific data since 1992, and we updated the evidence review to April 1996 (Ch. 16). The actual guideline is a single sheet that gives the main evidence statements and recommendations, and there is a separate 35 page evidence review.

At the time of writing, the *New Zealand acute low back pain guide* is the most up-to-date guide (ACC 1997). It was developed from the AHCPR (1994) clinical guidelines, supplemented by an extensive review of more recent evidence and the RCGP (1996) guidelines. Although the focus is still on acute pain, it places stronger emphasis on psychosocial factors and the prevention of chronic pain and disability. This led to a companion *Guide to assessing psychosocial yellow flags in acute low back pain* written by three internationally known clinical psychologists (Kendall et al 1997). This is the most comprehensive guide to these psychosocial issues now available and forms a bridge between acute and chronic pain.

Obtaining copies of guidelines

Supplies of these guidelines are available as follows:

Clinical practice guideline no. 14. Acute low back problems in adults. December 1994. Bigos S, Bowyer O, Braen G et al 1994 Acute low back problems in adults. Clinical practice guideline no. 14. AHCPR Publication No. 95–0642. Agency for Health Care Policy and Research, Public

Health Service, US Department of Health and Human Services, Rockville, MD

Available from: Government Printing Office, Superintendent of Documents, Washington, DC 20402

Clinical Standards Advisory Group report on back pain. December 1994. ISBN 0 11 321887 7. Price £14.95. (*Management guidelines for back pain included as an appendix*)

Available from: Her Majesty's Stationery Office, HMSO Publications Centre, PO Box 276, London SW8 5DT

Clinical guidelines for the management of acute low back pain. September 1996. Royal College of General Practitioners, London

Guidelines and evidence review available from: RCGP, 14 Princes Gate, Hyde Park, London SW7 1PU

New Zealand acute low back pain guide, and *Guide to assessing psychosocial yellow flags in acute low back pain*. January 1997. Accident Rehabilitation & Compensation Insurance Corporation of New Zealand and the National Health Committee, Wellington, NZ

Available from: ACC, PO Box 242, Wellington, New Zealand (e-mail: nhc@MOHWN.synet. net.nz; phone: 0-4-460-7700; internet: http: //www.nhc.govt.nz)

REFERENCES

ACC 1997 New Zealand acute low back pain guide. Accident Rehabilitation & Compensation Insurance Corporation of New Zealand and the National Health Committee, Wellington, NZ

AHCPR 1994 Management guidelines for acute low back pain. Agency for Health Care Policy and Research, US Department of Health and Human Services, Rockville MD

CSAG 1994 Report on back pain. Clinical Standards Advisory Group. HMSO, London

Farmer A 1993 Medical practice guidelines; lessons from the United States. British Medical Journal 307: 313–317

Feder G 1994 Editorial. Clinical guidelines in 1994. British Medical Journal 309: 1457–1458

Institute of Medicine (Field M J, Lohr K N, eds) 1992 Guidelines for clinical practice. From development to use. National Academy Press, Washington, DC

Kendall N A S, Linton S J, Main C J 1997 Guide to assessing psychosocial yellow flags in acute low back pain: risk factors for long-term disability and work loss. Accident Rehabilitation & Compensation Insurance Corporation

of New Zealand and the National Health Committee, Wellington NZ, p 1–22

Linton S J, Hallden K 1996 Risk factors and the natural course of acute and recurrent musculoskeletal pain: developing a screening instrument. In: Jensen T S, Turner J A, Wiesenfeld-Hallin Z (eds) 1997 Proceedings of the 8th World Congress on Pain. IASP Press, Seattle, p 527–536

Meeker W C 1995 The future impact of clinical practice guidelines. Proceedings of the Chiropractic Centennial Meeting, Washington, DC

NHS Executive 1994 Effective health care. Implementing clinical guidelines, number 8: can guidelines be used to improve clinical practice? NHS Executive, Leeds, p 1–12

RCGP 1996 Clinical guidelines for the management of acute low back pain. Royal College of General Practitioners, London

Sackett D L, Rosenberg W M C, Gray J A M, Haynes R B, Richardson W S 1996 Editorial. Evidence based medicine: what it is and what it isn't. British Medical Journal 312: 71–72

APPENDIX 17A: US Clinical practice guideline: acute low back problems in adults

Abstract

Findings and recommendations on the assessment and treatment of adults with acute low back problems – activity limitations due to symptoms in the low back and/or back-related leg symptoms of less than 3 months' duration – are presented in this clinical practice guideline. The following are the principal conclusions of this guideline:

• The initial assessment of patients with acute low back problems focuses on the detection of 'red flags' (indicators of potentially serious spinal pathology or other nonspinal pathology).

• In the absence of red flags, imaging studies and further testing of patients are not usually helpful during the first 4 weeks of low back symptoms.

• Relief of discomfort can be accomplished most safely with nonprescription medication and/or spinal manipulation.

• While some activity modification may be necessary during the acute phase, bed rest >4 days is not helpful and may further debilitate the patient.

• Low-stress aerobic activities can be safely started in the first 2 weeks of symptoms to help avoid debilitation; exercises to condition trunk muscles are commonly delayed at least 2 weeks.

• Patients recovering from acute low back problems are encouraged to return to work or their normal daily activities as soon as possible.

• If low back symptoms persist, further evaluation may be indicated.

• Patients with sciatica may recover more slowly, but further evaluation can also be safely delayed.

• Within the first 3 months of low back symptoms, only patients with evidence of serious spinal pathology or severe, debilitating symptoms of sciatica, and physiologic evidence of specific nerve root compromise which are corroborated on imaging studies can be expected to benefit from surgery.

• With or without surgery, 80% of patients with sciatica recover eventually.

• Nonphysical factors (such as psychologic or socioeconomic problems) may be addressed in the context of discussing reasonable expectations for recovery.

QUICK REFERENCE GUIDE FOR CLINICIANS

This *Quick Reference Guide for Clinicians* contains highlights from the *Clinical Practice Guideline* version of *Acute Low Back Problems in Adults*, which was developed by a private-sector panel of health care providers and consumers. The *Quick Reference Guide* is an example of how a clinician might implement the panel's findings and recommendations on the management of acute low back problems in working age adults. Topics covered include the initial assessment of patients presenting with acute low back problems, identification of red flags that may indicate the presence of a serious underlying medical condition, initial management, special studies and diagnostic considerations, and further management considerations. Instructions for clinical testing for sciatic tension, recommendations for sitting and unassisted lifting, tests for identification of clinical pathology, and algorithms for patient management are included.

Purpose and scope

Low back problems affect virtually everyone at some time during their life. Surveys indicate a yearly prevalence of symptoms in 50% of working age adults; 15–20% seek medical care. Low back problems rank high among the reasons for physician office visits and are costly in terms of medical care, lost productivity, and nonmonetary costs such as diminished ability to perform or enjoy usual activities. In fact, for persons under age 45, low back problems are the most common cause of disability.

Acute low back problems are defined as activity intolerance due to lower back or back-

Reproduced with permission from the US Agency for Health Care Policy and Research, Dec 1994.

related leg symptoms of less than 3 months', duration. About 90% of patients with acute low back problems spontaneously recover activity tolerance within 1 month. The approach to a patient with recurrent low back limitations is similar to that of a new acute episode.

The findings and recommendations included in the *Clinical Practice Guideline* define a paradigm shift away from focusing care exclusively on the pain and toward helping patients improve activity intolerance. The intent of this *Quick Reference Guide* is to bring to life this paradigm shift. The guide provides information on the detection of serious conditions that occasionally cause low back symptoms (conditions such as spinal fracture, tumor, infection, cauda equina syndrome or nonspinal conditions). However, treatment of these conditions is beyond the scope of this guideline. In addition, the guideline does not address the care of patients younger than 18 years or those with chronic back problems (back-related activity limitations of greater than 3 months' duration).

Initial assessment

- Seek potentially dangerous conditions.
- In the absence of signs of dangerous conditions, there is no need for special studies since 90% of patients will recover spontaneously within 4 weeks.

A focused medical history and physical examination are sufficient to assess the patient with an acute or recurrent limitation due to low back symptoms of less than 4 weeks' duration. Patient responses and findings on the history and physical examination, referred to as 'red flags' (Table 17A.1), raise suspicion of serious underlying spinal conditions. Their absence rules out the need for special studies during the first 4 weeks of symptoms when spontaneous recovery is expected. The medical history and physical examination can also alert clinicians to nonspinal pathology (abdominal, pelvic, thoracic) that can present as low back symptoms. Acute low back symptoms can then be classified into one of three working categories:

- potentially serious spinal condition – tumor, infection, spinal fracture or a major neurologic compromise such as cauda equina syndrome, suggested by a red flag
- sciatica – back-related lower limb symptoms suggesting lumbosacral nerve root compromise
- nonspecific back symptoms – occurring primarily in the back and suggesting neither nerve root compromise nor a serious underlying condition.

Medical history

In addition to detecting serious conditions and categorizing back symptoms, the medical history establishes rapport between the clinician and the patient. The patient's description of present symptoms and limitations, duration of symptoms, and history of previous episodes defines the basic problem. It also provides insight into concerns, expectations and nonphysical (psychologic and socioeconomic) issues that may alter the patient's response to treatment. Assessment tools such as pain drawings and visual analog pain-rating scales may help further document the patient's perceptions and progress.

A patient's estimate of personal activity intolerance due to low back symptoms contributes to the clinical assessment of the severity of the back problem, guides treatment, and establishes a baseline for recommending daily activities and evaluating progress.

Open-ended questions, such as those listed below, can gauge the need for further discussion or specific inquiries for more detailed information:

- What are your symptoms?
  — pain, numbness, weakness, stiffness?
  — located primarily in back, leg or both?
  — constant or intermittent?

- How do these symptoms limit you?
  — how long can you sit, stand, walk?
  — how much weight can you lift?

- When did the current limitations begin?
  — how long have your activities been limited? More than 4 weeks?

Table 17A.1 Red flags for potentially serious conditions

Possible fracture	Possible tumor or infection	Possible cauda equina syndrome
From medical history		
Major trauma, such as vehicle accident or fall from height	Age over 50 or under 20	Saddle anesthesia
	History of cancer	Recent onset of bladder dysfunction, such as urinary retention, increased frequency, or overflow incontinence
Minor trauma or even strenuous lifting (in older or potentially osteoporotic patient)	Constitutional symptoms, such as recent fever or chills or unexplained weight loss	
	Risk factors for spinal infection: recent bacterial infection (eg, urinary tract infection); IV drug abuse; or immune suppression (from steroids, transplant, or HIV)	Severe or progressive neurologic deficit in the lower extremity
	Pain that worsens when supine; severe night-time pain	
From physical examination		
		Unexpected laxity of the anal sphincter
		Perianal/perineal sensory loss
		Major motor weakness: quadriceps (knee extension weakness); ankle plantar flexors, evertors and dorsiflexors (foot drop)

— have you had any similar episodes previously?
— previous testing or treatment?

• What do you hope we can accomplish during this visit?

Physical examination

Guided by the medical history, the examination includes:

• general observation of the patient
• a regional back examination
• neurologic screening
• testing for sciatic nerve root tension.

The examination is mostly subjective since patient response or interpretation is required for all parts except reflex testing and circumferential measurements for atrophy.

Addressing red flags

Physical examination evidence of severe neurologic compromise that correlates with the medical history may indicate a need for immediate consultation. The examination may further modify suspicions of tumor, infection, or significant trauma. A medical history suggestive of nonspinal pathology mimicking a back problem may warrant examination of pulses, abdomen, pelvis or other areas.

Observation and regional back examination

Limping or coordination problems indicate the need for specific neurologic testing. Severe guarding of lumbar motion in all planes may support a suspected diagnosis of spinal infection, tumor, or fracture. However, given marked variations among persons with and without symptoms, range-of-motion measurements of the back are of limited value.

Vertebral point tenderness to palpation, when associated with other signs or symptoms, may be suggestive of but not specific for spinal fracture or infection. Palpable soft-tissue tenderness is, by itself, an even less specific or reliable finding.

Neurologic screening

The neurologic examination can focus on a few tests that seek evidence of nerve root impairment, peripheral neuropathy, or spinal cord dysfunction. Over 90% of all clinically significant lower extremity radiculopathy due to disc herniation involves the L5 or S1 nerve roots at the L4–5 or L5–S1 disc level. The clinical features of nerve root compression are summarized in Figure 17A.1.

Testing muscle strength. The patient's inability to toe walk (calf muscles, mostly S1 nerve root), heel walk (ankle and toe dorsiflexors, L5 and some L4 nerve roots), or do a single squat and rise (quadriceps muscles, mostly L4 nerve root) may indicate muscle weakness. Specific testing of the dorsiflexor muscles of the ankle or great toe (suggestive of L5 or some L4 nerve root dysfunction), and toe flexors (S1) is also important.

Circumferential measurements. Muscle atrophy can be detected by circumferential measurements of the calf and thigh bilaterally. Differences of less than 2 cm in measurements of the two limbs at the same level may be a normal variation. Symmetrical muscle bulk and strength are expected unless the patient has a neurologic impairment or a history of lower extremity muscle or joint problems.

Reflexes. The ankle jerk reflex tests mostly the S1 nerve root and the knee jerk reflex tests mostly L4; neither tests the L5 nerve root. The reliability of reflex testing can be diminished in the presence of adjacent joint or muscle problems. Up-going toes in response to stroking the plantar footpad (Babinski or plantar response) may indicate upper motor-neuron abnormalities (such as myelopathy or demyelinating disease) rather than a common low back problem.

Sensory examination. Testing light touch or pressure in the medial (L4), dorsal (L5) and lateral (S1) aspects of the foot (Fig. 17A.1) is usually sufficient for sensory screening.

Clinical tests for sciatic tension

The straight leg raising (SLR) test (Fig. 17A.2) can detect tension on the L5 and/or S1 nerve roots. SLR may reproduce leg pain by stretching nerve roots irritated by a disc herniation.

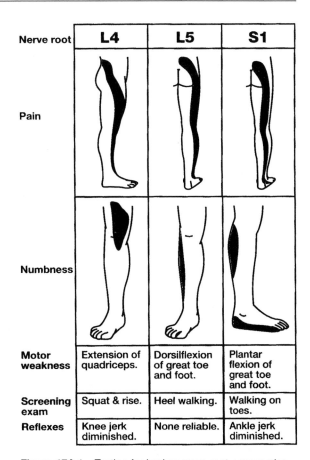

Nerve root	L4	L5	S1
Pain			
Numbness			
Motor weakness	Extension of quadriceps.	Dorsiflexion of great toe and foot.	Plantar flexion of great toe and foot.
Screening exam	Squat & rise.	Heel walking.	Walking on toes.
Reflexes	Knee jerk diminished.	None reliable.	Ankle jerk diminished.

Figure 17A.1   Testing for lumbar nerve root compromise.

Instructions for the SLR test

1. Ask the patient to lie as straight as possible on a table in the supine position.
2. With one hand placed above the knee of the leg being examined, exert enough firm pressure to keep the knee fully extended. Ask the patient to relax.
3. With the other hand cupped under the heel, slowly raise the straight limb. Tell the patient: 'If this bothers you, let me know and I will stop' (Fig. 17A.2a).
4. Monitor for any movement of the pelvis before complaints are elicited. True sciatic tension should elicit complaints before the hamstrings are stretched enough to move the pelvis.
5. Estimate the degree of leg elevation that elicits complaint from the patient. Then

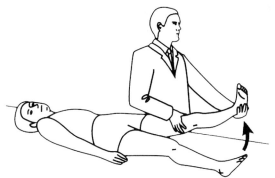

Figure 17A.2a Straight leg raising (SLR) test.

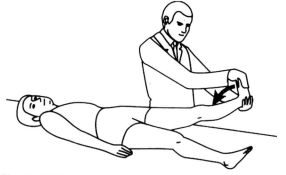

Figure 17A.2c

determine the most distal area of discomfort: back, hip, thigh, knee or below the knee (Fig. 17A.2b).

6. While holding the leg at the limit of straight leg raising, dorsiflex the ankle. Note whether this aggravates the pain. Internal rotation of the limb can also increase the tension on the sciatic nerve roots (Fig. 17A.2c).

Pain below the knee at less than 70° of straight leg raising, aggravated by dorsiflexion of the ankle and relieved by ankle plantar flexion or external limb rotation, is most suggestive of tension on the L5 or S1 nerve root relating to disc herniation. Reproducing back pain alone with SLR testing does not indicate significant nerve root tension.

Crossover pain occurs when straight raising of the patient's well limb elicits pain in the leg with sciatica. Crossover pain is a stronger indicator of nerve root compression than pain elicited from raising the straight painful limb alone.

Sitting knee extension (Fig. 17A.3) can also test sciatic tension. The patient with significant nerve root irritation tends to complain or lean backward to reduce tension on the nerve.

With the patient sitting on the table, both hips and knees flexed at 90°, slowly extend the knee as if evaluating the patella or bottom of the foot. This maneuver stretches nerve roots as much as a moderate degree of supine SLR.

Inconsistent findings and pain behavior

The patient who embellishes the medical history, exaggerates pain drawings, or provides responses on examination inconsistent with known physiology can be particularly challenging. A strongly positive supine SLR test without complaint on sitting knee extension and inconsistent responses on examination raise suspicion that nonphysical factors may be affecting the patient's responses. 'Pain behaviors' (verbal or

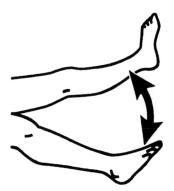

Figure 17A.2b

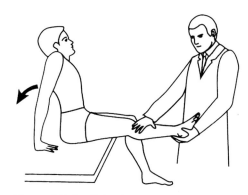

Figure 17A.3 Sitting knee extension test.

Algorithm 17A.1   Initial evaluation of acute low back problem.

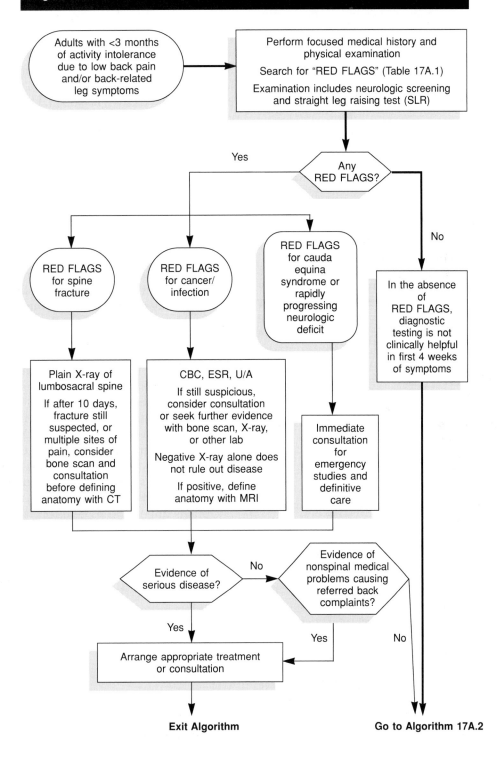

Exit Algorithm   **Go to Algorithm 17A.2**

nonverbal communication of distress or suffering) such as amplified grimacing, distorted gait or posture, moaning and rubbing of painful body parts may also cloud medical issues and even evoke angry responses from the clinician.

Interpreting inconsistencies or pain behaviors as malingering does not benefit the patient or the clinician. It is more useful to view such behavior and inconsistencies as the patient's attempt to enlist the practitioner as an advocate, or as a plea for help. The patient could be trapped in a job where activity requirements are unrealistic relative to the person's age or health. In some cases, the patient may be negotiating with an insurer or be involved in legal actions. In patients with recurrent back problems, inconsistencies and amplifications may simply be habits learned during previous medical evaluations. In working with these patients, the clinician should attempt to identify any psychologic or socioeconomic pressures that might be influenced in a positive manner. The overall goal should always be to facilitate the patient's recovery and avoid the development of chronic low back disability.

Initial care

- Education and reassurance
- Patient comfort
- Activity alterations.

Patient education

If the initial assessment detects no serious condition, reassure the patient that there is 'no hint of a dangerous problem' and that 'a rapid recovery can be expected'. The need for education will vary among patients and during various stages of care. An obviously apprehensive patient may require a more detailed explanation. Patients with sciatica may have a longer expected recovery time than patients with nonspecific back symptoms and thus may need more education and reassurance. Any patient who does not recover within a few weeks may need more extensive education and the reassurance that special studies may be considered if recovery is slow.

Patient comfort

Comfort is often a patient's first concern. Non-prescription analgesics will provide sufficient relief for most patients with acute low back symptoms. If treatment response is inadequate, as evidenced by continued symptoms and activity limitations, prescribed pharmaceutical or physical methods may be added. Comorbid conditions, side-effects, cost and provider/patient preference should guide the clinician's choice of recommendations. Table 17A.2 summarizes comfort options.

Oral pharmaceuticals

The safest, most effective medication for acute low back symptoms appears to be acetaminophen. Nonsteroidal anti-inflammatory drugs (NSAIDs), including aspirin and ibuprofen, are also effective although they can cause gastrointestinal irritation/ulceration or (less commonly) renal or allergic problems. Phenylbutazone is not recommended due to risks of bone marrow suppression. Acetaminophen may be used safely in combination with NSAIDs or other pharmacologic or physical therapeutics, especially in otherwise healthy patients.

Muscle relaxants seem no more effective than NSAIDs for treating patients with low back symptoms. Using them in combination with NSAIDs has no demonstrated benefit. Side-effects including drowsiness have been reported in up to 30% of patients taking muscle relaxants.

Opioids appear no more effective than safer analgesics for managing low back symptoms. Opioids should be avoided if possible and, when chosen, used only for a short time. Poor patient tolerance, risks of drowsiness, decreased reaction time, clouded judgement, and potential misuses/dependency have been reported in up to 35% of patients. Patients should be warned of these potential debilitating problems.

Physical methods

Manipulation, defined as manual loading of the spine using short or long leverage methods, is safe and effective for patients in the first month

Table 17A.2 Symptom control methods

RECOMMENDED		
Nonprescription analgesics Acetaminophen (safest) NSAIDS (aspirin[1], Ibuprofen[1])		
Prescribed pharmaceutical methods	**Prescribed physical methods**	
Nonspecific low back symptoms and/or sciatica	*Nonspecific low back symptoms*	*Sciatica*
Other NSAIDs[1]	Manipulation (in place of medication or a shorter trial if combined with NSAIDs)	
OPTIONS		
Nonspecific low back symptoms and/or sciatica	*Nonspecific low back symptoms*	*Sciatica*
Muscle relaxants[2,3,4] Opioids[2,3,4]	Physical agents and modalities[2] (heat or cold modalities for home programs only)	Manipulation (in place of medication or a shorter trial if combined with NSAIDs)
	Shoe insoles[2]	Physical agents and modalities[2] (heat or cold modalities for home programs only)
		Few days' rest[4]
		Shoe insoles[2]

[1]Aspirin and other NSAIDs are not recommended for use in combination with one another due to the risk of GI complications.
[2]Equivocal efficacy.
[3]Significant potential for producing drowsiness and debilitation; potential for dependency.
[4]Short course (few days only) for severe symptoms.

of acute low back pain without radiculopathy. For patients with symptoms lasting longer than 1 month, manipulation is probably safe but its efficacy is unproven. If manipulation has not resulted in symptomatic and functional improvement after 4 weeks, it should be stopped and the patient reevaluated.

Traction applied to the spine has not been found effective for treating acute low back symptoms.

Physical modalities such as massage, diathermy, ultrasound and cutaneous laser treatment, biofeedback, and transcutaneous electrical nerve stimulation (TENS) also have no proven efficacy in the treatment of acute low back symptoms. If requested, the clinician may wish to provide the patient with instructions on self-application of heat or cold therapy for temporary symptom relief.

Invasive techniques such as needle acupuncture and injection procedures (injection of trigger points in the back, injection of facet joints, injection of steroids, lidocaine or opioids into the epidural space) have no proven benefit in the treatment of acute low back symptoms.

Other miscellaneous therapies have been evaluated. No evidence indicates that shoe lifts are effective in treating acute low back symptoms or limitations, especially when the difference in lower limb length is less than 2 cm. Shoe insoles are safe and inexpensive options if requested by patients with low back symptoms who must stand for prolonged periods. Low back corsets and back belts, however, do not appear beneficial for treating acute low back symptoms.

Activity alteration

To avoid both undue back irritation and debilitation from inactivity, recommendations for alternate activity can be helpful. Most patients will not require bed rest. Prolonged bed rest (for more than 4 days) has potential debilitating effects, and its efficacy in the treatment of acute low back symptoms is unproven. Two to 4 days of bed rest are reserved for the patients with the most severe limitations (due primarily to leg pain).

Avoiding undue back irritation. Activities and postures that increase stress on the back also tend to aggravate back symptoms. Patients limited by back symptoms can minimize lifting stress by keeping any lifted object close to the navel. Twisting, bending and reaching while lifting also increase stress on the back. Sitting, though safe, may aggravate symptoms as well. Advise these patients to avoid prolonged sitting and to change positions often. A soft support placed at the small of the back, armrests to support some body weight, and a slight recline of the chair back may make required sitting more comfortable.

Avoiding debilitation. Until the patient returns to normal activity, aerobic (endurance) conditioning such as stationary biking, swimming or even light jogging may be recommended to help avoid debilitation from inactivity. An incremental, gradually increasing regimen of aerobic exercise (up to 20–30 minutes daily) can usually be started within the first 2 weeks of symptoms. Such conditioning activities have been found to stress the back no more than sitting for an equal time period on the side of the bed. Patients should be informed that any exercise may increase symptoms at first. If intolerable, some exercise alteration is usually helpful.

Conditioning exercises for trunk muscles are more mechanically stressful for the back than is aerobic exercise. Such exercises are not recommended for the first few weeks of symptoms, although they may later help patients regain and maintain activity tolerance.

There is no evidence to indicate that back-specific exercise machines are effective for treating acute low back problems. Neither is there evidence that stretching of the back helps patients with acute symptoms.

Work activities

When requested, clinicians may choose to offer specific instructions about activity at work for patients with acute limitations due to low back symptoms. The patient's age, general health, and perceptions of safe levels to sit, stand, walk or lift (noted on initial history) can help provide reasonable starting points for activity recommendations. Table 17A.3 provides a guide for recommendations about sitting and lifting. The clinician should make it clear to patients and employers that:

- even moderately heavy unassisted lifting may aggravate back symptoms
- any restrictions are intended to allow for spontaneous recovery or time to build activity tolerance through exercise.

Table 17A.3 Guidelines for sitting and unassisted lifting

	Symptoms						
	Severe	$\rightarrow$	Moderate	$\rightarrow$	Mild	$\rightarrow$	None
Sitting[1]	20 min	$\rightarrow$	$\rightarrow$	$\rightarrow$	$\rightarrow$	$\rightarrow$	50 min
Unassisted lifting[2]							
Men	20 lbs	$\rightarrow$	20 lbs	$\rightarrow$	60 lbs	$\rightarrow$	80 lbs
Women	20 lbs	$\rightarrow$	20 lbs	$\rightarrow$	35 lbs	$\rightarrow$	40 lbs

[1]Without getting up and moving around.
[2]Modification of NIOSH Lifting Guidelines, 1981, 1993. Gradually increase unassisted lifting limits to 60 lbs (men) and 35 lbs (women) by 3 months even with continued symptoms. Instruct patient to limit twisting, bending, reaching while lifting and to hold lifted object as close to the navel as possible.

Algorithm 17A.2 Treatment of acute low back problem on initial and follow-up visits.

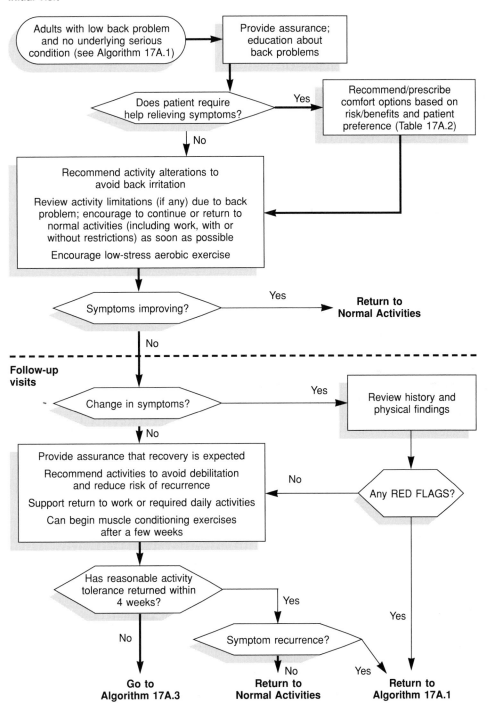

Activity restrictions are prescribed for a short time period only, depending upon work requirements (no benefits apparent beyond 3 months).

Special studies and diagnostic considerations

Routine testing (laboratory tests, plain X-rays of the lumbosacral spine) and imaging studies are not recommended during the first month of activity limitation due to back symptoms except when a red flag noted on history or examination raises suspicion of a dangerous or nonspinal condition. If a patient's limitations due to low back symptoms do not improve in 4 weeks, reassessment is recommended. After again reviewing the patient's activity limitations, history, and physical findings, the clinician may then consider further diagnostic studies and discuss these with the patient.

Timing and limits of special studies

Waiting 4 weeks before considering special tests allows 90% of patients to recover spontaneously and avoid unneeded procedures. This also reduces the potential confusion of falsely labeling age-related changes on imaging studies (commonly noted in patients older than 30 without back symptoms) as the cause of the acute symptoms. In the absence of either red flags or persistent activity limitations due to continuous limb symptoms, imaging studies (especially plain X-rays) rarely provide information that changes the clinical approach to the acute low back problem.

Selection of special studies

Prior to ordering imaging studies the clinician should have noted either of the following:

- the emergence of a red flag
- physiologic evidence of tissue insult or neurologic dysfunction.

Physiologic evidence may be in the form of definitive nerve findings on physical examination, electrodiagnostic studies (when evaluating sciatica), and a laboratory test or bone scan (when evaluating nonspecific low back symptoms).

Unquestionable findings that identify specific nerve root compromise on the neurologic examination (see Fig. 17A.1) are sufficient physiologic evidence to warrant imaging. When the neurologic examination is less clear, however, further physiologic evidence of nerve root dysfunction should be considered before ordering an imaging study. Electromyography (EMG) including H-reflex tests may be useful to identify subtle focal neurologic dysfunction in patients with leg symptoms lasting longer than 3–4 weeks. Sensory evoked potentials (SEPs) may be added to the assessment if spinal stenosis or spinal cord myelopathy is suspected.

Laboratory tests such as the erythrocyte sedimentation rate (ESR), complete blood count (CBC), and urinalysis (UA) can be useful as a screen for nonspecific medical diseases (especially infection and tumor) of the low back. A bone scan can detect physiologic reactions to suspected spinal tumor, infection, or occult fracture.

Should physiologic evidence indicate tissue insult or nerve impairment, discuss with a consultant selection of an imaging test to define a potential anatomic cause (CT for bone, MRI for neural or other soft tissue). Anatomic definition is commonly needed to guide surgery or specific procedures. Selection of an imaging test should also take into consideration any patient allergies to contrast media (myelogram) or concerns about claustrophobia (MRI) and costs. A discussion with a specialist on selection of the most clinically valuable study can often assist the primary care clinician to avoid duplication. Table 17A.4 provides a general comparison of the abilities of different techniques to identify physiologic insult and define anatomic defects. Missing from the table is discography, which is not recommended for assessing patients with acute low back symptoms.

In general, an imaging study may be an appropriate consideration for the patient whose limitations due to consistent symptoms have persisted for 1 month or more:

- when surgery is being considered for treatment of a specific detectable loss of neurologic function
- to further evaluate potentially serious spinal pathology.

Algorithm 17A.3 Evaluation of the slow-to-recover patient (symptoms >4 weeks).

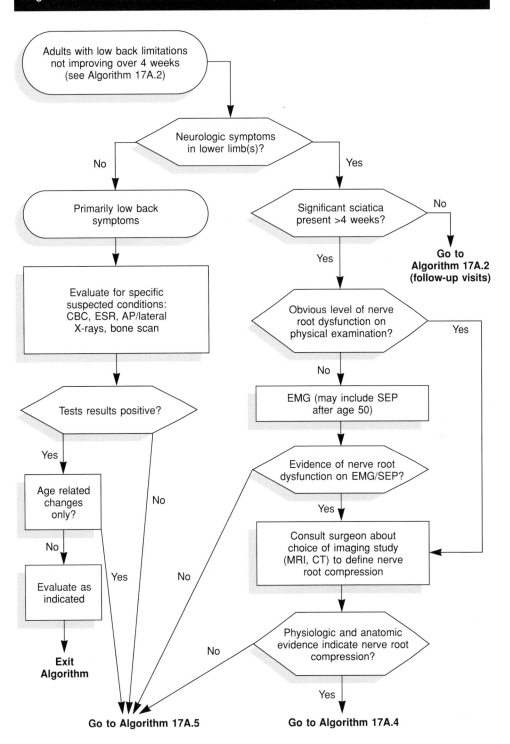

Table 17A.4 Ability of different techniques to identify and define pathology

Technique	Identify physiologic insult	Define anatomic defect
History	+	+
Physical examination		
Circumference		
measurements	+	+
Reflexes	++	++
Straight leg raising (SLR)	++	+
Crossed SLR	+++	++
Motor	++	++
Sensory	++	++
Laboratory studies? (ESR, CBC, UA)	++	0
Bone scan[1]	+++	++
EMG/SEP	+++	++
X-ray[1]	0	+
CT[1]	0	++++[2]
MRI	0	++++[2]
Myelo-CT[1]	0	++++[2]
Myelography[1]	0	++++[2]

[1]Risk of complications (radiation, infection, etc.): highest for myelo-CT, second highest for myelography, and relatively less risk for bone scan, X-ray and CT.
[2]False-positive diagnostic findings in up to 30% of people without symptoms at age 30.
Note: number of plus signs indicates relative ability to identify or define.

Reliance on imaging studies alone to evaluate the source of low back symptoms, however, carries a significant risk of diagnostic confusion, given the possibility of falsely identifying something that was present before symptoms began.

Management considerations after special studies

Definitive treatment for serious conditions (see Table 17A.1) detected by special studies is beyond the scope of this guideline. When special studies fail to define the exact cause of symptoms, however, no patient should receive an impression that the clinician thinks 'nothing is wrong' or that the problem could be 'in their head'. Reassure the patient that a clinical work-up is highly successful at detecting serious conditions, but does not reveal the precise cause of most low back symptoms.

Surgical considerations

Within the first 3 months of acute low back symptoms, surgery is only considered when serious spinal pathology or nerve root dysfunction obviously due to a herniated lumbar disc is detected. A disc herniation, characterized by protrusion of the central nucleus pulposis through a defect in the outer annulus fibrosis, may trap a nerve root causing irritation, leg symptoms and nerve root dysfunction. The presence of a herniated lumbar disc on an imaging study, however, does not necessarily imply nerve root dysfunction. Studies of asymptomatic adults commonly demonstrate intervertebral disc herniations that apparently do not entrap a nerve root or cause symptoms.

Therefore, nerve root decompression can be considered for a patient if all of the following criteria exist:

- Sciatica is both severe and disabling.
- Symptoms of sciatica persist without improvement for longer than 4 weeks or with extreme progression.
- There is strong physiologic evidence of a specific nerve root dysfunction with intervertebral disc herniation confirmed at the corresponding level and side by findings on an imaging study.

Algorithm 17A.4 Surgical considerations for patients with persistent sciatica.

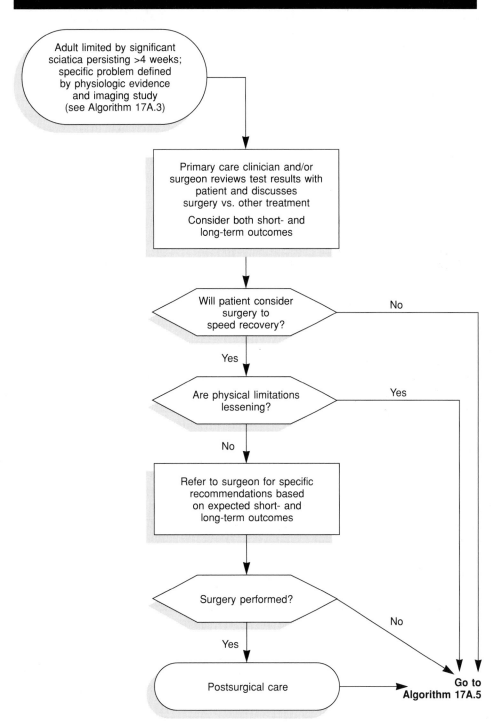

Patients with acute low back pain alone, without findings of serious conditions or significant nerve root compression, rarely benefit from a surgical consultation.

Many patients with strong clinical findings of nerve root dysfunction due to disc herniation recover activity tolerance within 1 month; no evidence indicates that delaying surgery for this period worsens the outcome. With or without an operation, more than 80% of patients with obvious surgical indications eventually recover. Surgery seems to be a luxury for speeding recovery of patients with obvious surgical indications, but benefits fewer than 40% of patients with questionable physiologic findings. Moreover, surgery increases the chance of future procedures with higher complication rates. Overall, the incidence of first-time disc surgery complications, including infection and bleeding, is less than 1%. The figure increases dramatically with older patients or repeated procedures.

Direct and indirect nerve-root decompression for herniated discs. Direct methods of nerve root decompression include laminotomy (expansion of the interlaminar space for access to the nerve root and the offending disc fragments), microdiscectomy (laminotomy using a microscope) and laminectomy (total removal of the laminae). Methods of indirect nerve root decompression include chemonucleolysis, which is the injection of chymopapain or other enzymes to dissolve the inner disc. Such chemical treatment methods are less efficacious than direct standard or microdiscectomy and have rare but serious complications. Any of these methods is preferable to percutaneous discectomy (indirect, mechanical disc removal through a lateral disc puncture).

Management of spinal stenosis. Usually resulting from soft tissue and bony encroachment of the spinal canal and nerve roots, spinal stenosis typically has a gradual onset and begins in older adults. It is characterized by nonspecific limb symptoms, called *neurogenic claudication* or *pseudoclaudication*, that interfere with the duration of comfortable standing and walking. The symptoms are commonly bilateral and rarely associated with strong focal findings on examination. Neurogenic claudication, however, can be confused or coexist with *vascular claudication*, in which leg pain also limits walking. The symptoms of vascular insufficiency can be relieved by simply standing still while relief of neurogenic claudication symptoms usually requires the patient to flex the lumbar spine or sit.

The surgical treatment for spinal stenosis is usually complete laminectomy for posterior decompression. Offending soft tissue and osteophytes that encroach upon nerve roots in the central spinal canal and foramen are removed. Fusion may be considered to stabilize a degenerative spondylolisthesis with motion between the slipped vertebra and adjacent vertebrae. Elderly patients with spinal stenosis who tolerate their daily activities usually need no surgery unless they develop new signs of bowel and bladder dysfunction. Decisions on treatment should take into account the patient's preference, lifestyle, other medical problems and risks of surgery. Surgery for spinal stenosis is rarely considered in the first 3 months of symptoms.

Except for cases of trauma-related spinal fracture or dislocation, fusion alone is not usually considered in the first 3 months of low back symptoms.

Further management considerations

Following diagnostic or surgical procedures, the management of most patients becomes focused on improving physical conditioning through an incrementally increased exercise program. The goal of this program is to build activity tolerance and overcome limitations due to back symptoms. At this point in treatment, symptom control methods are only an adjunct to making prescribed exercises more tolerable:

- Begin with low-stress aerobic activities to improve general stamina (walking, riding a bicycle, swimming and eventually jogging).
- Exercises to condition specific back and trunk muscles can be added a few weeks after. The back muscles may need to be in better condition than before the problem occurred. Otherwise, the back may continue to be painful and easily irritated by even mild activity. Following back surgery, recovery of activity tolerance may be delayed until protective

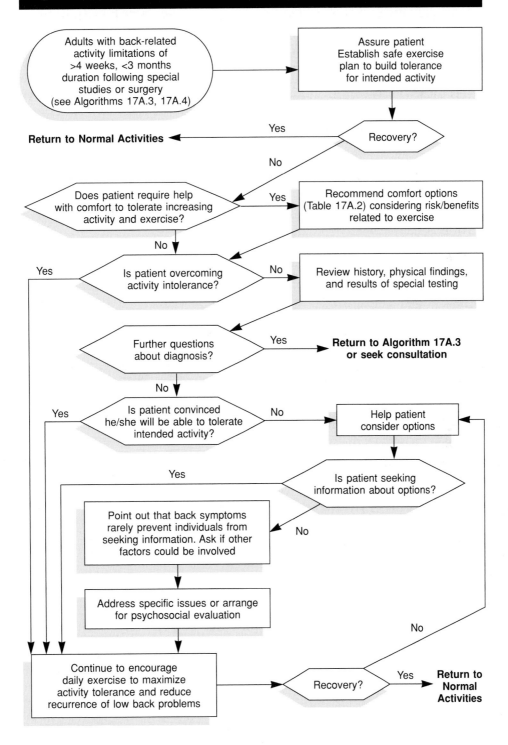

Algorithm 17A.5 Further management of acute low back problem.

muscles are conditioned well enough to compensate for any remaining structural changes.
- Finally, specific training to perform activities required at home or work can begin. The objective of this program is to increase the patient's tolerance in carrying out actual daily duties.

When patients demonstrate difficulty regaining the ability to tolerate the activities they are required (or would like) to do, the clinician may pose the following diagnostic and treatment questions:

- Could the patient have a serious, undetected medical condition? A careful review of the medical history and physical examination is warranted.
- Are the patient's activity goals realistic? Exploring briefly the patient's expectations, both short- and long-term, of being able to perform specific activities at home, work, or recreation may help the patient assess whether such activity levels are actually achievable.
- If for any reason the achievement of activity goals seems unlikely, what are the patient's remaining options? To answer this question, the patient is often required to gather specific information from friends, family, employers, or others. If on follow-up visits the patient has made no effort to gather such information, the clinician has the opportunity to point out that low back symptoms alone rarely prevent a patient from addressing questions so important to his or her future. This observation can lead to an open, nonjudgemental discussion of common but complicated psychosocial problems or other issues that often can interfere with a patient's recovery from low back problems. The clinician can then help the patient address or arrange further evaluation of any specific problem limiting the patient's progress. This can usually be accomplished as the patient continues, with the clinician's encouragement, to build activity tolerance through safe, simple exercises.

A summary of the guideline recommendations in presented in Table 17A.5.

Table 17A.5 Summary of guideline recommendations. The ratings in parentheses indicate the scientific evidence supporting each recommendation according to the following scale:
A = strong research-based evidence (multiple relevant and high-quality scientific studies);
B = moderate research-based evidence (one relevant, high-quality scientific study or multiple adequate scientific studies);
C = limited research-based evidence (at least one adequate scientific study in patients with low back pain);
D = panel interpretation of evidence not meeting inclusion criteria for research-based evidence.
The number of studies meeting panel review criteria is noted in each category

	Recommend	Option	Recommend against
History and physical examination (34 studies)	Basic history (B) History of cancer/infection (B) Signs/symptoms of cauda equina syndrome (C) History of significant trauma (C) Psychosocial history (C) Straight leg raising test (B) Focused neurologic examination (B)	Pain drawing and visual analog scale (D)	
Patient education (14 studies)	Patient education about low back symptoms (B) Back school in occupational settings (C)	Back school in nonoccupational settings (C)	
Medication (23 studies)	Acetaminophen (C) NSAIDs (B)	Muscle relaxants (C) Opioids, short course (C)	Opioids used >2 weeks (C) Phenylbutazone (C) Oral steroids (C) Colchicine (B) Antidepressants (C)
Physical treatment methods (42 studies)	Manipulation of low back during first month of symptoms (B)	Manipulation for patients with radiculopathy (C) Manipulation for patients with symptoms >1 month (C)	Manipulation for patients with undiagnosed neurologic deficits (D) Prolonged course of manipulation (D)

		Self-application of heat or cold to low back (C) Shoe insoles (C) Corset for prevention in occupational setting (C)	Traction (B) TENS (C) Biofeedback (C) Shoe lifts (D) Corset for treatment (D)
Injections (26 studies)		Epidural steroid injections for radicular pain to avoid surgery (C)	Epidural injections for back pain without radiculopathy (D) Trigger point injections (C) Ligamentous injections (C) Facet joint injections (C) Needle acupuncture (D)
Bed rest (4 studies)		Bed rest for 2–4 days for severe radiculopathy (D)	Bed rest >4 days (B)
Activities and exercise (20 studies)	Temporary avoidance of activities that increase mechanical stress on (D) Gradual return to normal activities (B) Low-stress aerobic exercise (C) Conditioning exercises for trunk muscles after 2 weeks (C) Exercise quotas (C)		Back-specific exercise machines (D) Therapeutic stretching of back muscles (D)
Detection of physiologic abnormalities (14 studies)	If no improvement after 1 month, consider: Bone scan (C) Needle EMG and H-reflex tests to clarify nerve root dysfunction (C) SEP to assess spinal stenosis (C)		EMG for clinically obvious radiculopathy (D) Surface EMG and F-wave tests (C) Thermography (C)
X-rays of L-S spine (18 studies)	When red flags for fracture present (C) When red flags for cancer or infection present (C)		Routine use in first month of symptoms in absence of red flags (B) Routine oblique views (B)
Imaging (18 studies)	CT or MRI when cauda equina, tumor, infection, or fracture strongly suspected (C) MRI test of choice for patients with prior back surgery (D) Assure quality criteria for imaging tests (B)	Myelography or CT-myelography for preoperative planning (D)	Use of imaging tests before 1 month in absence of red flags (B) Discography or CT-discography (C)
Surgical considerations (14 studies)	Discuss surgical options with patients with persistent and severe sciatica and clinical evidence of nerve root compromise after 1 month of conservative therapy (B) Standard discectomy and microdiscectomy of similar efficacy in treatment of herniated disc (B) Chymopapain, used after ruling out allergic sensitivity, acceptable but less efficacious than discectomy to treat herniated disc (C)		Disc surgery in patients with back pain alone, no red flags, and no nerve root compression (D) Percutaneous discectomy less efficacious than chymopapain (C) Surgery for spinal stenosis within the first 3 months of symptoms (D) Stenosis surgery when justified by imaging test rather than patient's functional status (D) Spinal fusion during the first 3 months of symptoms in the absence of fracture, dislocation, complications of tumor or infection (C)
Psychosocial factors	Social, economic, and psychologic factors can alter patient response to symptoms and treatment (D)		Referral for extensive evaluation/treatment prior to exploring patient expectations or psychosocial factors (D)

APPENDIX 17B: UK Management guidelines for back pain

The need for management guidelines

Back pain has affected human beings throughout recorded history and there is no evidence that the frequency and nature of back pain are any different today from what they were in the past. What is new is the scale of chronic disability, work loss and invalidity due to simple backache. There is increasing demand on health care and social security resources for back pain. Traditional medical treatment has failed to halt this epidemic and may even have contributed to it. There is a clear need to reconsider our whole approach to the management of low back pain and disability.

These management guidelines provide advice on overall strategies for managing back pain. Professional judgement must be used to decide on the most appropriate treatment methods for the individual patient.

The document refers to low back pain but the same principles apply to other regions of the spine.

The guidelines are based on the best scientific evidence now available. The US Back Pain Management Guidelines Panel, set up by the Agency for Health Care Policy and Research, has put a great deal of resources into collating this evidence. These UK management guidelines for back pain have been produced in collaboration with the US panel and are broadly similar to current US and Swedish guidelines.

They should be used as an outline and may need to be adapted to suit local needs and circumstances.

The importance of primary management

The importance of primary management of backache within the first 6 weeks cannot be over-emphasised. Once chronic back pain and disability are established, any form of treatment is more difficult and has a much lower chance of success. Early management sets the whole strategy and very largely determines the final outcome. It has a powerful influence on the

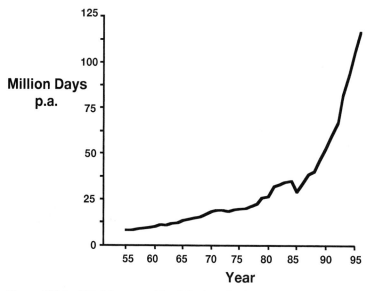

Figure 17B.1 UK sickness and invalidity benefits for back pain. The DSS data is mainly on chronic sickness.

Reproduced with permission from the UK Clinical Standards Advisory Group and HMSO, Dec 1994.

patient's and family's attitudes and beliefs about the problem and how it should be dealt with.

Backache has a good natural recovery rate. There is a 90% probability that an acute attack will settle, at least sufficient to return to work, within 6 weeks. Hence, there is a clear tendency towards natural recovery. However, the current statistics show that this should not be taken as grounds for complacency, inactivity or a policy of 'wait and see' on the part of health care professionals. The good natural history of backache is reassuring, but management must actively support and encourage recovery and act positively to prevent chronic pain and disability. Management must not do anything which interferes with natural recovery; iatrogenic disability must be avoided.

Main aims of primary management

Primary management of back pain has two main aims:

1. symptomatic control of pain
2. prevention of disability.

Pain and disability are not the same and should be clearly distinguished both conceptually and in clinical practice. However, control of pain and overcoming disability do go together: they are not alternatives. It is often not possible to provide complete relief of pain and it is not a question of waiting for pain relief and only then starting rehabilitation. Control of pain and overcoming disability must be achieved simultaneously and are mutually reinforcing. Lasting pain relief cannot be achieved unless chronic disability is prevented. The best method of achieving lasting pain relief is by returning to normal activity and to work, even if with some degree of persistent or recurrent pain and with some modification of these activities.

Responsibility for primary management

The main responsibility for preventing chronic low back pain and disability lies with the family doctor, occupational health service, physiotherapist, osteopath or chiropractor who is caring for the patient at this early stage. Early active rehabilitation is highly effective in preventing long-term pain and disability.

Active rehabilitation is the key

If the attack has not settled within 6 weeks, it is at risk of becoming chronic. Statistics show that the longer anyone is off with backache, the lower their chances of ever returning to work (Fig. 17B.2). Many physical, psychological and social factors may influence the duration of time off work, but whatever the cause the consequences can be disastrous. Once patients are off work for 6 months with backache they have only a 50% chance of returning to their previous job. Once they are off work for 2 years, or have lost their job because of back pain (which may happen very much earlier than 2 years), they will have great difficulty ever returning to any form of work. They are then likely to remain chronically disabled for many years, irrespective of their further treatment.

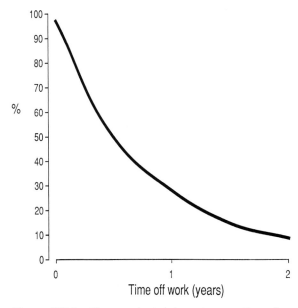

Figure 17B.2 Chances of return to work versus time off work.

Overview of management guidelines for acute back pain

Initial consultation
Diagnostic triage
- simple backache
- nerve root pain ⎫ urgent
- serious spinal pathology ⎭ referral

Early management strategy
Aims: symptomatic relief of pain
      prevent disability
- **Prescribe simple analgesia, NSAIDs**
  - avoid narcotics if possible and never more than two weeks
- **Arrange physical therapy if symptoms last more than a few days**
  - manipulation
  - active exercise and physical activity (modifies pain mechanisms, speeds recovery)
- **Advise rest only if essential: 1–3 days**
  - prolonged bed rest is harmful
- **Encourage early activity**
  - activity is not harmful
  - reduces pain
  - physical fitness beneficial
- **Practise psychosocial management; this is fundamental**
  - promote positive attitudes to activity and work
  - distress and depression
- **Advise absence from work only if unavoidable; early return to work**
  - prolonged sickness absence makes return to work increasingly difficult

Biopsychosocial assessment at 6 weeks
- Review diagnostic triage
- ESR and X-ray lumbosacral spine if specifically indicated
- Psychosocial and vocational assessment

Active rehabilitation programme
- Incremental aerobic exercise and fitness programme of physical reconditioning
- Behavioural medicine principles
- Close liaison with the workplace

Secondary referral
- Second opinion
- Rehabilitation
- Vocational assessment and guidance
- Surgery
- Pain management

Final outcome measure: maintain productive activity; reduce work loss

---

Diagnostic triage

A careful history and physical examination are essential in establishing rapport with the patient and providing reassurance and understanding of the best management strategy for simple backache. The first step in diagnosis is to determine that this is a musculoskeletal problem and to exclude nonspinal pathology such as renal, abdominal or gynaecological disease. The musculoskeletal assessment should then exclude serious spinal pathology, and should distinguish a nerve root problem from simple backache.

Diagnostic triage:

- simple backache
- nerve root pain
- possible serious spinal pathology.

The term simple backache has been used to describe the common 'mechanical' back pain that is musculoskeletal in origin and in which symptoms vary with different physical activities. Pain receptors are present in bone, joints, muscle, connective tissue, periosteum, the outer third of the intervertebral disc and in perivascular tissue. Pain receptors may be activated by mechanical strain, metabolites or inflammation. Clinically, simple backache is commonly related to mechanical strain or dysfunction, although it often appears to develop spontaneously. Simple backache may be very painful and often spreads as referred leg pain to one or both hips or thighs. However, the term simple backache also provides reassurance that the nerve roots and spinal cord are not compromised and that there is no evidence of more serious spinal pathology such as tumour or infection. Attempts at more precise diagnosis of simple backache based on theories of aetiology or pathology are not generally agreed by different specialities and tend to be unhelpful when deciding on management.

The term nerve root pain has been used in preference to sciatica to emphasise its underlying pathological basis and specific clinical features. Nerve root pain is commonly caused by a disc prolapse, spinal stenosis or surgical scarring. Permanent damage to the nervous system itself may also give rise to neuropathic pain. Nerve root pain commonly arises from a single nerve root and when more than one nerve root appears to be involved then a more widespread neurological disorder should be considered. In contrast to the referred leg pain described above, nerve root pain is relatively well localised, unilateral leg pain which at least approximates to a dermatomal distribution and commonly radiates into the foot or toes. It is often associated with numbness or paraesthesia in the same distribution. There may be specific signs of nerve irritation or localised motor, sensory or reflex signs of nerve root compression affecting the same dermatomal or myotomal distribution, though these are not essential for the diagnosis. When present, nerve root pain is usually the dominant clinical presentation.

The term serious spinal pathology has been used to include spinal tumour and infection, inflammatory disease such as ankylosing spondylitis, structural deformity such as scoliosis, and widespread neurological disorders. These may produce back pain or less commonly nerve root pain. The back pain is often constant, progressive and 'nonmechanical', in that it is unrelated to physical activity, although if structural failure occurs then mechanical back pain may also be produced. The major clinical presentation, diagnosis and management, however, concern the underlying spinal pathology.

The diagnostic triage forms the basis for decisions about referral, investigation and further management. It largely determines the further course and final outcome of treatment. Any errors in the initial diagnostic triage may have serious consequences.

Although the history must be thorough, if it is carefully focused on the following key elements it can be carried out within the average GP consultation time of 9 minutes. The main purpose of a brief examination is to check or corroborate the history, and should focus on specific signs of nerve root involvement or neurological compromise.

The main diagnostic indicators for simple back-ache, nerve root pain, 'red flags', cauda equina syndrome/widespread neurological disorder and inflammatory disorders are outlined below:

Simple backache

- Presentation generally age 20–55 years
- Lumbosacral region, buttocks and thighs
- Pain 'mechanical' in nature
  - varies with physical activity
  - varies with time
- Patient well
- Prognosis good
  - 90% recover from acute attack in 6 weeks

Nerve root pain

- Unilateral leg pain > back pain
- Pain generally radiates to foot or toes
- Numbness and paraesthesia in the same distribution
- Nerve irritation signs
  - reduced SLR which reproduces leg pain
- Motor, sensory or reflex change
  - limited to one nerve root
- Prognosis reasonable
  - 50% recover from acute attack within 6 weeks

Red flags: possible serious spinal pathology

- Age of presentation <20 or onset >55 years
- Violent trauma, e.g. fall from a height, RTA
- Constant, progressive, nonmechanical pain
- Thoracic pain
- PMH – Carcinoma
- Systemic steroids
- Drug abuse, HIV
- Systemically unwell
- Weight loss
- Persisting severe restriction of lumbar flexion
- Widespread neurology
- Structural deformity

If there are suspicious clinical features or if pain has not settled in 6 weeks, an ESR and plain X-ray should be considered:

- ESR > 25
- X-ray – vertebral collapse or bone destruction

Cauda equina syndrome/widespread neurological disorder

- Difficulty with micturition
- Loss of anal sphincter tone or faecal incontinence
- Saddle anaesthesia about the anus, perineum or genitals
- Widespread (>one nerve root) or progressive motor weakness in the legs or gait disturbance
- Sensory level

Inflammatory disorders (ankylosing spondylitis and related disorders)

- Gradual onset
- Marked morning stiffness
- Persisting limitation spinal movements in all directions
- Peripheral joint involvement
- Iritis, skin rashes (psoriasis), colitis, urethral discharge
- Family history

Emergency and urgent referrals

The initial diagnostic triage will identify the small number of patients requiring urgent and emergency referral to a hospital specialist. Guidelines for emergency and urgent referrals are set out below.

Emergency referral

Diagnosis. Acute spinal cord damage/acute cauda equina syndrome/widespread neurological disorder

Action. Emergency referral to a specialist with experience in spinal surgery within a matter of hours.

Urgent referrals (within a few weeks)

Diagnosis. Possible serious spinal pathology.

Action. Urgent referral for specialist investigation, generally to an orthopaedic surgeon or rheumatologist, depending on local availability.

Diagnosis. Possible acute inflammatory disorders.

Action. Urgent referral to a rheumatologist.

Diagnosis. Nerve root problem.

Action. Should generally be dealt with initially by the GP, providing there is no major or progressive motor weakness. Early referral may be required for additional acute pain control. If it is not resolving satisfactorily after 6 weeks, the patient should then be referred urgently for appropriate specialist assessment and investigation.

Diagnostic imaging

X-rays should be used as advised in the Royal College of Radiologists guidelines.

No routine need for X-ray

Unnecessary irradiation should be avoided. Standard X-rays of the lumbosacral spine involve about 120 times the dose of radiation for a chest X-ray. X-rays are not usually required in the initial management of acute back pain in patients between the ages of 20 and 55 years. Acute back pain is usually caused by conditions that cannot be diagnosed by plain X-rays. Pain correlates poorly with degenerative changes found on X-rays: these X-ray findings are usually normal, age-related changes and should not be labelled 'arthritis'.

When to arrange X-rays

AP and lateral X-rays of the lumbosacral spine are required if there is a question of possible serious spinal pathology. If thoracic pain is

Table 17B.1 Summary: diagnostic triage and referral

	Initial management	By 4–6 weeks
Possible serious spinal pathology	Urgent/emergency referral for specialist investigation	
Nerve root problem	General practitioner ?Refer for acute pain control ?Physiotherapy ??Osteopathy/chiropractic	Urgent surgical referral
Simple backache	General practitioner ?Physiotherapy ?Osteopathy/chiropractic ??Refer for acute pain control	Psychosocial and vocational assessment Active rehabilitation for return to work

present, thoracic X-rays may also be required. X-rays of the lumbosacral spine may be performed for simple backache if symptoms and disability are not improving after 6 weeks. It should always be remembered that lumbar spinal radiography involves one of the highest radiation doses of any plain radiographic procedure, and that the yield of positive findings is very low.

What X-rays cannot show

It is important to remember that serious pathology can exist in the presence of normal X-rays. It takes time for such disease processes to produce bony destruction and false–negative X-rays are common in the early stages of both tumour and infection. If there are clinical 'red flags' of possible serious spinal pathology, then a negative X-ray does not exclude infection or tumour and referral and investigation should proceed.

X-rays should not delay urgent referral

If the patient is being referred urgently for specialist investigation, it may be better to let the specialist arrange the necessary X-rays. Referral should not be delayed while awaiting X-rays.

Other imaging techniques

Diagnostic imaging with CT or MRI provides detailed anatomical information of serious spinal pathology and for the preoperative planning of nerve root problems. Their use in simple backache is less well established. Because of their high false positive rates due to normal age-related changes, they are not suitable for diagnostic screening.

After comprehensive clinical assessment and plain X-rays, a bone scan may provide a better second-line test for serious spinal pathology.

Primary management of simple backache

Most acute backache is probably of soft tissue origin. Although it is often not possible to identify the exact origin of the pain, there is now good evidence on which to base the musculoskeletal principles of management.

Information and advice

There is general agreement that patients should be given accurate information about back pain and about the structure and function of the back. Avoid serious labels like 'arthritis of the spine'; reassure the patient that age-related X-ray changes are normal. Medical information and advice may have lasting effects on the patient's and family's attitudes and beliefs about the problem and how it should be managed. This information and advice should be designed to reduce apprehension and encourage progressive mobilisation and rehabilitation.

Patients should be given simple, practical advice on how to avoid excessive loads on the back while performing everyday activities. Advice should be tailored to the patient's individual life and work. Three key areas of information to cover are:

- expectations about rapid recovery but also possible recurrence of symptoms
- safe and proven methods of symptom control
- safe and reasonable activity modifications.

Responsibility for management

Most acute and recurrent episodes of simple backache are managed by the person themselves or by the GP. Primary management may also commonly involve an occupational health service or a physiotherapist, osteopath or chiropractor. Hospital specialist referral is generally neither required nor helpful.

Recurrence of simple backache

The history, examination and initial diagnostic triage provide the basis for reassurance that the patient's condition is simple backache with no evidence of a trapped nerve or of any more serious underlying pathology. Simple backache should be a benign, self-limiting condition.

However, while 90% of acute or recurrent attacks settle within 6 weeks, 60% of people may have at least one recurrence within the next year. These recurrent attacks may become nearly as much a cause for clinical concern and work loss as chronic pain. Recurrent attacks do tend to settle over 3–5 years, but frequent recurrence may require secondary referral and management similar to chronic pain.

Age and simple backache

Patients should be reassured that back pain does not generally increase with age. Simple backache generally peaks in the middle decades of life and tends to become less frequent in later life.

Early management strategy

There is increasing evidence that the approach outlined below improves the natural history of simple backache and reduces recurrence. On the available evidence, the best early management strategy consists of:

Prescribe simple analgesia, NSAIDs
- avoid narcotics if possible and never for more than 2 weeks

Arrange physical therapy if symptoms last more than a few days
- manipulation
- active exercise and physical activity
  — modifies pain and mechanisms, speeds recovery

Advise rest only if essential: 1–3 days maximum
- prolonged bed rest is harmful

Encourage early activity
- activity is not harmful
- reduces pain
- physical fitness beneficial

Practise psychosocial management, this is fundamental
- promote positive attitudes to activity and work
- awareness and management of distress and depression

Avoiding loss of work

The most important consequence of backache is loss of time from work and even loss of employment. The aim of management must be to maintain productive activity and minimise work loss. Back pain may restrict physical activity and activities may need to be modified at the acute stage. However, it is important to avoid iatrogenic disability.

Whenever possible, every effort should be made to keep the patient at work. Symptomatic measures to control pain should be used to help the patient stay active. Simple, practical advice should be given on how to modify physical activities. If an occupational health service is available it may be able to assist at work. A patient at work should not be advised to stop work except on the rare occasion when there is clear evidence that remaining at work is likely to cause lasting physical harm. There is rarely any clear clinical basis for advising a patient to change their job or to give up work because of simple backache. The consequences of medical advice about work must be considered very carefully and discussed in detail with the patient.

The prognosis for successful treatment and rehabilitation is poorer in patients who are unemployed or who have lost their job due to back pain. Management should then concentrate on providing symptomatic relief and on restoration of physical activity levels and whatever form of productive activity is available to the patient. However, medical treatment cannot solve the social problems of unemployment and it is important to avoid making the problem a medical one and thereby adding all the long-term consequences of assignment to invalidity status.

Managing nerve root pain

Most acute episodes of nerve root pain resolve naturally without requiring surgery. For the first 6 weeks, management follows the same principles as simple backache, but progress is likely to be slower. Adequate analgesia is particularly important initially. A higher proportion of patients may require initial bed rest which may be required for up to 1 or 2 weeks. There is no evidence to support bed rest for more than 2 weeks even for severe nerve root pain, but the harmful effects of more prolonged bed rest are well recognised in standard medical and nursing teaching. Mobilisation and rehabilitation then follow the same principles as simple backache but progress is generally slower.

Symptomatic measures

(a) Medication Simple analgesics are adequate for most patients. Medication should be given on a regular basis for a fixed duration to control pain, and not intermittently p.r.n.

Guidelines for medication are:

- Paracetamol up to 4 g per day in divided doses.
- If inadequate on its own, paracetamol may be used in combination tablets with codeine (Co-codamol), dihydrocodeine (Co-dydramol) or dextropropoxyphene (Co-proxamol).
- Nonsteroidal anti-inflammatory drugs (NSAIDs) may be used, particularly if there is marked stiffness. The simplest and safest NSAID is ibuprofen. Aspirin is still a useful alternative. NSAIDs should be avoided if the patient has dyspepsia, or may be combined with anti-ulcer treatment. When there is marked muscle spasm, analgesics or NSAIDs may be combined with a muscle relaxant such as methocarbamol or baclophen.
- When there is marked psychological distress, analgesics or NSAIDs may be combined with a sedative such as benzodiazepine (Diazepam). These should generally only be used for short periods and are rarely required for more than 2 weeks.
- Narcotics such as morphine and pethidine are only rarely indicated and generally only for a few days. Opioid derivatives or alternatives such as Meptazinol, Nefopam, Bupramorphine or Pentazocine may be considered instead for short periods. If any of these drugs are required for more than 2 weeks, urgent specialist opinion should be sought.

(b) Manipulation There is considerable evidence that manipulation can provide short-term symptomatic benefit in some patients with acute back pain of less than 1 month's duration and without nerve root pain. Manipulation may be equally effective in dealing with recurrent attacks.

There is more limited evidence for the effectiveness of manipulation in patients with chronic low back pain. There is limited evidence available on the use of manipulation in patients with nerve root pain. Manipulation should not be used in patients with severe or progressive neurological deficit in view of the rare but serious risk of neurological complication. Serious neurological conditions should always be excluded before considering manipulation.

Rest vs. active exercise

Avoid bed rest

There is strong evidence against the use of bed rest for more than 1–3 days for acute back pain. Bed rest may be used for up to 1–2 weeks for nerve root pain but there is no evidence to support its use for longer periods. In general, bed rest may be better regarded as a potentially harmful and undesirable consequence of back pain rather than a treatment. Prolonged or repeated bed rest should be avoided. There is no evidence for bed rest in hospital rather than at home.

Promote exercise

There is strong evidence for an active exercise and rehabilitation approach to back pain. The particular type of exercise may be less important. This is largely based on extensive evidence in chronic low back pain, but both theoretical principles and several controlled trials suggest that the earlier it is commenced the better – probably within the first 2 weeks and possibly within a few days for acute back pain. The same principles may apply to nerve root pain after the first 1 or 2 weeks.

Some temporary increase in pain is common at first, as occurs with most musculoskeletal conditions, but the patient should be reassured that hurt and harm are not the same and that such symptoms are normal at this stage. This is not a reason for reverting to passive management. There is no evidence that active exercise and early return to work increases the risk of recurrence. On the contrary, patients treated with active exercise and early return to work have fewer recurrences, less additional time off work and less health care over the following two years.

Aerobic, endurance exercises such as walking, cycling and swimming are effective to improve physical fitness and modify pain mechanisms. They also produce minimal mechanical stress to the back and are most easily tolerated by most patients during the first two weeks. Strengthening exercises for abdominal and back muscles may be gradually increased, particularly after the first two weeks. There is little evidence to support any specific type of back exercise. The exercise programme must be active and must promote the patient's own physical activity and responsibility. Exercises should start from a tolerable level and then be increased by planned increments, rather than depending on reports of pain.

Biopsychosocial assessment at 6 weeks

If managed properly, most patients with simple backache should have recovered sufficiently to return to work before 6 weeks, even if with some residual or recurrent symptoms. Those patients who have not returned to work by 6 weeks should be reassessed more thoroughly to find out why. The initial diagnostic triage should be rechecked.

There is also clear evidence that chronic disability due to simple backache is often associated with psychological and social factors. These commonly develop as a secondary consequence of continued pain and failed treatment, but may then become even more important than the original physical problem (Fig. 17B.3). Psychosocial factors should be considered carefully in all patients who are still off work after 6 weeks. If the patient has any previous history of psychological or social problems, or if there

are any psychosocial 'yellow flags', psychosocial factors should be considered at an earlier stage. A simple psychosocial history should then be part of the initial clinical assessment.

Psychosocial assessment can be carried out by the family doctor or therapist and does not necessarily require referral to a psychologist. However, it is important that the family doctor and therapist be aware of and consider these issues.

An overview of biopsychosocial assessment

> *Bio-*
> - review diagnostic triage
>   — nerve root problem
>   — serious spinal pathology
> - ESR and plain X-ray
> *Psycho-*
> - attitudes and beliefs about back pain
>   — fear avoidance beliefs about activity and work
>   — personal responsibility for pain and rehabilitation
> - Psychological distress and depressive symptoms
> - Illness behaviour
> *Social*
> - Family?
>   — attitudes and beliefs about the problem
>   — reinforcement of disability behaviour
> - Work
>   — physical demands of job
>   — job satisfaction
>   — other health problems causing time off or job loss
>   — nonhealth problems causing time off or job loss

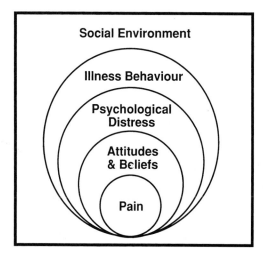

Figure 17B.3 A biopsychosocial model of low back disability.

Risk factors for chronicity

The risk factors for chronicity are:

- Previous history of low back pain
- Total work loss (due to low back pain) in past 12 months
- Radiating leg pain
- Reduced straight leg raising
- Signs of nerve root involvement
- Reduced trunk muscle strength and endurance
- Poor physical fitness
- Self-rated health poor
- Heavy smoking
- Psychological distress and depressive symptoms
- Disproportionate illness behaviour
- Low job satisfaction
- Personal problems – alcohol, marital, financial
- Adversarial medicolegal proceedings.

Low educational attainment and heavy physical occupation slightly increase the risk of low back pain and chronicity but markedly increase the difficulty of rehabilitation and retraining.

Multidisciplinary rehabilitation programme

The risk factors for chronicity show that as pain and disability become chronic, biopsychosocial factors become increasingly important. For this reason, purely physical treatment for chronic pain based on the disease model has a low success rate.

Traditional medical treatment not enough

Traditional medical treatment has certainly not solved our present epidemic of low back disability. Chronic pain and disability is a complex biopsychosocial problem which is perhaps better regarded as 'activity intolerance'. The main strategy should now be to 'de-medicalize' symptoms and to regard the problem as one of rehabilitation.

Importance of a multidisciplinary approach

Clinical management should place equal emphasis on both the physical and psychosocial aspects of chronic pain and disability. A number of common elements can be identified from successful trials in chronic back pain. These are:

- incremental exercise and fitness programme of physical reconditioning
- behavioural medicine principles with functional objectives
- close liaison with the workplace.

Varying levels of treatment

These principles can be implemented at several levels of intensity. Many of the principles have been achieved by a sole, part-time physical therapist working at the acute stage in a small workplace. All of the principles have been achieved effectively by a small research team consisting of a rehabilitation physician, a physical therapist and a psychologist working at the subacute stage in an occupational setting. In the case of chronic back cripples, comprehensive pain management programmes may require a large multidisciplinary team of medical and health care specialists. These principles should form the basis of management of back pain by every family doctor, physiotherapist, osteopath, chiropractor or occupational health service.

Additional options for symptomatic relief

A large number of therapeutic options may be considered to provide symptomatic relief. However, there is no good scientific evidence that these options produce lasting benefits or that they change the natural history of back pain or sciatica. They should not be regarded as treatments in themselves but rather as symptomatic measures – the focus should be on active exercise and rehabilitation.

Therapeutic options for symptomatic relief are only valuable to the extent that they facilitate active exercise and rehabilitation. If symptoms and disability are not improved within 6 weeks, alternative or additional symptomatic and rehabilitative measures should be considered.

Additional therapeutic options for symptomatic relief include:

- Drugs
  — analgesics
  — NSAIDs
  — muscle relaxants
  — antidepressants in low doses

- Injections
  — trigger point injections
  — epidural injections
  — sclerosant injections
  — facet injections

- Physical modalities
  — heat/cold
  — SWD and other electrotherapies
  — TENS
  — acupuncture
  — biofeedback
  — lumbosacral support
  — sitting lumbar support
  — shock relieving shoe insoles

Symptomatic measures to avoid

The treatments listed below should not be used. There is no evidence that they are of any benefit in low back pain or sciatica. They are also associated with harmful effects or risks which outweigh any potential benefit. In every case simpler and safer alternatives exist.

Do not use these treatments:

- Bed rest with traction
- Narcotics for more than 2 weeks
- Benzodiazepines (Diazepam) for more than 2 weeks
- Systemic steroids
- Colchicine
- Manipulation under general anaesthesia
- Plaster jacket.

Secondary referral

If the patient with simple backache has not returned to work within 3 months, then primary care management has failed. Chronic pain and disability are then likely. If the patient has not returned to work within 3 months, if symptoms are not controlled, or if the patient has frequent recurrent attacks, then secondary referral should be considered. The aims of any secondary referral should be clearly identified and specified in the referral request.

The aims of the secondary referral may include:

- second opinion for investigation, diagnosis, advice on management and reassurance
- rehabilitation
- vocational assessment and guidance
- surgery
- pain management.

Final outcome measure: maintain productive activity; reduce work loss

The primary aim of management is to control pain and prevent disability: the result is to return the patient to normal function. The measure of successful management is the extent to which these are achieved.

Control of pain and prevention of disability go together. In the short term, relief of pain and distress and satisfaction with care may seem more important to the patient. Nevertheless, in the long term chronic disability is just as important and damaging as chronic pain. Moreover, return to normal function and to work are associated with reduced pain, while chronic pain and unemployment in themselves lead to psychosocial dysfunction. In the final outcome, the extent to which the patient returns to normal function is the best measure of control of pain.

Low back disability affects patients in many ways: restriction in activities of daily living, loss of productive activities and work loss. All are important, and management should set goals appropriate to the individual patient. In the previously disabled, the young, the elderly, housewives and the unemployed, the aim may be to return to their normal function and to productive activities. In the previously disabled and in chronic pain patients, realistic goals may fall short of that ideal. But for the working patient, loss of time from work with all its financial, psychological and social ill-effects on the individual and the family is the most

Algorithm 17B.1   Diagnostic triage of a patient presenting with low back pain with or without sciatica.

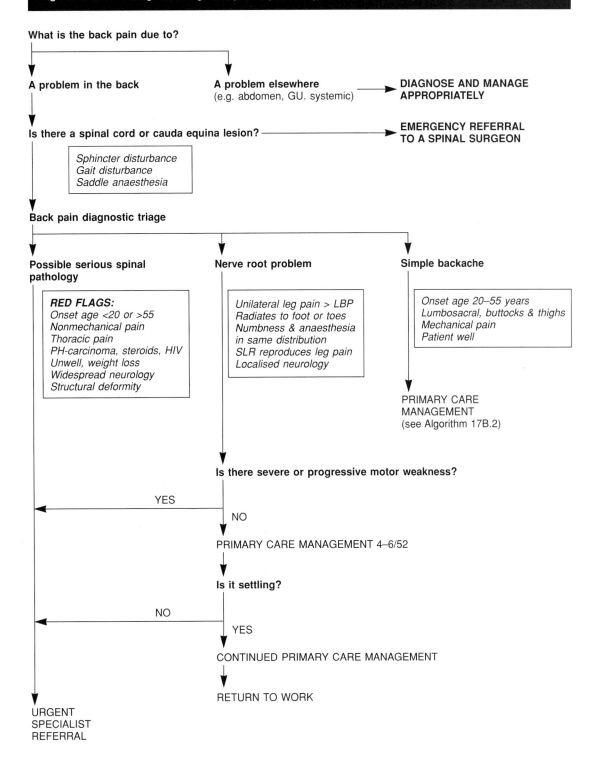

What is the back pain due to?

A problem in the back

A problem elsewhere
(e.g. abdomen, GU. systemic) → **DIAGNOSE AND MANAGE APPROPRIATELY**

Is there a spinal cord or cauda equina lesion? → **EMERGENCY REFERRAL TO A SPINAL SURGEON**

> *Sphincter disturbance*
> *Gait disturbance*
> *Saddle anaesthesia*

Back pain diagnostic triage

Possible serious spinal pathology

> **RED FLAGS:**
> *Onset age <20 or >55*
> *Nonmechanical pain*
> *Thoracic pain*
> *PH-carcinoma, steroids, HIV*
> *Unwell, weight loss*
> *Widespread neurology*
> *Structural deformity*

Nerve root problem

> *Unilateral leg pain > LBP*
> *Radiates to foot or toes*
> *Numbness & anaesthesia*
> *in same distribution*
> *SLR reproduces leg pain*
> *Localised neurology*

Simple backache

> *Onset age 20–55 years*
> *Lumbosacral, buttocks & thighs*
> *Mechanical pain*
> *Patient well*

PRIMARY CARE
MANAGEMENT
(see Algorithm 17B.2)

Is there severe or progressive motor weakness?

YES

NO

PRIMARY CARE MANAGEMENT 4–6/52

Is it settling?

NO

YES

CONTINUED PRIMARY CARE MANAGEMENT

RETURN TO WORK

URGENT
SPECIALIST
REFERRAL

Algorithm 17B.2 Primary care management of simple backache.

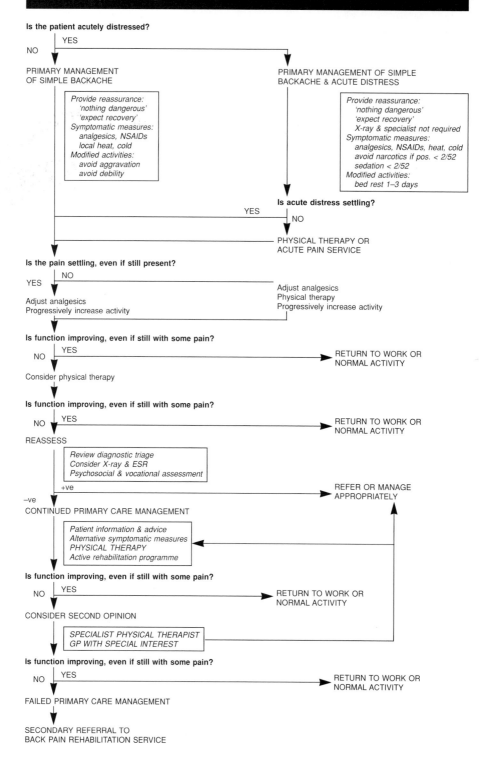

Is the patient acutely distressed?

NO — YES

PRIMARY MANAGEMENT
OF SIMPLE BACKACHE

> Provide reassurance:
>   'nothing dangerous'
>   'expect recovery'
> Symptomatic measures:
>   analgesics, NSAIDs
>   local heat, cold
> Modified activities:
>   avoid aggravation
>   avoid debility

PRIMARY MANAGEMENT OF SIMPLE
BACKACHE & ACUTE DISTRESS

> Provide reassurance:
>   'nothing dangerous'
>   'expect recovery'
>   X-ray & specialist not required
> Symptomatic measures:
>   analgesics, NSAIDs, heat, cold
>   avoid narcotics if pos. < 2/52
>   sedation < 2/52
> Modified activities:
>   bed rest 1–3 days

Is acute distress settling?

YES — NO

PHYSICAL THERAPY OR
ACUTE PAIN SERVICE

Is the pain settling, even if still present?

YES — NO

Adjust analgesics
Progressively increase activity

Adjust analgesics
Physical therapy
Progressively increase activity

Is function improving, even if still with some pain?

NO — YES

Consider physical therapy

RETURN TO WORK OR
NORMAL ACTIVITY

Is function improving, even if still with some pain?

NO — YES

REASSESS

> Review diagnostic triage
> Consider X-ray & ESR
> Psychosocial & vocational assessment

RETURN TO WORK OR
NORMAL ACTIVITY

+ve

–ve

CONTINUED PRIMARY CARE MANAGEMENT

> Patient information & advice
> Alternative symptomatic measures
> PHYSICAL THERAPY
> Active rehabilitation programme

REFER OR MANAGE
APPROPRIATELY

Is function improving, even if still with some pain?

NO — YES

CONSIDER SECOND OPINION

> SPECIALIST PHYSICAL THERAPIST
> GP WITH SPECIAL INTEREST

RETURN TO WORK OR
NORMAL ACTIVITY

Is function improving, even if still with some pain?

NO — YES

FAILED PRIMARY CARE MANAGEMENT

RETURN TO WORK OR
NORMAL ACTIVITY

SECONDARY REFERRAL TO
BACK PAIN REHABILITATION SERVICE

important consequence of back pain. For the community, work loss is the most important measure of the social impact of back pain on employers, productivity, the economy and social costs. Success in halting the present epidemic of low back disability depends on reducing work loss. For all these reasons, how soon the patient returns to work, and then remains at work, is the single most important measure of low back disability. It is also the easiest and most objective to measure.

Work loss and return to work are also highly dependent upon work-related and socioeconomic factors outwith medical control. Despite this, medical management of back pain can never be judged successful unless it reduces work loss.

What matters to the patient with backache is both control of pain and returning to normal function. The single most important measure of achieving this is work loss.

APPENDIX 17C: UK Clinical guidelines for the management of acute low back pain

Contributing organisations

- Royal College of General Practitioners
- Chartered Society of Physiotherapy
- Osteopathic Association of Great Britain
- British Chiropractic Association
- National Back Pain Association

These brief clinical guidelines and their supporting base of research evidence are intended to assist in the management of acute back pain. They present a synthesis of up-to-date international evidence and make recommendations on case management.

These guidelines have been constructed by a multi-professional group and subjected to extensive professional review.

Recommendations and evidence relate primarily to the first 6 weeks of an episode, when management decisions may be required in a changing clinical picture.

They are intended to be used as a guide by the whole range of health professionals in the NHS and in private practice who advise people with acute back pain.

Diagnostic triage

Diagnostic triage is the differential diagnosis between:

- simple backache (nonspecific low back pain)
- nerve root pain
- possible serious spinal pathology.

Simple backache: specialist referral not required

- Presentation 20–55 years
- Lumbosacral, buttocks & thighs

- 'Mechanical' pain
- Patient well.

Nerve root pain: specialist referral not generally required within first 4 weeks, provided resolving

- Unilateral leg pain worse than low back pain
- Radiates to foot or toes
- Numbness & paraesthesia in same distribution
- SLR reproduces leg pain
- Localised neurological signs.

Red flags for possible serious spinal pathology: prompt referral (less than 4 weeks)

- Presentation under age 20 or onset over 55
- Nonmechanical pain
- Thoracic pain
- Past history – carcinoma, steroids, HIV
- Unwell, weight loss
- Widespread neurology
- Structural deformity.

Cauda equina syndrome: immediate referral

- Sphincter disturbance
- Gait disturbance
- Saddle anaesthesia.

The evidence is weighted as follows:

*** Generally consistent finding in a majority of acceptable studies.

** Either based on a single acceptable study, or a weak or inconsistent finding in some of multiple acceptable studies.

* Limited scientific evidence, which does not meet all the criteria of 'acceptable' studies.

Reproduced with permission from The Royal College of General Practitioners, 1996.

Principal recommendations

Assessment

- Carry out diagnostic triage (see above)
- X-rays are not routinely indicated in simple backache
- Consider psychosocial factors.

Drug therapy

- Prescribe analgesics at regular intervals, not p.r.n.
- Start with paracetamol. If inadequate, substitute NSAIDs (e.g. ibuprofen or diclofenac) and then paracetamol-weak opioid compound (e.g. codydramol or coproxamol) Finally, consider adding a short course of muscle relaxant (e.g. diazepam or baclofen)
- Avoid narcotics if possible.

Bed rest

- Do not recommend or use bed rest as a treatment for simple back pain
- Some patients may be confined to bed for a few days as a consequence of their pain but this should not be considered a treatment.

Advice on staying active

- Advise patients to stay as active as possible and to continue normal daily activities
- Advise patients to increase their physical activities progressively over a few days or weeks
- If a patient is working, then advice to stay at work or return to work as soon as possible is probably beneficial.

Manipulation

- Consider manipulative treatment within the first 6 weeks for patients who need additional help with pain relief or who are failing to return to normal activities.

Back exercises

- Patients who have not returned to ordinary activities and work by 6 weeks should be referred for reactivation/rehabilitation.

Evidence

Assessment

* Diagnostic triage forms the basis for referral, investigation and management.
* Royal College of Radiologists Guidelines.
*** Psychosocial factors play an important role in low back pain and disability and influence the patient's response to treatment and rehabilitation.

Drug therapy

** Paracetamol effectively reduces acute low back pain.
*** NSAIDs effectively reduce simple backache. Ibuprofen and diclofenac have lower risks of GI complications.
** Paracetamol-weak opioid compounds are effective when NSAIDs or paracetamol alone are inadequate.
*** Muscle relaxants effectively reduce acute back pain.

Bed rest

*** Bed rest for 2–7 days is worse than placebo or ordinary activity and is not as effective as alternative treatments for relief of pain, rate of recovery, return to daily activities and work.

Advice on staying active

*** Advice to continue ordinary activity can give equivalent or faster symptomatic recovery from the acute attack and lead to less chronic disability and less time off work.

Manipulation

*** Within the first 6 weeks of onset, manipulation can provide short-term improvement in pain and activity levels and higher patient satisfaction.
** The evidence is inconclusive that manipulation produces clinically significant improve-ment in chronic low back pain.
** The risks of manipulation are very low in skilled hands.

Back exercises

*** It is doubtful that specific back exercises produce clinically significant improvement in acute low back pain.
** There is some evidence that exercise programmes and physical reconditioning can improve pain and functional levels in patients with chronic low back pain, and there are also theoretical arguments for starting this by 6 weeks.

Key patient information points

Simple backache

Give positive messages.

- There is nothing to worry about. Backache is very common.
- No sign of any serious damage or disease. Full recovery in days or weeks – but may vary.
- No permanent weakness. Recurrence possible – but does not mean reinjury.
- Activity is helpful, too much rest is not. Hurting does not mean harm.

Nerve root pain

Give guarded positive messages.

- No cause for alarm. No sign of disease
- Conservative treatment should suffice – but may take a month or two
- Full recovery expected – but recurrence possible.

Possible serious spinal pathology

Avoid negative messages.

- Some tests are needed to make the diagnosis
- Often these tests are negative

- The specialist will advise on the best treatment
- Rest or activity avoidance until appointment to see specialist.

Patient booklet

The above messages can be enhanced by an educational booklet given at consultation. *The Back Book* is an evidence-based booklet developed for use with these guidelines, and is published by HMSO (ISBN 011 702 0788).

Key audit points

- Consideration of 'red flag' symptoms
- Discourage bed rest
- Recommendation to return to normal activities
- Specific aims for physical therapy.

Key implementation points

- Local ownership is important. Guidelines should be placed in local context but not at the expense of changing the principal recommendations.
- Multiple methods of implementation are more likely to be effective than single methods. These can include peer groups, audit feedback, facilitators and educational outreach.

APPENDIX 17D: New Zealand Acute low back pain guide

Background

This guide has been developed from the comprehensive publication *Clinical Practice Guideline – Acute Low Back Problems in Adults: Assessment and Treatment* (AHCPR), which was distributed by ACC and the National Health Committee in January 1996. The participation of various professional groups, through submissions and a health professionals' hearing, enabled an expert panel to develop this guide. The guide reflects current best practice in New Zealand and will be reviewed as new evidence becomes available. The expert panel recommends that this guide should have its first review within 2 years of publication.

Any further comments and submission of new evidence for the National Health Committee and ACC should be made through the appropriate professional association.

No references are provided in this document. Comprehensive lists of references are available in the documents detailed in the acknowledgement at the end of this guide.

Acute low back pain is:

- common
- self-limiting in most people
- best managed by good assessment, explanation (and reassurance), advice about staying active and expectations of recovery
- best managed (where necessary) with simple analgesics and/or manipulation
- best managed by advice against bed rest for more than 2 days.

Recurrent low back pain is:

- fairly common
- probably best treated in a similar way to acute low back pain episodes.

Chronic low back pain is:

- a major cause of disability that can leave a person miserable and unemployable

Reproduced with permission from the Accident Rehabilitation & Compensation Insurance Corporation of New Zealand and the National Health Committee, Wellington, New Zealand, 1997.

- very difficult to treat
- almost certainly easier to prevent than treat
- often associated with psychosocial risk factors.

This guide:

- *promotes* better management of acute low back pain to prevent chronicity
- *simplifies* the history and examination of people with acute low back pain making it easier to identify:
  - people without signs of serious disease, who should be reassured, treated symptomatically and encouraged to remain active
  - people who should be referred for appropriate specialist opinion on the basis of red or yellow flags
- *suggests* timeframes for recovery from an acute episode of low back pain, so that people not fitting this 'normal' pattern can be identified
- *identifies* psychosocial risk factors for chronic back pain
- *suggests* strategies for better management for people at risk of chronic low back pain or those not recovering as expected
- *aims* to change the attitudes of treatment providers and the public about acute low back problems. Excess disability can result from:
  - reliance on a narrow medical model of pain
  - discouragement of self care strategies and failure to instruct the patient in self-management
  - sanctioning of disability and not providing interventions that will improve function
  - over-investigation and perpetuation of belief in the 'broken part hypothesis'.

Evidence

This guide is based on a review of the best available scientific evidence for improved clinical outcomes, in accordance with the approach to systematic reviews recommended by the international Cochrane Collaboration.

The advice in the guide is based on 'at least moderate research evidence', where moderate research evidence is defined as one relevant

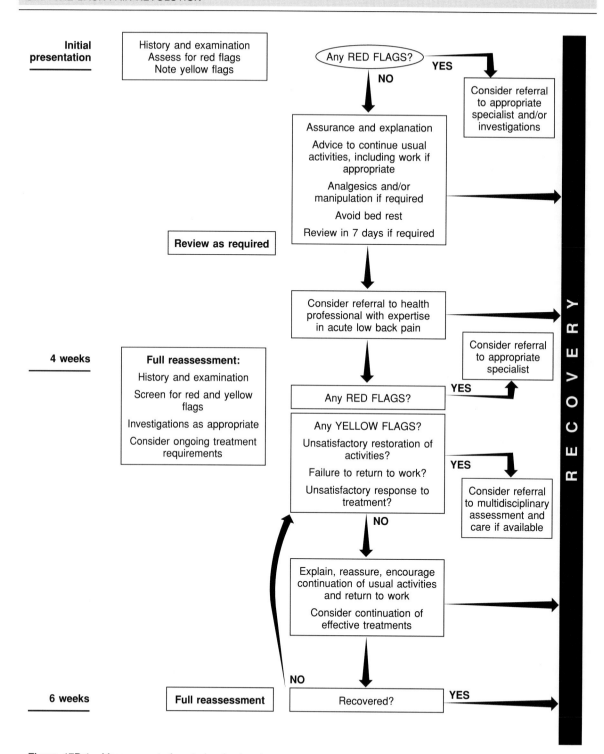

Figure 17D.1   Management of acute low back pain.

high quality scientific study or multiple adequate scientific studies of an acceptable design. Randomised controlled trial studies of therapy or prospective cohort studies of assessment and natural history, meeting specific criteria, are internationally recognised as acceptable evidence.

Evidence for some treatment options such as biofeedback is unlikely to become available in view of their cost and limited application to the management of acute low back pain. Acceptable evidence may become available for some other treatment options and will be described in future editions of the guide.

Best practice advice

The 'best practice' advice given in the management of acute low back pain flowchart (Fig. 17D.1) and in the summary of management options (Box 17D.3) is *not* intended to be read as a rigid prescription. The advice is intended to offer flexibility and choice, so that clinical judgement can be made according to patients' circumstances, supported by the best available evidence for improved clinical outcome.

Definitions

Acute low back problems: activity intolerance due to lower back or back and leg symptoms lasting less than 3 months.

Chronic low back problems: activity intolerance due to lower back or back and leg symptoms lasting more than 3 months.

Recurrent low back problems: episodes of acute low back problems lasting less than 3 months but which recur after an interval free of low back symptoms sufficient to restrict activity or function.

Natural history

Most severe back pain and severe activity limitation improves considerably in a few days or at most a few weeks, but milder symptoms may persist longer, often for a few months.

Initial assessment

A good *history* must be taken to identify:

- the risk factors for serious disease (red flags, see below)
- how limiting the symptoms are
- similar previous episodes
- any factors that might limit an early return to usual activities, including work (this includes screening for yellow flags – see p. 317 and accompanying booklet (Appendix 17E).

The *clinical examination* aims to identify any neurological deficit (note that over 90% of all clinically significant lower limb radiculopathy due to disc herniation involves the L5 or S1 nerve root at the L4/5 or L5/S1 disc level). Pointers in the history may indicate the need for a more general examination, particularly if red flags for serious or systemic disease (such as cancer) are suspected.

Red flags

The following approach to investigations and referral is recommended:

- Patients with persistent neurological deficit and pain should be referred to the appropriate specialist.
- Patients with red flags should be investigated appropriately and referred if investigations are abnormal. Referral may still be appropriate at 4 weeks, even if investigations are normal.

Box 17D.1 Red flags for potentially serious conditions

- Features of cauda equina syndrome (especially urinary retention, bilateral neurological symptoms and signs, saddle anaesthesia)
  — this requires very urgent referral
- Significant trauma
- Weight loss
- History of cancer
- Fever
- Intravenous drug use
- Steroid use
- Patient aged over 50 years
- Severe, unremitting night-time pain
- Pain that gets worse when patient is lying down

- Patients with no red flags and normal neurological examination should only have full blood count, ESR and plain X-rays of the lumbar spine if they have not recovered at 4–6 weeks or if there are other indications.

Abnormal investigations may justify referral to an appropriate specialist.

- At 6 weeks, patients with no red flags, normal investigations and persistent symptoms should be referred to a specialist or specialist team if available. Multidisciplinary teams may be more effective in preventing pain and disability.

Intervention between 4 and 8 weeks after acute low back problems start is most likely to help prevent chronic low back problems. Patients with low back symptoms persisting beyond 12 weeks have a rapidly reducing rate of return to normal activity.

Note: yellow flags. It may be useful to conduct a preliminary screening for important psychosocial factors (yellow flags) at the time of initial presentation. Potential yellow flags should be more comprehensively and formally assessed at the 4 and 6 week full reassessments, if the patient is not making expected progress. Refer to page 317 and the Guide to Assessing Psychosocial Yellow Flags in Acute Low Back Pain (Appendix 17E).

Investigations

A full blood count and ESR should be performed only if there are any red flags. Other tests may be indicated depending on the clinical situation.

Plain X-rays of the lumbar spine are indicated if any of the red flags are present but not otherwise in the first 4 weeks. The value of plain X-rays to some treatment providers in developing a management plan must be balanced against the radiation exposures involved.

As 30% of people *without* low back symptoms will have significant abnormalities on MRI and CT scans of the lumbar spine, these investigations should be reserved for people being worked up for surgery or where a specific pathology (such as cancer or infection) is strongly suspected.

Assurance and explanation

It is important to let the patient know that, if a full history and examination have uncovered no suggestion of serious problems, no further investigations are needed. They should be advised to stay as active as possible and continue usual daily activities.

Activity alteration and work activities

Bed rest for more than 2 days should be discouraged, as it has been shown to impair recovery. It is recommended that patients should increase physical activity progressively according to a timetable rather than be guided by pain level. Activities and postures may need to be modified in the short term, and suitable advice provided.

It is important to discuss work activities, especially those involving heavy lifting, bending or twisting, that may have contributed to the original problems. Alternative duties and/or workplace design may need to be discussed with the worker and/or employer.

Symptom control

Effective interventions to control symptoms of acute low back pain include:

- *Analgesics*. If patients need their pain symptoms controlled, paracetamol and nonsteroidal anti-inflammatory drugs have been shown to be effective.
- *Manipulation*. Manual loading of the spine using short or long leverage methods is safe and effective in the first 4–6 weeks of acute low back symptoms.

Treatments to relieve low back pain that do not include an appropriate emphasis on return to usual activity may inadvertently encourage the patient to fear moving or using their back. It is important to combine symptom control with encouragement to promote activity, including returning to work.

Advice on staying active

Advice to continue ordinary activity usually results in more rapid symptomatic recovery from an acute episode, and leads to less chronic disability and less time off work when compared to 'traditional' medical treatment. Traditional medical treatment has inappropriately focused on analgesics only as required, advice to rest and 'letting pain be your guide' for return to usual activity. All of these have been shown to delay recovery.

Progressive reactivation over a short period of days or a few weeks, combined with behavioural management of pain, makes little difference to the rate of initial recovery of pain and disability, but leads to less chronic disability and work loss.

Advice on a planned return to normal work within a short time may lead to shorter periods of work loss and less time off work.

Education

Educating patients about low back symptoms provides assurance. This can lead to improved feelings of well-being, reduced health service use and improved use of self-management strategies. Education as part of a 'back school' at the workplace may be effective. The efficacy of back schools in nonoccupational settings has yet to be demonstrated by randomised controlled trials.

Review

The clinician is responsible for making sure that the episode resolves as expected. Follow-up will depend on the clinical situation, including the severity of symptoms, the presence of any neurological deficit, history of previous episodes and other medical and/or psychosocial factors. A reasonable approach for most patients is a review by the end of the first week, unless symptoms have completely resolved. It may be appropriate to arrange an earlier review, to reinforce the message to keep active and avoid prolonged bed rest.

Yellow flags

Yellow flags and red flags can be thought of as:

- yellow flags = psychosocial risk factors
- red flags = physical risk factors.

Yellow flags are factors that may increase the risk of developing, or perpetuating, long-term disability and work loss associated with low back pain. Identification of risk factors can inform appropriate cognitive and behavioural management strategies to achieve functional outcome goals.

The accompanying *Guide to Assessing Psychosocial Yellow Flags in Acute Low Back Pain* (see Appendix 17E) provides:

- a method of screening for psychosocial factors that are likely to increase the risk of an individual with acute back pain developing prolonged pain and disability causing work loss and associated loss of quality of life
- a systematic approach to assessing psychosocial factors, including a screening questionnaire
- suggested strategies for better management by primary care treatment providers for those with acute back pain who are 'at risk'.

The primary aim of management is to *control pain* and *prevent disability*. Identifying 'at risk' individuals makes prevention of long-term problems possible in most cases, with benefits far outweighing the risks of over-identification.

The presence of psychosocial risk factors does not mean that the back pain is any less real nor does it reduce the need for symptom control.

Most 'at risk' individuals can be effectively managed by their usual treatment provider, without the need for referral to a psychologist. These patients will require strategies that are effectively integrated with requirements for analgesia and physical modalities to enable them to remain active and return to ordinary activities.

Box 17D.2 Psychosocial yellow flags – main categories

Clinical assessment of yellow flags may identify the risk of long-term disability, distress and work loss due to:
- Attitudes and beliefs about back pain
- Behaviours
- Compensation issues
- Diagnostic and treatment issues
- Emotions
- Family
- Work

Referral

All patients with symptoms and/or signs of cauda equina syndrome should be referred urgently to an appropriate specialist. The presence of red flags and/or abnormal tests indicates the need to consider referral or at least fuller investigation. Certain red flags (such as severe pain at night or weight loss) should lead to full investigation and/or referral being considered, even if the tests are normal.

Leg pain

Patients with pain radiating from the back down one leg as far as the ankle, with or without neurological signs, have a higher chance of a disc herniation as the cause of their low back problems. Nevertheless, the natural history of back-related leg pain is benign in most patients and these patients should be managed as shown in Figure 17D.1 unless there is unremitting, severe pain or increasing neurological deficit. Caution should be exercised in advising manipulation if there is any neurological deficit.

Surgery

Surgery is not indicated for nonspecific low back pain. Where there is no improvement, some patients with back-related leg pain and a defined disc lesion may recover more rapidly with surgery. Note that the long-term results of surgery for back-related leg pain are no better than conservative management. Patient preferences will be important in any decision about surgical intervention.

Full reassessment

Most patients with episodes of acute low back pain should have largely recovered within 4 weeks. Some studies suggest that as many as 90% of affected people will have resumed their normal activities in this time. All patients who have not regained usual activity after 4 weeks should be formally reassessed then and again at 6 weeks. The assessment should include retaking the history and examination, and looking for red or yellow flags, neurological deficit and any evidence of systemic disease. Treatment providers must consider whether continuing treatment will accelerate recovery or simply prolong the 'traditional' medical model.

Comment on multidisciplinary teams

There is clear evidence that multidisciplinary teams or networks are effective in managing chronic back pain. The evidence for their effectiveness in unresolved episodes of acute low back pain is yet to be determined. The expert panel has recommended the use of multidisciplinary team management for episodes of acute low back pain unresolved at 6 weeks in line with international opinion.

Who might be in the multidisciplinary teams?

They might include health professionals with appropriate training in musculoskeletal disorders, psychosocial assessment, vocational management and other relevant specialities. These teams may not be embodied in a discrete organisation, but may reflect a close collaborative team approach for the assessment and comprehensive management of 'at risk' patients by professionals from various disciplines with specific skills working together. This is particularly true of rural areas where access to specialist teams would otherwise be a treatment barrier to those needing prompt specialist intervention.

What is the role of multidisciplinary teams?

The lead treatment provider may require support from a multidisciplinary team to integrate all components of the comprehensive evaluation and management plan. This support could provide input into key clinical decisions and promote service coordination. Multidisciplinary teams are able to:

1. make an objective review of progress to date and a comprehensive evaluation of the presenting problem, emphasising the early identification of barriers to progress that have so far gone unnoticed

2. develop a comprehensive management plan including:
   - integration of all components of the evaluation into the decision-making process
   - an outline of expected milestones with time frames
   - incorporation of strategies for dealing with any barriers that are identified
   - options for continued lack of progress
3. provide treatment, only for the most complex or resistant cases.

Recommended treatment options

Box 17D.3 provides a summary of management options based on the available evidence for improved clinical outcomes. The evidence was reviewed by an expert panel who felt that it was more helpful to focus on the availability of evidence rather than to make recommendations about the treatments that must or must not be used.

Caution should be exercised in recommending treatment options for which the evidence of improved clinical outcomes is lacking or inconclusive. Treatment providers who wish to provide best practice care can now choose treatments for which there is good evidence for improved clinical outcomes.

Box 17D.3 Summary of management options for an episode of acute low back pain based on the evidence available at present

---

At least moderate research **evidence for improvement** *in clinical outcomes*
- Advice to stay active and continue usual activities
- Paracetamol
- NSAIDs (nonsteroidal anti-inflammatory drugs)
- Manipulation – in the first 4 to 6 weeks only

At least moderate research **evidence of no improvement** *in clinical outcomes*
- Bed rest for more than 2 days
- TENS (trancutaneous electrical nerve stimulation)
- Traction
- Specific back exercises
- Education pamphlets about low back symptoms

At least moderate research evidence of potential harm from the treatments below which should **not** *be used for an episode of acute low back pain*
- Use of narcotics or diazepam (especially for more than 2 weeks)
- Bed rest with traction
- Manipulation under general anaesthesia
- Plaster jacket

Insufficient research evidence for any improvement in clinical outcomes
- Conditioning exercises for the trunk muscles
- Aerobic conditioning
- Epidural steroid injections
- Workplace back schools
- Acupuncture
- Shoe lifts
- Corsets
- Biofeedback
- Physical modalities (includes ice, heat, short wave diathermy, massage, ultrasound)

APPENDIX 17E: New Zealand Guide to assessing psychosocial yellow flags in acute low back pain

What this guide aims to do

This guide complements the *New Zealand Acute Low Back Pain Guide* and is intended for use in conjunction with it. This guide describes 'yellow flags' – psychosocial factors that are likely to increase the risk of an individual with acute low back pain developing prolonged pain and disability causing work loss, and associated loss of quality of life. It aims to:

• provide a method of screening for psychosocial factors
• provide a systematic approach to assessing psychosocial factors
• suggest strategies for better management of those with acute low back pain who have 'yellow flags' indicating increased risks of chronicity.

This guide is not intended to be a rigid prescription and will permit flexibility and choice, allowing the exercise of good clinical judgement according to the particular circumstances of the patient. The management suggestions outlined in this document are based on the best available evidence to date.

What are psychosocial yellow flags?

'Yellow flags' are factors that increase the risk of developing, or perpetuating long-term disability and work loss associated with low back pain.

Psychosocial 'yellow flags' are similar to the 'red flags' in the *New Zealand Acute Low Back Pain Guide* (see Appendix D).

Yellow and red flags can be thought of in this way:

• yellow flags = psychosocial risk factors
• red flags = physical risk factors.

Reproduced with permission from the Accident Rehabilitation & Compensation Insurance Corporation of New Zealand and the National Health Committee, Wellington, New Zealand.

Identification of risk factors should lead to appropriate intervention. Red flags should lead to appropriate medical intervention; yellow flags to appropriate cognitive and behavioural management.

The significance of a particular factor is relative. Immediate notice should be taken if an important red flag is present, and consideration given to an appropriate response. The same is true for the yellow flags.

Assessing the presence of yellow flags should produce two key outcomes:

• a decision as to whether more detailed assessment is needed
• identification of any salient factors that can become the subject of specific intervention, thus saving time and helping to concentrate the use of resources.

Red and yellow flags are not mutually exclusive – an individual patient may require intervention in both areas concurrently.

Why is there a need for psychosocial yellow flags for back pain problems?

Low back pain problems, especially when they are long-term or chronic, are common in our society and produce extensive human suffering. New Zealand has experienced a steady rise in the number of people who leave the work force with back pain. It is of concern that there is an increased proportion who do not recover normal function and activity for longer and longer periods.

The research literature on risk factors for long-term work disability is inconsistent or lacking for many chronic painful conditions, except low back pain, which has received a great deal of attention and empirical research over the last 5 years. Most of the known risk factors are psychosocial, which implies the possibility of appropriate intervention, especially where specific individuals are recognised as being 'at risk'.

Who is 'at risk'?

An individual may be considered 'at risk' if they have a clinical presentation that includes one or more very strong indicators of risk, or several less important factors that might be cumulative.

Definitions of primary, secondary and tertiary prevention

It has been concluded that efforts at every stage can be made towards prevention of long-term disability associated with low back pain, including work loss.

Primary prevention: elimination or minimisation of risks to health or well-being. It is an attempt to determine factors that cause disabling low back disability and then create programmes to prevent these situations from ever occurring.

Secondary prevention: alleviation of the symptoms of ill health or injury, minimising residual disability and eliminating, or at least minimising, factors that may cause recurrence. It is an attempt to maximise recovery once the condition has occurred and then prevent its recurrence. Secondary prevention emphasises the prevention of excess pain behaviour, the sick role, inactivity syndromes, reinjury, recurrences, complications, psychosocial sequelae, long-term disability and work loss.

Tertiary prevention: rehabilitation of those with disabilities to as full function as possible and modification of the workplace to accommodate any residual disability. It is applied after the patient has become disabled. The goal is to return to function and patient acceptance of residual impairment(s); this may in some instances require work site modification.

The focus of this guide is on secondary prevention, which aims to prevent:

- excess pain behaviour, sick role, inactivity syndromes
- reinjury, recurrences
- complications, psychosocial sequelae, long-term disability, work loss.

Definitions

Before proceeding to assess yellow flags, treatment providers need to carefully differentiate

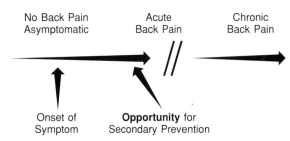

Figure 17E.1 Secondary prevention.

between the presentations of acute, recurrent and chronic back pain, since the risk factors for developing long-term problems may differ even though there is considerable overlap.

Acute low back problems: activity intolerance due to lower back or back and leg symptoms lasting less than 3 months.

Recurrent low back problems: episodes of acute low back problems lasting less than 3 months but recurring after a period of time without low back symptoms sufficient to restrict activity or function.

Chronic low back problems: activity intolerance due to lower back or back and leg symptoms lasting more than 3 months.

Goals of assessing psychosocial yellow flags

The three main consequences of back problems are:

- pain
- disability, limitation in function including activities of daily living
- reduced productive activity, including work loss.

Pain

Attempts to prevent the development of chronic pain through physiological or pharmacological interventions in the acute phase have been relatively ineffective. Research to date can be summarised by stating that inadequate control of acute (nociceptive) pain *may* increase the risk of chronic pain.

Disability

Preventing loss of function, reduced activity, distress and low mood is an important, yet distinct goal. These factors are critical to a person's quality of life and general well-being. It has been repeatedly demonstrated that these factors can be modified in patients with chronic back pain. It is therefore strongly suggested that treatment providers must prevent any tendency for significant withdrawal from activity being established in any acute episode.

Work loss

The probability of successfully returning to work in the early stages of an acute episode depends on the quality of management, as described in this guide. If the episode goes on longer, the probability of returning to work reduces. The likelihood of return to any work is even smaller if the person loses their employment, and has to reenter the job market.

Prevention

Long-term disability and work loss are associated with profound suffering and negative effects on patients, their families and society. Once established they are difficult to undo. Current evidence indicates that to be effective, preventive strategies must be initiated at a much *earlier* stage than was previously thought. Enabling people to keep active in order to maintain work skills and relationships is an important outcome.

Most of the known risk factors for long-term disability, inactivity and work loss are psychosocial. Therefore, the key goal is to identify yellow flags that increase the risk of these problems developing. Health professionals can subsequently *target* effective early management to prevent onset of these problems.

Please note that it is important to avoid pejorative labelling of patients with yellow flags as this will have a negative impact on management. Their use is intended to encourage treatment providers to *prevent* the onset of long-term problems in 'at risk' patients by interventions appropriate to the underlying cause.

How to judge if a person is 'at risk'

A person may be at risk if:

- there is a cluster of a few very salient factors
- there is a group of several less important factors that combine cumulatively.

There is good agreement that the following factors are important and consistently predict poor outcomes:

- presence of a belief that back pain is harmful or potentially severely disabling
- fear-avoidance behaviour (avoiding a movement or activity due to misplaced anticipation of pain) and reduced activity levels
- tendency to low mood and withdrawal from social interaction
- an expectation that passive treatments rather than active participation will help.

Suggested questions (to be phrased in treatment provider's own words):

- Have you had time off work in the past with back pain?
- What do you understand is the cause of your back pain?
- What are you expecting will help you?
- How is your employer responding to your back pain? Your coworkers? Your family?
- What are you doing to cope with back pain?
- Do you think that you will return to work? When?

How to assess psychosocial yellow flags

- If large numbers need to be screened quickly there is little choice but to use a questionnaire. Problems may arise with managing the potentially large number of 'at risk' people identified. It is necessary to minimise the number of false positives (those the screening test identifies who are not actually at risk).
- If the goal is the most accurate identification of yellow flags prior to intervention, clinical assessment is preferred. Suitably skilled clinicians with adequate time must be available.

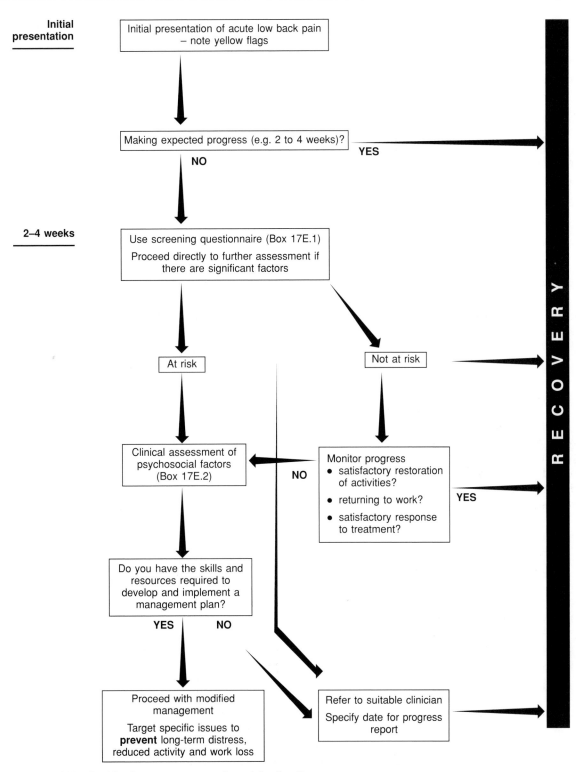

Figure 17E.2 Deciding how to assess psychosocial yellow flags.

Today's Date ___/___/___

Name _____   ACC Claim Number _____

Address _____   Telephone (___) _____ (home)

_____   (___) _____ (work)

Job Title (occupation) _____   Date stopped work for this episode ___/___/___

These questions and statements apply if you have aches or pains, such as back, shoulder or neck pain. Please read and answer each question carefully. Do not take too long to answer the questions. However, it is important that you answer every question. There is always a response for your particular situation.

1. What year were you born?   19 ___

2. Are you: ☐ male   ☐ female

3. Were you born in New Zealand? ☐ yes   ☐ no

4. Where do you have pain? Place a ✓ for all the appropriate sites.

   ☐ neck   ☐ shoulders   ☐ upper back   ☐ lower back   ☐ leg

   2 X count ▭

5. How many days of work have you missed because of pain during the past 18 months? Tick (✓) one.

   ☐ 0 days [1]   ☐ 1–2 days [2]   ☐ 3–7 days [3]   ☐ 8–14 days [4]   ☐ 15–30 days [5]

   ☐ 1 month [6]   ☐ 2 months [7]   ☐ 3–6 months [8]   ☐ 6–12 months [9]   ☐ over 1 year [10]

   ▭

6. How long have you had your current pain problem? Tick (✓) one.

   ☐ 0–1 weeks [1]   ☐ 1–2 weeks [2]   ☐ 3–4 weeks [3]   ☐ 4–5 weeks [4]   ☐ 6–8 weeks [5]

   ☐ 9–11 weeks [6]   ☐ 3–6 months [7]   ☐ 6–9 months [8]   ☐ 9–12 months [9]   ☐ over 1 year [10]

   ▭

7. Is your work heavy or monotonous? Circle the best alternative.

   | 0 | 1 | 2 | 3 | 4 | 5 | 6 | 7 | 8 | 9 | 10 |

   Not at all   *Extremely*

   ▭

8. How would you rate the pain that you have had during the past week? Circle one.

   | 0 | 1 | 2 | 3 | 4 | 5 | 6 | 7 | 8 | 9 | 10 |

   No pain   *Pain as bad as it could be*

   ▭

9. In the past 3 months, on average, how bad was your pain? Circle one.

   | 0 | 1 | 2 | 3 | 4 | 5 | 6 | 7 | 8 | 9 | 10 |

   No pain   *Pain as bad as it could be*

   ▭

10. How often would you say that you have experienced pain episodes, on average, during the past 3 months? Circle one.

   | 0 | 1 | 2 | 3 | 4 | 5 | 6 | 7 | 8 | 9 | 10 |

   Never   *Always*

   ▭

11. Based on all the things you do to cope, or deal with your pain, on an average day, how much are you able to decrease it? Circle one.

   | 0 | 1 | 2 | 3 | 4 | 5 | 6 | 7 | 8 | 9 | 10 |

   Can't decrease it at all   *Can decrease it completely*

   10–x ▭

12. How tense or anxious have you felt in the past week? Circle one.

   | 0 | 1 | 2 | 3 | 4 | 5 | 6 | 7 | 8 | 9 | 10 |

   Absolutely calm and relaxed   *As tense and anxious as I've ever felt*

   ▭

Figure 17E.3 Acute low back pain screening questionnaire (Linton & Hallden 1996)

13. How much have you been bothered by feeling depressed in the past week? Circle one.

    0   1   2   3   4   5   6   7   8   9   10

  Not at all   *Extremely*

14. In your view, how large is the risk that your current pain may become persistent? Circle one.

    0   1   2   3   4   5   6   7   8   9   10

  No risk   *Very large risk*

10−x

15. In your estimation, what are the chances that you will be working in 6 months? Circle one.

    0   1   2   3   4   5   6   7   8   9   10

  No chance   *Very large chance*

10−x

16. If you take into consideration your work routines, management, salary, promotion possibilities and work mates, how satisfied are you with your job? Circle one.

    0   1   2   3   4   5   6   7   8   9   10

  Not at all   *Completely*

  satisfied   *satisfied*

Here are some of the things which other people have told us about their back pain. For each statement please circle one number from 0 to 10 to say how much physical activities, such as bending, lifting, walking or driving would affect your back.

17. Physical activity makes my pain worse.

    0   1   2   3   4   5   6   7   8   9   10

  Completely   *Completely*

  disagree   *agree*

18. An increase in pain is an indication that I should stop what I am doing until the pain decreases.

    0   1   2   3   4   5   6   7   8   9   10

  Completely   *Completely*

  disagree   *agree*

19. I should not do my normal work with my present pain.

    0   1   2   3   4   5   6   7   8   9   10

  Completely   *Completely*

  disagree   *agree*

Here is a list of 5 activities. Please circle the one number which best describes your current ability to participate in each of these activities.

20. I can do light work for an hour.

    0   1   2   3   4   5   6   7   8   9   10

  Can't do it because   *Can do it without pain*

  of pain problem   *being a problem*

10−x

21. I can walk for an hour.

    0   1   2   3   4   5   6   7   8   9   10

  Can't do it because   *Can do it without pain*

  of pain problem   *being a problem*

10−x

22. I can do ordinary household chores.

    0   1   2   3   4   5   6   7   8   9   10

  Can't do it because   *Can do it without pain*

  of pain problem   *being a problem*

10−x

23. I can go shopping.

    0   1   2   3   4   5   6   7   8   9   10

  Can't do it because   *Can do it without pain*

  of pain problem   *being a problem*

10−x

24. I can sleep at night.

    0   1   2   3   4   5   6   7   8   9   10

  Can't do it because   *Can do it without pain*

  of pain problem   *being a problem*

10−x

Sum

- The two-stage approach shown in Figure 17E.2 is recommended if the numbers are large and skilled assessment staff are in short supply. The questionnaire can be used to screen for those needing further assessment (see Fig. 17E.3). In this instance, the number of false negatives (those who have risk factors, but are missed by the screening test) must be minimised.
- To use the screening questionnaire, see Box 17E.1.
- To conduct a clinical assessment for acute back pain, see Box 17E.2.

Clinical assessment of yellow flags involves judgements about the relative importance of factors for the individual. Box 17E.2 lists factors under the headings of 'attitudes and beliefs about back pain', 'behaviours', 'compensation issues', 'diagnosis and treatment', 'emotions', 'family' and 'work'.

These headings have been used for convenience in an attempt to make the job easier. They are presented in alphabetical order since it is not possible to rank their importance. However, within each category the factors are listed with *the most important at the top*.

Please note, clinical assessment may be supplemented with the questionnaire method (i.e. the acute low back pain screening questionnaire – Fig. 17E.3, Box 17E.1) if that has not already been done. In addition, treatment providers familiar with the administration and interpretation of other pain-specific psychometric measures and assessment tools (such as the pain drawing, the multidimensional pain inventory, etc) may choose to employ them. Become familiar with the potential disadvantages of each method to minimise any potential adverse effects.

The list of factors provided here is not exhaustive and for a particular individual the order of importance may vary. *A word of caution*: some factors may appear to be mutually exclusive, but are not in fact. For example, partners can alternate from being socially punitive (ignoring the problem or expressing frustration about it) to being overprotective in a well intentioned way (and inadvertently encouraging extended rest and withdrawal from activity, or excessive treatment seeking). In other words, both factors may be pertinent.

Box 17E.1 Scoring instructions for the acute low back pain screening questionnaire (see Fig. 17E.3; Linton & Hallden 1996)

- For Question 4, count the number of pain sites and multiply by 2
- For Questions 6, 7, 8, 9, 10, 12, 13, 14, 17, 18 and 19 the score is the number that has been ticked or circled
- For Questions 11, 15, 16, 20, 21, 22, 23 and 24 the score is 10 minus the number that has been ticked or circled
- Write the score in the shaded box beside each item – Questions 4 to 24
- Add them up, and write the sum in the box provided – this is the total score

Note: the scoring method is built into the questionnaire.

Interpretation of scores
Questionnaire scores greater than 105 indicate that the patient is 'at risk'.
This score produces:

- 75% correct identification of those not needing modification to ongoing management
- 86% correct identification of those who will have between 1 and 30 days off work
- 83% correct identification of those who will have more than 30 days off work

The use of this questionnaire in New Zealand
A prospective study is under way to determine the validity of the cut-off score of 105 in New Zealand using a local sample. Information regarding any amendment to this scoring system will be provided as soon as it becomes available.

What can be done to help somebody who is 'at risk'?

These suggestions are not intended to be prescriptions, or encouragement to ignore individual needs. They are intended to assist in the prevention of long-term disability and work loss.

Suggested steps to better early behavioural management of low back pain problems

1. Provide a *positive expectation* that the individual will return to work and normal activity. Organise for a regular expression of interest from the employer. If the problem persists beyond 2 to 4 weeks, provide a 'reality based' warning of what is going to be the

Box 17E.2 Clinical assessment of psychosocial yellow flags

Attitudes and beliefs about back pain
- Belief that pain is harmful or disabling resulting in fear-avoidance behaviour, e.g., the development of guarding and fear of movement
- Belief that all pain must be abolished before attempting to return to work or normal activity
- Expectation of increased pain with activity or work, lack of ability to predict capability
- Catastrophising, thinking the worst, misinterpreting bodily symptoms
- Belief that pain is uncontrollable
- Passive attitude to rehabilitation

Behaviours
- Use of extended rest, disproportionate 'downtime'
- Reduced activity level with significant withdrawal from activities of daily living
- Irregular participation or poor compliance with physical exercise, tendency for activities to be in a 'boom–bust' cycle
- Avoidance of normal activity and progressive substitution of lifestyle away from productive activity
- Report of extremely high intensity of pain, e.g., above 10, on a 0–10 Visual Analogue Scale
- Excessive reliance on use of aids or appliances
- Sleep quality reduced since onset of back pain
- High intake of alcohol or other substances (possibly as self-medication), with an increase since onset of back pain
- Smoking

Compensation issues
- Lack of financial incentive to return to work
- Delay in accessing income support and treatment cost, disputes over eligibility
- History of claim(s) due to other injuries or pain problems
- History of extended time off work due to injury or other pain problem (e.g. more than 12 weeks)
- History of previous back pain, with a previous claim(s) and time off work
- Previous experience of ineffective case management (e.g. absence of interest, perception of being treated punitively)

Diagnosis and treatment
- Health professional sanctioning disability, not providing interventions that will improve function
- Experience of conflicting diagnoses or explanations for back pain, resulting in confusion
- Diagnostic language leading to catastrophising and fear (e.g. fear of ending up in a wheelchair)
- Dramatisation of back pain by health professional producing dependency on treatments, and continuation of passive treatment
- Number of times visited health professional in last year (excluding the present episode of back pain)
- Expectation of a 'techno-fix', e.g. requests to treat as if body were a machine
- Lack of satisfaction with previous treatment for back pain
- Advice to withdraw from job

Emotions
- Fear of increased pain with activity or work
- Depression (especially long-term low mood), loss of sense of enjoyment
- More irritable than usual
- Anxiety about and heightened awareness of body sensations (includes sympathetic nervous system arousal)
- Feeling under stress and unable to maintain sense of control
- Presence of social anxiety or disinterested in social activity
- Feeling useless and not needed

Family
- Over-protective partner/spouse, emphasising fear of harm or encouraging catastrophising (usually well-intentioned)
- Solicitous behaviour from spouse (e.g. taking over tasks)
- Socially punitive responses from spouse (e.g. ignoring, expressing frustration)
- Extent to which family members support any attempt to return to work
- Lack of support person to talk to about problems

Work
- History of manual work, notably from the following occupational groups
  — fishing, forestry and farming workers
  — construction, including carpenters and builders
  — nurses
  — truck drivers
  — labourers
- Work history, including patterns of frequent job changes, experiencing stress at work, job dissatisfaction, poor relationships with peers or supervisors, lack of vocational direction
- Belief that work is harmful; that it will do damage or be dangerous
- Unsupportive or unhappy current work environment
- Low educational background, low socioeconomic status
- Job involves significant biomechanical demands, such as lifting, manual handling heavy items, extended sitting, extended standing, driving, vibration, maintenance of constrained or sustained postures, inflexible work schedule preventing appropriate breaks
- Job involves shift work or working 'unsociable hours'
- Minimal availability of selected duties and graduated return to work pathways, with unsatisfactory implementation of these
- Negative experience of workplace management of back pain (e.g. absence of a reporting system, discouragement to report, punitive response from supervisors and managers)
- Absence of interest from employer

Remember the key question to bear in mind while conducting these clinical assessments is *'What can be done to help this person experience less distress and disability?'*

likely outcome (e.g. loss of job, having to start from square one, the need to begin reactivation from a point of reduced fitness, etc.).

2. Be directive in scheduling *regular reviews of progress*. When conducting these reviews shift the focus from the symptom (pain) to function (level of activity). Instead of asking 'how much do you hurt?', ask 'what have you been doing?'. Maintain an interest in improvements, no matter how small. If another health professional is involved in treatment or management, specify a date for a progress report at the time of referral. Delays will be disabling.

3. *Keep the individual active and at work* if at all possible, even for a small part of the day. This will help to maintain work habits and work relationships. Consider reasonable requests for selected duties and modifications to the work place. After 4 to 6 weeks, if there has been little improvement, review vocational options, job satisfaction, any barriers to return to work, including psychosocial distress. Once barriers to return to work have been identified, these need to be targeted and managed appropriately. Job dissatisfaction and distress cannot be treated with a physical modality.

4. *Acknowledge difficulties* with activities of daily living, but avoid making the assumption that these indicate all activity or any work must be avoided.

5. Help to *maintain positive cooperation* between the individual, an employer, the compensation system and health professionals. Encourage collaboration wherever possible. Inadvertent support for a collusion between 'them' and 'us' can be damaging to progress.

6. *Make a concerted effort to communicate that having more time off work will reduce the likelihood of a successful return to work.* In fact, longer periods off work result in reduced probability of ever returning to work. At the 6 week point *consider suggesting vocational redirection, job changes*, the use of 'knight's move' approaches to return to work (same employer, different job).

7. Be alert for the presence of individual beliefs that he/she should stay off work until treatment has provided a 'total cure'; watch out for expectations of *simple 'techno-fixes'*.

8. Promote *self-management and self-responsibility*. Encourage the development of self-efficacy to return to work. Be aware that developing self-efficacy will depend on *incentives and feedback* from treatment providers and others. If recovery only requires development of a skill such as adopting a new posture, then it is not likely to be affected by incentives and feedback. However, if recovery requires the need to overcome an aversive stimulus such as fear of movement (kinesiophobia) then it will be readily affected by incentives and feedback.

9. Be prepared to ask for a second opinion, provided it does not result in a long and disabling delay. Use this option especially if it may help clarify that further diagnostic work-up is unnecessary. *Be prepared to say 'I don't know'* rather than provide elaborate explanations based on speculation.

10. Avoid confusing the *report of symptoms* with the presence of emotional distress. Distressed people seek more help, and have been shown to be more likely to receive ongoing medical intervention. Exclusive focus on symptom control is not likely to be successful if emotional distress is not dealt with.

11. *Avoid suggesting* (even inadvertently) that the person from a regular job may be able to *work at home*, or in their own business because it will be under their own control. This message, in effect, is to allow pain to become the reinforcer for activity – producing a deactivation syndrome with all the negative consequences. Self-employment nearly always involves more hard work.

12. Encourage people to recognise, from the earliest point, that *pain can be controlled and managed* so that a normal, active or working life can be maintained. Provide *encouragement for all 'well' behaviours* – including alternative ways of performing tasks, and focusing on transferable skills.

13. If barriers to return to work are identified and the problem is too complex to manage, referral to a multidisciplinary team as described in the *New Zealand Acute Low Back Pain Guide* (see Appendix D) is recommended.

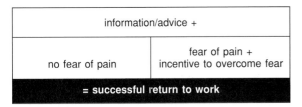

information/advice +	
no fear of pain	fear of pain + incentive to overcome fear
= successful return to work	

Figure 17E.4

What are the consequences of missing psychosocial yellow flags?

Under-identifying 'at risk' patients may result in inadvertently reinforcing factors that are disabling. Failure to note that specific patients strongly believe that movement will be harmful may result in them experiencing the negative effects of extended inactivity. These include withdrawal from social, vocational and recreational activities.

Cognitive and behavioural factors can produce important physiological consequences, the most common of which is muscle wasting.

Since the number of earlier treatments and length of the problem can themselves become risk factors, most people *should* be identified the second time they seek care. Consistently missing the presence of yellow flags can be harmful and usually contributes to the development of chronicity.

There may be significant adverse consequences if these factors are overlooked.

What are the consequences of over-identifying psychosocial yellow flags?

Over-identification has the potential to waste some resources. However, this is readily outweighed by the large benefit from helping to prevent even one person developing a long-term chronic back problem.

Some treatment providers may wonder if identifying psychosocial risk factors, and subsequently applying suitable cognitive and behavioural management can produce adverse effects. Certainly if the presence of psychosocial risk factors is misinterpreted to mean that the prob-

lem should be translated from a physical to a psychological one, there is a danger of the patient losing confidence in themselves and their treatment provider(s).

There are unlikely to be adverse consequences from the over-identification of yellow flags.

The presence of risk factors should alert the treatment provider to the possibility of long-term problems and the need to *prevent* their development. Specialised psychological referrals should only be required for those with psychopathology (such as depression, anxiety, substance abuse, etc), or for those who fail to respond to appropriate management.

Quick reference guide to assessing psychosocial yellow flags in acute low back pain

Differentiate acute, recurrent and chronic low back pain

Acute low back problems: activity intolerance due to lower back or back and leg symptoms lasting less than 3 months.

Chronic low back problems: activity intolerance due to lower back or back and leg symptoms lasting more than 3 months.

Recurrent low back problems: episodes of acute low back problems lasting less than 3 months' duration but recurring after a period of time without low back symptoms sufficient to restrict activity or function.

Key goal

To identify risk factors that increase the probability of long-term disability and work loss with the associated suffering and negative effects on patients, their families and society. This assessment can be used to target effective early management and prevent the onset of these problems.

The acute pain screening questionnaire

Useful for quickly screening large numbers. Interpret the results in conjunction with the history and clinical presentation. Be aware of, and take into account, reading difficulties and different cultural backgrounds.

Clinical assessment

There is good agreement that the following factors are important, and consistently predict poor outcomes:

- presence of a belief that back pain is harmful or potentially severely disabling
- fear-avoidance behaviour and reduced activity levels
- tendency to low mood and withdrawal from social interaction

- an expectation of passive treatment(s) rather than a belief that active participation will help.

Suggested questions (to be phrased in your own style)

- Have you had time off in the past with back pain?
- What do you understand is the cause of your back pain?
- What are you expecting will help you?
- How is your employer responding to your back pain? Your co-workers? Your family?
- What are you doing to cope with back pain?
- Do you think that you will return to work? When?

18

Information for patients

Patients with back pain want information and advice about their problem. von Korff & Saunders (1996) asked primary care patients at a health maintenance organization about their goals when they saw the doctor. They found that patients wanted to understand:

- the likely course of their back pain and associated activity limitations
- how to manage their back pain
- how to return to usual activities quickly
- how to minimize the frequency and severity of recurrences.

These concerns ranked higher than seeking a cause for their back pain or a diagnosis. Both the American and British clinical guidelines emphasize the need to give patients accurate and up-to-date information to help them deal with the problem. Deyo & Diehl (1986) showed that good communication and explanation lead to greater patient satisfaction with care.

There is a wealth of material available for patients with back pain: hundreds of leaflets and booklets and dozens of books. Unfortunately, they are almost all based on traditional ideas about spinal disease and old-fashioned management. If we are going to change clinical management, patient material must be up to date and in line with current clinical guidelines. The message is more likely to get through if patients get the same information and advice from all members of the health care team (Box 18.1). Any written material must reinforce that. However, leaflets and booklets on their own have a limited effect. They are simply an aid to supplement information and advice from the doctor and therapist.

Such material is now available to accompany both the American and British clinical guidelines. The main messages are the same, but it is interesting to compare the content and emphasis. The American material is based on the evidence up to 1992 for the AHCPR (1994) guidelines. It is a balance between traditional medical teaching about spinal disorders and the new approach. The British booklet includes additional evidence available by 1996 and gives a stronger message about staying active. It also makes a deliberate attempt to 'de-medicalize' the problem.

Box 18.1 Information and advice from health professionals

It is important that all doctors, therapists and any other health professionals give consistent advice, in line with clinical guidelines and any patient information leaflets.

- REASSURE that there is no serious damage or disease
- EXPLAIN back pain as a symptom that the back is 'not working properly'
- AVOID labeling as injury, disc trouble, degeneration or wear and tear
- REASSURE about good natural history, providing you stay active, but with accurate information about recurrent symptoms and how to deal with them
- ADVISE to use simple, safe treatments to control symptoms
- ENCOURAGE staying active, continuing daily activities as normally as possible, and staying at work. This gives the most rapid and complete recovery and less risk of recurrent problems
- AVOID 'let pain be your guide'
- ENCOURAGE patients to take responsibility for their own continued management

'Simple backache should not cripple you unless you let it.'

REFERENCES

AHCPR 1994 Clinical Practice Guideline Number 14. Acute low back problems in adults. Agency for Health Care Policy and Research, US Department of Health and Human Services, Rockville, MD
CSAG 1994 Report on back pain. Clinical Standards Advisory Group. HMSO, London
Deyo R A, Diehl A K 1986 Patient satisfaction with medical care for low back pain. Spine 11: 28–30

RCGP 1996 Clinical guidelines for the management of acute low back pain. Royal College of General Practitioners, London
Roland M, Waddell G, Moffett J K, Burton K, Main C, Cantrell T 1996 The back book. The Stationery Office, London
von Korff M, Saunders K 1996 The course of back pain in primary care. Spine 21: 2833–2839

APPENDIX 18A: US Patient guide: Understanding acute low back problems

The *Clinical Practice Guideline for Acute Low Back Problems in Adults* included material for patients. The *Patient Guide* was a brief presentation of the main conclusions of the guideline, written in simple language for patients. The full guideline also included four handouts for the doctor to give to different patients. I have included the AHCPR material in its original form and resisted the temptation to change or edit it.

About the back and back problems

The human spine (or backbone) is made up of small bones called vertebrae. The vertebrae are stacked on top of each other to form a column. Between each vertebra is a cushion known as a disc. The vertebrae are held together by ligaments, and muscles are attached to the vertebrae by bands of tissue called tendons.

Openings in each vertebra line up to form a long hollow canal. The spinal cord runs through this canal from the base of the brain. Nerves from the spinal cord branch out and leave the spine through the spaces between the vertebrae.

The lower part of the back holds most of the body's weight. Even a minor problem with the bones, muscles, ligaments, or tendons in this area can cause pain when a person stands, bends, or moves around. Less often, a problem with a disc can pinch or irritate a nerve from the spinal cord, causing pain that runs down the leg, below the knee, called sciatica.

Purpose

This booklet is about acute low back problems in adults. If you have a low back problem, you may have symptoms that include:

- pain or discomfort in the lower part of the back
- pain or numbness that moves down the leg (sciatica).

Reproduced with permission from the US Agency for Health Care Policy and Research.

Low back symptoms can keep you from doing your normal daily activities or doing things that you enjoy.

A low back problem may come on suddenly or gradually. It is acute if it lasts a short while, usually a few days to several weeks. An episode that lasts longer than 3 months is not acute.

If you have been bothered by your lower back, you are not alone. Eight out of 10 adults will have a low back problem at some time in their life. And most will have more than one episode of acute low back problems. In between episodes, most people return to their normal activities with little or no symptoms.

This booklet will tell you more about acute low back problems, what to do, and what to expect when you see a health care provider.

Causes of low back problems

Even with today's technology, the exact reason or cause of low back problems can be found in very few people. Most times, the symptoms are blamed on poor muscle tone in the back, muscle tension or spasm, back sprains, ligament or muscle tears or joint problems. Sometimes nerves from the spinal cord (see Fig. 18A.1) can be irritated by 'slipped' discs causing buttock or leg pain. This may also cause numbness, tingling, or weakness in the legs.

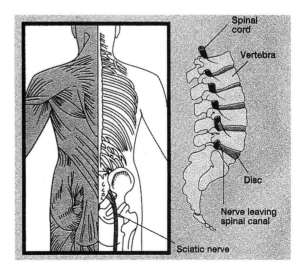

Figure 18A.1 Muscles of the back and the spine.

People who are in poor physical condition or who do work that includes heavy labor or long periods of sitting or standing are at greater risk for low back problems. These people also get better more slowly. Emotional stress or long periods of inactivity may make back symptoms seem worse.

Low back problems are often painful. But the good news is that very few people turn out to have a major problem with the bones or joints of the back or a dangerous medical condition.

Things to do about low back problems

Seeing a health care provider

Many people who develop mild low back discomfort may not need to see a health care provider right away. Often, within a few days, the symptoms go away without any treatment.

A visit to your health care provider is a good idea if:

- your symptoms are severe
- the pain is keeping you from doing things that you do every day
- the problem does not go away within a few days.

If you also have problems controlling your bowel or bladder, if you feel numb in the groin or rectal area, or if there is extreme leg weakness, call your health care provider right away.

Your health care provider will check to see if you have a medical illness causing your back problem (chances are you will not). Your health care provider can also help you get some relief from your symptoms.

Your health care provider will:

- ask about your symptoms and what they keep you from doing
- ask about your medical history
- give you a physical exam.

Talking about your symptoms

Your health care provider will want to know about your back problem. Here are some exam-ples of the kinds of questions he or she may ask you. You can write down the answers in the space below each question:

When did your back symptoms start?

_____

_____

_____

Which of your daily activities are you not able to do because of your back symptoms?

_____

_____

_____

Is there anything you do that makes the symptoms better or worse?

_____

_____

_____

Have you noticed any problem with your legs?

_____

_____

_____

Around the time your symptoms began, did you have a fever or symptoms of pain or burning when urinating?

_____

_____

_____

Talking about your medical history

Be sure to tell your health care provider about your general health and about illnesses you have had in the past. Here are some questions your health care provider may ask you about your medical history. You can write your answers in the space below each question:

Have you had a problem with your back in the past? If so, when?

_____

_____

_____

What medical illnesses have you had (for example, cancer, arthritis, or diseases of the immune system)?

_____

_____

_____

Which medicines do you take regularly?

_____

_____

_____

Have you ever used intravenous (IV) drugs?

_____

_____

Have you recently lost weight without trying?

_____

_____

You should also tell your health care provider about anything you may be doing for your symptoms: medicines you are taking, creams or ointments you are using, and other home remedies.

Having a physical exam

Your health care provider will examine your back. Even after a careful physical examination, it may not be possible for your health care provider to tell you the exact cause of your low back problem. But you most likely will find out that your symptoms are not being caused by a dangerous medical condition. Very few people (about 1 in 200) have low back symptoms caused by such conditions. You probably won't need special tests (p. 337) if you have had low back symptoms for only a few weeks.

Getting relief

Your health care provider will help you get relief from your pain, discomfort, or other symptoms. A number of medicines and other treatments help with low back symptoms. The good news is that most people start feeling better soon.

Proven treatments

Medicine often helps relieve low back symptoms. The type of medicine that your health care provider recommends depends on your symptoms and how uncomfortable you are.

• If your symptoms are mild to moderate, you may get the relief you need from an over-the-counter (nonprescription) medicine such as acetaminophen, aspirin, or ibuprofen. These medicines usually have fewer side-effects than prescription medicines and are less expensive.

• If your symptoms are severe, your health care provider may recommend a prescription medicine.

For most people, medicine works well to control pain and discomfort. But any medicine can have side-effects. For example, some people cannot take aspirin or ibuprofen because it can cause stomach irritation and even ulcers. Many medicines prescribed for low back pain can make people feel drowsy. These medicines should not be taken if you need to drive or use heavy equipment. Talk to your health care provider about the benefits and risks of any medicine recommended. If you develop side-effects (such as nausea, vomiting, rash, dizziness), stop taking the medicine, and tell your health care provider right away.

Your health care provider may recommend one or more of the following to be used alone or along with medicine to help relieve your symptoms:

• _Heat or cold applied to the back._ Within the first 48 hours after your back symptoms start, you may want to apply a cold pack (or a bag of ice) to the painful area for 5 to 10 minutes at a time. If your symptoms last longer than

48 hours, you may find that a heating pad or hot shower or bath helps relieve your symptoms.

• *Spinal manipulation.* This treatment (using the hands to apply force to the back to 'adjust' the spine) can be helpful for some people in the first month of low back symptoms. It should only be done by a professional with experience in manipulation. You should go back to your health care provider if your symptoms have not responded to spinal manipulation within 4 weeks.

Keep in mind that everyone is different. You will have to find what works best to relieve your own back symptoms.

Other treatments

A number of other treatments are sometimes used for low back symptoms. While these treatments may give relief for a short time, none has been found to speed recovery or keep acute back problems from returning. They may also be expensive. Such treatments include:

• traction
• TENS (transcutaneous electrical nerve stimulation)
• massage
• biofeedback
• acupuncture
• injections into the back
• back corsets
• ultrasound.

Physical activity

Your health care provider will want to know about the physical demands of your life (your job or daily activities). Until you feel better, your health care provider may need to recommend some changes in your activities. You will want to talk to your health care provider about your own personal situation. In general, when pain is severe, you should avoid:

• heavy lifting
• lifting when twisting, bending forward, and reaching
• sitting for long periods of time.

The most important goal is for you to return to your normal activities as soon as it is safe. Your health care provider and (if you work) your employer can help you decide how much you are able to do safely at work. Your schedule can be gradually increased as your back improves.

Bed rest

If your symptoms are severe, your health care provider may recommend a short period of bed rest. However, bed rest should be limited to 2 or 3 days. Lying down for longer periods may weaken muscles and bones and actually slow your recovery. If you feel that you must lie down, be sure to get up every few hours and walk around – even if it hurts. Feeling a little discomfort as you return to normal activity is common and does not mean that you are hurting yourself.

About work and family

Back problems take time to get better. If your job or your normal daily activities make your back pain worse, it is important to communicate this to your family, supervisor, and coworkers. Put your energy into doing those things at work and at home that you are able to do comfortably. Be productive, but be clear about those tasks that you are not able to do.

Things you can do now

While waiting for your back to improve, you may be able to make yourself more comfortable if you:

• Wear comfortable, low-heeled shoes.
• Make sure your work surface is at a comfortable height for you.
• Use a chair with a good lower back support that may recline slightly.
• If you must sit for long periods of time, try resting your feet on the floor or on a low stool, whichever is more comfortable.
• If you must stand for long periods of time, try resting one foot on a low stool.

• If you must drive long distances, try using a pillow or rolled-up towel behind the small of your back. Also, be sure to stop often and walk around for a few minutes.

• If you have trouble sleeping, try sleeping on your back with a pillow under your knees, or sleep on your side with your knees bent and a pillow between your knees.

Exercise

A gradual return to normal activities, including exercise, is recommended. Exercise is important to your overall health and can help you to lose body fat (if needed). Even if you have mild to moderate low back symptoms, the following things can be done without putting much stress on your back:

• walking short distances
• using a stationary bicycle
• swimming.

It is important to start any exercise program slowly and to gradually build up the speed and length of time that you do the exercise. At first, you may find that your symptoms get a little worse when you exercise or become more active. Usually, this is nothing to worry about. However, if your pain becomes severe, contact your health care provider. Once you are able to return to normal activities comfortably, your health care provider may recommend further aerobic and back exercises.

If you are not getting better

Most low back problems get better quickly, and usually within 4 weeks. If your symptoms are not getting better within this time period, you should contact your health care provider.

Special tests

Your health care provider will examine your back again and may talk to you about getting some special tests. These may include X-rays, blood tests, or other special studies such as an MRI (magnetic resonance imaging) or CT (computerized tomography) scan of your back.

These tests may help your health care provider understand why you are not getting better. Your health care provider may also want to refer you to a specialist.

Certain things, such as stress (extra pressure at home or work), personal or emotional problems, depression, or a problem with drug or alcohol use can slow recovery or make back symptoms seem worse. If you have any of these problems, tell your health care provider.

About surgery

Even having a lot of back pain does not by itself mean you need surgery. Surgery has been found to be helpful in only 1 in 100 cases of low back problems. In some people, surgery can even cause more problems. This is especially true if your only symptom is back pain.

People with certain nerve problems or conditions such as fractures or dislocations have the best chance of being helped by surgery. In most cases, however, decisions about surgery do not have to be made right away. Most back surgery can wait for several weeks without making the condition worse.

If your health care provider recommends surgery, be sure to ask about the reason for the surgery and about the risks and benefits you might expect. You may also want to get a second opinion.

Prevention of low back problems

The best way to prevent low back problems is to stay fit. If you must lift something, even after your back seems better, be sure to:

• keep all lifted objects close to your body
• avoid lifting while twisting, bending forward and reaching

You should continue to exercise even after your back symptoms have gone away. There are many exercises that can be done to condition muscles of your body and back. You should talk to your health care provider about the exercises that would be best for you.

When low back symptoms return

More than half of the people who recover from a first episode of acute low back symptoms will have another episode within a few years. Unless your back symptoms are very different from the first episode, or you have a new medical condition, you can expect to recover quickly and fully from each episode.

While your back is getting better

It is important to remember that even though you are having a problem with your back now, most likely it will begin to feel better soon. It is important to keep in mind that you are the most important person in taking care of your back and in helping to get back to your regular activities.

It may also help you to remember that:

● Most low back problems last for a short amount of time and the symptoms usually get better with little or no medical treatment.

● Low back problems can be painful. But pain rarely means that there is serious damage to your back.

● Exercise can help you to feel better faster and prevent more back problems. A regular exercise program adds to your general health and may help you get back to the things you enjoy doing.

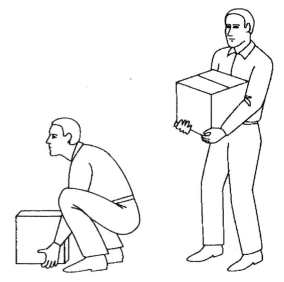

Figure 18A.2   Safe lifting and carrying positions.

APPENDIX 18B: US Clinical practice guidelines: patient discussion handouts

Explanation of handouts

Four discussion handouts for patients are provided. They are sufficiently specific to address a full range of patient concerns. The patient's focus tends to change during treatment. Early concerns may focus on comfort, or fear of potentially dangerous causes of low back pain. Later, questions about special studies, procedures, and diagnoses may arise. The few patients having trouble overcoming their activity limitations may have to consider the relative benefits either of conditioning more vigorously or of changing their activity goals. These handouts are not intended to stand alone for all patients. Rather, they are designed to foster the clinician's discussions with patients about important issues, as needed.

• The first discussion handout is intended to prepare the patient for treatment recommendations. It can be provided to all patients if no serious condition is detected (probably at the first visit).
• The second discussion handout, which is only useful for the 10% of patients who are slowest to recover, helps patients understand about the use of special studies and the potential for diagnostic confusion.
• The third discussion handout is for the same 10% of patients when they are facing further treatment. It helps the patient understand the change in focus from merely treating symptoms and avoiding debilitation to building activity tolerance through safe exercises.
• The last discussion handout is only for those patients who, for whatever reasons, are experiencing difficulties in overcoming their activity limitations. It allows the clinician to help the patient develop an understanding of available options. If the patient is failing to overcome his or her limitations and seeks no

Reproduced with permission from the US Agency for Health Care Policy and Research.

other alternatives, the clinician has an avenue to further address potential nonphysical (e.g., psychologic and socioeconomic) pressures that can accompany activity limitations due to low back symptoms.

HANDOUT 1: BACK PROBLEMS?

The news is good. Your clinician has not found any dangerous causes for your back problem. Almost everyone has a low back problem at some time. In only one person out of 200 does the problem have a serious cause. A medical history and physical examination alone are very good at detecting these uncommon cases.

You should recover soon. Nine out of 10 persons with low back problems recover within 1 month, and most recover even sooner. Therefore, an X-ray of your back or other tests at this time would only waste your time. If your recovery happens to be slower than normal, your clinician will then look further for a reason.

Even with back symptoms, you may be able to continue your usual activities. But you might have to slow your pace. Strenuous activity or heavy lifting could give you trouble. If you work outside the home, much depends on the kind of work you do. Office work may require few changes. On the other hand, if your job involves heavy labor – like a furniture mover – you will probably have trouble working as usual right away.

Age also makes a difference. As we age, so do our spines. Activities that require speed and strength become harder to do. This happens to many people by age 30, to most people by age 40, and to nearly everyone by age 50. Consider your age as you plan your daily tasks when recovering from a back problem.

You can ease your discomfort safely. Your clinician will suggest safe ways for you to be more comfortable as you recover. But staying in bed is usually not the best thing. More than a few days in bed actually weakness your back and could cause your symptoms to last longer. Neither bed rest, medications, nor any other remedies should be expected to do away with *all* the discomfort. It is important to be up and around as much as possible even if you are uncomfortable. The sooner you return to normal daily activities, the sooner your symptoms will disappear.

You may need to make changes in your daily activities

Sitting may not be comfortable. Sitting is not dangerous, but it puts more stress on the back than standing. While recovering, try to spend less time sitting. To make sitting easier, support the curve of your lower back with a towel or small pillow. If possible, use a chair or other seat with a slightly reclining back.

Lifting. Keep anything you must lift close to the belly button. Lifting a carton of milk or orange juice at arm's length can stress your back more than lifting 30 pounds held close to the body. Also try not to bend forward, twist, or reach when lifting.

Exercising can help your back. Your health care provider may suggest safe exercises such as walking, swimming, or riding a stationary bike. If done correctly, these exercises do not stress the back any more than does sitting on the side of your bed (which is not dangerous). What exercising does is keep your back muscles from becoming weakened by not enough activity. In addition, exercise is good for your general health, can speed your recovery, and may help protect you from future back problems. As your symptoms lessen, daily exercise will make it easier for you to resume your normal activities.

Points to remember

- There is no hint of a serious problem.
- Your back symptoms are the kind that usually disappear within a month. Expect a rapid recovery.
- No medications or other treatments, including home remedies, can be expected to relieve all the discomfort immediately.
- You may need to change some daily activities to keep from irritating your back. But stay active enough to keep from weakening your muscles.

- If you are one of the few who is slow to recover, your clinician will look for the reason. Even if you are slow to recover, there is little chance of a serious reason for your back problem.

HANDOUT 2: SEEKING A REASON FOR SLOW RECOVERY...

Special tests may be needed. If your back problem is slow to recover, your health care provider may consider special studies (tests) to find the reason. They may include blood tests, or an imaging study may be needed to view your spine. Nerve tests may help identify certain leg problems. The chances are good that your problem will not be serious. In only one person out of 200 do low back problems have a serious cause.

Why wait to do special studies? You may have read or heard of tests like MRI, CAT scan, or myelogram. These are special imaging studies. They use special equipment to provide different views of body structures like your spine. You may wonder why your health care provider did not order these tests in the first place. There is a good reason. Imaging studies can be confusing. By themselves, they cannot tell the difference between possible causes of a back problem and common changes in the spine because of aging.

As we grow older, the spine changes. Almost half the population has aging changes in the spine as early as age 35. Yet most people who have such changes will not have a back problem lasting longer than 1 month. Remember that nine out of 10 people who have low back problems recover within 1 month. For these persons, imaging studies are unnecessary and confusion can be avoided. The tests could show a condition that is really not a problem and has no connection to back symptoms.

Imaging studies are seldom used alone. Surgery is never based on imaging studies alone. The studies could find something that is not really the cause of your problem. Before deciding whether imaging studies are needed, your health care provider should review your physical examination carefully. He or she may also do other kinds of tests to find evidence of a problem. Ask your health care provider to explain what tests are needed for you.

Box 18B.1 lists a number of terms that are commonly used to describe (diagnose) the cause of low back symptoms. However, scientific studies have not been able to show a connection between these diagnoses and back symptoms. In addition, there is no evidence that these conditions benefit from surgery or other specialized forms of treatment.

Box 18B.1 Common diagnoses used to explain back symptoms

- Annular tear
- Fibromyalgia
- Spondylosis
- Degenerative joint disease
- Disc derangement/disruption
- Adult spondylosis
- Disc syndrome
- Lumbar disc disease
- Sprain
- Dislocation
- Myofasciitis
- Strain
- Facet syndrome
- Osteoarthritis of the spine
- Subluxation

When is surgery a choice? If your back symptoms affect your legs and are not getting better, a herniated lumbar disc (what many people call a 'slipped disc') may be the reason. The disc can press on a nerve root in your back and can either irritate the nerve or affect its function. If tests show strong evidence that this is happening, surgery to take the pressure off of the nerve may speed your recovery.

If your health care provider tells you that surgery is a possibility, ask about your choices. Ask what would happen without surgery. Before agreeing to surgery, get a second opinion from another health care provider. Also, ask about the tests that were done to suggest that surgery is the best approach for your back symptoms. Box 18B.2 lists some conditions or diagnoses that sometimes benefit from surgery or other special treatment.

Tests cannot always tell you the cause of your symptoms. Medical science cannot always explain

---

Box 18B.2 Diagnoses that may benefit from surgery or other treatment

- *Leg pain due to herniated lumbar disc.* Surgery is sometimes used to relieve the pressure on the nerve and can speed recovery if the diagnosis is based on strong evidence. Surgery should not be expected to make the back brand new
- *Leg pain due to spinal stenosis.* Spinal stenosis is an uncommon cause of walking limitation in the elderly. It is very rare under the age of 60. Surgery to take pressure off the nerves can improve walking distance and leg pain
- *Leg pain with spondylolisthesis.* Spondylolisthesis is measurable slippage of one vertebra upon another. In extremely rare cases, the slippage may be great enough to affect nerve root function. Surgery is sometimes used to take pressure off of the nerve and to fuse the vertebrae to prevent future slippage
- *Fracture or dislocation.* Surgery is commonly used to repair a fracture or dislocation if the fracture or dislocation affects the spinal nerves
- *Spinal arthritis.* If the condition is verified by a positive blood test and is not osteoarthritis or degenerative joint disease, nonsteroidal anti-inflammatory drugs (NSAIDs), such as ibuprofen, may be used

---

the exact cause of most common low back symptoms. But medical science is very good at finding out if you have a dangerous condition causing your symptoms. If your problem is not caused by a serious condition, you can continue looking forward to recovery.

Exercise is important. Remember to continue to exercise as you were instructed by your health care provider and as described in Handout 1. It is important not to neglect your muscles. Exercise regularly!

Points to remember

- Special studies are not needed for early detection and care of low back problems.
- Special studies can mislead if used alone. They can give additional information about a problem if used with other evidence.
- If your health care provider suggests surgery, ask what the evidence is for surgery. Ask about your choices and what would happen without surgery. Get a second opinion from another health care provider. Your surgeon will understand how important it is for you to be sure.

HANDOUT 3: OVERCOMING YOUR BACK PROBLEM

By now your health care provider has given you the news that you can comfortably begin to get back to your daily activities. Even if you required surgery, you can now safely begin a specific, gentle exercise program to condition your body and your back muscles. This program will increase your back's ability to help you do the things you want and need to do.

Start with a simple, safe exercise such as walking, stationary bicycling, or swimming to build your general stamina. If you have been inactive, you may need to begin slowly and gradually increase your activity each day. Your health care provider will make specific recommendations for safe exercises that do not stress your back any more than sitting on the side of your bed. Exercise helps because it:

- trains the muscles that protect your back
- conditions your whole body
- stimulates the body to make its own powerful pain killers
- allows you to do more things more comfortably.

You also will find out what you can do easily and what takes more effort.

Reality about back problems. Although your recovery seems slow, your symptoms will continue to decrease unless you are inactive. However, your back may never feel as 'young' as it once did. This happens to many of us by age 30, most by age 40, and just about everyone by age 50. Back problems often are the *first* sign of aging. You may have noticed that few professional athletes can continue competing beyond age 40. While some people may be able to resume strenuous activity after back problems as they get older, it usually needs to be at a slower pace. Most people need to 'shift gears' and make changes in goals and activities as they grow older. Even at a slower pace, exercise will help you to be able to tolerate more of your daily activities.

Once you have had an activity-limiting back problem that lasts more than a few weeks, there is a 40–60% chance of having another back problem within the next few years. However, symptoms usually are not as severe in future episodes as in the first episode.

Success. As you begin to recover, the goal is to try to prevent back problems from returning or, if they do return, from being severe. Success will depend upon two factors. The first is the condition of your protective muscles. The second is the activities you ask your back to tolerate.

Ignoring either of these factors usually means more back problems. For example, a coal miner can expect further problems because mining is so demanding on the back. By contrast, a member of royalty who never needs to stress his or her back but does no conditioning exercises also can expect regular back problems. How well *you* do in the future will depend on what kind of condition you are in and what you ask your back to do. The more easily you and your protective muscles tire, the greater the chance that your symptoms will return. Taking action to condition the protective muscles of your back can reduce your future problems.

Safe exercises that are good for you and your back. Although exercises such as walking, stationary bicycling, or swimming are safe, you may feel some discomfort when you *first* start. After muscles become better conditioned, the soreness goes away. For example, during the winter when the weather is bad and many of us might stay indoors and be less active, the muscles of the back can lose their conditioning. When the first day of spring arrives and many of us go out to garden, the back may begin to ache when the out-of-condition protective muscles easily tire. Continuing such work daily over a few days or weeks *reconditions* the protective muscles so that they don't tire quite so easily, and the soreness disappears.

Remember that an increase in discomfort in an already painful back is common. But safe exercises (that involve less stress on the back than sitting on the side of the bed) should not harm your back. The shorter the time since beginning the conditioning, the greater the chance of increased soreness.

Conditioning requires regular activity. Regular activity is essential to obtain the conditioning effect to protect your back. Conditioning is achieved by building up to 30 minutes of continuous walking, stationary cycling, or swimming at a targeted heart rate (Box 18B.3) or through jogging for 20 minutes. Conditioning works best if combined with your normal, daily activities both at home and at work. Stay as active as possible and exercise every day.

Box 18B.3 Building exercise tolerance

1. Try to maintain your daily activity as close to your normal level as possible
2. As soon as possible begin walking, riding a stationary bicycle, or swimming. Choose what works for you
3. Gradually build up to 30 minutes of activity without stopping
4. Once you can tolerate 30 minutes of activity, establish a target heart rate that will help you to condition your muscles, heart, and respiratory system
5. Then, your health care provider may also recommend some exercises for your back muscles

---

Your health care provider may have suggested ways to modify your daily chores to reduce the chance of irritating your back. Such changes at home or work are usually temporary. They are intended to give you time to improve the condition of your protective back muscles so that you can resume most normal activities. Table 18B.1 offers guidelines to your health care provider on work recommendations to allow you reasonable time to recondition your back. Long-term activity tolerance varies greatly from person to person. Age and overall health are important factors, too. Regular, mild exercise may be enough for some. Others may be able to return to vigorous activities at a slower pace.

Points to remember

- Both your level of physical condition and the stresses you put on your back will determine how often you will have problems and how severe they become.
- Conditioning usually requires daily work and commitment.
- Be sure your activity goal is realistic and you know what it will take to achieve it. Once

Table 18B.1 Guidelines for sitting and unassisted lifting

	Symptoms			
	Severe → Moderate	→ Mild	→ None	
Sitting[1]	20 min → →	→ →	→ 50 min	
Unassisted lifting[2]				
Men	20 lbs → 20 lbs	→ 60 lbs → 80 lbs		
Women	20 lbs → 20 lbs	→ 35 lbs → 40 lbs		

[1]Without getting up and moving around.
[2]Modification of NIOSH Lifting Guidelines, 1981, 1993. Gradually increase unassisted lifting limits to 60 lbs (men) and 35 lbs (women) by 3 months even with continued symptoms. Limit twisting, bending, and reaching. Always lift close to belly button.

you are over your back symptoms or after a month of general conditioning training, your health care provider may suggest that you begin doing back muscle, trunk, or extremity exercises to gain further tolerance for specific tasks.

- If you have great difficulty resuming your previous daily routine, you may need to consider whether your old routine is realistic for you now.

HANDOUT 4: WHEN EXERCISE IS NOT HELPING

By now, your health care provider has made every effort to seek a medical reason for your continued activity limitation. You are well into the exercise program intended to condition your back for the activities you need to do. Unfortunately, for some people success is less easy and slower to achieve. If this is the case, there are many things to consider.

Age is important. Few middle-aged persons have a back that is as strong as it was at age 18. Medical science presently cannot reverse the aging process that limits activities requiring both speed and strength. Young people may find it hard to accept these limitations. Older people commonly find it difficult to give up or alter activities they have been doing for a long time.

Some people continue to look for a 'cure' when progress is slow. Such efforts rarely succeed. Consider a basketball star like Larry Bird. Money was surely no object in seeking a cure for his back problem. He could afford the most expensive medical care and conditioning programs. Nevertheless, he was forced to retire at age 34. His back could no longer tolerate the physical stress of basketball.

How many athletes in strenuous sports can compete beyond age 35 or 40? Very few! Most of us must adjust our activities as we age, regardless of occupation or level of physical condition, many by age 30, most by age 40, and just about all of us by age 50. Some people can continue strenuous activities into their older years, especially if they are able to do it at their own pace. Others may need to consider change.

Be realistic. Ask yourself three key questions about your daily activity requirements:

- Can a reasonable exercise program overcome my back problem?
- Will it be possible to continue a more time-consuming exercise program and my usual daily requirements long term?
- Is there any way I can change my activity requirements now or in the future?

If a reasonable exercise program is not helping you, there are several options: (1) You can choose to put up with discomfort and expect some setbacks; (2) you can begin a more time-consuming conditioning program; (3) you can change the pace of doing difficult activities. This may include a job change. People may use a combination of the three approaches.

Considering a job change is difficult, especially if back problems continue to limit your ability to do your work. Again, ask yourself this important question: 'Is my activity goal realistic, or do I need to look at my options?' A review now might help you avoid a similar dilemma in the near or distant future, when increased age may work against you. Being a few years older sometimes makes a big difference in the chance of changing jobs. Some creative planning could benefit you now, or in the future, especially if your job activities present a problem.

When considering a job or career change, it is important to gather information from many sources. Some possibilities include private career counsellors, local or State employment officers, and veterans' or consumer groups. You may also want to talk to someone working in the field.

Information is your ally. Whether or not you explore job opportunities alone or with professional help, remember this important point: *Only you can find a way to adjust your life, your job, or your plans in a way that is right for you.*

Availability

The AHCPR guidelines are available from the Government Printing Office, Superintendent of Documents, Washington DC 20404. Telephone (202) 512–1800 for price and ordering information.

APPENDIX 18C: The Back Book (UK)

A group of us wrote this patient booklet to go with the RCGP (1996) guidelines. The authors were a family doctor, an osteopath, a physical therapist, a rehabilitation specialist, a clinical psychologist and an orthopedic surgeon. Several of us were in the groups who prepared the CSAG (1994) and RCGP (1996) clinical guidelines. The booklet is strictly evidence-based and in line with current concepts. We put a great deal of effort into making it easy to read. The message is sharply focused and uncompromising: the spine is strong; not a disease; benign natural history; rest is bad, activity is good; self-coping is the answer, doctors are not. We played down the traditional content of anatomy, ergonomics and back-specific exercises.

THE BACK BOOK

The best and most up-to-date advice on how to:

- Deal with backache yourself
- Recover quickly and keep moving
- Stay active and avoid disability
- Help yourself to lead a normal life.

Based on the latest medical evidence.

The new approach to back pain

Back pain has always been very common and we have learned a great deal about it. There has been a revolution in thinking about back care, and we now approach it in a different way.

Most people can and do deal with back pain themselves most of the time. This booklet gives you the best and most up-to-date advice on how to deal with it, avoid disability and recover quickly. It is based on the latest research.

There are a lot of things you can do to help yourself

Reproduced with permission from Roland et al 1996.

Back facts

- Back pain or ache is usually not due to any serious disease.
- Most back pain settles quickly, at least enough to get on with your normal life.

Back pain need not cripple you unless you let it!

- About half the people who get backache will have it again within a couple of years. But that still does not mean that it is serious. Between attacks most people return to normal activities with few if any symptoms.
- It can be very painful and you may need to reduce some activities for a time. But rest for more than a day or two usually does not help and may do more harm than good. So keep moving.
- Your back is designed for movement. The sooner you get back to normal activity the sooner your back will feel better.
- The people who cope best are those who stay active and get on with their life despite the pain.

Causes of back pain

Your spine is one of the strongest parts of your body. It is made of solid bony blocks joined by discs to give it strength and flexibility. It is reinforced by strong ligaments. It is surrounded by large and powerful muscles which protect it. It is surprisingly difficult to damage your spine.

People often have it wrong about back pain.

In fact: It is surprisingly difficult to damage your spine

- Most people with back pain or backache do not have any damage in their spine.
- Very few people with backache have a slipped disc or a trapped nerve. Even then a slipped disc usually gets better by itself.
- Most X-ray findings in your back are normal changes with age. That is not arthritis – it is normal, just like grey hair.

Back pain is usually not due to anything serious

In most people we cannot pinpoint the exact source of backache. It can be frustrating not to know exactly what is wrong. But in another way it is good news – that you do not have any serious disease or any serious damage in your back.

Most back pain comes from the muscles and ligaments and joints in your back. They are simply not moving and working as they should. Or you can think of your back as 'out of condition'. So what you need to do is get your back working properly again.

Stress can also increase the amount of pain we feel. Tension can cause muscle spasm and the muscles themselves can become painful.

People who are physically fit generally have less back pain, and recover faster if they do get it.

So the answer to backache is to get your back moving and working properly again. Get back into condition and physically fit.

It's your back – get going!

Rest or active exercise?

The old fashioned treatment for back pain was prolonged rest. But bed rest for more than a day or two is the worst treatment for backache, because:

Bed rest is bad for backs

- Your bones get weaker
- Your muscles get weaker
- You get stiff
- You lose physical fitness
- You get depressed
- The pain feels worse
- It is harder and harder to get going again.

No wonder it didn't work! We no longer use bed rest to treat any other common condition. It is time to stop bed rest for backache. The message is clear: bed rest is bad for backs.

Of course you might need to do a bit less when the pain is bad. You might be forced to have a day or two in bed at the start. But the most important thing is to get moving again as soon as you can.

Exercise is good for you

Use it or lose it

Your body must stay active to stay healthy. It thrives on use.

Regular exercise:

- gives you stronger bones
- develops fit active muscles
- keeps you supple
- makes you fit
- makes you feel good
- releases natural chemicals which reduce pain.

Even when your back is sore, you can make a start without putting too much stress on your back:

- walking
- exercise bike
- swimming.

Walking, using an exercise bike, or swimming all use your muscles and get your joints moving. They make your heart and lungs work and are a start to physical fitness.

When you start to exercise you may need to build up gradually over a few days or weeks. You should then exercise regularly and keep it up – fitness takes time.

Different exercises suit different people. Find out what suits your back best. Rearrange your life to get some exercise every day. Try walking instead of going by car or bus. Some of the easiest to get back to are walking, swimming, cycling and smooth rhythmic exercises. The important thing is general exercise and physical fitness.

Athletes know that when they start training their muscles can hurt. That does not mean that they are doing any damage. The same applies to you and your back.

No-one pretends exercising is easy. Pain killers and other treatments can help to control the pain to let you get started. It often does hurt at first, but one thing is sure: the longer you put off exercise, the harder and more painful it will be. There is no other way. You have a straight choice: rest or work through your pain to recovery.

Staying active

Dealing with an acute attack

What you do depends on how bad your back feels.

Remember, your back isn't badly damaged. You can usually:

- use something to control the pain
- modify your activities
- stay active and at work.

You may have good days & bad days – that's normal

If your pain is more severe you may have to rest for a few days. You might need stronger pain killers from your doctor, and you might even have to lie down for a day or two. But only for a day or two; don't think of rest as treatment. Too much rest is bad for your back. The faster you get going the sooner you will make your back feel better.

You should build up your activities and your exercise tolerance over several days or a few weeks. But the faster you get back to normal activities and back to work the better, even if you still have some pain and some restrictions. If you have a heavy job, you may need some help from your workmates. Simple changes can make your job easier. Talk to your foreman or boss.

Control of pain

There are many treatments which can help back pain. They may not remove the pain completely, but they should control it enough for you to get active. These treatments help to control the pain, but they do not cure your back. It is up to you to get going and get your back working again

Pain killers: Paracetamol or soluble aspirin are the simplest and safest pain killers. It may surprise you, but they are still often the most effective for backache. Take two tablets every 4–6 hours. Or you can use anti-inflammatory tablets like ibuprofen.

You should usually take the pain killers for a day or two but you may need to take them for a few weeks. Take them regularly and do not wait till your pain is out of control. Do not take aspirin or ibuprofen if you have indigestion or an ulcer problem.

Heat or cold. In the first 48 hours you can try a cold pack on your back for 5–10 minutes at a time – a bag of frozen peas wrapped in a towel. Other people prefer heat – a hot water bottle, a bath or a shower.

Spinal manipulation. Most doctors now agree that manipulation can help. It is best within the first 6 weeks. Manipulation is carried out by osteopaths, chiropractors, some physiotherapists

	Some ways to help your pain	Some things may make your pain worse
Lifting	Know your own strength: lift what you can handle Always lift and carry close to your body Bend your knees and make your legs do the work Don't twist your back – turn with your feet	Lifting without thinking
Sitting	Use an upright chair Try a folded towel in the small of your back Get up and stretch every 20–30 minutes	A low, soft chair Lack of back support Long periods in one position
Standing	Try putting one foot on a low box or stool Have your working surface at a comfortable height	Long periods in one position
Driving	Adjust your seat Try a folded towel in the small of your back	Long drives without a break
Activity	20–30 minutes walking, cycling or swimming every day Gradually increase physical activity	Sitting around all day Never exercising: being unfit
Sleeping	Some people prefer a firm mattress – or try boards beneath your mattress	Staying in bed too long
Relax	Learn how to reduce stress Use relaxation techniques	Worry: being tense

and a few doctors with special training. It is safe if it is done by a qualified professional.

Other treatments: Many other treatments are used and some people feel that they help. It is up to you to find out what helps you.

Stress and muscle tension. If stress is a problem you need to recognize it at an early stage and try to do something about it. It is not always possible to remove the cause of stress, but it is quite easy to learn to reduce its effects by breathing control, muscle relaxation and mental calming techniques.

How to stay active

You can do most daily activities if you think about them first.

The basic idea is not to stay in one position or do any one thing for more than 20–30 minutes without a break. Then try to move a little further and faster every day.

What do you find helps you?

1 _____

2 _____

3 _____

4 _____

5 _____

What do you find makes your pain worse?

1 _____

2 _____

3 _____

4 _____

5 _____

When to see your doctor

You can deal with most back pain yourself, but there are times when you should see your doctor.

What doctors can and can't do

Doctors can diagnose and treat the few serious spinal diseases. But they have no quick fix for simple back pain. You must be realistic about what you can expect from your doctor and therapist:

- They can reassure you that you do not have any serious disease.
- They can try various treatments to help control your pain.
- They can advise you on how you can best deal with the pain and get on with your life.

It is natural to worry that back pain might be due to something serious. Usually it isn't. But you may still feel the need to check. That is one of the most important things that your doctor can do for you.

Doctors can support and help you but it's your back and it is up to you to get it going!

Warning signs

If you have severe pain which gets worse over several weeks instead of better, or if you are unwell with backache, you should see your doctor.

Here are a few symptoms which are all very rare, but if you do have back pain and suddenly develop any of these symptoms you should see a doctor straight away:

- difficulty passing or controlling urine
- numbness around your back passage or genitals
- numbness, pins and needles or weakness in both legs
- unsteadiness on your feet.

Don't let that list worry you too much.

Remember that back pain is rarely due to any serious disease

It's your back

Backache is not a serious disease and it should not cripple you unless you let it. We have tried to show you the best way to deal with back-ache. The important thing now is for you to get on with your life. How your backache affects you depends on how you react to the pain and what you do about it yourself.

There is no instant answer. You will have your ups and downs for a while – that is normal. But this is what you can do for yourself.

Two types of sufferer

One who *avoids* activity and one who *copes*.

☹ The *avoider* gets frightened by the pain and worries about the future.

- The *avoider* is afraid that hurting always means further damage – it doesn't.
- The *avoider* rests a lot, and waits for the pain to get better.

☺ The *coper* knows that the pain will get better and does not fear the future.

- The *coper* carries on as normally as possible.
- The *coper* deals with the pain by being positive, staying active and staying at work.

Who suffers most?

☹ *Avoiders* suffer the most. They have pain for longer, they have more time off work and they can become disabled.

☺ *Copers* suffer less at the time and they are healthier in the long run.

So how do I become a *coper* and prevent unnecessary suffering?

Follow these guidelines – you really can help yourself

☺ Live life as normally as possible. This is much better than staying in bed.

- Keep up daily activities – they will not cause damage. Just avoid really heavy things.
- Try to stay fit – walking, cycling or swimming will exercise your back and should make you feel better. And continue even after your back feels better.
- Start gradually and do a little more each day so you can see the progress you are making.

- Either stay at work or go back to work as soon as possible. If necessary, ask if you can get lighter duties for a week or two.
- Be patient. It is normal to get aches or twinges for a time.

☹ Don't just rely on pain killers. Stay positive and take control of the pain yourself.

- Don't stay at home or give up doing things you enjoy.
- Don't worry. It does not mean you are going to become an invalid.
- Don't listen to other people's horror stories – they're usually nonsense.
- Don't get gloomy on the down days.

Be positive and stay active,
you will get better quicker and have less trouble later.

Remember

- Back pain is common but it is rarely due to any serious disease.
- Even when it is very painful that usually does not mean there is any serious damage to your back. Hurt does not mean harm.
- Mostly it gets better with little or no medical treatment.
- Bed rest for more than a day or two is usually bad for your back.
- Staying active will help you get better faster and prevent more back trouble.
- The sooner you get going, the sooner you will get better.
- Regular exercise and staying fit helps your general health and your back.
- You have to run your own life and do the things you want to do. Don't let your back take over.

That's the message from the latest research – you really can help yourself

Availability

The Back Book is available from The Stationery Office, St Crispins, Duke Street, Norwich NR3 1PD or bookshops (ISBN 0–11–702078–8, price £1.25). Prices for bulk orders are available on application.

Table 18C.1 Patients' acceptance of *The Back Book*

Very easy to read	88%
Information clear and interesting	100%
Gives new and helpful information*	90%
Believe most of what it says	90%
Would tell a friend or family to read it	100%
Length is about right	86%
Think it will help people	100%

*Only four patients said they 'knew most of the information anyway'.

PILOT STUDIES OF *THE BACK BOOK*

Burton et al (1996) tested this booklet in 124 primary care patients attending an osteopath or a community physical therapy department. Almost all the patients found the booklet very easy to read, interesting, believable and helpful, and said they would recommend it to family or friends (Table 18C.1). Despite some professional concern, neither workers nor primary care patients took offense at the concept of avoiders and copers. They also absorbed the main messages (Table 18C.2).

We then looked at how the booklet changed patients' beliefs about back pain and compared this with a non-randomized group of patients who saw the osteopath but did not receive the booklet (Table 18C.3).

The Back Book offers a very different type of patient information, which challenges traditional teaching and advice about how to deal with back pain. The pilot studies show that patients readily understand and accept this new approach and that such a simple booklet can shift their beliefs. We are now carrying out a proper randomized controlled trial to test if it can actually change what patients do.

Table 18C.2 The most important messages that patients took from *The Back Book*

Message	Percentage of readers
Exercise is good	63%
Normal activity is good	41%
Too much rest is bad	31%
Positive attitudes are helpful	22%

Table 18C.3 Shift in scores on Back Beliefs Questionnaire (BBQ): comparing with and without the booklet

	Mean BBQ score ± SD		
	Before	After	P
Booklet + osteopath (n = 31)	29.0 (7.4)	33.8 (6.6)	<0.001
Osteopath only (n = 26)	30.0 (6.4)	31.9 (6.2)	NS

REFERENCES

Burton A K, Waddell G, Burtt R, Blair S 1996 Patient educational material in the management of low back pain in primary care. Bulletin of the Hospital for Joint Diseases 55: 138–146

19

Approaches to chronic low back pain

There is a growing consensus as to how we can improve our management of acute and subacute low back pain, even if we still have a long way to go to put it into practice. This is what this book is all about, for prevention is certainly better and probably easier than cure for chronic pain and disability. But I admit that no matter how much we improve acute care, we will always have some failures. And because of the scale of the problem, even a small failure rate will produce a large number of chronic pain patients. There is also a large pool of existing patients with chronic low back pain who will continue to need care.

The definition of chronic

The usual definition of chronic low back pain is simply pain that continues for more than 3 months. However, as many as 6–10% of adults may have persistent or recurrent back pain which meets that definition. Many of them lead more or less normal lives with only minor modification of their daily activities. They deal with their symptoms themselves and do not seek health care. They have little disability and they are working. They are certainly not 'chronic pain patients' (Fig. 19.1).

The real problem is the 1–2% of adults who have chronic intractable low back pain and disability (Box 19.1). They have been off work for many months or years and have often lost their job. They use more than 80% of all health care for back trouble and the only common feature is that it has failed to give lasting relief.

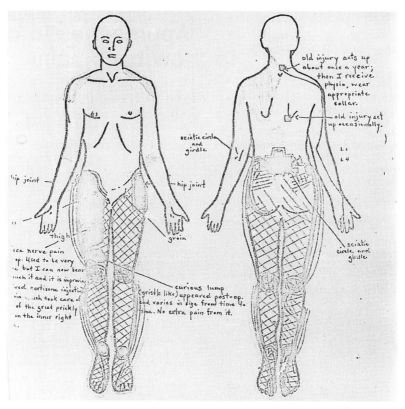

Figure 19.1 Chronic intractable low back pain.

Box 19.1 Features exhibited by most patients with chronic intractable pain

- Persistent pain which may be out of proportion to physical findings
- Progressive inactivity at home, socially and at work, with secondary physical deconditioning
- Disturbed mood; distressed
- Unhelpful beliefs
- Increasing requests for and use of medications or invasive medical procedures
- Treatment failures and side-effects
- Additional stress due to the impact on their family and financial situation
- Anger and hostility.

These are the chronic pain patients for whom we have no simple or easy answer. Remember McGill's curve (Fig. 7.6, p. 110)? These are the patients who are well down the slippery slope.

Health care may have a continuing impact on this situation. The patient, his or her family and health care providers often believe that these problems would all disappear if only they could find a cure for the pain. Such patients may continue to 'doctor shop' for a purely medical answer, but this rarely leads to the magic cure. Instead, this whole approach may actually add to the problem. Health professionals, by continued investigations and physical treatments, may reinforce unhelpful beliefs and behavior. It all takes time, often months or years, during which chronic pain and disability become established. It discourages the patients from taking a more active role in dealing with their pain and in rehabilitation. Side-effects of medication or surgery may increase pain and disability. The patient, the family and health professionals conspire unconsciously to make the problem worse.

Clinical experience and the epidemiology show that we have no good medical answer to chronic low back pain and disability. Perhaps we should look at some alternative approaches to see what we may learn about improving clinical management.

We will look first at treatment for low back pain of more than 3 months' duration. Then we will look at two main approaches to chronic intractable pain:

- pain management
- functional restoration.

Pain management is a psychologic approach that tries to help patients deal better with their pain and so reduce its impact on their lives. Functional restoration is a rehabilitation approach that focuses on disability rather than pain. These two approaches are not mutually exclusive, but they may each teach us different philosophies and principles. Finally, we will consider how we may apply these approaches in routine practice.

TREATMENT FOR LOW BACK PAIN OF MORE THAN 3 MONTHS' DURATION

There is a vast array of treatments for chronic low back pain, but little good evidence on what works. Indeed, the sheer range of treatments may say something about how ineffective most of them are. van Tulder et al (1996) have carried out the most up-to-date and systematic review of this entire field. They defined chronic low back pain quite simply as pain for more than 12 weeks. They found 80 randomized controlled trials (RCTs) of all forms of treatment for chronic low back pain, but many were of poor quality. I am grateful to them for permission to summarize their conclusions.

Drug therapy

van Tulder et al (1996) found moderate evidence that NSAIDs give short-term pain relief, and suggested that we may use them to aid rehabilitation. There are very few RCTs of analgesics or muscle relaxants in chronic low back pain.

Six trials suggested that antidepressants do not provide effective pain relief for chronic low back pain. Turner & Denny (1993) found no significant effect on pain, use of analgesics or functional disability. However, a much larger review of antidepressants in other types of neuropathic pain suggested that they may provide some pain relief (McQuay et al 1996). They may help patients with clinical features of depression.

Epidural steroid injections (see also Koes et al 1995)

Epidural steroid injections give better short-term pain relief than placebo, for patients who have root pain. However, there is no difference between injections of steroids and local anesthetic alone. Epidural injections do not appear to be effective for chronic low back pain alone.

Manipulation

Most other reviewers conclude that the strongest evidence for manipulation is in acute low back pain. However, van Tulder et al (1996) also found nine RCTs of manipulation for chronic low back pain. They concluded that there is strong evidence that manipulation is more effective than placebo, and that there is moderate evidence that it is more effective than most other treatments to which it has been compared.

Traction

There is only one small RCT which showed no significant effect on pain or disability.

Orthoses

There is only one poor-quality RCT which showed no benefit.

TENS

Three RCTs, two of which are of high quality, gave conflicting results. One of the high-quality trials showed short-term pain relief; the other showed no effect. There is no evidence that TENS has any long-term effect.

Acupuncture

There are six RCTs in chronic low back pain, but most are of poor quality and the results are conflicting. Ter Riet et al (1990) carried out a more comprehensive review of acupuncture for all types of chronic pain. They also concluded that most of the studies are of poor or mediocre quality and that the efficacy of acupuncture is still in doubt.

EMG biofeedback

There are five small, low-quality, RCTs in chronic low back pain, four of which reported negative results. This limited evidence suggests that EMG biofeedback is not effective for chronic low back pain.

Exercise therapy

van Tulder et al (1996) found 16 RCTs of exercise therapy for chronic low back pain, although many are of poor quality. Faas (1996) has also reviewed exercise therapy. van Tulder et al concluded that a small majority of these trials, including all three high-quality trials, showed positive results. However, their review did not distinguish specific back exercises from general rehabilitation programs. Faas (1996) looked at six RCTs of specific back exercises in chronic low back pain. Two high-quality RCTs showed that an intensive program of dynamic extension exercises was better than mild exercise (Hansen et al 1993, Manniche et al 1991). One RCT showed that a fitness program was better than home exercises (Frost et al 1995). Intensive exercise showed better overall results at 3–6 months. After 12 months, however, there was little difference, except in a subgroup of patients who maintained intensive exercise and physical fitness.

Back school

Zachrisson-Forsell (1981) started the original 'Swedish back school' and Bergquist-Ullman & Larsson (1977) published the first results. The main aim was education to give better knowledge and understanding, and so enable people to deal better with their own back pain. Four lessons of 45 minutes each dealt with the anatomy and function of the back, ergonomics and activities of daily living. The original back school also taught isometric abdominal exercises, and most back schools still include some form of exercise program. They encourage patients to increase their activity level. Most back schools are run by a physical therapist, often with a special interest and enthusiasm. They teach patients in small groups of about six to twelve. There are now many hundreds of such back schools throughout the US and Europe. The content varies widely, but usually includes teaching of anatomy, biomechanics and skills in daily activities, with an exercise regime.

van Tulder et al (1996) found 10 RCTs of some form of back school for back pain, but only two were of high quality (Harkapaa et al 1989–90, Hurri 1989). Both the high-quality trials showed positive results compared with no treatment. The other, lower-quality trials comparing back schools with various other treatments showed conflicting results. They concluded that there is strong evidence that intensive back schools in an occupational setting can be effective, at least in Scandinavia. Because many programs include so much, there is little evidence on the value of the educational component alone. There is limited evidence on the value of other forms of back school, in nonoccupational settings, in other countries.

van Tulder et al (1996) concluded that there is strong evidence in favour of manipulation, back schools and exercise therapy for patients with chronic low back pain lasting more than 3 months. However, this is mainly for their short-term effects. There is moderate evidence that NSAIDs may provide short-term symptomatic relief. There is little evidence for most other forms of treatment, partly because of the limited number of trials and partly because of their poor quality. What evidence there is suggests that many of these other treatments are ineffective. There is little evidence that any treatment has much long-term impact on the natural history of chronic low back pain. Table 19.1 summarizes these findings.

Scheer et al (1997) recently carried out a very careful and thorough review of occupational outcomes. They found little evidence that any form of treatment for chronic low back pain has much effect on working capacity and return to work.

PSYCHOLOGIC APPROACHES TO PAIN MANAGEMENT

As the limitations of medical treatment for chronic pain were realized in the 1960s and 1970s, psychologists began to develop alternative approaches. Most pain management programs still deal mainly with chronic patients who have exhausted more traditional medical care, and at least 50% have back pain. However, a few programs are beginning to look at the possibility of applying these approaches at an earlier stage. Turner (1996) has argued that all health professionals should be aware of these psychologic principles and apply them to the management of patients with chronic, or indeed even acute, low back pain.

Pain management starts from the assumption that pain is worthy of assessment and treatment in its own right, in contrast with the medical focus on pain simply as a signal of disease or injury. If psychologic and behavioral factors can perpetuate and aggravate pain and disability, then dealing with these issues may help. Even if we have no medical cure for the underlying physical cause of these patients' pain, we should still be able to help them deal with their present situation. Thus,

the aim of pain management is not to reduce pain *per se*, but rather to develop patients' responsibility for their own pain and to help them to control and manage it. This should reduce the impact of pain on their life, help them to be more active, and improve their quality of life (Gatchel & Turk 1996, Main & Spanswick 1998).

We will look at three main psychologic approaches to chronic pain:

- behavioral approaches
- cognitive and cognitive-behavioral approaches
- approaches based on psychophysiology.

Behavioral approaches focus on changing patients' pain behavior. More cognitive approaches focus on mental events – how patients think about and cope with their pain. However, there is no such thing as a purely cognitive approach and most pain management now combines cognitive and behavioral approaches. Psychophysiologic approaches are generally based on the feedback between mental stress and muscle tension. Conceptually, these three approaches are quite different. In practice, however, most pain management combines elements of these approaches to varying degrees.

Behavioral management

This was the first modern psychologic approach to chronic pain, and is probably still the most influential (Fordyce 1976).

Behavioral psychologists focus on pain behavior rather than on the subjective experience of pain. They concentrate on actions and behaviors that they can observe, and are less interested in reports of pain, because these are purely subjective and difficult to measure. They argue that behavior is governed mainly by its consequences. Positive or negative reinforcement from the environment determines whether pain behavior continues, whatever the original cause of the pain. The effects depend partly on the strength of the social reinforcement and are often temporary, so reinforcement must be repeated. Reinforcement tends to be specific to

Table 19.1 Summary of the evidence on effective treatment for chronic low back pain. (After van Tulder et al 1996, with permission)

Effective treatment for low back pain >3 months' duration	Short-term effect	Long-term effect
NSAIDs	+	−
Manipulation	+	−
Intensive exercises	+	+/−
Back schools	+/−	+/−

+, strong or moderate evidence.

the situation, so patterns of behavior learned in one setting may not continue in a different situation.

Fordyce et al (1968) were first to apply these behavioral principles to pain. They accepted that acute pain is due to tissue damage but argued that soft tissue injury should heal within a fixed time. On the basis of collagen healing, this may be about 6 weeks. They then addressed chronic pain that persists beyond the expected healing time mainly as a behavioral issue.

Assessment looks for pain behaviors by which other people know that the patient is in pain, such as limping, resting in bed or taking medication. It looks for direct positive reinforcers such as encouragement and support of these behaviors by family or health professionals. It looks for avoidance behavior, and for negative reinforcement or blocks to well behavior. We must interview the patient and his or her spouse or partner, and observe how they interact. We should also ask about the information and advice they have had from health professionals, or at least their understanding and interpretation of that advice.

Behavioral therapy tries to shape and change behavior by manipulating the social context in which pain and pain behaviors occur. It tries to extinguish pain behavior by withdrawal of its reinforcements. At the same time, it develops healthy behavior by positive reinforcement. It sets specific goals,:

- increase mobility and social activity
- reduce medication use
- reduce health care use.

It removes positive reinforcers such as medications, sympathetic attention, bed rest and release from daily activities and duties. And staff and families are taught to ignore pain behavior. It encourages and reinforces well behavior. It usually involves an incremented exercise program and increasing daily activities. Patients take analgesics and exercise on a fixed timetable. They receive analgesics at regular times, not in response to pain or on demand. Rest and attention are used to reinforce meeting exercise targets, but are withheld

for failure to meet the quota. Graphs and records provide patients with feedback on their progress.

Training involves the patient's partner and family so that they continue the same management at home. Family members become aware of how they have reinforced pain behaviors, and how they should instead reinforce well behaviors. All other health professionals involved in the patient's continuing care must take the same approach. Otherwise, progress will be sabotaged by those who reinforced pain behavior in the first place!

Critics argue that a purely behavioral approach ignores more subjective mental, emotional and psychologic factors and the complex interactions between them. It defines successful treatment purely in terms of reduced pain behavior, but we may question whether that really means less pain or disability (Sternbach 1984).

Cognitive and cognitive-behavioral approaches

Partly in response to these criticisms of the behavioral approach, cognitive approaches place more emphasis on mental events. The gate control theory of pain established the importance of thoughts in modulating pain. Thoughts influence feelings and behavior and this belief led to the cognitive approach (Turk et al 1983):

- psychologic techniques to help patients identify, monitor and change maladaptive thoughts, feelings and behaviors
- teaching pain management skills that patients can apply in their daily lives.

Cognitive therapy is a specific kind of psychotherapy. Psychotherapy is usually given by a trained therapist in a series of one-to-one sessions, and is particularly helpful for emotional problems. Cognitive therapy started for depressed patients, who often have distorted thinking about their situation. Patients could learn which thoughts were a feature of their depression and how certain thoughts could trigger changes in mood. Gaining control over such thoughts led to improvement. We have already noted the similarities between chronic pain patients and depressed patients, so it was logical to try this approach for chronic pain. Cognitive therapy may still be performed on a one-to-one basis, but it is now more frequently part of a pain management program.

Cognitive therapy deals primarily with patients' thoughts and feelings about their pain:

- the meaning of the pain to the patient, their fears and beliefs
- beliefs about how to deal with the pain
- expectations of treatment
- coping skills and strategies.

There are several stages to cognitive therapy (Turk et al 1983):

- Help patients to rethink their beliefs about the pain, and what they do about it. This also depends on building confidence in their own ability and skills.
- Teach patients to use mental techniques to reduce the pain experience
  — stop unhelpful thoughts
  — change the focus of attention
  — redefine pain as a different sensation.
- Teach patients to manage stress more effectively, and to use these skills to help cope with their pain and exacerbations.
- Patients practice and consolidate these skills, with special attention to situations that can lead to relapse.

The behavioral and cognitive approaches are conceptually totally different, but in practice they are really only different perspectives on the pain experience (Sternbach 1984). Cognitive therapy tries to change mental approaches to pain, but its aim is to use that to change behavior. Even if there could be such a thing as a purely cognitive program, it would still use changed behavior as the main measure of outcome and the reinforcement of the patient's beliefs. We may caricature the behavioral approach as social manipulation to produce a reflex response, but that is not completely true either. Active involvement, learning and self-help are fundamental. Changed pain behavior also changes and reinforces the patient's thinking about the pain.

Cognitive-behavioral approaches combine these ideas (Turk et al 1983, Gatchel & Turk 1996). They help patients to restructure the way they think about their pain and at the same time change their pattern of behavior. The goal is to address all the psychologic aspects of the pain problem. Cognitive-behavioral programs:

- encourage the patient to recognize the link between thoughts, emotions and behavior
- help the patient to identify and change unhelpful thoughts, feelings and behavior
- help the patient to acquire mental skills, and the ability and confidence to use them on their own
- use behavioral methods to promote change; however, they use changed behavior to provide feedback on the patient's fears and beliefs – 'learning by doing'
- are active, time-limited and structured
- use a wide range of treatment strategies and techniques, either individually or in groups.

Approaches based on psychophysiology

Psychophysiology looks at the relation between mental events and neuromuscular activity. For example, stress may lead to autonomic arousal, increased muscle tension or vascular changes, and so influence pain. Few people now believe in such psychosomatic mechanisms as a common *cause* of back pain. However, local neuromuscular activity may play a part in chronic pain (Flor & Birbaumer 1994). Psychophysiologic treatments aim to reduce autonomic arousal and muscle tension, and so reduce pain. Some of these techniques overlap with cognitive approaches, but they are more focused on the psychophysiologic mechanisms.

Psychophysiologic techniques include (Turner & Chapman 1982, Main 1992, Main & Spanswick 1998):

- relaxation techniques
- breathing control
- hypnosis
- meditation
- biofeedback.

These techniques may be of potential value to many chronic pain patients. However, it would be better if we could identify the role of psychophysiologic factors in individual patients and then plan specific treatment for them (Main & Spanswick 1998).

Modern pain management

Most pain management now combines cognitive, behavioral and psychophysiologic techniques (Loeser et al 1990, Main 1992, Main & Spanswick 1998).

The common features are:

- a new understanding of pain and disability
- a positive, optimistic mental approach
- aim to combat demoralization: increase confidence
- largely group therapy, but also individual counseling
- active patient participation and responsibility
- skills acquisition and training
- patient takes over management of his or her pain and life
- involvement of spouse or partner.

Results of pain management

Flor et al (1992) reviewed 65 reports of multidisciplinary treatment for chronic low back pain. They concluded quite optimistically that these programs can improve pain, mood and quality of life, and that these effects are stable over time. Overall, they found that patients who receive such treatment improve 30% more than controls. They claimed that it could also reduce medication and health care use and help patients to return to work. Unfortunately, their review included very few RCTs. Most of the studies were of poor quality with inadequate controls. Turk & Rudy (1991) had already pointed out that most studies neglected the major problems of chronic pain patients failing to comply with treatment, dropping out and relapsing.

More recently, van Tulder et al (1996) carried out a much more critical, systematic review. They found 11 RCTs of various forms of cognitive-behavioral therapy for chronic low back pain. Although these were at least RCTs, they still felt that the methodologic quality was low. Eight of the 11 trials showed positive results. Four trials by Turner's group showed positive results compared with waiting list controls. However, Turner herself has pointed out that, although these results were statistically significant, the effect was weak. Five other trials showed positive results compared with other conservative treatments, such as traditional care, physical therapy or exercises. van Tulder et al (1996) were much more cautious in their conclusions:

There is limited evidence that cognitive-behavioral therapy is an effective treatment for chronic low back pain with good short-term results. There is no evidence that one particular type of cognitive-behavioral therapy is more effective than others.

Scheer et al (1997) also recently carried out a systematic review of occupational outcomes. They found little evidence that pain management programs return patients with chronic low back pain to work.

Many of these psychologic approaches are theoretically good and the published results are encouraging if not conclusive, but there are still major questions. At present, there is little evidence to suggest a long-term advantage of any particular approach, or even to suggest that these approaches are much better than good advice, education and exercise. How can we select which patients are most likely to benefit from which form of treatment? The principles look good, but how can we implement them in clinical practice? Can we integrate them into routine health care, medication regimes, physical therapy, rehabilitation and vocational rehabilitation? The ideal management strategy should probably combine health care and physical and psychosocial rehabilitation. However, we have no evidence at present that these approaches actually work in primary care.

FUNCTIONAL RESTORATION

In functional restoration, 'the focus is no longer on diagnosis or treatment but on promoting and maximizing functional abilities in the face of on-going pain and other symptoms' (Teasell & Harth 1996).

Mayer & Gatchel (1988) developed this approach in Dallas in the early 1980s. Like the advocates of pain management, they were dissatisfied with traditional medical treatment. However, they felt that pain clinics simply accepted the pain and just tried to reduce the patient's complaints. Their approach started with new technology that could measure dynamic trunk function (Fig. 19.2), and showed the importance of deconditioning. It also provided a tool to monitor progress. However, this is not just a method of assessment. It led to a whole new approach to the problem, its assessment and its management.

Mayer & Gatchel (1988) stressed that chronic pain is a complex biopsychosocial problem and emphasized the limitations of clinical assessment and diagnosis. To overcome this, they shifted the focus from subjective complaints of pain to objective assessment of function. The general view is that these programs 'essentially ignore the complaint of pain and instead focus on improving the patient's capacity for movement and for tasks specific to his or her occupation'. However, Mayer & Gatchel argue that they do not completely ignore pain. They point out that improved function often leads to less pain. In contrast, subjective expressions of pain usually do not improve unless there is improved function. They do deal with psychologic concerns, although mainly as 'barriers to recovery'. I think it is fair to say that it is a behavioral approach, and draws on the work of Fordyce (1976). Patients receive education and are encouraged to take responsibility for their own care and to reduce their dependence on health care.

One of the main hallmarks of the functional restoration approach is the use of objective measures of function. Mayer & Gatchel used range of movement, static and dynamic strength, endurance, effort and aerobic capacity. They also simulated tasks of daily living and work. The most novel element, however, was dynamic measurement of trunk strength using the new iso-machines. For the first time, this gave an objective measure of trunk function actually during physical activity (Fig. 19.2). It also provided very graphic feedback of progress. There have been two main claims about these machines. First, that they measure 'real' physical impairment associated with low back pain and that this measure is objective, reliable and valid. Second, that only maximal effort can produce a consistent recording and so these machines can assess 'effort'. It is often implied that this can detect malingerers, and therefore that iso-machines can function as 'spinal lie detectors'. Critical reviews have cast doubt on these claims (Newton & Waddell 1993). These machines do produce objective, reliable measures that can monitor progress and provide valuable feedback during rehabilitation. However, they measure performance, not strength or capacity. That performance bears little relationship to pain, disability or capacity for work. There is also no evidence to support the claim that these machines can assess 'effort'

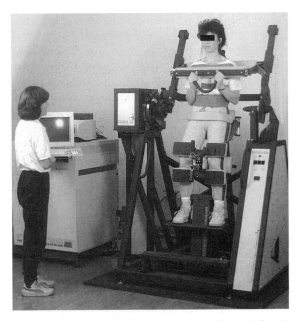

Figure 19.2 Isokinetic assessment on the Cybex II Trunk Flexion–Extension device.

or 'malingering' (Newton et al 1993). It is now clear that we should not over-interpret the results of such assessment.

Iso-machines offer a powerful tool for rehabilitation research, but they may not be indispensable. There are several current efforts to develop low-tech, low-cost methods of functional restoration.

Functional restoration programs are usually full-time for 3–4 weeks. The core is an intensive program of incremented physical activity, and the goal is physical reconditioning based on sports medicine principles. Subjective reports of symptoms are ignored, and there are no passive treatment modalities. Assessment of progress and the continued program depend on objective measures of function instead of subjective reports of pain.

A complete functional restoration program needs an interdisciplinary team of health professionals. This team is led by a physician who can address medical concerns and provide clinical direction. Physical therapists guide the reconditioning program. Occupational therapists provide training in task performance and assist the patient to deal with socioeconomic problems of disability and rehabilitation. Psychologists help patients and other team members to understand and deal with barriers to recovery.

Mayer & Gatchel (1988) stressed the importance of return to work as the main outcome measure. Return to work is objective, and reflects the cost of low back disability to society and third party payers. Cutler et al (1994) discussed the problems of assessing return to work, but it remains one of the most important measures of the impact of low back pain on the individual and society. For all these reasons, it is the most appropriate and best measure of the success of functional restoration.

The results of functional restoration

The first published results were most impressive, and a review by Cutler et al (1994) concluded that functional restoration does return patients to work. Teasell & Harth (1996) carried out a much more penetrating and critical review. Teasell presented this to the Royal Australasian College of Surgeons in May 1997, and I am grateful to him for much of this analysis.

The first two studies of functional restoration by Mayer et al (1985) and Hazard et al (1989) claimed success rates of 85 and 81% return to work. These results have had great influence and are still quoted. However, it is worth looking at these studies in some detail.

Mayer et al (1985) studied 199 patients with chronic low back pain referred to their functional restoration program. They presented the results in three groups of patients. Group 1 was 116 patients who completed the program. Group 2 was 72 patients whom they did not admit to the program because they were refused third party funding. They used this group as the 'treatment comparison group'. Group 3 was 11 patients who were admitted to the program but who dropped out before completing it. Table 19.2 compares return to work in the three groups.

Functional restoration

- The focus is on function rather than pain
- Physical (and psychologic) deconditioning plays a major role in chronic low back pain and disability
- A 'functional restoration' approach to rehabilitation
- Objective measurement of dynamic function and monitoring of progress
- Sports medicine principles
- Psychologic support to disability management and rehabilitation
- The most important outcome measure is return to work

Table 19.2 The original functional restoration results (based on data from Mayer et al 1985, 1987)

Group	Return to work 1 year	Return to work 2 years
1. Functional restoration program	85%	87%
2. No funding	39%	41%
3. Drop-outs	13%	25%
1 + 3. Drop-outs included	70%	69%

These results look very impressive, but we should not accept them at face value. The authors used group 2 as a comparison or control group, but this was not a randomized study. Group 2 was a selected group of patients whom the insurers refused to fund. They were not comparable. Nor are the drop-outs in group 3 a comparison group. These are actually failures of the program who should be included in the treatment group. If we do that (Table 19.2), the success rate falls to 70%. Also, 13% of the original group of patients were lost to follow-up by 1 year, and 20% by 2 years.

Hazard et al (1989) repeated that study, with an almost identical functional restoration program. They studied 90 consecutive patients with 97% follow-up at 1 year. They looked at the results in the same way as Mayer et al and obtained almost identical figures. Eighty-one per cent of patients who completed the program were working at 1 year. Only 29% of those who were denied access to the program because of lack of funding were working at 1 year. Again, the major limitation to this study was the lack of an adequate control group and the pre-selection of patients. Neither of these studies provided much detail on the nature and demands of the patients' occupations. All the same criticisms apply to a multicenter study of functional restoration in 11 US centers (Burke et al 1994).

Oland & Tveiten (1991) tried to replicate Mayer et al's work in Norway. They studied 66, mostly unskilled, blue collar workers who had been off work for 13 months. Their treatment program lasted 4 weeks, with aggressive exercises, group education sessions, consultations with a psychiatric nurse, and vocational counseling. They had 100% follow-up. Only 32% returned to work at 6 months, and by 18 months this had fallen to 23%. They had no control group, but these results were in marked contrast to those of Mayer et al (1985) and Hazard et al (1989).

As you might expect, these differences led to heated debate. Gatchel et al (1992) suggested possible reasons for the Norwegian results:

- inadequate assessment and treatment of deconditioning
- use of passive treatment techniques
- lack of adequate and integrated psychosocial interventions
- differences in the patient population.

Oland & Tveiten (1991) themselves suggested differences:

- patient selection in the US studies
- more psychologists in the US clinics
- differences in the health and social security systems.

This debate led to two proper RCTs of functional restoration (Alaranta et al 1994, Mitchell & Carmen 1990). Alaranta et al (1994) tested a functional restoration program in Finland. They studied 293 patients, aged 30–47 years, who all had low back pain for more than 6 months. Most had been off work for several months. Their full-time, in-patient program lasted 3 weeks. It included an intensive fitness, muscle strengthening and endurance exercise program, and patients continued an exercise program on their own. They had no passive physical therapy modalities. They had intensive psychosocial training but there was no specific vocational rehabilitation. The approach and goals of this program were very similar to those of Mayer & Gatchel (1988), even if the detail varied. The control group had the same length of treatment, which was mainly physical therapy, and the authors estimated that the intensity of exercise was about 40–50%. The control group had no psychosocial training.

This study had 98% follow-up at 1 year. At 3 months, the functional restoration patients improved their range of movement, muscle strength and endurance. However, these improvements were greater in men than in women and fell off by 12 months. Self-reports of physical performance and disability improved in males and females and were maintained at 12 months. These improvements in physical performance were similar to those reported by Mayer et al (1988). Both the treatment and control groups showed variable improvements in their psychologic status. However, there was *no* difference between the treatment and control groups in the number of health care visits or in the amount of sick leave in the following year (Table 19.3).

The other RCT of functional restoration for low back pain was carried out in Canada (Mitchell & Carmen 1990). The Ontario Workers' Compensation Board (WCB) was very impressed by the early published results and pilot studies in Ontario were promising, so they set up functional restoration clinics across the province. Mitchell & Carmen (1990) studied 542 injured workers at two of these clinics in Toronto. All patients were funded by the Ontario WCB and none were refused treatment because of lack of funding. There was no preselection of patients. All the patients were working full-time before their injury and had been off work for 3–6 months before starting treatment. All had 'elements of inappropriate illness behavior with continued pain'. They randomly allocated the patients into equal groups. The first group received an extensive functional restoration program lasting 8–12 weeks, with 40 treatment days lasting 7 hours/day. The program consisted of:

- an active exercise routine using a sports medicine approach
- an individualized goal-oriented program
- intensive psychologic support.

The control group were sent back to their primary care provider for routine management in the community. This study had 100% follow-up. At 1 year, 79% of the treatment group were working full-time, compared with 78% of the control group. There was no difference.

The Institute for Work and Health has studied the more recent performance of these Ontario WCB rehabilitation clinics (Sinclair et al 1997). They followed a further group of about 2000 injured workers for 1 year. The rehabilitation program made no difference to any subjective measures such as pain, disability or quality of life. However, patients at the intensive rehabilitation program stayed off work an average of 7 days *longer*, presumably because they were attending the program. Average medical costs were almost double. This study offers a few possible explanations of these findings. Over the years there has been considerable change in when workers reach the program. Many now come at an earlier stage when they may be more likely to get better quite quickly, with or without treatment. For political reasons, the WCB has also banned any direct contact between the rehabilitation physicians and the patient's workplace.

These Finnish and Canadian trials raise questions about functional restoration. These were both reasonable programs, which took typical, unselected workers. They were proper randomized controlled trials, and show the weakness of the Mayer et al (1985) and Hazard et al (1989) studies on selected patients without proper control groups. They show conflicting results in pain, self-report disability and physical performance. The most striking finding, however, is the lack of effect on sick leave or return to work. Mayer et al and Hazard et al were treating selected patients, even if it is difficult to define them clinically. The Canadian patients certainly showed chronic illness behavior. A

Table 19.3 The Finnish RCT of functional restoration for chronic low back pain (based on data from Alaranta et al 1994)

	Functional restoration	Control rehabilitation program
Reduction in health care		
Visits to physicians	−74%	−67%
Visits to physical therapists	−69%	−77%
Mean days sick leave		
Previous year	58 days	59 days
Following year	34 days	37 days

surprisingly high proportion of the control groups in Finland and Canada did return to work. The other important difference is that neither the Finnish nor the Canadian programs included vocational rehabilitation, which may be a major factor in the success of functional restoration and needs more study. The different social, economic and work environments in different countries may also have an impact.

Conclusion

Functional restoration remains an important rehabilitation principle. It is a well-established and successful approach for conditions such as stroke and spinal cord injury. Functional restoration for chronic low back pain looks promising, but there is a lack of good evidence that it does actually return patients to work. These programs are expensive and labor-intensive, and we need further proper trials. Until we have these, it would seem reasonable to use the principles of functional restoration, but there is little evidence to justify setting up such programs. We also need to be clear about our goals for these patients.

A COMPARISON OF DIFFERENT APPROACHES TO CHRONIC PAIN

Main & Benjamin (1995) made a useful comparison of these approaches to chronic pain (Tables 19.4–19.6). Traditional medical care is usually on a one-to-one health professional–patient basis.

The focus is on diagnosis and treatment of the cause of pain, and assumes that if we cure the pain, we will automatically restore normal function.

Back schools are primarily educational, working on the principle that better information will help the person to take better care of their back. They emphasize improving physical function, but there is little psychologic or vocational content.

Functional restoration focuses on return to work and tries to 'normalize' back function. It ignores biomedical issues and pays little attention to pain. It is a behavioral approach and addresses psychologic issues mainly as 'barriers to recovery'.

Pain management aims to improve quality of life but pays little attention to biomedical issues or return to work. It has a high psychologic content and emphasis on self-help.

A CLINICAL PRACTICE GUIDELINE FOR CHRONIC PAIN SYNDROME PATIENTS (condensed from Sanders et al 1996, with permission)

How can we apply these ideas to our routine management of the patient with chronic low back pain? When we consider the effort that has gone into guidelines for acute low back pain, it is surprising that there are no chronic guidelines. The *New Zealand Yellow Flags Guide* looks at the transition from acute to chronic, but all the back pain guidelines stop short of chronic pain.

Table 19.4 A general comparison of different approaches to chronic pain (from Main & Benjamin 1995, with permission from Oxford University Press)

	General medical approach	Back schools	Functional restoration programs	Pain management programs
Stage in illness	Acute/chronic	Pre acute Subacute	Chronic	Chronic
General aim	Treatment	Prevention	Rehabilitation	Improve quality of life
Occupational emphasis	Minor	Moderate	Major	Minor/moderate
Professional contact	Individual/ multidisciplinary	Multidisciplinary/ group	Multidisciplinary/ individual	Interdisciplinary/ group

Table 19.5 A comparison of philosophy of care (from Main & Benjamin 1995, with permission from Oxford University Press)

	General medical approach	Back schools	Functional restoration programs	Pain management programs
Education	None	Major	Moderate/major	Major
Patient involvement in:				
treatment	None	Major	Major	Major
decision making	None	Minor	Minor	Major
Emphasis on self-help	None	Major	Major	Major
Emphasis on return to work	Minor	Minor	Major	Minor

Table 19.6 A comparison of treatment goals (from Main & Benjamin 1995, with permission from Oxford University Press)

	General medical approach	Back schools	Functional restoration programs	Pain management programs
Pain reduction	Major	Minor	Minor	Minor
Increase mobility	Minor	Moderate	Major	Major
Increase strength	Minor	Minor	Major	Minor
Reduce distress	None	Minor	None/minor	Major
Reduce invalidism	None	Minor	Moderate	Major
Give coping skills	None	Moderate	Minor	Major

Sanders et al (1996) made a first attempt at a guideline for chronic intractable pain. It is not specifically for low back pain, although that accounts for the majority of these patients. It excludes cancer pain. The American Pain Society set up this project, but did not accept the guideline, and it was then adopted by the Academy of Physical Medicine and Rehabilitation. I think it is fair to say that this is a rehabilitation view of the problem, which reflects the background of its authors. It draws heavily on the principles of pain management and functional restoration that we have already discussed in this chapter. The guideline was written mainly for pain programs, but the authors suggest that all health professionals dealing with these patients should apply as many of these principles as possible.

Treatment goals

The goals for treating patients with chronic pain include:

- reduce the misuse of medications (prolonged use of opioids or sedative-hypnotics in more than recommended daily doses) and invasive medical procedures
- maximize and maintain physical activity
- return to productive activity at home, socially and/or at work
- increase the patient's ability to manage pain and related problems
- reduce subjective pain intensity
- reduce or stop the use of health care services for pain
- assist to resolve any medicolegal issues and allow case settlement

- minimize treatment costs without sacrificing quality of care.

There should be a strong emphasis on increasing patients' level of function and their ability to manage their symptoms, even if it is not possible to reduce their pain.

Clinical evaluation

These patients need thorough assessment to plan their management. Medical evaluation should include a detailed medical history, review of medical records and test results, and physical examination. Psychologic evaluation should include developmental history, mental status examination, and analysis of behavior and function. It may also include further psychologic testing to clarify or quantify symptoms and disability. Physical functional evaluation at the onset of treatment should include active and passive range of movement, muscular strength and stamina assessment, and evaluation of activities of daily living. If return to work is a realistic goal or there is a disability claim, these patients also need a vocational and disability evaluation.

Clinical evaluation and assessment of progress should continue throughout treatment. Update the management plan regularly to achieve as many of the treatment goals as possible.

There should be close communication between all health professionals who care for the patient, to coordinate their management.

Treatment

There is no clear evidence as to which treatments are most effective to achieve these goals. On the basis of the available evidence, Sanders et al (1996) recommended that the following treatments should be available.

Medication.

- Most patients should be tried or continued on NSAIDs and/or antidepressant medication for pain control.
- The use of opioids and sedative-hypnotics should be limited, and avoided if possible.

Some patients may require very occasional use of these medications for acute exacerbations, but only in the recommended daily dose for 1–10 days. Until better evidence is available, these drugs should be used with extreme caution.

- Primary alcohol or drug abuse should be treated before patients are admitted to the pain rehabilitation program.

Physical and occupational therapy. These patients need active physical and occupational therapy. Again, the goal is reactivation and improved function. Patients should be taught awareness of body mechanics and ergonomics. They should have an active exercise program to gradually improve general fitness, strength, coordination, range and flexibility of motion, and posture. Passive modalities should only be used in a secondary, supportive role to aid active rehabilitation. Occupational therapy may assist patients to improve their daily independence and to return to work. Whenever possible, patients should be given an active exercise program at the start of treatment, which they can continue independently at home.

Psychologic support. These patients need psychologic support to deal with their pain, assist in pain management, and overcome barriers to progress. Each patient should have an individual treatment plan that may include individual and group sessions.

Vocational and disability management. If return to work is a realistic possibility, treatment should include vocational and disability management. This may involve the following elements:

- multidisciplinary assessment of the pain problem
- job site analysis and initiation of job specific reconditioning
- vocational evaluation to assess ability to perform vocational tasks and possible transferable skills
- evaluation of residual functional capacity and impairment levels.

Invasive treatment. As an adjunct to the primary treatments, there may be a role for more invasive methods in selected patients.

Nerve blocks and trigger point injections can assist pain control during the initial phase of rehabilitation, and enable patients to start active exercise. They should be for a strictly limited time and only if the patient shows improvement in *function*. They should not be used in isolation just for symptom relief.

More invasive medical procedures. Spinal surgery is not helpful for most chronic pain patients unless there are clear indications of a new, surgically treatable lesion. Repeated spinal surgery in these patients is rarely indicated or successful. Implanted spinal devices, continuous infusion devices and brain stimulation have low to modest long-term effectiveness, and are also invasive and expensive. They cannot be recommended for chronic pain patients at this time.

Future directions

Many of these approaches seem reasonable, and they offer a basis for management of these difficult patients. However, noone has a good answer to chronic intractable low back pain and disability. In view of the enormous human and social costs, we urgently need more research into effective methods of chronic pain management and rehabilitation. This also reinforces my plea for better understanding and management of all low back pain to prevent many of these people ever becoming chronic back cripples.

REFERENCES

Alaranta H, Rytokoski U, Rissanen A et al 1994 Intensive physical and psychosocial training program for patients with chronic low back pain. A controlled clinical trial. Spine 19: 1339–1349

Bergquist-Ullman M, Larsson U 1977 Acute low back pain in industry. Acta Orthopaedica Scandinavica (supplement) 170: 1–117

Burke S A, Harms-Constas C K, Aden P S 1994 Return to work/work retention outcomes of a functional restoration program. A multi-center, prospective study with a comparison group. Spine 17: 1880–1886

Cutler R B, Fishbain D A, Rosomoff H L, Abdel-Moty E, Khalil T M, Rosomoff R S 1994 Does non-surgical pain center treatment of chronic pain return patients to work? A review and meta-analysis of the literature. Spine 19: 643–652

Faas A 1996 Exercises: which ones are worth trying, for which patients, and when? Spine 21: 2874–2879

Flor H, Birbaumer N 1994 Acquisition of chronic pain: psychophysiologic mechanisms. American Pain Society Journal 3: 119–127

Flor H, Fydrich T, Turk D C 1992 Efficacy of multidisciplinary pain treatment centers: a meta-analytic review. Pain 49: 221–230

Fordyce W E 1976 Behavioural methods for chronic pain and illness. Mosby, St Louis

Fordyce W E, Fowler R S, Lehmann J F, Delateur B J 1968 Some implications of learning in problems of chronic pain. Journal of Chronic Disease 21: 179–190

Frost H, Klaber Moffet J A, Moser J S, Fairbank J C T 1995 Randomised controlled trial for evaluation of fitness programme for patients with chronic low back pain. British Medical Journal 310: 151–154

Gatchel R J, Mayer T G, Hazard R G, Rainville J, Mooney V 1992 Functional restoration. Pitfalls in evaluating efficacy (editorial). Spine 17: 988–995

Gatchel R J, Turk D C 1996 Psychological approaches to pain management. Guilford Publications, New York

Hansen F R, Bendix T, Skow P et al 1993 Intensive, dynamic back muscle exercises, conventional therapy or placebo control treatment of low back pain. Spine 18: 98–107

Harkapaa K, Jarvikoski A, Mellin G, Hurri H 1989–90 A controlled study on the outcome of inpatient and outpatient treatment of low-back pain. Scandinavian Journal of Rehabilitation Medicine 21: 81–89, 91–95; 22: 181–194

Hazard R G, Fenwick J W, Kalisch S M, Redmond J, Reeves V, Reid S, Frymoyer J W 1989 Functional restoration with behavioural support: a one year prospective study of patients with chronic low back pain. Spine 14: 157–161

Hurri H 1989 The Swedish back school in chronic low back pain. Part I. Benefits. Scandinavian Journal of Rehabilitation Medicine 21: 33–40

Koes B W, Scholten R J P M, Mens J M A, Bouter L M 1995 Efficacy of epidural steroid injections for low-back pain and sciatica: a systematic review of randomized clinical trials. Pain 63: 279–288

Loeser J D, Seres J L, Newman R I 1990 Interdisciplinary, multimodal management of chronic pain. In: Bonica J J (ed) The management of pain, 2nd edn. Lea & Febiger, Philadelphia, ch 100, p 2107–2120

Main C J 1992 Psychological treatment. In: Jayson M I V (ed) The lumbar spine and back pain, 4th edn. Churchill Livingstone, Edinburgh, ch 26, p 487–505

Main C J, Benjamin S 1995 Psychological treatment and the health care system; the chaotic case of back pain. Is there a need for a paradigm shift? In: Mayou R, Bass C Sharpe (eds) Treatment of functional somatic symptoms. Oxford University Press, Oxford, ch 12, p 214–230

Main C J, Spanswick C C (eds) 1998 Textbook on interdisciplinary pain management. Churchill Livingstone, Edinburgh, in press

McGill C M 1968 Industrial back programmes: a control program. Journal of Occupational Medicine 10: 174–178

McQuay H J, Tramer M, Nye B A, Carroll D, Wiffen P J, Moore R A 1996 A systematic review of antidepressants in neuropathic pain. Pain 68: 217–227

Manniche C, Lundberg E, Christensen I, Bensen I, Hesselsoe G 1991 Intensive dynamic exercises for chronic low back pain: a clinical trial. Pain 47: 53–63

Mayer T G, Gatchel R J 1988 Functional restoration for spinal disorders: the sports medicine approach. Lea & Febiger, Philadelphia, p 1–321

Mayer T, Gatchel R, Kishino N et al 1985 Objective assessment of spine function following industrial injury. A prospective study with comparison group and one-year follow-up. Spine 10(6): 482–493

Mayer T G, Gatchel R J, Mayer H, Kisnino N D, Keeley J, Mooney V 1987 A prospective two year study of functional restoration in industrial low back injury. Journal of the American Medical Association 258: 1763–1767

Mitchell R I, Carmen G M 1990 Results of a multicenter trial using an intensive active exercise program for the treatment of acute soft tissue and back injuries. Spine 15: 514–521

Newton M, Thow M, Somerville D, Henderson I, Waddell G 1993 Trunk strength testing with iso-machines. Part II Experimental evaluation of the Cybex II Back Testing System in normal subjects and patients with chronic low back pain. Spine 18: 812–824

Newton M, Waddell G 1993 Trunk strength testing with iso-machines. Part I Review of a decade of clinical evidence. Spine 18: 801–811

Oland G, Tveiten G 1991 A trial of modern rehabilitation for chronic low-back pain and disability: vocational outcome and effect on pain modulation. Spine 16: 457–459

Sanders S H, Rucker K S, Anderson K O et al 1996 Guidelines for program evaluation in chronic non-malignant pain management. Journal of Back and Musculoskeletal Rehabilitation 7: 19–25

Scheer S J, Watanabe T K, Radack K L 1997 Randomized controlled trials in industrial low back pain. Part 3. Subacute/chronic pain interventions. Archives of Physical Medicine and Rehabilitation 78: 414–423

Sinclair S, Hogg-Johnson S, Mondloch M V, Shields S A 1997 Evaluation of effectiveness of an early, active intervention program for workers with soft tissue injuries. Spine 22: 2919–2931

Sternbach R A 1984 Behaviour therapy. In: Wall P D, Melzack R (eds) Textbook of pain. Churchill Livingstone, Edinburgh, ch 3, p 800–805

Teasell R W, Harth M 1996 Functional restoration: returning patients with chronic low back pain to work – revolution or fad? Spine 21: 844–847

ter Riet G, Kleijnen J, Knipschild P 1990 Acupuncture and chronic pain: a criteria-based meta-analysis. Journal of Clinical Epidemiology 43: 1191–1199

Turk D C, Meichenbaum D H, Genest M 1983 Pain and behavioural medicine. A cognitive-behavioural perspective. Guilford Press, New York

Turk D C, Rudy T E 1991 Neglected topics in the treatment of chronic pain patients: relapse, noncompliance and treatment adherence. Pain 44: 5–28

Turner J A 1996 Educational and behavioral interventions for back pain in primary care. Spine 21: 2851–2859

Turner J A, Chapman C R 1982 Psychological interventions for chronic pain, a critical review. I Relaxation, training and biofeedback. Pain 12: 1–21

Turner J A, Denny M C 1993 Do anti-depressant medications relieve chronic low back pain? Journal of Family Practice 37: 545–553

van Tulder M W, Koes B W, Bouter L M 1996 Conservative treatment of chronic low back pain. A mega-analysis of 80 randomized trials of 14 interventions. In: van Tulder M W, Koes B W, Bouter L M (eds) Low back pain in primary care. Institute for Research in Extramural Medicine, Amsterdam, p 245–285

Zachrisson-Forsell M 1981 The back school. Spine 6: 104–106

20

UK health care for backs

Health professionals spend their working lives treating individual patients, and it is difficult to see the broad picture of health care. Let us now try to look at it from a different perspective. What are the health care resources devoted to back pain? Let us look first at the UK, where the National Health Service (NHS) may make it easier to see the whole picture.

Remember the background of need (Ch. 5). There are now 55 million people in Britain, but back trouble mainly affects adults, and the number of people aged 16 or over is 44 million. Twenty-seven million are employed: 15 million men and 12 million women, although many, particularly women, only work part-time. Thirty-seven per cent of adults have back pain lasting at least 24 hours each year, i.e. about 16 million people. Ten million or more of them have back pain lasting at least 2 weeks each year. Three to four per cent of those aged 16–44 years, and 5–7% of those aged 45–64 years, say that their back trouble is a 'chronic illness'.

So, who gets health care for back pain in the UK? Who do they see? And what happens to them?

In the UK, back pain accounts for:
- 4% of all family doctor consultations
- 5% of elective referrals to medical specialists
- 15% of state sickness benefits.

The National Health Service

The health care system in Britain is very different from that in the US. The NHS provides 97–98% of all health care in Britain. The NHS was started in 1948 with the basic principle that care should be free when you need it and should be funded from taxation. The NHS now gets 6.1% of the GNP, which is about the lowest in the Western world. Health care costs are rising faster than inflation, so the underfunding is getting worse. It is not possible to meet unrestrained demand with limited resources and the result is waiting lists. You often wait 2–7 days for an appointment to see a family doctor. It may take weeks or even months to see a therapist. It takes months – sometimes many months – to see a specialist. You may then join another waiting list for surgery and in some places that will take more than a year. Recent political reforms and patient charters are pushing down waiting times and stopping the worst excesses, but waiting lists are still a major problem. On the whole, the NHS is quite good at seeing urgent and emergency cases. The problem is how to provide an adequate service for the large numbers of 'routine' patients – and much back pain is regarded as routine.

Access to NHS service is through your family doctor or general practitioner. Everyone in Britain has a GP and many people stay with the same GP for years. In theory, and often in practice, GPs know their patients. They know their medical histories and their social and family background. The GP is the 'gate keeper' who controls referral to a specialist and the choice of specialist, although patients can request referral and a second opinion. Access to physiotherapy – the British term for physical therapy – is also through the GP. Osteopathy and chiropractic are not available at present on the NHS, although this may change. The only way to bypass your GP for NHS treatment is through a hospital accident and emergency (A & E) department. Each year nearly half a million people attend A & E departments with back pain. These departments are really meant for 'accident and emer-

gency' cases but people can walk in off the street. This may sometimes give a more direct route to hospital services, but at other times that attempt is rebuffed.

All NHS staff, therapists and MDs alike, are salaried. So there is no direct financial incentive to NHS investigation or treatment.

Private medicine only provides 2–3% of all health care in Britain. It includes medical specialists (MDs), who usually work both in the NHS and in private practice, some physiotherapists, and all chiropractors and osteopaths. Private medical specialists in the UK function very much as in the US. In the UK, however, patients usually get their GP to refer them to a private medical specialist and do not self-refer. Physiotherapy practice in the UK is very similar to physical therapy in the US. Chiropractors in the UK have very similar training, professional status and practice as in the US, but they are far fewer. Osteopaths, however, are very different. In the US, a DO is more or less the same as an MD and functions very much as any other physician, whether in family practice or as a medical specialist. In the UK, however, osteopaths function much more like chiropractors. Most patients go directly to any of these private therapists and few GPs refer patients to them. Access to private therapy is usually within a matter of days, which is one of its major advantages over the NHS. Many private health care insurance schemes do cover osteopathy or chiropractic, but only if authorized by a GP or medical specialist. So in practice, most patients consult and pay for an osteopath or chiropractor themselves.

Patients also attend their GP for sick certificates. Employers, private insurance and state benefits all demand sick certificates from an MD. Registered osteopaths and chiropractors can legally issue sick certificates, but they rarely do. Since 1982, patients have been able to sign their own sick certificates for up to 7 days.

Health care statistics

We can get information about health care from patients or from medical records, but these sources are very different. They ask different questions and give different results. They have different problems and errors:

Population surveys depend on patients' own memory of health care. The answers are subjective and there is no cross-check. The answers vary with the exact wording of the questions. The questions usually define a time period, often of 1 year, but the longer the period, the less accurate the answers. If a patient has had a lot of trouble, he or she is more likely to answer 'yes', even if his or her treatment was actually before the time period of the question. Many questions simply ask 'Have you seen ...?' or 'Have you had ...?', but perhaps back pain was not the main reason for consulting. Patient and doctor may have different ideas of what the consultation was about. The patient may indeed have back pain, but the doctor may not think that was the main reason for consulting. For all these reasons, population surveys probably over-estimate health care for back pain; or they may over-estimate serious health problems but under-estimate minor problems because people forget.

Medical records have other problems. They focus on medical diagnosis or at least the clinical problem, but this does not always reflect the patient's concerns or reason for consulting. They record the main problem but may not include all secondary symptoms or problems. Patients with back pain do often have other problems and the doctor must judge which to record as the main problem. Medical records are often sparse and the coding of data is crude. For example, it is often difficult to separate low back problems from neck problems in official UK statistics. These statistics depend on large numbers of clerical staff collecting and sorting data. With all these potential problems, it is not surprising that most NHS statistics have an error of at least 15% and sometimes much more. Data also comes from different sources and methods and may not be comparable. They reflect official interest and do not give a complete picture. The Department of Social Security, for example, records state benefits paid, which is not the same as work loss or sickness. Most official UK figures omit all private health care. For all these reasons, official statistics probably under-estimate health care for back pain.

The true figure probably lies between these two estimates. Or they may tell us different things. Medical records may give a better estimate of health care resources used mainly for back pain, while population surveys may give a better estimate of total perceived need for health care for back pain.

The other major problem is that official statistics are often several years out of date. Most health care use for back pain is increasing over time, so we must place all data in its correct time frame.

This chapter offers an overview of health care for back pain in Britain. If you wish more detailed statistics and references you should see Waddell (1994). The largest recent national population survey on health care for back problems in the UK is Mason (1994). The best and most comprehensive medical record data is the Fourth National Morbidity Survey in General Practice (McCormick et al 1995).

- Population surveys and official health care statistics give different results
- People's reports in population surveys overestimate health care use
- Official NHS statistics have an error of up to 15% and underestimate health care use

---

WHO CONSULTS?

No health worker dealing with back pain should ever forget that most people deal with it themselves most of the time. The Consumers' Association (1985) found that of those British people who had ever had back pain, about one-third had sought care in the previous year; one-third had had treatment at some time in the past but not in the previous year; and one-third had never seen anyone about it. Mason (1994) found that half of those with back pain in the previous year had sought health care for it in that year.

There is no imperative about health care for back pain. It is not life-threatening and noone has to get treatment. Nor is it only a question of severity of pain. People with more severe and more prolonged pain are more likely to seek help, while those with less severe and shorter periods of pain are more likely to deal with it themselves (Tables 20.1 and 20.2). But a surprising number of people who say that their pain is very severe and present all or most of the year still do not seek any health care – 18% of those who say they have 'unbearable pain' have never seen a doctor.

Table 20.1 How severity of pain affects consulting in the UK (based on data from Consumer's Association 1985)

	Seen GP in the past year	No health care in the past year
Duration of back pain in the past year		
None	12	211
Part of the year	132	310
All or most of the year	126	79
Severity of back pain on a scale 0–10		
0–4	48	190
4–7	111	141
7–10	99	59

Table 20.2 How severity of pain affects consulting in the US (based on data from the *Nuprin Pain Report* (Taylor & Curran 1985))

Severity of back pain on a scale 0–10	Percentage who have ever consulted a doctor
Slight 0–3	39%
Moderate 4–6	51%
Severe 7–9	74%
Unbearable 10	82%

The *South Manchester Study* (Croft et al 1994) also found little difference in the back pain described by people who saw their GP and those who dealt with it on their own (Table 20.3). The greatest difference was that more of those who were off work saw their doctor, which may just reflect the need to see a doctor for a sick certificate.

What people do about back pain depends as much on the person as on their medical state. The *Nuprin Pain Report* found that people with more stress are more likely to seek medical help. It is a matter of how they view the problem, how they react and how they try to deal with it. Many factors affect whether they seek health care (Mechanic 1968):

- severity of symptoms
- effect on quality of life
- fear and anxiety
- attitudes and beliefs about backache and what they should do about it
- family and fellow workers' attitudes and beliefs
- expectations and experience of health care for backache
- availability, social costs and benefits of health care
- need for sick certification to stay off work.

There are many steps in seeking health care:

- recognize symptoms
- self-treatment
- communication with family and fellow workers
- assess symptoms

Table 20.3 Nature of low back pain and disability in adults who have had pain in the past year (from the *South Manchester Study*, with permission)

	Adults with back pain who have not consulted*	Adults who have consulted their GP*
Continuous pain	18%	31%
Pain down leg	46%	36%
More than 3 months of pain in the past year	37%	38%
Restricted activity	44%	55%
Needed bed rest	18%	20%
Off work due to low back pain	8%	23%

*Percentages of those with back pain.

- express concern
- assume sick role
- assess treatment options
- choice of treatment
- consultation
- investigation and treatment
- assess how treatment affects symptoms
- recovery and rehabilitation.

Patients with chronic pain may recycle through some of these steps again and again.

Different patients may have very different reasons for consulting. The same patient may have different reasons at different times. Recognizing and meeting their needs may be the key to a successful consultation and patient satisfaction.

Most people deal with back pain themselves most of the time
- Only about a quarter or a third of people who have back pain each year consult a doctor
- There is little difference in the back pain described by those who consult a doctor and those who deal with it themselves
- Many factors influence the decision to seek health care for back pain

---

GP consultation

Eighty-five per cent of people who seek any health care for backache in the UK see their GP (Consumers' Association 1985, Mason 1994). The other 15% seek private health care only. For all health reasons, 78% of the population of the UK see their GP each year: 43 million people see their GPs some 130 million times (McCormick et al 1995).

Although back pain is one of the two or three most common bodily symptoms, it is not one of the most common reasons for seeing a doctor in the UK. Respiratory conditions are by far the most common reason for seeing a GP, accounting for 19% of men and 30% of women each year. Genitourinary problems are nearly as common in women. Next come problems with the nervous system and sense organs, other injuries, ill-defined symptoms and signs, skin conditions, infectious diseases,

and only then back pain and other musculoskeletal conditions. In men, back pain comes eighth and in women it comes tenth.

Over the last 40 years, there has been a steady increase in the number of people who see their GP with back pain (Fig. 20.1). The best and most up-to-date figures are from the Fourth National Morbidity Study, which found that 7.4% of the population – 9.2% of adults – saw their GP with back pain each year, i.e. 4 million people. Mason (1994) obtained a much higher figure of 16% of adults who said that they had seen their GP with back pain in the previous year, but remember the differences between medical records and population surveys.

CSAG (1994) was only able to make a rough estimate of the total number of GP visits for back pain, mainly because of doubt about how often patients return. We now have much better

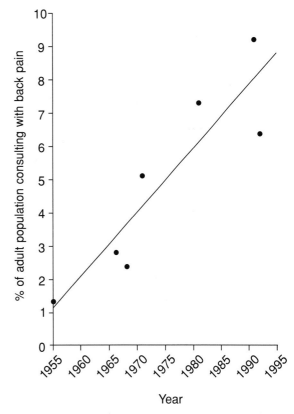

Figure 20.1 Trends in family doctor consultation rates for back pain in the UK.

data from the Fourth National Morbidity Study, which found that each person who saw their GP with back pain attended an average of 1.6 times. It varied from 1.4 times for sprains and strains of the back to 2.0 times for disc disorders. In the *South Manchester Study*, 40% of those who attended with back pain saw their GP again within 3 months. However, only 25% came again with back pain and the other 15% with some other complaint. If 4 million people attend their GP an average of 1.6 times, there are about 6.5 million GP consultations for back pain each year in the UK. So just over 4% of all GP consultations in the UK are for back pain.

GPs visit at least 10% of these 4 million people at home because the pain is so acute (Croft et al 1994, McCormick et al 1995). Compare that with the rarity of 'domiciliary visits' in the US!

Consulting rates vary with sex and age. Most studies show the same pattern as the Fourth National Morbidity Study (Table 20.4). Women consult slightly more than men, with back pain as for all health reasons. Consulting rates for back pain increase from early adult life, with a peak in late middle life and a slight fall in older age.

Table 20.5 shows current GP diagnosis of back problems in the UK. Remember that medical diagnosis of nonspecific low back pain follows fads and fashions and has little to do with pathology.

There is some variation in diagnosis with age. Sprains and strains are most common in the young. Osteoarthritis of the spine increases with age. Intervertebral disc disorders peak at 45–64 years. This may to some extent reflect the age range of different pathologies, but it probably also depends on diagnostic beliefs and customs.

FORMS OF TREATMENT
GP treatment

Mason (1994) asked patients what their GP did for their back pain (Table 20.6). The *South Manchester Study* also compared people who saw their GP with those who dealt with their own back pain (Table 20.7).

Most medical treatment for back pain was passive. The most common treatment was analgesics and anti-inflammatory agents, which GPs gave to nearly two-thirds of patients. More than half of those who saw their GP said they were told to have bed rest. GPs issued sick certificates to stay off work to almost a quarter of those who came to see them with back pain. There is no doubt that consulters got more treatment, but we cannot tell if this reflects their medical state, the kind of people who consult, or the advice their GP gave them.

This is very similar to a survey of 430 Scottish GPs in 1985. Twenty-four per cent said that they 'always', and 42% 'usually', prescribed simple pain killers, 43% sometimes prescribed anti-inflammatory agents, and 10% would add a muscle relaxant, usually diazepam. Forty-eight per cent of these GPs said that they advised bed rest for a week, and 10% advised longer periods of rest. A quarter of GPs advised other treatments. Eleven per cent would refer patients to a physiotherapist, although only 7% would actually prescribe exercise. Nine per cent would advise patients to see an osteopath, but only two out of 430 GPs did manipulation themselves.

GPs arranged X-rays for 13% of patients within 3 months (Croft et al 1994) or about 20% within a year (Mason 1994). Only 3% of patients with back pain had any blood tests. The *South Manchester Study* found that only 2% got physiotherapy within 3 months of their first visit to their GP. Mason (1994) found that about 12% of all those with back pain had physiotherapy in the past year, but most of this was probably for chronic pain.

Table 20.4 GP consulting rates for back pain per annum as a percentage of the population (based on data from the Fourth National Morbidity Study)

Age	Male	Female
5–15	1.1	1.3
16–24	4.7	6.0
25–44	8.2	9.6
45–64	10.5	12.6
65–74	8.7	10.6
75–84	8.2	9.9
All ages	6.7	8.1

Table 20.5 GP diagnosis of back disorders (based on data from the Fourth National Morbidity Study)

Diagnosis	Percentage of population consulting	Average number of consultations
Ankylosing spondylitis and related disorders	0.10	1.8
Spondylosis and allied disorders (or 'osteoarthritis of the spine')	1.19	1.7
Intervertebral disc disorders	0.39	2.0
Other disorders of cervical region	0.91	1.3
Sciatica*	1.20	
Backache and lumbago*	2.52	
Sprains and strains	2.12	1.4

*Together these are 'other & unspecified disorders of the back'.

Table 20.6 What GP did for back pain (from Mason 1994, with permission)

What GP did	Percentage of those consulting
Gave medication	64
Gave advice	37
Gave sick certificate	22
X-ray	22
Referred to hospital doctor	19
Referred to physiotherapist	12
Referred to osteopath or chiropractor	3
Said could not do anything	7

Table 20.7 Treatment for back pain in the past year reported by GP consulters and nonconsulters with back pain (from the *South Manchester Study*, with permission)

	GP consulters	Nonconsulters*
Medication	61%	19%
Avoid lifting	80%	40%
Bed rest	56%	21%
Heat	56%	25%
Local cream or sprays	56%	36%
Exercises	27%	14%

*Expressed as a percentage of those with back pain.

Earlier reports suggested that 9–17% of patients who saw their GP with back disorders were referred to a specialist. Mason (1994) found that about 20% of those who had seen their GP in the past year said that their GP had referred them to a hospital specialist. This more recent figure of 20% fits with total NHS statistics. Many of these patients are then referred more than once, so the total number of specialist referrals each year is about a third of the number of new GP attendances.

- Most people who consult their family doctor with back pain are reassured, advised to rest and prescribed analgesics
- If their pain persists more than a few months, they will probably get a plain X-ray
- About 20% will be referred to a medical specialist, but most later rather than sooner. They are then often referred again and again
- If their pain persists more than a few months, they will probably be referred for physiotherapy

Therapy

About 2.3 million people in the UK get some form of physical therapy for back pain each year. The average course of physiotherapy, osteopathy or chiropractic is about six to seven sessions. However, a small minority of patients continue to attend for months or even years. Table 20.8 details the UK statistics for these three forms of therapy for back pain. To some extent these figures simply reflect the numbers of the three kinds of therapists. Remember that only physiotherapy is available at present to NHS patients. The striking fact is that private practitioners now provide more than half of all physical therapy for back pain in the UK. Few NHS staff realize this.

Hospital outpatient clinics

In the UK, NHS patients see medical specialists in hospital outpatient clinics.

The *South Manchester Study* gives the most detailed information on the current position. They found that the four 'back pain specialties' were orthopedics, rheumatology, pain clinics

Table 20.8 UK staffing and workload of various forms of therapy for back pain

Type of therapy	Number of therapists[a]	Percentage of time spent on back pain	Number of patients treated for back pain each year[b]
NHS			
Physiotherapy	12 000	10%	1.0 million
Private			
Physiotherapy	2200	?	0.3 million
Osteopathy	2500	67%	0.7 million
Chiropractic	1000	50%	0.3 million
		Total private =	1.3 million

[a]Estimated number working, in full-time equivalents.
[b]Based on 1993 data, before the CSAG (1994) report.

and neurosurgery. Every patient whose back pain was due to a spinal problem or a mechanical problem in his or her back went to one of these departments. Small numbers of patients going to other specialties had 'back pain at least in part the reason for referral'. In all these patients, however, the symptom of back pain was a minor part of some other problem. GP triage between primary back disorders and other nonspinal disease does seem to be reasonably accurate.

Of the four back pain specialties, orthopedics has by far the largest clinics and about half the patients with back trouble attend there (Table 20.9). That is where patients with back pain go. Looking at it from another perspective, back pain is a large part of the outpatient workload of each of the four back pain specialties (Table 20.10).

At Hope Hospital, 28% of new patients with back disorders were seen within 3 months, and

83% were seen within 6 months. In a national survey, 29% of all routine orthopedic outpatients were seen within 4 months. To my personal knowledge, however, some orthopedic departments give patients with back pain a lower priority on a slower waiting list, so they may wait longer than average.

The *South Manchester Study* also obtained clinical detail on these outpatients referred to hospital. Their back pain was severe and long-standing. Ninety-one per cent had back pain for more than 3 months in total in the past year; 73% had continuous rather than recurrent pain; 62% had other medical problems as well as back pain. Despite apparently being new referrals, 36% had seen a specialist before with back problems. Only 10% were in full-time work outside the home. Half said they had lost or changed their job because of their back, and 63% were 'not working because of ill health or disability'.

Table 20.9 Percentage of patients with back pain seen in each specialty clinic (from the *South Manchester Study*, with permission)

Clinic	Hope Hospital	Stockport hospitals
Orthopedic	48	61
Rheumatology	22	14
Pain	7	8
Neurosurgery	6	–
General medicine	8	6
Urology and gynecology	8	10
General surgery	2	–
Psychiatry	–	2
Total patients with any back pain	100%	100%

Table 20.10 Back pain as a proportion of the total workload of specialty clinics: proportion of new patients at each clinic who present with back pain (from the *South Manchester Study*, with permission)

Clinic	Hope Hospital	Stockport hospitals
General orthopedic (excluding knee and hand clinics)	45%	28%
Rheumatology	36%	27%
Pain	41%	52%
Neurosurgery	21%	–

At the clinic, 35% had X-rays and 34% were given blood tests. The most common treatments were physiotherapy for 38% and further medication for 25%. Thirty-one per cent got a return appointment to the same clinic and 15% were referred on to another hospital specialist.

Mason (1994) provides the best national data about outpatient clinics. About 10% of adults with back pain said they had attended hospital with their back in the past year. This means that about 1.6 million people attend outpatient clinics each year with back pain, which is close to estimates from official figures. Back pain is the reason for about 5% of all new outpatient visits in all adult specialties in NHS hospitals.

What do specialist consultations achieve?

Coulter et al (1989, 1991) studied GP referrals to NHS outpatient clinics. Table 20.11 shows the reasons GPs gave for referring patients with back pain. In my practice, reassuring the patient or GP is a more common reason than these GPs admit. But the striking thing is that GPs do seem to have realistic expectations and do not often refer these patients looking for a magic cure.

Table 20.11 Reasons GPs gave for referring patients with back pain to a specialist (based on data from Coulter et al 1989)

Reason	Percentage
For advice on management	29%
To establish diagnosis	25%
For treatment	18%
To take over management	14%
For specific investigation	3%
To reassure patient	3%
To reassure GP	3%
Other	5%

The GPs referred 20% of these patients within 6 months of their first visit with back pain. But they treated 59% of them for at least 2 years before their first specialist referral. So it seems that GPs use specialist referral as a last rather than a first resort. However, 46% of these GP referrals had already seen a specialist before with back trouble, and for 8% this was at least their fourth specialist referral. So when GPs do refer patients with back pain to a specialist, they then often refer them again and again.

Coulter et al (1989) also looked at the outcome of these referrals. What actually happened was very different from what the GP was looking for. Seventy-five per cent of patients got treatment, although that was the GP's reason for referral in only 29% of cases. Sixty-nine per cent of those sent for reassurance or advice only actually got some form of treatment. Many of these patients then had multiple clinic appointments and 33% were still attending their GP 5 years later with back pain.

The *South Manchester Study* interviewed the patients at Hope Hospital 3 months after their outpatient visit. Most said they had no change in their condition and 91% still had backache. Almost half had been a little (29%) or very disappointed (19%) with their clinic visit. Remember that Hope Hospital is a regional centre with many problem cases who will respond poorly to treatment, so these figures probably do not reflect the national pattern. But it is still a depressing picture.

CSAG (1994) reviewed current NHS services for back pain in the UK. We visited eight districts in different parts of the country. At each visit we met GPs and hospital specialists and heard about their experience. We looked at

- Most patients attending hospital specialists have chronic low back pain and disability
- Many of them are not working
- They have often seen other specialists before
- Specialist treatment achieves little and leaves many patients dissatisfied

standards of care and compared them with UK clinical guidelines (Ch. 17). Most people at the meetings welcomed the guidelines, but few districts felt that they met these standards at present. We heard many common criticisms of present services:

- Everyone agrees that diagnostic triage is fundamental to referral. But family doctors cannot put this into practice because there are no different NHS services for patients with different kinds of back trouble. The main problem is that, in practice, we do not separate patients with serious spinal disease and nerve root problems from those with simple backache.
- Most specialist services are designed to investigate and treat patients with serious spinal disease, nerve root problems and those who may require surgery. Emergency and urgent referrals of these patients are usually dealt with satisfactorily. Routine referrals of these patients suffer long delays due to waiting lists caused by large numbers of patients with simple backache.
- These specialty services are usually inappropriate for patients with simple backache and provide them with a very poor service.
- There are no NHS services specifically designed for patients with simple backache, apart from a few isolated examples.
- Only half the districts feel that spinal X-rays for back pain follow the Royal College of Radiology guidelines. Too many patients still have repeat X-rays because previous X-rays or reports are not available due to simple clerical inefficiency. Some GPs want direct access to spinal imaging, but it seems that they often use this simply as a mechanism to by-pass specialist waiting lists. Most agree that this is not the ideal way to run a service.

- There is very variable access to physiotherapy. Some districts have direct GP access, while others set criteria for referral or use specialist clinics and their waiting lists as a filter to control demand. Waiting times for physiotherapy vary greatly. Few NHS patients with back pain actually receive any form of physical therapy at the acute stage.
- Many health professionals feel that the system creates the chronic pain patient. It is still common practice to give analgesics and send patients home for bed rest without information or advice about their problem. There are too many delays before patients get any active treatment. They are then sent to the wrong specialist, often with unrealistic expectations of a cure. Delayed access may lead to chronic pain and by that time they may also have lost their job.
- We heard frequent comment about the 'revolving door' of specialist care for chronic back pain. Patients wait months to see a specialist and then find that he has nothing to offer. A typical example is waiting to see a surgeon with simple backache that is not a surgical problem. Then they have to wait all over again to see another specialist, with the same result. Or they are passed from one specialist to another.
- Pain services in the UK are usually the last resort for patients with chronic intractable pain. They often have long waiting lists. Most NHS pain clinics are run by anesthesiologists and the main treatment offered is medication and regional anesthesia. Many GPs and other specialists feel that present NHS pain services are of limited value for patients with back problems.
- GPs are under a lot of pressure to give sick certificates. Sometimes this is for social rather than health reasons, to get state benefits. Many GPs feel that this is a particular problem with back pain where they find it difficult to assess fitness for work. Some feel that it would be better to separate sick certification from health care.

Many GPs and specialists are dissatisfied with present specialist services for back pain. Patients also are disillusioned.

- There is lack of triage between possible spinal pathology, nerve root problems and simple backache
- Most specialist services are designed for the investigation and treatment of patients with serious spinal pathology, nerve root problems, and those who require consideration of surgery
- These specialist services provide an inappropriate and ineffective service for patients with simple backache
- There are very few services designed to meet the needs of patients with simple backache

X-rays

Nine per cent of people with back pain say that they have had an X-ray of their back in the past year (Mason 1994). That would be about 1.5 million plain X-rays of the lumbar spine in 1993, which is close to NHS estimates. GPs arrange about 0.6 million of these and specialists about 0.9 million. That is 3% of all medical and dental X-rays, but because of the high dose of lumbar X-rays it is about 15% of total medical radiation.

In 1989 there were 54 000 CT scans of the lumbar spine in the UK. The number of CT scanners has doubled since then and throughput has also risen. There were very few MRI scanners in routine NHS use in 1989. Although the number is rising, there are still more CT than MRI scans of the lumbar spine. In total, more than 100 000 people in the UK now have spinal imaging each year (National Radiation Protection Board data).

Up till now, most spinal imaging in Britain was carried out at the request of a specialist. Some experts still argue that we should only image patients with back pain after a surgeon has made a clinical decision that they may require surgery. In practice, imaging is now often used as part of assessment and diagnosis. A few centers in the UK now provide direct GP access to spinal imaging. And I now see the first few NHS patients who arrive at my clinic with their MRI scan in their hand looking for

an operation. Britain may be heading down the same slippery slope as the US, although I hope it is not yet too late to stop this.

Hospitalization

There were about 100 000 hospital admissions for back problems in Britain in 1993. These patients occupied 770 000 bed-days. There were another 30 000 day case admissions. So about 130 000 people had some form of 'inpatient' hospital treatment.

Table 20.12 shows where they went. About half were in the surgical specialties of orthopedics and neurosurgery, but only 14.8% of these patients had a surgical operation. 85% of admissions were for investigation, bed rest and 'conservative treatment'. Most NHS bed occupancy for back problems is 'nonsurgical hospitalization'.

Figure 20.2 shows the rising number of admissions for back problems during the 1980s. This has now plateaued, due to increasing pressure to reduce NHS bed occupancy.

Surgery

In 1982 there were about 9000 disc operations and another 2000 spinal fusions in England and Wales (OHE 1985). The annual figures show a steady increase since (Table 20.13). By 1993, it was estimated that there were about 24 000 surgical operations on the spine throughout the UK. There were 33 000 other 'procedures' most of which were epidural or paraspinal injections.

REGIONAL VARIATION

There is little evidence of much regional variation in low back pain or disability across the

Table 20.12 Hospital in-patients for back disorders in Scotland 1992 (based on data from the Scottish Health Services, Information and Statistics Division)

Specialty	Discharges	Bed-days	Average stay
Orthopedics	4012	30 550	7.6
Neurosurgery	1364	7683	5.6
Other specialties	4932	44 452	9.0
Total	10 308	82 685	8.0

Number of
Admissions

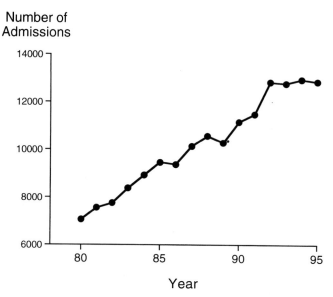

Year

Figure 20.2 Trends in number of patients admitted to hospital with spinal diagnoses (Scotland, 1980–1995) (based on data from the Scottish Health Services, Information and Statistics Division).

UK, but there is a lot of difference in health care. Porter & Hibbert (1986) looked at patients with back pain in four GP practices in different parts of the UK. The number who had ever had an X-ray varied from 23 to 44%, those who had ever seen an orthopedic surgeon varied from 13 to 55%, and those who had ever been off work varied from 46 to 90% – and that was in a very small sample of four practices! Some GPs and practices must vary much more, either way.

Most studies show a higher GP consulting rate for back pain in the north of England and Scotland, where the GP is also more likely to prescribe medication. People with back pain in

the south-east and south-west are more likely to feel that their GP cannot do anything for back pain and are less likely to receive NHS physiotherapy. Those in London, the south-east and the south-west are more likely to attend an osteopath. Those in the south-east and the south-west are more likely to attend a chiropractor.

CSAG (1994) found wide variation in access to NHS specialists in different parts of the UK. Numbers of orthopedic surgeons, rheumatologists, neurosurgeons and pain clinics vary greatly in different areas. Routine waiting times for a specialist appointment vary from about 6 weeks to more than 1 year. Patients in London, the Midlands and the south-east are more likely to see a private specialist. Those in the north of England and Scotland are more likely to receive hospital in-patient treatment. Referral patterns depend on the individual specialists in the area, local custom and waiting times. Who you see and how long you wait depend on where you live. This in turn determines the treatment you receive and the waiting times may decide your outcome.

All these patterns probably simply reflect the availability of NHS and private services for

Table 20.13 Surgical operations for back disorders in England 1989–1990 (based on NHS in-patient statistics)

Operation	Number
Cervical disc operations	1869
Fusion	503
Thoracic spine	532
Lumbosacral disc operations	12 040
Fusion	1164
Deformity	857
Fracture – dislocation	258
Total	17 223

back pain. The greatest differences however, as in the US, seem to be between individual GP practices and hospitals. These differences depend partly on socioeconomic factors, but they probably depend most of all on how individual GPs and specialists practice.

There is also some variation in health care for back pain with social class (Table 20.14). Mason (1994) showed the same pattern, but gave more clinical detail. Social classes IIIM–V have more GP visits, specialist referrals, X-rays and physiotherapy. Social classes I–II are more likely to see an osteopath or chiropractor privately but are also more likely to deal with the problem on their own without professional health care.

TOTAL HEALTH CARE USE

Benn & Wood (1975) made one of the first attempts to estimate the size of the problem of back pain in the UK, using data from the 1950s and 1960s. At that time they found that about 2.7% of people consulted their GP with back disorders each year. Of these, 1 in 2.3 would see a hospital specialist, 1 in 4 would get a spinal support, 1 in 30 would be admitted to hospital, and 1 in 200 would have a disc operation. They pointed out that this pattern of health care looks very different to people with back pain and to health professionals. Few people with back pain in the UK received any specialist treatment, but the specialist only saw a select few of those with back pain.

The Office of Health Economics (OHE) (1985) looked at total health care for back pain in the UK in the mid-1980s (Fig. 20.3). In their published figure they gave the number for surgery as 'less than 10 000 cases?' but their own text and original sources suggest that the correct figure is 11 000. We can make a similar summary of health care use for back pain in the UK in 1993 (Fig. 20.4).

Some of the figures for 1985 and 1993 are not directly comparable. The data is from different sources, the definitions are different, and some of the estimates are of variable quality. If you really want to look at the details, you

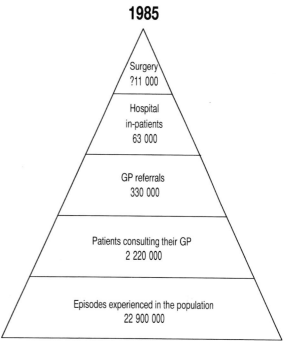

Figure 20.3 Estimated health care for back pain in the UK in 1985. (From OHE 1985, with permission.)

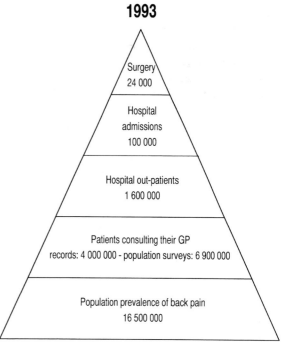

Figure 20.4 Estimated health care for back pain in Britain in 1993. (Updated from CSAG 1994.)

Table 20.14 GP consulting rates for back pain by social class (based on data from the Third National Morbidity Survey 1981–82)

Social class	Standardized ratios all ages	
	Male	Female
I & II (professional and managerial)	72	85
IIINM (skilled nonmanual)	92	92
IIIM (skilled manual)	110	115
IV & V (partly skilled and unskilled)	134	110
Average (all social classes)	100	100

should go back to the original sources. In general, however, CSAG had much more comprehensive data by 1993 than the earlier OHE estimates. For example, the OHE estimate of 'episodes in the population' just assumed that GPs saw 10% of all attacks. We now have good population survey data for prevalence. Over the past 40 years there has been a steady rise in the number of people who visit their GP with backache. The rise in the number going to specialists came later in the last decade. The number of patients admitted to hospital has risen slightly, but the average length of stay has fallen so total bed occupancy is much the same. The number of operations has more than doubled in the last decade.

We can now summarize health care for back pain in the UK. Most people with back pain in the UK deal with it themselves most of the time. If they seek medical care, most go first to the NHS. GP records suggest that about 4 million people consult primarily for back pain each year, which is 9% of the adult population. In population surveys, 6.9 million say that back pain was one of the reasons they attended their GP's surgery in the previous year. 1.6 million of these patients attend a hospital specialist. 1.5 million have X-rays and more than 100 000 have a CT or MRI of the lumbar spine. 1.0 million have NHS physiotherapy. 480 000 attend hospital A & E departments. 100 000 are admitted to hospital and a further 30 000 are treated as day cases. 24 000 have a spinal operation.

But many people with back pain in Britain seek private health care. Each year about 0.5 million people see a private medical special-ist for back pain. 0.3 million attend a private physiotherapist, 0.7 million an osteopath and 0.3 million a chiropractor. Fifteen per cent of patients who seek health care for back pain stay away from the NHS altogether and depend entirely on the private sector. More than half of the therapy for back pain is private. As far as I know, back pain is the only common condition where this is true. Access to and satisfaction with NHS services for back pain are so bad that many patients vote with their feet and their wallets.

THE COST OF BACK PAIN

Coyle & Richardson (1994) and Moffett et al (1995) estimated NHS costs of health care for back pain in the UK in 1993. Using the more accurate numbers of GP consultations from the Fourth National Morbidity Survey, it was probably closer to £420 million. There are many problems associated with such estimates and they have a considerable range of error. But depending on how you look at it, this is either a great deal of money or not nearly enough to meet the need. The total cost of back pain

Table 20.15 Estimated costs of back pain in UK in 1993 (adapted from Coyle & Richardson 1994)

Resource	Best estimate (£ millions)
GP consultations[a]	70
Prescribed drugs	48
Outpatient consultations	72
Physiotherapy	63
X-rays	45
In-patient bed-days (including surgery)	106
A & E attendances	17
Total NHS costs[a]	**421**
Private medical consultations	35
Private therapy	144
Nonprescription analgesics	18
Local government costs	23
Non-NHS health costs	**220**
Work loss: lost production[b]	3800
DSS benefits	1400
Total[a]	**5841**

[a]Corrected from Coyle & Richardson's (1994) estimate to allow for the new data on number of GP consultations.
[b]The estimate for lost production is very approximate.

in the UK, including work loss and state benefits, is very approximately £6 billion, and that is rising by £0.5 billion every year (see Table 20.15).

CONCLUSION

Back pain in UK accounts for:

- 4% of all GP consultations
- 5% of all NHS specialist referrals
- 15% of all state sickness benefits
- 1.2% of total NHS spending.

Yet back disorders only get 1.2% of total NHS spending. Worse still, we spend that money in the wrong way. There is wide agreement that our present services for back pain are inappropriate and ineffective. We fail to provide the best possible care and waste limited and expensive resources. Patients, GPs and specialists alike are dissatisfied with the present system (CSAG 1994).

There is wide agreement on the need for change and on what is wrong with our present NHS services for back pain. Up till now, there has been much less will to do anything about it, especially if it involved changing established professional practice or spending money.

REFERENCES

Benn R T, Wood P H N 1975 Pain in the back: an attempt to estimate the size of the problem. Rheumatology and Rehabilitation 14: 121–128

Consumers' Association 1985 Back pain survey. Consumers' Association, London

Coulter A, Noone A, Goldacre M 1989 General practitioners' referrals to specialist outpatient clinics. British Medical Journal 299: 304–306

Coulter A, Bradlow J, Martin-Bates C 1991 Outcome of general practitioner referrals to specialist out-patient clinics for back pain. British Journal of General Practice 41: 450–453

Coyle D, Richardson G 1994 The cost of back pain. In: The epidemiology of back pain. Annex to the Clinical Standards Advisory Group's report on back pain. HMSO, London, p 65–72

Croft P, Joseph S, Cosgrove S et al 1994 Low back pain in the community and in hospitals. A report to the Clinical Standards Advisory Group of the Department of Health. Prepared by the Arthritis & Rheumatism Council, Epidemiology Research Unit, University of Manchester

There are more detailed references and sources in CSAG (1994) and Waddell (1994).

CSAG 1994 Report on back pain. Clinical Standards Advisory Group. HMSO, London, p 1–89

McCormick A, Fleming D, Charlton J 1995 Morbidity statistics from general practice. Fourth national study 1991–1992. Office of Population Censuses and Surveys Series MB5 No. 3. HMSO, London, p 1–366

Mason V 1994 The prevalence of back pain in Great Britain. Office of Population Censuses and Surveys Social Survey Division. HMSO, London, p 1–24

Mechanic D 1968 Medical sociology. Free Press, New York

Moffett J K, Richardson G, Sheldon T A, Maynard A 1995 Back pain: Its management and cost to society. Discussion paper 129 Centre for Health Economics, York, p 1–67

OHE 1985 Back pain. Office of Health Economics, London

Porter R W, Hibbert C S 1986 Back pain and neck pain in four general practices. Clinical Biomechanics 1: 7–10

Waddell G 1994 The epidemiology of back pain. Annex to the Clinical Standards Advisory Group's report on back pain. Her Majesty's Stationery Office, London: 1–64

21

US health care for back pain

The health care system in the US is very different from the UK and that affects the treatment Americans receive for back pain.

Almost all health care in the US takes place in independent professional practices (Box 21.1). Payment for different patients is from many sources: private health insurance, worker's compensation and government programs. But between 15 and 25% of Americans have little or no health insurance. This system produces wide variation in treatment for a problem like back pain where any health care is a matter of choice.

Box 21.1   US health care for back pain

There are two independent health care systems for back pain in the US:

- 60% seek orthodox medical care
  —40% is mainly in primary medical care
  —20% is specialist care
- 40% seek chiropractic care instead

We must also see health care for back pain in its US context. Of course American patients do not get simple backache. They all have low back pain, and can often tell of their medical state in great detail. Carey et al (1995) found that 47% of Americans with chronic back pain thought they had disc disease. This is partly a matter of linguistics, but it also reflects cultural attitudes to back pain, health and health care.

BACK PAIN AND DISABILITY IN THE US

The US population in 1992 was 255 million: 124 million men and 131 million women. Clinical back pain mainly affects adults aged 18 and over, of whom there are 190 million in the US.

Despite some claims, most of the evidence suggests that back pain in the US is more or less the same as in the rest of the Western world. Many authors quote Deyo & Tsui-Wu (1987) for a 1 year prevalence of 10.3% and a lifetime prevalence of 13.8% in the US, compared with 40–60% in Europe, but that does not compare like with like. Many US surveys try to pick out 'significant' or 'disabling' back pain. Deyo & Tsui-Wu used the National Health and Nutrition Examinations Survey (NHANES) which only included back pain that lasted 'most days for at least two weeks'. Another US survey only considered back pain that caused days in bed or led to health care. These are clearly only the more severe cases of back pain. Those US studies that ask more open questions about back pain get very similar results to European studies (Taylor & Curran 1985, von Korff et al 1988, Frymoyer 1988).

About 70–85% of Americans have back pain at some time in their life. The *Nuprin Pain Report* (Taylor & Curran 1985) was a telephone survey of 1254 Americans aged 18 years or more. Fifty-six per cent said they had back pain in the last year. Only headache was more common in 73%. Ninety per cent of those with frequent back pain had multiple pains, but 50% of them said back pain was the 'most troublesome'. Most people have mild and self-limiting episodes, but recurrences were common. Twenty-two per cent had only occasional backache for 1–5 days in the previous year and it had very little effect on their daily life. 34% had pain for 6 days or more. 25% of those with back pain said it interfered with their routine activities, work or sleep for 1 or more days in the year.

von Korff et al (1988) also found that 41% of adults aged 26–44 years had back pain in the previous 6 months. Most people had occasional short attacks of pain over a long period. Their pain was usually mild or moderate and did not limit activities. However, about a quarter of those with any back pain said they had it on more than half the days and that it did cause some limitation of their activities. Andersson (1991) found that back problems were the most common cause of activity limitation in people below the age of 45 and the fourth most common in those aged 45–64 years. Seven per cent of adults reported a disability due to their back or due to both their back and other joint problems. On average, this limited their activities for about 23 days each year. Eight per cent of those with back pain had lost time from work for an average of 8 days each year.

These various figures suggest that between 7 and 14% of US adults have some disability due to back pain for a least 1 day each year. That is about 15–25 million people. Just over 1% of Americans are permanently disabled by back pain and another 1% are temporarily disabled by back pain at any one time. That is 5 million people.

Back injuries also make up about two-fifths of all work-related injuries in the US. There are now about 1 million compensation claims for work-related back injuries each year.

Guo et al (1995) looked at total work loss due to back pain in the US. They used data from 30 000 workers in the 1988 National Health Interview Survey. They estimated that 22.4 million workers lost 149 million days per annum in the US. About 2.1% of all workers said they had ever lost or changed a job because of back pain. This survey only looked at those who had back pain every day for a week or more in the previous year, so these estimates may be slightly low. These figures are also now 10 years old.

- There are about 190 million Americans age 18 and over
- 50–60% of them get some back pain each year
- More than 20 million US workers lose about 150 million days from work because of back pain each year. They make about 1 million compensation claims for work-related back injuries each year
- About 1 million Americans are permanently disabled, and another 1 million temporarily disabled by back pain at any time

Information available on health care

Deyo et al (1994) have reviewed the sources of data on US health care for back pain.

The National Centre for Health Statistics carries out a number of Federal surveys that cover the entire US. The National Health and Nutrition Examination Surveys (NHANES) were carried out in 1971–75, 1976–80 and 1988–94. These got health histories and carried out physical examinations of many thousands of adults. The National Health Interview Survey asks questions about health status and health care use but performs no physical examinations. The National Ambulatory Medical Care Survey gives annual data on visits to office-based physicians. The National Hospital Discharge Survey gives annual data on hospital discharges across the US. Health insurance data such as Workers' Compensation, Medicare and Medicaid cover selected groups of patients. Local studies such as those in Washington State and North Carolina can collect much more clinical detail, but we can only apply them with care to the whole country.

The major problem with most of these surveys is access. You cannot simply go to a library and look up the facts you want. It takes expert knowledge and considerable effort even to get the raw data base on computer disc. You then have to set up and learn the system before you can begin the analysis. In practice, we must depend on expert research groups to do this for us. Fortunately, there are now a number of published papers that provide this data in user-friendly form.

We must also recognize the limitations of these data bases. Most of the surveys are now out of date. Some are more than 10 years old by the time they are analyzed and published. Most of the surveys are for administrative purposes and we must be careful using the data to answer questions for which it was not designed. Often, the information that we want is simply not there. The data is also open to bias. There may be selection of the patients, the questions and the presentation of the data. There is a major problem with missing data and that may produce further bias. However, we should not be too pessimistic. Provided we are cautious, we can build up a reasonable picture of health care for back pain in the US.

- Large, national, population surveys give very limited biomedical information. Clinical surveys can give much more biomedical information, but are usually of selected groups of patients
- The data is very difficult to access, and we must depend on experts to extract it
- *Much of this data on US health care for back pain is now about 10 years out of date.*

WHO SEEKS HEALTH CARE AND WHO DO THEY SEE?

Always remember that there are two different systems of health care for back pain in the US. Conventional medicine and chiropractic medicine are completely independent and competing. About 60–70% of Americans who seek health care for back pain use conventional medicine, but about a third use chiropractic medicine instead, which deals with about 40% of all episodes. There are fundamental differences in philosophy and practice between these two health care systems, although they share some treatments in common.

The *Nuprin Pain Report* (Taylor & Curran 1985) found that about 70% of those with 'more than occasional' back pain had seen a medical doctor at some time. von Korff et al (1988) found that 66% of those with any back pain in the previous 6 months had consulted at some time. These figures suggest that at least 25% of all Americans seek medical care for back pain at some time in their lives.

In the *Nuprin Pain Report,* 12.5% of US adults said that they had sought medical care for back pain in the previous year. However, as we saw in the last chapter, such survey data is likely to overestimate reality. Using health records from 1974 to 1982, Shekelle et al (1995a) estimated that there were 9.1 episodes of care for back pain per 100 person-years. Each person had an average of 1.5 episodes of care during the period of their study. That would mean about 6% of US adults per annum sought health care for back pain, which gives a lower estimate of about 12 million people each year. Medical doctors were the main providers of care for 7.2 million people, and chiropractic doctors were the main providers for the other 4.8 million. A number of other studies support Shekelle's estimates and there does not seem to have been much change since then. Data for first visits from Hart et al (1995) suggests that about 5.6 million people saw a physician in 1990 with a primary diagnosis of back pain. If we include those who had back pain as a secondary reason for the visit, this gives a figure of 8.9 million people. AAOS (1996) gives a figure of just over 6 million new visits to office-based physicians for back disorders in 1993. The *Nuprin Pain Report* and Eisenberg et al (1993) give similar figures for the number who attend a chiropractor.

Many authors describe back pain as the first or second most common reason for all physician office visits in the US, quoting Cypress (1983). She found that back pain was the reason for 3% of all visits to a physician and the second most common presenting symptom. It was the most common symptom in males aged 25–64 and females aged 35–64. It was the most common reason for seeing an osteopathic physician, orthopedic surgeon, neurosurgeon and occupational medicine physician. It was the second most common reason for seeing a general or family physician. However, that data is now 20 years old and there are problems with its diagnostic coding.

Hart et al (1995) provide more complete data on office visits from the National Ambulatory Medical Care Surveys of 1988–1990. These are large surveys of office-based physicians across the US. They exclude a few who are not in private practice, and Hart et al considered that their figures were a slight under-estimate. The greatest problem is that they do not include chiropractors. Note also that this data refers to numbers of visits, while Shekelle et al looked at numbers of patients. Back pain was the primary diagnosis for 2.8% of all office visits, and this proportion stayed constant through the decade. Visits for back pain rose from 12 million in 1980–1981 to 15 million in 1989–1990, but that is the same increase as for all health reasons. If we include those patients for whom back pain was a secondary reason for the visit

then it was 4.5%, or 24 million visits, each year. Back pain was the only complaint or diagnosis in 49%. It was the first of multiple complaints in 28% and the second or third complaint in 23%. Back pain is now the fifth most common reason for an office visit to a physician in the US (Table 21.1).

Back pain is also the most common reason for seeking alternative medicine. 36% of those with back pain have sought some form of alternative medicine in the past year. The number seeking chiropractic care has doubled in the last 15–20 years.

Shekelle et al (1995a) looked at 'episodes of health care'. Of those who sought any health care for back pain, 71% had only a single episode of care over a 3- or 5-year period; 16% had two episodes, 9% had three episodes, and 3% had four episodes. Only 1% of these patients had five episodes of health care or more in the 3- or 5-year period. Half of all episodes of health care for back pain lasted 1 week or less, and two-thirds lasted 1 month or less; only 8% lasted more than 6 months. Note that this is not the duration of symptoms but the period during which people received health care. Many people may continue to have some symptoms for a much longer time but do not seek further health care.

Who do they see?

Cypress (1983), Deyo & Tsui-Wu (1987), Shekelle et al (1995a,b) and Hart et al (1995) all show a similar pattern of consulting for back pain (Table 21.2). About two-thirds of medical care for back pain is in the primary care specialties of family practice, osteopathic medicine and

Table 21.1 Reasons for physician office visits in 1989–1990 (from Hart et al 1995, with permission)

Reason for visit	Percentage of all visits
Hypertension	5.5%
Pregnancy	5.2%
General medical examination and well care	4.1%
Acute upper respiratory infection	3.3%
Back pain	2.8%

Table 21.2 Number of adults consulting each year and who they visit

	Number (millions)
Total patients consulting (medical records)	12 (4.7%)
Medical doctor:total	7.2
Primary care	4.7
Specialist	2.5
(referred from another doctor)	(45%)
Chiropractor	4.8
Main provider of care	
Chiropractor	4.8
General/family physician (MD)	3.8
Osteopathic doctor (DO)	0.9
Orthopedic surgeon	1.0
Other medical specialist	1.5

general internal medicine. One-third is provided by medical specialists, particularly by orthopedic surgeons.

Table 21.3 shows the specialty market share of back pain visits and the proportion that back pain forms of each specialty's case load. Most patients go directly to family doctors, DOs and internists. Some patients are then referred to a specialist. But in the US, unlike in the UK, many patients go directly to a specialist of their choice without any previous medical screening. That applies to 55% of those who go to orthopedic surgeons, 27% to neurosurgeons and 26% to neurologists.

Table 21.4 shows back pain diagnosis by specialty. The case mix may vary between specialties and that reflects both referral patterns and pathology. However, we should interpret these figures with caution. In most nonspecific back pain, it is not possible to make any firm diagnosis. Physicians often simply provide a label, which may reflect their specialty leaning rather than actual pathology.

However, that only reflects the very broad differences between the specialties. Much more important, each doctor may have an individual *diagnostic signature*. That may produce much greater variation between doctors within each profession, and may be quite idiosyncratic.

There is some uncertainty about whether patients who go to a chiropractor are comparable to those who go to a physician. One study suggests that they may have less pain and disability (Nviendo et al 1996), but other studies suggest that they have about the same. Most patients who attend a chiropractor have recur-

Table 21.3 Specialty market share and workload of back pain (based on data from Hart et al 1995)

Specialty	Percentage market share of all back pain visits	Back pain as a percentage of specialty office visit caseload
General/family physician		
MD	30	2.6
DO	11	5.4
Internal medicine	14	2.4
Orthopedic surgery	25	11
Neurosurgery	7	35
Neurology	4	10

Table 21.4 Back diagnosis by specialty (based on data from Hart et al 1995)

	General/ family practice	Orthopedic surgery	Neurosurgery
Nonspecific LBP	76%	40%	19%
Herniated disc	3%	20%	46%
Degenerative changes	10%	19%	6%

rent pain and one-third have seen a chiropractor before. Just over half attend within 3 weeks of onset of their back pain, but one-quarter have had pain for more than 6 months. Carey et al (1995) also found that those seeking chiropractic care were in better general health, were more likely to have good health insurance and had less severe pain. Use of chiropractic varies most with region of the country and availability of practitioners. Whites are more likely to attend a DC or DO. The poorly educated are more likely to attend a family doctor (MD). Shekelle et al (1995b) found that chiropractors are more likely to give patients a specific diagnosis such as 'sacroiliac injury', 'disc displacement' and 'disc dislocation'. MDs are more likely to give a vague diagnosis such as 'pain in the back' and 'back injury'.

Hart et al (1995) and Shekelle et al (1995b) both give information on average numbers of visits (Table 21.5). Family doctors (MDs) have the lowest number of return visits, while DOs and surgeons have more, and chiropractors have by far the highest number. Shekelle et al (1995b) also give data on costs (Table 21.5). The cost of health care per episode depends on the number of visits, the cost per visit, drug costs, investigations and hospitalization. Surgeons are by far the most expensive, mainly because of high-tech investigations and hospitalization. Perhaps surprisingly, chiropractic may not be cheaper than primary medical care. In Shekelle's study, low chiropractic costs per visit, low investigation costs and no hospital costs were balanced by the large number of chiropractic visits per episode. However, some chiropractors dispute these figures, and argue they are not comparing like with like.

Family practice and chiropractic are potentially the cheapest and most cost-effective types of health care for an episode of nonspecific low back pain. Most of the high costs of medical care are due to investigations and hospitalization, much of which may be unnecessary. If family practice could reduce these, it would be by far the cheapest. Conversely, many chiropractic visits may be unnecessary. If chiropractic could control the number of visits per episode, it would be the cheapest and possibly also the most cost-effective.

Shekelle et al (1995b) used RAND data from 1974 to 1982, but preliminary results from Nviendo et al (1996) showed little change in the relative costs of chiropractic and family medicine. However, Shekelle et al only looked at direct MD and chiropractic costs. When the MD also orders physical therapy, the total cost may be greater than a chiropractor who provides the complete course of treatment (Stano & Smith 1996). None of these estimates allows for clinical outcomes and we still do not have good data on the cost effectiveness of different health care for back pain.

WHAT HAPPENS TO THEM?

The average medical consultation for back pain in primary care lasts 15 minutes. The average first chiropractic visit is about 30 minutes and the return visit is about 15 minutes.

Table 21.6 shows what happens to patients with back pain when they visit different providers. Once again, allow for case mix.

MDs and DOs are very alike in US family practice, but there are some differences with back pain. MDs take more X-rays and prescribe

Table 21.5 Number and relative costs of visits to each specialty (based on data from Shekelle et al 1995 a and b)

Specialty	Mean number of visits/episode	Mean cost/visit (in 1982 $)	Total cost/episode (in 1982 $)
Chiropractor	10.4	$19.45	$281
Family doctor			
MD	2.3	$20.21	$199
DO	5.3	$22.18	$388
Internist	3.4	$21.85	$332
Orthopedic surgeon	5.0	$38.53	$531

Table 21.6 Percentage of visits at which each treatment ordered (based on data from Hart et al 1995)

Specialty	X-ray	Drugs	Physical therapy
General/family medicine			
MD	13	60	16
DO	6	45	30
General/internal medicine	18	57	32
Orthopedic surgery	28	35	23
Neurosurgery	21	26	13*
Chiropractic	50	?	–

*27% admitted to hospital after initial visit; all other specialties, 0–2%.

more drugs for back pain. DOs order more physical therapy, and more than 50% recommend manipulation for back pain compared with less than 7% of MDs.

In contrast to medical care, chiropractic is entirely outpatient, nonsurgical and 'drug-free'. Shekelle et al (1995b) confirmed that no patient under chiropractic care had hospitalization or surgery during the period of their study. Surprisingly, drug costs of patients under chiropractic care were no lower, although it is not clear to what extent these drugs were prescribed by the chiropractor, by a primary care doctor or self-prescribed. Chiropractors also now order as many X-rays and scans for back pain as primary care physicians.

Cherkin et al (1994a) carried out a fascinating study of how different medical specialists would investigate and treat back pain. They described three hypothetical patients with acute back pain, acute back pain with sciatica and chronic low back pain. There was little agreement on the use of diagnostic tests. Rheumatologists were more likely to order blood tests. Neurosurgeons and neurologists were more likely to order imaging. Neurologists and physiatrists were more likely to order EMGs. Physiatrists were also more likely to order psychologic evaluation. Investigations seemed to vary more with the specialty of the doctor than with the clinical condition of the patient. They concluded that 'who you see is what you get'. Once again, the *diagnostic signature* may produce much greater individual variation.

In the second part of the study, Cherkin et al (1995) looked at treatment for these three patients. Bed rest, back exercises and physical therapy were most frequent for all three patients. Patients with acute back pain or sciatica were more likely to be prescribed bed rest. Patients with chronic pain were more likely to be prescribed back exercises and physical therapy. Contrary to current guidelines, 59% of physicians prescribed more than 3 days' bed rest for acute sciatica, 30% for acute back pain, and 17% for chronic back pain. The mean bed rest was 5.8 days for acute sciatica, 4.5 days for acute back pain and 5 days for chronic back pain. Neurologists and neurosurgeons were no more likely to prescribe bed rest, but if they did, they gave longer periods of 7.5 days for all three patients. Emergency medicine physicians were most likely to order bed rest, imaging and surgical referral (Table 21.7). They used high-tech and costly interventions too early, without clinical indications and contrary to the AHCPR guidelines. However, on the contrary, 10% would refer the patient with acute back pain and 28% would refer the patient with chronic back pain to a rehabilitation specialist.

There is little direct evidence, but there is considerable anecdotal evidence that the *treatment signature* of individual doctors may produce the greatest variation of all.

What physicians say they would do in a questionnaire may not be quite the same as what they actually do in practice. So it is also worth seeing what patients report about their treatment. The *Nuprin Pain Report* (Taylor &

Table 21.7 Treatment prescribed by emergency room physicians (based on data from Elam et al 1995)

	Acute back pain <1 week without sciatica	Chronic back pain without sciatica
Bed rest	76%	57%
CT	4%	8%
MRI	9%	16%
Refer to surgical specialist	41%	52%

Curran 1985) found that 75% of those with back pain had taken nonprescription analgesics in the previous year; two-thirds of them had taken more than one course. Most patients who had ever back pain for at least 2 weeks had used multiple treatments (Table 21.8).

Carey et al (1995, 1996) investigated care seeking among people with chronic disabling low back pain in North Carolina (Table 21.9). These were the most severe cases. Fifty-three per cent felt that their general health was poor, and 34% were permanently disabled from working. The number of days spent in bed varied widely, with a median of 3 days but a mean of over 25 days. Three out of 269 people said they had spent all or nearly all of the previous 365 days in bed because of back pain. So most people, even those with chronic low back pain, had only brief spells in bed but a very few were more or less bed-bound. Many of these patients had seen multiple health care providers in the previous year, and most had three or four treatments in that time.

Carey et al reported a high use of imaging. 17% had an X-ray, 37% had a CT scan and 25% had an MRI scan during the previous year. 19%

Table 21.8 Patients' report of treatment received during 1976–1980 (based on data from Deyo & Tsui-Wu 1987)

Treatment	Ever used
Rest	81%
Local heat	74%
Aspirin	58%
Stiff mattress	58%
Exercises and physical therapy	41%
Brace	27%
Traction	21%
Diathermy	17%

Table 21.9 Treatment received by patients with severe chronic low back pain and disability in 1992 (from Carey et al 1995, with permission)

Treatment	Percentage of patients in past year
Pain medication	92%
Bed rest	65%
Back exercises	64%
Massage	42%
Corset or brace	35%
Back injections	32%
Ultrasound	27%
Physical therapy	26%
Spinal manipulation	22%
TENS	18%
Traction	8%

had a myelogram or discogram. Ten per cent had back surgery, which is slightly higher than the true surgery rate in North Carolina so there may be some selection bias and over-reporting in this sample. Nevertheless, this study shows the extensive use of medical technology and passive treatment modalities in these chronic patients.

> 'Who you see is what you get.'
>
> The choice of investigations and treatments for back pain depends more on the specialty of the doctor than the condition of the patient's back.
> Individual doctors vary even more within each specialty:
>
> - individual *diagnostic signature*
> - individual *treatment signature*

Physical therapy

Hart et al (1995) found that physical therapy was ordered at 21% of medical visits for back pain in 1990. That would mean about 1.5 million people with back pain get physical therapy each year in the US. At least 25% of all physical therapy is for low back pain. Jette et al (1994) found that 99% of physical therapy patients with back pain were referred by a doctor. At least until 1990, hardly any Americans went directly to physical therapy, although there are some suggestions that this may be changing in the last few years. About half the patients attend within 1 month of onset of pain but about 40% have chronic pain for more than 3 months. They are mainly white and middle-aged, and there are equal numbers of men and women. The average course of physical therapy is 10–11 visits over about 5 weeks. In 1990 that cost $767.

Battie et al (1994) gave Cherkin's three patient vignettes to physical therapists. There are striking professional differences in beliefs about the cause of nonspecific low back pain. Physicians believe the most common cause is muscle strain. Chiropractors believe it is vertebral subluxation. And physical therapists believe it is disc problems and muscle strain. When it comes to diagnostic coding, however, they all use 'sprains and strains' (ICD 846 and 847), which are the diagnostic codes for which they are most likely to be paid.

Physical therapists believe the goals of treatment for back pain are to reduce pain (90%), improve range of movement (57%), increase strength (35%), reduce muscle spasm (22%) and improve posture (22%) (Jette et al 1994). For Cherkin's three patients, therapists usually gave a combination of education, passive modalities and some form of back exercises.

Jette et al (1994) reported actual practice, from a national survey of physical therapists in 1989–1990. Seventy-six per cent of patients with back pain were prescribed back exercises, 76% got modalities, 34% got manual therapy and only 6% got functional training. The McKenzie system was most popular and 85% of its practitioners believed it to be effective.

Jette & Jette (1996) and Jette & Delitto (1997) present the most up-to-date information from a further survey in 1993–1994 (Table 21.10).

Table 21.10 Treatments recorded by physical therapists for back pain during 1993–1994 (based on data from Jette & Jette 1996)

Treatment	Percentage of patients with back pain
Flexibility exercises	84%
Strengthening exercises	81%
Heat modalities	81%
Endurance exercises	52%
Manual therapy	39%
Cold modalities	19%

Ninety-six per cent of patients got a combination of treatments, most often flexibility exercises, strengthening exercises and heat. Many therapists start at the acute stage with mainly passive modalities and manual therapy to relieve pain. Then, as pain becomes less, they progress to more active treatment such as aerobic exercises. However, the data from this study suggests that may be more to do with the therapist's routine of treatment rather than the clinical course of the individual patient.

This study also related treatments to outcome. Patients who received passive treatments with heat or cold had worse outcomes. Flexibility and strengthening exercises made no difference to outcomes. Patients who were prescribed endurance exercises had better outcomes. These findings all agree with the scientific evidence. Manual therapy made no difference to outcomes, which is contrary to the scientific evidence. However, at the acute stage, 27% of these patients received 'mobilization' while only 3.7% received 'manipulation'. The lack of effect on outcomes may raise questions about the form of mobilization given by physical therapists. There are limitations to this type of survey, and we should not over-interpret these results. There is no data on patient characteristics or on which patients received different treatments. Obviously, the therapist had some reason for giving different treatments to different patients and they may not be comparable. Most patients got multiple treatments, which makes it difficult to disentangle their effects. Nevertheless, it does appear that a great deal of physical therapy for back pain in

1993–1994 was still educational advice, passive modalities and specific back exercises – this despite the scientific evidence that these are all ineffective. More encouraging is the fact that there is much greater use of endurance exercises, and the survey confirms the value of that approach on a national scale. Ehrmann-Feldman et al (1996) offered suggestive evidence that patients who receive physical therapy within a month of onset are more likely to return to work within 60 days.

Physician beliefs and patient satisfaction

Bush et al (1993) found that primary care physicians had little confidence in their ability to treat back pain. 'I lack the diagnostic tools or knowledge to effectively assess patients with back pain'. 'There is little I can do to prevent patients with acute back pain from developing chronic back pain'. 'I am very uncomfortable treating patients with low back pain'.

Chiropractors are much more confident about their training and their ability to help patients with back pain (Cherkin et al 1988). They are more comfortable and less frustrated by back pain, which is just as well as it is two-thirds of their practice! Despite the philosophic basis of chiropractic medicine, the chiropractors in this study firmly believed that back pain depends on physical factors that they can and should diagnose. Family doctors (MDs) were less certain about the physical basis of back pain and their ability to assess it. Medical doctors and physical therapists placed more emphasis on the role of psychosocial factors in chronic pain and disability. Most practitioners agreed that job factors are also important, although DOs and DCs rated them less highly.

Battie et al (1994) found that only 8% of physical therapists felt well prepared and ready to manage low back pain when they first entered practice. Even experienced therapists had doubts about their ability to affect recovery. Seventy-five per cent felt that they could help patients with acute sciatica. Only 50–65% felt that they could help patients with acute,

recurrent or chronic low back pain without sciatica. Half the therapists agreed that: 'Patients with low back pain often have unrealistic expectations about what therapists can do for them'. 'I often feel frustrated by patients with low back pain who want me to fix them'.

Deyo & Diehl (1986) found that about one-third of patients with acute low back pain felt they did not get an adequate explanation of their problem. They still did not understand what was wrong. These patients remained more worried about serious illness and felt they should have had more tests. They were less satisfied with their doctor and less likely to want to see the same doctor again.

Bush et al (1993) found that patients were reasonably satisfied with their health providers and treatment but less satisfied with the information they received. When physicians were more confident, their patients were more satisfied with the information they gave. Bush et al suggested that the main reason for consulting a physician with back pain may be to seek information and reassurance. These patients may not expect a cure and have little need for empathy. Rather, they want to learn about their low back pain, what to expect and what they can do about it. If they get the information they want, they will be more satisfied with their care. Several studies have found that chiropractic patients are more satisfied with the chiropractor's explanations and with their care. Perhaps for that reason, a higher proportion of chiropractic patients continue to attend the same practitioner.

von Korff et al (1994) studied 44 primary care physicians and how they managed patients with low back pain. Practice style varied in the amount and intensity of medical intervention (Table 21.11). Some physicians ordered less medication on a time-contingent basis, advised patients to stay active and put more emphasis on self-care. Others ordered more opioids and sedatives on a pain-contingent basis, and more and longer bed rest. The latter group were also more likely to raise the question of further investigation and possible surgery.

Table 21.11 Physician practice styles (based on data from von Korff et al 1994)

Percentage of patients receiving	Low interventionist	Moderate	High interventionist
Sedatives or hypnotics	22%	27%	44%
Extended use	3%	5%	8%
Opioids	17%	31%	43%
Extended use	2%	4%	6%
Multiple medications	3%	11%	20%
Bed rest	16%	29%	40%
Extended use	4%	8%	15%

von Korff et al then looked at how physician practice style affected patient outcomes. Patients of low interventionist physicians were more satisfied with the information they received. Despite getting fewer analgesics, they had similar pain relief and there was no difference in long-term outcome. They returned to daily activities faster and had less activity limitation at 1 month although there was no significant difference by 1 year. They had lower health care costs for back pain over the next year. The benefits are clear. A low interventionist practice style can give faster return to normal activity at lower cost, with no difference in pain relief, patient satisfaction or long-term outcomes.

Hospitalization

Back problems were the seventh leading cause for hospitalization in the US in 1988. Non-surgical hospitalization for back pain was the fourth most common medical reason after heart failure and shock, angina and psychoses.

National Hospital Discharge Surveys show that nonsurgical hospitalizations fell from 580 500 in 1979 to 265 500 in 1990 (Taylor et al 1994). This reflects change in medical practice. There was some change from inpatient myelography to noninvasive imaging and outpatient investigation, but most of the change was probably due to insurers introducing review criteria for payment.

Cherkin & Deyo (1993) studied 337 000 nonsurgical hospitalizations for low back pain in 1988. The mean age of these patients was 50 years, and 23% were over 65 years. There were equal numbers of males and females.

Thirty-one per cent were admitted from the emergency room. Eleven per cent had pain for less than 1 day, 27% for 1–7 days, 30% for 1–6 weeks, and 32% for more than 6 weeks. The median length of stay was 4 days but a quarter stayed in hospital more than 1 week. Forty-three per cent were under the care of a family physician or internist; 30% were under an orthopedic surgeon; 10% were under a neuro-surgeon, and 17% were under other specialties. The discharge diagnosis was nonspecific back pain in 35%, a herniated disc in 31% and degenerative changes in 15%.

About half were admitted for imaging studies, a quarter for pain control and a quarter for both reasons. While in hospital, 72% were prescribed bed rest and 22% received traction. 83% were given narcotics and 71% were given sedatives, and 55% of patients got these by the parenteral route. Forty-nine per cent of these patients had previous hospitalization for back pain and 30% had previous back surgery. Twenty per cent were subsequently readmitted for surgery and 8% for further nonsurgical hospitalization within the next year. Psychosocial problems were very common: 20% of records noted psychologic problems and a further 28% had no carer at home. The circumstances of admission and discharge diagnoses suggest that 70–80% of these patients had no clear medical indication for hospitalization. Rather, it reflects psychosocial pressure on physicians and the lack of adequate outpatient alternatives for acute pain relief.

We need a new medical and social consensus on the role of hospitalization for back pain. Cherkin & Deyo (1993) suggested that valid medical reasons for hospitalization include severe or increasing neurology, major trauma and serious spinal pathology. Nonmedical reasons might include difficulty ambulating and lack of a carer at home, especially in elderly patients. Rural patients living long distances from medical care and investigations may need accommodation, but that does not need to be in hospital. There is already a trend to outpatient investigations. There is also a need for alternative methods of providing outpatient acute pain relief.

Low back surgery

Back and neck operations are the third most common form of surgery in the US. Only caesarean section and tubal ligation are more common.

National Hospital Discharge Surveys show that low back operations increased from 147 500 in 1979 to 279 000 in 1990 (Taylor et al 1994). Surgery rates rose in all age groups, but the greatest rise was in the elderly. For those under age 65, the rate rose from 113 to 152 per 100 000. For older patients, it rose from 51 to 188 per 100 000 – nearly four-fold. The rate of fusion doubled, for no clear reason. The greatest increase was in surgery for spinal stenosis, which rose eight-fold from 7.8 to 61.4 per 100 000. This was probably due to greater awareness of the condition and greater availability of imaging and surgery.

Taking both nonsurgical and surgical cases, the total number of Americans admitted to hospital with back problems fell from 728 000 in 1979 to 544 500 in 1990. The latest figures for 1993 show that it is unchanged at 575 000 (AAOS 1996).

REGIONAL VARIATION

There has been great debate about regional variation in health care for back pain. 'Marked regional variations ... imply a lack of consensus about appropriate assessment and treatment of low back problems, suggesting that some patients may be receiving inappropriate or sub-

optimal care' (AHCPR 1994). Much of the concern is about the escalating cost of health care. 'Health care reform has assumed an aura of inevitability, with cost containment a major goal of the reform movement' (Volinn et al 1994).

There is little evidence of any regional variation in back pain. The *Nuprin Pain Report* found identical prevalence in different parts of the country. Deyo & Tsui-Wu (1987) suggested there might be a lower prevalence of chronic back pain in the north-east, but despite this found no regional variation in disability or work loss.

There is a great deal of regional variation in health care for back pain. Shekelle et al (1995a) found that the numbers seeking health care for back pain each year varied between 4.5 and 7.5% in different centers. Deyo & Tsui-Wu (1987) and Hart et al (1995) found that people with back pain in the north-east are least likely to consult a physician. There is also regional variation in whom they consult. Those in the north-east are more likely to go to family doctors and orthopedic surgeons. There is more use of chiropractic in the west and less in the north-east.

There is nearly twofold variation in hospitalization and surgery rates in different regions of the country. Nonsurgical hospitalization, myelography rates and surgery rates are all highest in the south and lowest in the west and north-east (Table 21.12). Sixteen per cent of spinal operations involve fusion in the midwest, but only 11% in the north-east.

The smaller the areas we compare, the greater the variations in health care for back pain. It varies up to two-fold between the main regions of the country, up to about 10-fold

Table 21.12 Regional variation in hospital treatment; annual rates per 100 000 adults (based on data from Taylor et al 1994)

	Nonsurgical hospitalization	Spinal surgery
West	104	113
North-east	162	131
Mid-west	191	157
South	204	171

between different centers, and most of all between individual practitioners. Volinn et al (1992) found nearly 15-fold variation in spinal surgical rates between Washington State counties in 1985. By 1990, after much professional education, nonsurgical hospitalization rates varied from 38 to 97/100 000 and surgery rates from 153 to 300/100 000 in the same areas (Taylor et al 1995). Those centers with the highest surgery rates also had the highest nonsurgical hospitalization rates. So nonsurgical hospitalization is not a substitute for surgery. Rather, both hospital admission and surgery appear to reflect a more interventionist practice style.

We should keep this regional variation in perspective. Back pain is no different from any other medical condition. The variation for back pain is about average and much less than for many other common health problems. However, as AHCPR points out, the amount of variation does imply lack of consensus. Patients and physicians may simply feel that they have to 'do something' but they are still not sure what to do. Volinn et al (1992) tried to analyze 28 possible influences on this variation, with little success. Occupational factors and the number of surgeons in each area did affect surgical rates, but to a limited extent. They could only suggest once again that the variation depends mainly on 'physician practice style'.

If there is so much variation, how do we decide what is appropriate or 'correct' care? Is medical care rationed in low rate areas, or overused in high rate areas, or both? We simply do not have the data at present to answer this. There is no direct evidence that too little or too much care for back pain produces better or worse outcomes, or affects the amount of pain and disability in the population. If we cannot show what kind of care is effective, it is tempting to ask if expensive interventions are justified. If all regions had the same rates of hospitalization and surgery for back pain as those with the lowest rates, that might save $500 million in health care costs each year. That is certainly true, but that does not mean it is right.

We might also compare current practice with agreed standards or guidelines, and that can produce impressive figures. By this argument, we might reduce plain radiographs by 50%, most conservative treatments by 80%, imaging by 50%, disc surgery by 50% and fusion by up to 90%. But are these figures real, and does this mean anything? It depends on who sets the 'standards', and how well they reflect scientific evidence or simply current consensus. Guidelines and health care use are quite different things. The supporters of most of these procedures produce clinical evidence to suggest that current rates are actually too low. At present, we simply do not have the information to decide what should be the 'correct' level of health care for back pain.

The answers to these dilemmas depend on research in three areas (Volinn et al 1994):

- outcomes of treatment for low back pain, effectiveness and cost-effectiveness
- patient preferences
- doctor and patient decision-making, practice style and how to change practice to achieve the first two goals.

HEALTH CARE FOR BACK PAIN IN THE US

Let me try to summarize health care for back pain in the US.

About 110 million US adults have some low back pain each year and 20 million have back pain lasting 2 weeks or more. There is no evidence that the prevalence of back pain in the US is changing or much different from that in Europe. About 12 million Americans seek health care for back pain each year. Back pain is now the fifth most common reason for visiting a physician in the US and accounts for 2.8% of physician office visits. That is a total of about 15 million visits each year. The number of visits rose about one-quarter over the past decade, but that is the same as the increase in all health care.

Health care for back pain in the US is a curious mixture of dramatic contrasts. The majority of Americans still deal with back pain themselves most of the time and get on with their lives more or less normally. Then there are two completely different health care systems for back pain in the US: conventional medicine and chiropractic medicine. Sixty per cent of people who seek health care for back pain choose medical care, and 40% choose chiropractic instead.

Medical care has two very different patterns. Forty per cent of patients with back pain get treatment mainly in primary medical care. But about 20% get treatment from medical specialists with a great deal of high-tech and high-cost investigations and interventions. A total of 575 000 patients are now hospitalized each year for back disorders, and 300 000 of them have a spinal operation. Nonsurgical hospitalization has come under scrutiny and has fallen by more than half in the past decade. Over the same period the number of spinal operations has nearly doubled. Nearly 5 million Americans make about 50 million visits to chiropractors each year. This had doubled in the previous decade, and some recent estimates suggest that it may now be even higher. There are also about 15 million visits to physical therapists.

It is likely that many American patients move between the different health care systems for back pain, although we do not know what influences their choices. The *Nuprin Pain Report* (Taylor & Curran 1985) found that about one-third of patients said they had only seen one doctor with their back pain. A quarter had seen two and 40% had seen three or more doctors,

although it is not clear over what period. Deyo & Tsui-Wu (1987) found that patients with at least 2 weeks of back pain had seen an average of 1.66 physicians. About one-third of those who attend a medical doctor have also used some form of complementary medicine in the past year. About one-half of those who see a specialist are referred from primary medical care. We can combine these figures to get a very rough estimate of the complete picture (Table 21.13).

Remember, the scientific evidence shows that many of the treatments still in common use for back pain are ineffective. So it is not surprising that the choice of provider appears to make little difference to clinical outcomes. And despite enormous and rising costs of health care for back pain, we have little evidence on the cost-effectiveness of different kinds of care.

There are no good figures for the cost of back pain in the US, although there is no doubt it is expensive. It is difficult to get an accurate estimate because of the way health care is organized and funded and the lack of national data. It is also difficult to estimate trends. There is increasing use of high-tech and high-cost investigations and interventions, but we do not know the impact of managed care. Frymoyer & Durett (1997) estimated direct medical costs to be $33 billion in 1994, but unfortunately tried to extrapolate this from 1972 to 1978 data. Indirect costs may be two to four times the direct costs but Frymoyer & Durett were unable to reach any definite figure.

Table 21.13 Estimated overlap between different health care systems in the US (millions per annum)

	Deal with it themselves	Chiropractic	Primary medical care	Medical specialist
Total	100	4.8	4.7	2.5
Alone		3.2	1.8	?

Chiropractic + primary care 1.6

Referred from primary care to specialist 1.3

Other health providers ?

US vs. UK

How does health care for back pain in the US compare with that in the UK (Waddell 1996)?

Perhaps surprisingly, more people in the UK seek health care for back pain (Table 21.14), which probably reflects free access to the National Health Service (NHS). The RAND Health Insurance Experiment in the US showed that free access may increase use of health care for back pain by up to 28%.

In the UK, 99% of all health care is by the NHS, and access to investigations, therapy and specialists is via the family doctor. In the US, health care is in private practices. More US patients with back pain see a medical specialist and many patients self-refer directly to a specialist. In the US there are many more chiropractors than in the UK and they provide about 40% of the health care for back pain. There are fewer chiropractors in the UK, but the numbers are growing.

Table 21.15 compares treatments and costs of back pain in the two countries. Medical care for back pain in the UK is mainly in primary care and consists of rest, analgesics, plain X-rays and physical therapy. It is high-volume, low-tech and low-cost. It is often long delayed and only 2% of NHS patients receive physical

Table 21.15 A comparison of treatment for back pain in the US and the UK (number of patients per annum) (from Waddell 1996, with permission)

	US	UK
Treatment		
Physical therapy	1.5 million	1.3 million
Plain X-ray	4 million	1.5 million
Spinal CT and MRI	1.8 million	100 000
Nonsurgical hospitalization	265 500	76 000
Spinal operation	279 000	24 000
Fusion	45 500	<2000
Cost		
Health care costs	$33 billion	$1 billion
Total cost to society	>$100 billion?	$9 billion

therapy within 3 months of onset of their pain. Dissatisfaction with NHS services for back pain is so high that 55% of patients with back pain seek private therapy instead. Primary medical care and treatment for back pain in the US are very similar to those in the UK. But more American patients see medical specialists with high rates of CT, MRI and surgery. This specialist care is high-tech and high-cost. Orthopedics is the main medical specialty in both countries, but US and UK orthopedic surgeons do different things for back pain. In the US, about one in five of the patients who go to see an orthopedic or neurosurgeon will sooner or later

Table 21.14 Millions of adults consulting each year and who they visit (based on data from Waddell 1996)

	US	UK
Total population	255	55
Adults >18 years	190	44
Patients consulting (and as % of adults)		
Population surveys	24 (12.2%)	6.9 (15.7%)
Medical records	12 (6.1%)	4.5 (10.2%)
Medical doctor	7.2	4.0
Primary care	4.7	4.0
Specialist	2.5	1.6
(Referred from another doctor)	(45%)	(100%)
Chiropractor	4.8	0.3
Main provider of care		
General/family physician (MD)	3.1	4.0
Chiropractor	4.8	0.3
Osteopath (DO)	0.9	0.7
Orthopedic surgeon	1.0	0.8
Other medical specialist	2.2	0.7

have spinal surgery. In the UK, less than 3% of those who see a surgeon will ever have an operation. British patients go to an orthopedic surgeon for a second opinion and advice, and orthopedic principles then influence their management. American patients go to surgeons for an operation and the US has the highest rate of spinal surgery in the world (Table 21.16).

US vs. UK – a caricature

- US medical care for back pain is fragmented, too specialized, too invasive and too expensive
- NHS care for back pain in the UK is more cohesive, but under-funded, too little, and too late
- Despite the very different health care systems, there is little evidence that they make much difference to the social impact of back pain in the two countries.

Table 21.16 International back surgery rates compared with the US for 1988 (based on data from Cherkin et al 1994b)

	Ratio to US rate
US	1.0
Netherlands	0.73
Denmark	0.64
Finland	0.56
Norway	0.49
Canada	0.49
Australia	0.44
New Zealand	0.40
Sweden	0.33
UK	0.19

REFERENCES

AAOS 1996 Physician visits and hospitalization for back and neck conditions by major diagnostic grouping 1993. American Academy of Orthopaedic Surgeons, Rosemont, IL

AHCPR 1994 Clinical Practice Guideline Number 14. Acute low back problems in adults. Agency for Health Care Policy and Research, US Department of Health and Human Services, Rockville, MD

Andersson G B J 1991 The epidemiology of spinal disorders. In: Frymoyer J W (ed) The adult spine: principles and practice. Raven Press, New York, ch 8, p 107–146

Battie M C, Cherkin D C, Dunn R, Clol M A, Wheeler K J 1994 Managing low back pain: attitudes and treatment preferences of physical therapists. Physical Therapy 74: 219–226

Bush T, Cherkin D, Barlow W 1993 The impact of physician attitudes on patient satisfaction with care for low back pain. Archives of Family Medicine 2: 301–305

Carey T S, Evans A T, Hadler N M et al 1996 Acute severe low back pain. A population-based study of prevalence and care-seeking. Spine 21: 339–344

Carey T S, Garrett J, Jackman A, McLaughlin C, Fryer J, Smuckler D R 1995 The outcomes and costs of care for acute low back pain among patients seen by primary care practitioners, chiropractors and orthopaedic surgeons. New England Journal of Medicine 333: 913–917

Cherkin D C, MacCornack F A, Berg A O 1988 Managing low back pain – a comparison of the beliefs and behaviors of family physicians and chiropractors. Western Journal of Medicine 149: 475–480

Cherkin D C, Deyo R A 1993 Non-surgical hospitalization for low-back pain: is it necessary? Spine 18: 1728–1735

Cherkin D C, Deyo R A, Wheeler K, Ciol M A 1994a Physician variation in diagnostic testing for low back pain. Arthritis and Rheumatism 37: 15–22

Cherkin D C, Deyo R A, Loeser J D, Bush T, Waddell G 1994b An international comparison of back surgery rates. Spine 19: 1201–1206

Cherkin D C, Deyo R A, Wheeler K, Ciol M A 1995 Physician views about treating low back pain. The results of a national survey. Spine 20: 1–10

Cypress B K 1983 Characteristics of physician visits for back symptoms: A national perspective. American Journal of Public Health 73: 389–395

Deyo R A, Diehl A K 1986 Patient satisfaction with medical care for low back pain. Spine 11: 28–30

Deyo R A, Taylor V M, Diehr P et al 1994 Analysis of auto-mated administrative and survey databases to study patterns and outcomes of care. Spine 19: 2083S–2091S

Deyo R A, Tsui-Wu Y-J 1987 Descriptive epidemiology of low back pain and its related medical care in the United States. Spine 12: 264–268

Ehrmann-Feldmann D, Rossignol M, Abenhaim L, Gabrielle D 1996 Physician referral to physical therapy in a cohort of workers compensated for low back pain. Physical Therapy 76: 150–157

Eisenberg D M, Kessler R C, Foster C et al 1993 Unconventional medicine in the United States. New England Journal of Medicine 328: 246–252

Elam K C, Cherkin D C, Deyo R 1995 How emergency physicians approach low back pain: choosing costly options. Journal of Emergency Medicine 13: 143–150

Frymoyer J W 1988 Back pain and sciatica. New England Journal of Medicine 318: 291–300

Frymoyer J W, Durett C L 1997 the economics of spinal disorders. In: Frymoyer J W (ed) The adult spine, 2nd edn. Lippincott-Raven, Philadelphia, p 143–150

Guo H-R, Tanaka S, Cameron L L et al 1995 Back pain among workers in the United States: national estimates and workers at high risk. American Journal of Industrial Medicine 28: 591–602

Hart L G, Deyo R A, Cherkin D C 1995 Physician office visits for low back pain. Frequency, clinical evaluation, and treatment patterns from a U.S. national survey. Spine 20: 11–19

Jette A M, Delitto A 1997 Physical therapy treatment choices for musculoskeletal impairments. Physical Therapy 77: 145–154

Jette D U, Jette A M 1996 Physical therapy and health outcomes in patients with spinal impairments. Physical Therapy 76: 930–945

Jette A M, Smith K, Haley S M, Davis K D 1994 Physical therapy episodes of care for patients with low back pain. Physical Therapy 74: 101–110

Nviendo J, Haas M, Goldberg B 1996 Cost-effectiveness of chiropractic and medical treatment for acute and chronic recurrent low back pain. Proceedings of the FCER International Conference on Spinal Manipulation, Bournemouth, England, p 87–88

Shekelle P G, Markovich M, Louie R 1995a An epidemiologic study of episodes of back pain care. Spine 20: 1668–1673

Shekelle P G, Markovich M, Louie R 1995b Comparing the costs between provider types of episodes of back pain care. Spine 20: 221–227

Stano M, Smith M 1996 Chiropractic and medical costs of low back care. Medical Care 34: 191–204

Taylor H, Curran N M 1985 The Nuprin pain report. Louis Harris and Associates, New York

Taylor V M, Deyo R A, Cherkin D C, Kreuter W 1994 Low back pain hospitalization. Recent United States trends and regional variations. Spine 19: 1207–1213

Taylor V M, Deyo R A, Goldberg H, Ciol M, Kreuter W, Spunt B 1995 Low back pain hospitalizations in Washington State: recent trends and geographical variations. Journal of Spinal Disorders 8: 1–7

Volinn E, Mayer J, Diehr P, Van Koevering D, Connell F A, Loeser J D 1992 Small area analysis of surgery for low back pain. Spine 17: 575–581

Volinn E, Turczyn K M, Loeser J D 1994 Patterns in low back pain hospitalizations: implications for the treatment of low back pain in an era of health care reform. Clinical Journal of Pain 10: 64–70

Von Korff M, Barlow W, Cherkin D, Deyo R A 1994 Effects of practice style in managing back pain. Annals of Internal Medicine 121: 187–195

Von Korff M, Dworkin S F, Le Resche L A et al 1988 An epidemiologic comparison of pain complaints. Pain 32: 173–183

Waddell G 1996 Low back pain: a twentieth century health care enigma. Spine 21: 2820–2825

22

Future health care for back pain

I must make it clear that this is a personal view, although I have used ideas and material from many sources. I am particularly grateful to the Clinical Standards Advisory Group subcommittee on back pain (CSAG 1994). However, I would emphasize that this is simply a starting point for research and development into future health care for back pain.

There is growing acceptance of the need to change our clinical management for back pain. This whole book presents the argument and the evidence for such an approach. We are slower to realize that to put this new approach into practice we must also change the health care delivery system to make it possible. Let us try to work out how we should change professional practice and the health care system to do this (Box 22.1).

I fully recognize that the proposals in Box 22.1 still need to be tested in practice, although there are a few successful pilot schemes. You may disagree with these suggestions, and it is possible that some of them will turn out to be wrong. But it is not enough for you to argue that you have always practiced a different way and you just know that you are right. These proposals are based on the best evidence that we have at present. If you want to justify your different way of practice, you will need to have a convincing argument and in due course produce the evidence that it works. None of us can simply defend the status quo or evade the need to improve health care for back pain.

Box 22.1 A basis for future health care for back pain

- A biopsychosocial view of low back pain and disability
- We now have considerable evidence for a new approach to the clinical management of back pain, as in recent guidelines
- Current health care for back pain does not meet these guidelines
- Trends of low back disability show that current management and health care have failed to solve the problem

---

Let us put this discussion of health care for back pain into perspective with an epidemiologic view (Croft et al 1997).

- *Primary prevention* of back pain would be ideal, but there is little evidence that we can prevent back pain. General health measures could include reducing smoking and increasing regular exercise and fitness, although it is doubtful how much impact they would have. It may be possible to reduce the risk for specific occupational groups, but there is little evidence at present as to the effectiveness of an ergonomic approach.
- *Secondary prevention:* concentrate on active treatment of episodes to reduce recurrences and chronicity. There is good evidence that this can produce short-term benefits, but little evidence on its long-term benefits or effect on the natural history. As a corollary, concentrate services on those at high risk of chronic pain and disability. This needs more research. Croft et al (1997) gave secondary prevention cautious support but felt that it needs further research.
- *Tertiary prevention:* rehabilitation to reduce the impact of back pain on life and activity, including work. There is reasonable evidence that this can improve clinical outcomes, but little evidence that it improves working capacity. In a sense, this approach also admits defeat, that it is not possible to prevent chronic pain and disability.

THE PROBLEMS WITH PRESENT HEALTH CARE FOR BACK PAIN

There is growing dissatisfaction with health care for back pain throughout the Western world. Many treatments still in common use are ineffective, yet they continue to consume large amounts of health care resources. Much routine management is directly contrary to current clinical guidelines. These guidelines suggest how we could improve clinical management, but practice is slow to change. Equally important, patients can only get the health care that is actually available.

When we presented the CSAG report to a group of British family doctors, one of them accosted us angrily with his dilemma:

These proposals on how to treat back pain are all very well. I agree with most of them. But I can't do that. My local physiotherapy department has a 3 month waiting list. The only place I can refer patients with back pain is to the orthopedic clinic. I know these patients don't have a surgical problem, and that the orthopedic surgeon won't do anything for them, but I don't have any alternative!

I heard a different version of the same dilemma at a recent meeting in the US:

I agree that we do too many MRI scans for back pain. But my patients know all about scans and they want to know what's wrong. The radiologists tell everyone MRI is the best investigation. My patients expect to go and see a surgeon, and if I don't refer them they will just go themselves. The surgeons don't want to miss anything and are afraid they might be sued if they do. Then if the scan shows anything, both patient and surgeon are hooked and can't see past it. You say that MRI doesn't help the management of ordinary back pain, but how can I stop them? I sometimes feel as if that scanner drives my whole clinical practice!

Leave aside the rights or wrongs of these two examples. The common message is that treatment will always be constrained by the services available and by referral patterns. As Cherkin showed, who you see is what you get. The basic problem is that there is a mis-match between what patients with back pain need and the health care that is available for them. If we want to change clinical practice, we must change the health care system to provide the resources and referral patterns required for the new management.

Patients with simple backache have very different needs from those with serious spinal disease. I believe that many of our present problems come from our failure to distinguish and provide for these different needs. We refer them all to the same specialists and clinics. We do not separate patients with nonspecific low back pain from those with serious spinal pathology or nerve root problems. Most medical specialists rightly focus on the investigation and treatment of serious spinal pathology and neurologic problems. That is their expertise, and it is a vital service for the small minority of patients with such problems. But these patients are few in the multitude of patients with back pain. The problem is that the present medical system simply does not provide appropriate resources or services for patients with simple backache. At the same time, patients with simple backache may swamp specialist services. In some countries, this may cause delay for those who do need and can benefit from specialist investigation and treatment. More often, patients with simple backache receive inappropriate and even harmful investigations and treatment that are really designed for different problems. Even when such treatment is simply ineffective rather than directly harmful, it may cause more subtle harm. It perpetuates the focus on disease and on passive, mechanical treatment. It creates unrealistic expectations of symptomatic cure. Delays and protracted treatment also defer more effective management and lead directly to chronic pain and disability. In some cases it may have been better not to have had that referral or treatment at all.

Expensive specialist and hospital investigations and treatments also consume a large portion of the health care dollars spent on back pain. There is much ineffective and wasteful use of health care resources for back pain, and we could spend that money much better in other ways.

The relative balance of these difficulties varies in each health care system. They all share the basic flaw of failing to separate simple backache from specific pathology.

A NEW HEALTH CARE SYSTEM FOR BACK PAIN

How would we need to reorganize the health care system to deliver the kind of care recommended in the guidelines? We should be able to find common principles of a good service for patients with back pain, even if the system will always differ in each country. Most specialist services for serious spinal pathology, nerve root problems and spinal surgery are satisfactory, provided patients are referred and seen without delay. The key problem is to provide a better service for the large number of patients with simple backache. The main aim is to deliver better health care for these patients, but these proposals should also lead to more efficient and cost-effective use of resources.

First, let us consider the basic principles for such a service. Then let us apply these principles to the primary care services needed to manage simple backache, and to a 'back pain rehabilitation service' for those patients who do not settle with primary care management.

Principles of services for back pain

Diagnostic triage
Diagnostic triage forms the basis of appropriate referral and the division of responsibility between primary care and specialist services.

Diagnostic triage and decisions about referral take place at the point of first contact in primary care. Primary care clinicians must detect the few patients with specific pathology among the vast majority with simple backache. Deyo & Phillips (1996) compared this to searching for the proverbial needle in a haystack. Because of the primary care filter, specialists have a much easier task to search for the needles in a smaller stack of hay.

Primary care clinicians must also distinguish between what sometimes seem to be two very different groups of patients with nonspecific back pain. Most patients seem to get better no matter what we do, and need little more than reassurance and advice. We need to identify as early as possible the few who are at risk of developing chronic pain and disability.

Diagnostic triage is generally accurate, but is so fundamental to all these proposals that continuing education is essential.

Division of responsibility between primary care and medical specialist services

There should be a much clearer division of responsibility between primary care and specialist services. This applies both to clinical management and to the provision of services.

Primary care. Management of nonspecific low back pain is, and should be, mainly in primary care (Box 22.2). Specialist services are mainly responsible for the investigation and treatment of patients with serious spinal pathology, nerve root problems that do not settle, and those who require consideration of surgery. Services for those patients with simple backache who fail to settle with routine primary care management should be quite separate from traditional specialist services. There should be a shift of resources from medical specialist services to support management of simple backache in primary care.

Box 22.2 Primary care

- Family medicine
- Osteopathic medicine
- Chiropractic medicine
- Physical therapy
- Occupational health

The aim should be to manage, investigate and treat patients with simple backache as far as possible in primary care. The facilities they require are most appropriate to primary care. These patients do not need medical specialist or hospital facilities. The family doctor or occupational health professional should be aware of the patient's family and work background and can adjust advice and management to suit. We need professional and patient education to

change attitudes and accept that simple backache is really a primary care problem.

Better primary care management of simple backache depends on a shift of resources to primary care. It also requires better undergraduate training and continuing education of primary care health professionals who look after patients with back pain.

Specialist services. Specialists provide two distinct services to patients with back pain. Their main role is the investigation and treatment of patients with specific pathology. They may also provide a secondary service for patients with failed primary care management of simple backache. These two services should be quite distinct, with separate referral patterns, resources and funding.

The main 'spinal disorders' specialties are orthopedic surgery, rheumatology, neurology and neurosurgery. The first priority of these acute specialities should be to provide a rapid and efficient service for those patients who need their expertise and facilities. Acute orthopedic services should focus on patients who need investigation of possible serious spinal pathology or nerve root problems that are not settling. Acute rheumatology services should focus on patients who need investigation of possible serious spinal pathology or inflammatory disorders. Neurology and neurosurgery should provide a service to patients who need investigation and management of neurologic problems or spinal surgery.

The other role is to provide a secondary service for patients with simple backache who do not get better with primary care management. Some specialists and departments do at present provide a very good service for such patients, incorporating many of the present ideas. However, most routine visits to medical specialists do not meet these needs, which is why many patients and family doctors are dissatisfied with these visits for back pain.

The reasons why patients go to a specialist are often different from what actually happens to them (Coulter et al 1991). Any referral of a patient with simple backache to a specialist should have clear and explicit goals. The referring doctor, the patient and the specialist should all agree these goals, which may include confirming the diagnosis, pain control, rehabilitation or vocational assessment. The choice of specialist, the facilities they provide and outcome measures should reflect these goals. There is no point referring a patient to a surgeon and judging the outcome of surgery if what that patient really needs is rehabilitation, retraining or re-employment.

Time-scale of management

Time is vital. Health care for back pain must always take account of the passage of time and the risks of chronic pain and disability. The natural history of back pain is that it is a recurrent problem and recovery may not mean the complete absence of pain. Residual symptoms may remain or pain may recur. The key question is the duration of time off work. There are three main stages (Fig. 22.1) in which the needs for health care are very different.

In the first few weeks most people have a very good chance of recovering rapidly. Indeed, most people with back pain do not seek any professional health care. Most of those who do seek help have very simple health needs:

- reassurance that they do not have any serious disease
- simple, safe symptomatic measures such as medication
- advice to stay as active as possible.

A few patients with more severe pain and distress may require additional symptomatic measures such as manipulation. In view of the good natural history, however, the most important principle at this stage is: 'First, do no harm'. Avoid iatrogenic disability. Do not make the problem a medical one. The main strategy at this stage should be to keep professional intervention to a minimum. There is even an argument that we should discourage any health care for most back pain and instead encourage people to deal with it themselves. If we are going to provide any health care at this stage, we must audit its impact critically.

For the 10% or so who do not recover and return to work within a few weeks, the needs of health care change rapidly. Now, time is of the essence. Waiting for natural recovery lets the patient slide passively and unobtrusively into chronic pain and disability. All the evidence suggests that the first 3–6 weeks are crucial. Too much current health care for back pain is way beyond that time frame. All health

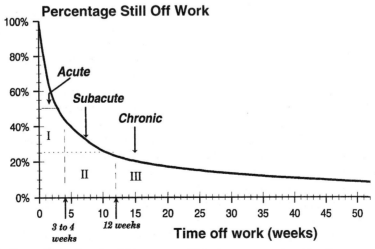

Figure 22.1 Time is of the essence. Clinical management and health care delivery must take account of time. (From Frank et al 1996, with permission.)

professionals dealing with back pain should be much more aware of the dangers of time. There should be a major shift in resources to provide effective management at the subacute stage. Prevention would be much better and probably easier than the present relatively ineffective and wasteful treatment of chronic pain and disability.

Once someone is off work for 3–6 weeks with nonspecific low back pain:

- Time is of the essence
- They are at rapidly increasing risk of chronic pain and disability
- The priority of health care must be to get them back to normal activity and work as fast as possible

---

At the chronic stage, health care resources for established pain and disability should be redirected to pain management and rehabilitation.

Equal emphasis on pain and disability

At present, most health care resources for back pain are for symptomatic treatment. We need a major increase in resources for rehabilitation.

Pain and disability are equally important, and we must manage them both simultaneously. We cannot wait until pain has gone before starting rehabilitation. The best method of achieving lasting relief of pain is to get the patient back to normal activity as soon as possible. We should devote much more effort and resources to the assessment and management of disability and to rehabilitation. We must also organize the service so that access to these resources is readily available to every patient with back pain.

- Low back pain and disability are closely linked and equally important
- Too much current treatment for back pain is purely symptomatic
- We must provide more resources for rehabilitation

Shared responsibility

Back pain is a common bodily symptom that most people deal with themselves most of the time. Health care should help to control symptoms and assist recovery, but that may not mean the complete absence of pain. Residual symptoms may remain or pain may recur. The natural history of nonspecific low back pain is a recurrent problem. Patients rightly have rising expectations of health care, but they must also be realistic. Some will always need help with acute symptoms, and a minority may need prolonged periods of care. But health care can never be the permanent solution to a symptom like back pain. Patients must share responsibility with the doctor or therapist for their own recovery. Patients themselves must take responsibility for their own continued management, and in most cases the sooner they do this, the better.

- Most back pain is an everyday bodily symptom
- There is no magic medical answer for simple backache
- Patients must share responsibility for dealing with their back pain

---

Audit and outcome measures

The aims of clinical management are to provide symptomatic relief and prevent disability. Effectiveness depends on the extent to which we achieve both these aims. Clinical outcome measures include pain, distress, analgesic intake, activities of daily living, capacity for work and health care use. But the most important measure of successful health care for back pain, for the patient and for society, is return to work. We do now have some evidence on the effectiveness of various therapies for back pain. However, the epidemiology of low back disability raises serious doubts about the social impact of health care for back pain. All our professions need much more rigorous audit of health care delivery and clinical outcomes for patients with back pain.

Sick certification

The aim of health care is to control pain and restore the patient to normal activity. That is quite different from, and sometimes in direct conflict with, the need for medical certification for sickness benefits or compensation. Responsibility for clinical management should perhaps be separate from decisions about compensation, in which case the doctor who is caring for the patient should not be the one to decide about sick certification.

Key elements for a primary care service for back pain

If we are going to manage nonspecific low back pain in primary care, we must provide the necessary health care facilities to make this possible (see Box 22.3). These support services should be in primary care or provided by direct access to specialists or hospital services. The key issue is that they should be under the direct control and remain the responsibility of the primary health care provider. The exact form of such a service will vary in each health care system, and will depend on local needs and resources, and patient preferences.

Box 23.3 A primary care service for back pain

- A primary health care provider
- Radiologic services
- Symptomatic control of pain
- Rehabilitation
- Educational material
- An acute pain relief service
- A second opinion
- *A multidisciplinary back pain rehabilitation service*

The primary health care provider

I know it is not currently politically correct, but I am sufficiently old-fashioned to believe that patients still get the best care if one health professional takes final responsibility for their management. Other members of the health care team may play vital roles, but the primary health care provider should take personal responsibility for:

- Clinical assessment. Investigation if appropriate
- Diagnostic triage and referral to the appropriate specialist if required

- Providing or arranging symptomatic relief
- Providing accurate and up-to-date information and advice
- Arranging rehabilitation and coordinating return to work or vocational rehabilitation if required.

Radiologic services

There should be direct primary care access to plain X-rays and bone scans, provided we are always conscious of the role and limitations of these tests. They provide little information about simple backache. There is a strong argument that imaging is inappropriate to the primary care management of simple backache. CT and MRI have high false-positive rates in asymptomatic people, particularly with increasing age, which makes them unsuitable for screening tests. CSAG (1994) argued that these are specialist investigations which should be used for patients with possible serious spinal pathology or those who are being worked up for surgery. There is less argument that we should order both plain X-rays and imaging on clear clinical indications according to radiologic guidelines. There is considerable concern on both sides of the Atlantic about the overuse of these investigations in nonspecific low back pain. X-rays of the spine involve high doses of irradiation. Overinvestigation with imaging leads directly to overtreatment. We should audit the use of radiology in nonspecific low back pain.

Symptomatic measures

One of the primary roles of health care is the relief of pain, and patients will always need symptomatic measures. Simple, safe measures such as temporary modification of activities, medication and the application of heat or cold are adequate for most acute patients.

In view of the evidence that is now available, we should organize services to make manipulation available as an option for all patients with back pain. Osteopathic physicians, chiropractors, osteopaths and an increasing number of physical therapists have professional training and expertise in manipulation. A few medical practitioners also have some training. Some forms of manipulation or mobilization are now widely available, but the techniques used and levels of skills vary widely. We need further research on which forms of manual therapy are most effective for which patients. We also need to audit levels of education, skills and the delivery of manual therapy.

There is then a wide range of further symptomatic options, even if there is little scientific evidence that they are effective.

Symptomatic modalities are not an end in themselves, and probably have little effect on the long-term natural history of back pain. Their main purpose is to provide temporary control of pain, thus allowing patients to increase their activity level and rehabilitate.

- Patients need symptomatic measures to relieve or control their pain
- Symptomatic measures do not cure the problem
- The main aim of symptomatic measures is to let patients get active

Rehabilitation

Rehabilitation facilities should be available for all patients at risk of chronic pain and disability, and particularly those still off work after 3–6 weeks. Physical therapy has a key role in rehabilitation. Referral patterns, physical therapy facilities and organization should reflect this. At present, rehabilitation is often regarded as a tertiary service after 'medical treatment' is complete or has failed. All health care for back pain should stress rehabilitation, and this should start from the acute stage in primary care. To provide these facilities, a major reorganization of services is required, with a shift of resources.

We also need much more research to develop more effective and cost-effective methods of rehabilitation for back pain. And we need to develop ways of delivering them in primary care.

Educational material

Printed and visual educational material should be available that is in line with current guidelines. All members of the primary health care team should give the same information and advice.

An acute pain relief service

Most patients with simple backache get adequate relief of pain from medication or manipulative therapy. Some patients with nerve root pain or, more rarely, simple backache may require further help for the control of acute pain and psychologic distress.

There are a few pilot schemes for acute pain relief for back pain, often linked to chronic pain services or an acute post-operative pain service. This type of service should be much more generally available. It would be a much more appropriate and cost-effective service for these patients than hospitalization or inappropriate surgical consultations. Such an acute pain service would require specific resources and referral arrangements. Patients should be seen within 48 hours of telephone referral to a locally agreed, named contact. The acute pain service is most likely at present to be provided from hospital resources on an outpatient or day case basis.

Second opinion

Some patients and primary care providers may feel the need for a second opinion, particularly if pain and disability are not settling as quickly as they wish. This may reassure both patient and provider and give extra support on:

- assessment, diagnostic triage and psychosocial assessment
- further symptomatic control
- active exercise, rehabilitation and return to work.

On the principle of managing back pain in primary care, this second opinion should ideally remain in the primary care setting. There are at least two ways of providing this:

- *A family doctor with a special interest and expertise in back pain or musculoskeletal disorders.* A family doctor has the ideal skills and is in the ideal situation to provide this service. It is important that family doctors retain a broad clinical practice, but many do now also develop a special interest. Back pain is such a common problem that some family doctors do now have such a special interest in back pain, musculoskeletal medicine or manipulative medicine. Some run special clinics, particularly in large group practices or health maintenance organizations.
- *A chiropractor, osteopath or physical therapist with specialist training and expertise in the assessment and management of back pain.* Many patients find this more satisfactory than a visit to a medical specialist. However, in some health care systems, the role and status of the practitioner or therapist must change if they are to fulfil this need. Every specialist must record and report their assessment, opinion and advice on management, which might be a condition of contract and payment.

Responsibility for overall clinical management would remain with the primary care provider, but the practitioner offering a second opinion would take professional responsibility for the treatment he or she gave. Perhaps most importantly, everyone must accept that this practitioner has the status of an expert or specialist. Some practitioners do now fulfil these criteria and there is emerging acceptance of this role.

A back pain rehabilitation service

Better early management and better primary care services should greatly reduce the number of patients who need further referral. Ideally, we should be able to manage all patients with simple backache in primary care. However, no matter how much we improve management

and services, there will always be some patients with persistent pain and disability. There is a point at which we must accept that primary care management is failing and that some patients need further help.

CSAG (1994) considered how to reorganize secondary services to best meet the needs of these patients. We got wide support for the idea of a 'back pain rehabilitation service', (Box 22.4). This should be a dedicated service because of the numbers of patients and the resources it requires. These are multidisciplinary in nature and cut across specialty and organizational boundaries. The service should have completely separate aims, resources and referral patterns from medical specialty services for patients with serious spinal pathology or nerve root problems. The service should be clearly identified and named as a back pain rehabilitation service.

Box 22.4 A dedicated, multidisciplinary, back pain rehabilitation service

- Led by a specialist with expertise in back pain rehabilitation
- Distinct referral patterns
- Organization, staffing and resources focusing on pain management and rehabilitation
- Facilities for:
  — diagnostic triage and investigation
  — clinical, psychologic and occupational assessment
  — pain control
  — manipulative therapy
  — an active exercise, functional restoration and rehabilitation program
  — counseling
  — occupational or vocational rehabilitation

In principle, we could locate the service wherever the resources are available. Ideally, on the principle of managing simple backache in primary care, we should locate it in primary care. To get patients back to work, it might best be in the workplace as part of an occupational health service. These options should be the subject of future research. However, the multidisciplinary resources that such a service needs are rarely available at present in either primary care or occupational health. The staff, resources and organization may at present be most available and supplied most efficiently from a specialist or hospital service.

The service should be multidisciplinary in nature and approach, although the exact range of staff might vary with local needs and resources. Ideally, the service should have the facilities to provide: diagnostic triage and investigation; clinical, psychologic, and occupational assessment; pain control facilities; manipulative therapy; an active exercise, functional restoration and rehabilitation program; counseling; and occupational or vocational rehabilitation.

The major emphasis of the service should be on pain management and rehabilitation. The choice of staff should match this aim. These needs are mainly low-tech, low-cost and high-volume in nature, and the organization, staffing and resources should reflect that. CSAG did not recommend a multidisciplinary group of high-tech medical specialties.

The service should be led by an experienced practitioner. Both patients and family doctors expect and demand high-quality, expert service. The nominated person should be able to take final professional responsibility for the service. His or her contract should specify that responsibility and the person should have adequate time in his or her job description. At present, the person is most likely to be a medical specialist from orthopedic surgery, rheumatology, rehabilitation medicine, pain management, orthopedic or musculoskeletal medicine. However, in future he or she might better come from family medicine, osteopathic medicine, chiropractic medicine, behavioral medicine or physical therapy. Whatever the practitioner's background, his or her main commitment and responsibility must be to the overall management and rehabilitation of back pain. His or her job is not to provide individual specialty skills or techniques.

Many of the resources required for such a service already exist, and are already provided piecemeal to patients with back pain. It is largely a matter of more efficient organization of these resources. This is also likely to be more cost-effective. Medical specialty input to the service should be on a sessional basis, e.g. pain relief techniques. Primary care staff of family doctors, chiropractors, osteopaths, physical therapists and counselors can and should do much of the work. The back pain rehabilitation service should work closely with local primary care services and contribute to continuing professional education. Close links will also facilitate referral and coordination with primary care management. There should be a major emphasis on self-help to prepare patients for their own continued management. Group therapy and support groups are useful in principle and cost-effective. The service should liaise with employers and occupational health services to help patients return to work as soon as possible. There may be links and shared resources with an acute pain service or pain management program. The main physical resources are clinic space, physical and manual therapy and occupational therapy facilities, and low-cost rehabilitation equipment.

Conclusion

To change clinical management for back pain, we must reorganize the health care system to provide these new services. We must change referral patterns to match patient rather than professional needs. We need different numbers of different kinds of health professionals for back pain. We must shift health care resources and change how we spend health care dollars for back pain. Unless we change the system, we will not achieve real change in the health care that we deliver to patients with back pain.

CHANGE IN PROFESSIONAL PRACTICE

New clinical management and a new health care system for back pain means that we must all change our professional practice. We must change what we do and how we use our time with patients with back pain. This applies to physicians, chiropractors, physical therapists and osteopaths alike.

A biopsychosocial approach

We all share common philosophic ideals for health care. Despite that, most orthodox and alternative health professionals still think and practice according to an outdated biomedical model:

- pain as a signal of injury and tissue damage
- search for a structural cause and cure
- purely symptomatic treatment
- a mechanical 'fix'
- taking over responsibility and control from the patient.

Too often, we all focus too much on pain and the search for a biologic cause and cure, to the exclusion of all else.

A biopsychosocial approach offers the tools to put our common philosophic ideals into practice. It demands a whole new way of thinking. We must assess and deal with:

- the biologic basis of low back pain and disability
- the patient's attitudes and beliefs, emotions and behavior
- social, work and economic impact and influences.

These are all equally important to planning management. This is a much more difficult and challenging type of professional practice, but it opens a whole new vista on back pain.

Triage

One of the first priorities is to make sure there is no serious disease. The primary health care provider usually carries out initial assessment and triage. In some countries and situations, a physical therapist may do this.

Once we rule out serious disease, we should stop the frenzied search for structural pathology. Once we are sure this is nonspecific low back pain, we must approach it more as a matter of disturbed function.

One of the major implications of triage is referral to appropriate care. All health professionals must have a clear idea about which patients for whom our care is appropriate.

More important and more difficult, we must recognize and admit that there are patients for whom our care is not appropriate and refer them to someone else. This is particularly true of simple backache.

Information and advice

Too often, we all give patients the wrong message about back pain. Most of what we say and do – our investigations and diagnosis, and our information and advice to patients – reflects and reinforces the biomedical model. It is about:

- anatomy, discs, trapped nerves, degeneration and mechanical dysfunction
- injury and fear of reinjury
- biomechanics, ergonomics
- physical treatment.

Too often, we label back pain patients with a serious disease, and at the same time offer unconvincing platitudes and unrealistic advice. Too often, patients get conflicting information and advice.

Patients need accurate and honest information, in line with the biopsychosocial model and current guidelines. We should all speak the same language and give the same message. We should think about how our information and advice affect not only patients' backs but also their beliefs and what they do about their pain. We must direct our advice to the goals of rehabilitation and helping patients to take over the care of their own backs.

Information and advice

- Reassurance that there is no serious disease or damage
- A simple explanation of physical dysfunction
- Accurate information about the natural history of back pain
- Encouragement to stay active and continue normal life and work.

Symptomatic modalities

We must provide the best pain control we can, but we must be realistic that all it gives is temporary relief. Most symptomatic treatments have little, if any, lasting effect on recovery from the acute attack or the natural history of back pain. Many health professionals need to reduce the amount of time, effort and resources they put into passive modalities. When we use these modalities, it should be to provide temporary relief of pain with the clear understanding that it is to facilitate rehabilitation.

Rehabilitation

We must place equal importance and spend equal time assessing and dealing with disability. We must consider how all that we say and do, our advice, every treatment, and our whole management affects the patient's function as well as their pain. Too often, in the name of symptomatic treatment, we actually prescribe disability.

Instead, our treatment should support patients to continue their normal activities and to stay at work, or return to work as soon as possible. Our main aim must be to help patients get on with their lives, and that is also the measure of our success. This is a very different agenda from just dealing with physical disease. All health professionals dealing with back pain must be at least aware of and preferably involved in rehabilitation. For some of us, this may mean learning new skills and further training. Liebenson (1996), in his book on *Rehabilitation of the Spine*, shows how to integrate rehabilitation into chiropractic. He points out that manual medicine and rehabilitation make natural partners in musculoskeletal health care.

The importance of work

At present, most health professionals regard their job as health care. We assume that if we make patients better, they will automatically return to normal activity and work. As a result, we pay little direct attention to work issues. Few of us have much knowledge of or any contact with our patient's workplace.

If we are to put equal emphasis on disability, however, work is of paramount importance. We must all think about, ask about, and understand our patient's work situation and demands. We must try to keep patients at work or get them back to work as rapidly as possible. We should more readily and more often pick up the phone and contact their employers or supervisors or the occupational health service to coordinate return to work (Fig. 22.2). Most of all, we should always be conscious of the impact of work loss on our patients and the risk of long-term incapacity.

Health care is not complete or wholly successful, and we have not fulfilled our professional responsibility, until we get our patients back to work.

Sharing responsibility

Too often, health professionals are guilty of taking over control. Occasional patients with back pain continue to attend for months or

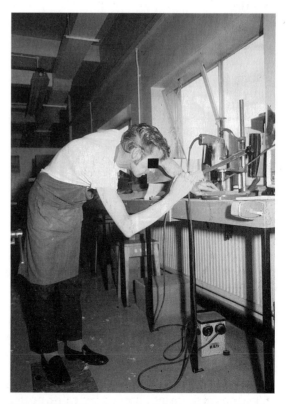

Figure 22.2 'Work for all, for those with low back pain as well.' Return to normal activities and work is the ultimate measure of successful health care for back pain.

> **The longer someone is off work with back pain, the lower their chance of returning to work**
>
> - The minute someone stops work with back pain, there is a risk of 1–10% that they will go on to long-term incapacity
> - Once they are off work for 3–6 months, the risk is 50%
> - By 1–2 years, they are virtually unemployable, irrespective of the physical state of their back or further health care

even years. All our specialties are guilty of this. If patients are to take responsibility for their own backs, we must be willing to relinquish control.

That means one of the measures of success is when patients do take over their own management and no longer need our health care. I am not suggesting that we should deny treatment or set any arbitrary time limit. But in one sense, as long as patients continue to attend, our management has not been wholly successful. There is no evidence that regular 'maintenance therapy' is of any value in the natural history of back pain. It goes against the basic principle that patients should take a large measure of responsibility for their own back pain. Whatever the claimed symptomatic benefit, continuing to attend a health professional may simply perpetuate the illness.

Change in practice

This all means a very different kind of professional practice. It means that we must change how we assess patients, what we say to them and how we treat them.

All of us may argue defensively that we are already making these changes. I agree. Some physicians, chiropractors, physical therapists and osteopaths are now putting these principles into practice. But too often these are isolated examples, or the change is only cosmetic. Different professions commit different sins and need to make different changes. You should recognize what applies to you. All our professions still have a long way to go to put the new management for back pain into routine practice.

This may mean major and fundamental change in our professional practice. At best, it is a challenge. At worst, it is a threat. It can exact a heavy price. I know, perhaps better than most, what that means. I have spent my professional life as an orthopedic surgeon. It has been a good life, and I am proud of what I have done. But I have to admit that surgery is not the answer for back pain, and change what I do. The needs of our patients must over-ride our professional pride.

Knowing what we need to change is one thing. Actually changing professional practice and patient behavior is quite another. There is a great deal of inertia and resistance to change and I can already hear some howls of professional anguish.

There is also sometimes an element of vested interest in maintaining the professional status quo. I had a sudden wicked impulse during the opening ceremony of the 8th World Congress on Pain. I wanted to jump up and address the 4300 pain professionals who had gathered from around the world:

We have wonderful news. Someone has just discovered the cure for pain. It is 100% effective, has no side-effects and only costs a cent. Isn't that wonderful? Human beings need never suffer any more pain. So we might as well cancel this congress. Oh – and you are all out of a job.

I resisted the temptation. I do not know if I would have been lynched or crucified. Of course, health professionals do genuinely have the best interests of their patients at heart. It is just that sometimes we assume that our interests are the same as those of our patients and we may lose sight of what is actually happening to them. We have so much faith and commitment to our own professional activities that we just assume that they *must* be doing our patients good. There is an old saying that health professionals need patients more than patients need us. With back pain, that may be true.

Most health professionals do genuinely believe in most of these ideas for better patient care. The problem is putting these philosophic principles into daily practice. Too often, it is easier just to get on with the job of mechanics.

It is much more difficult and threatening to try to change what we do. It is much easier for me as a surgeon to deal with discs and scans and surgical techniques than to struggle with the complex biopsychosocial problems of chronic low back pain and disability. Yet to serve our patients best, we must all escape from our professional shackles.

There is now an extensive literature on ways of trying to change professional practice (Davis et al 1992, RCGP 1995). Helping professionals to change takes careful planning, enthusiasm and persistence. Different professionals have differing attitudes to new ideas and guidelines, and vary greatly in their willingness to change. It depends on whether they are convinced that change is necessary and worthwhile. They may be influenced by professional opinion leaders and by peer pressure. They must come to feel that these are their ideas, with 'ownership' of the new practice. It will depend on the ease or difficulty of change, and whether they have the necessary skills and abilities to change. There should be local strategies and broad agreement on how to implement the change. Practical reminders during each consultation should focus on the management of the individual patient. Audit, peer review and feedback may reinforce the new practice. The more cynical would suggest that health professionals, just like donkeys, may also respond to the carrot or the stick of financial incentives.

Most of that is about change imposed from outside, and much of the evidence suggests that is not very effective. Real change comes from within and depends on new ideas that spark our imagination and change the way we think. Optimistically, I believe the time for that revolution in thinking may have come for back pain.

FUTURE RESEARCH AND DEVELOPMENT

Priorities for health research should match patients' and society's needs. Back pain is now a major cause of human suffering and disability, health care use and cost to society. By any criteria, back pain should be a high priority for research funding.

Box 22.5 lists the main areas of biomedical research from a 1980 symposium on idiopathic back pain. These priorities are equally valid today. Continued basic research is vital. It is the hope for better understanding of the cause and treatment of back pain.

We need much more basic research into the physical basis of non-specific low back pain. We must relate this to clinical findings in the individual patient, and differentiate syndromes within nonspecific low back pain. We must find which treatments are effective for which types of back pain, and develop a rational basis for choosing the best treatment for each patient. We must develop effective methods of dealing with the important psychosocial issues and more effective methods of rehabilitation.

Within the last decade, randomized controlled trials of all treatments for back pain have given us our present evidence base and clinical guidelines. However, we still need many more high quality RCTs. In future, the Cochrane Collaboration should collate that evidence and make it available on-line for instant access (Bombardier et al 1997).

However, that is only one kind of research, which reflects the interests of basic scientists, pain specialists and spinal surgeons. But there are other kinds of research that are just as important. We also need health services research into how we can actually deliver better care. How can we provide the most effective and cost-effective health care with finite resources in the trenches of daily practice? How well does our health care actually meet the needs of our patients with nonspecific low back pain?

Until recently, there was little primary care research into back pain, but that situation has now changed. In the past decade there has been an explosion of chiropractic research, mainly in the US. In the last 5 years a flourishing primary care research has emerged, particularly in the US, the UK, the Netherlands and Israel. The first international forum for primary care research on low back pain was in Seattle in October 1995. Sixty leading researchers in the field came from nine countries. One of the main goals of the forum was to draft an agenda for primary care research. All those

coming to the meeting had to submit a written list of their most important research questions. At the end of the two day meeting we discussed these issues, and then each cast five votes to those we felt were most important. Box 22.6 lists the top 20 research questions (Borkan & Cherkin 1996).

Box 22.5   Research priorities from the 1980 symposium on idiopathic low back pain sponsored by the National Institute of Arthritis, the American Academy of Orthopedic Surgeons and the Orthopaedic Research Society (White & Gordon 1982). (From Borkan & Cherkin 1996, with permission)

Epidemiology, natural course, and psychologic and psychiatric aspects
- Identification of risk factors that initiate or perpetuate LBP
- Identification of characteristics of patients without LBP
- Evaluation of strength testing and training techniques as preventive measures
- Evaluation of the role of smoking, drinking and other off-the-job activities on LBP

Anatomy and ultrastructure of the lumbosacral spine
- Study of elderly asymptomatic individuals with degenerated discs
- Investigation of regional inflammation
- Use of animal models to study a number of variables, such as intraosseous pressure on nociceptive nerve endings and intraspinal pathways

Biomechanics
- Study of the effect of different variables on the mechanical behavior of the spine
- Development of validated mathematical models of the spine, its components and the whole trunk
- Complete analysis of the spine's material properties

Biochemistry of the supporting structures
- Investigation of the relationships between biochemical structure and mechanical function of components of the spinal unit
- Study whether biochemical breakdown products have the capacity to stimulate nociceptive nerve endings
- Anatomic, ultrastructural, radiographic and biochemical analysis of lumbar discs

Neuromechanisms
- Investigation of nociceptors and nociceptive stimuli in bone, ligaments and other deep tissues of the spinal unit
- Examination of the effects of various chemical substances present in lesions resulting from LBP injuries on the mediation of nociceptors

Development of animal models
- Study of mechanical and biologic variables in chemically or mechanically damaged nerves and ganglia
- Study of the role of endorphins, particularly in the placebo response
- Study of the trunk muscle activity and trigger points

Box 22.6   Research priorities from the first international forum for primary care research on low back pain (LBP) (with the number of votes in brackets). (From Borkan & Cherkin 1996, with permission)

---

1. Can different varieties or subgroups of LBP (including chronic LBP) be indentified and, if they can, what criteria can be used to differentiate among them? (30)
2. What can be done to contain and reverse the epidemic of LBP disability and cost in developed countries? (17)
3. What psychosocial interventions are effective in LBP? (15)
4. What are the most effective ways of changing the way primary care practitioners deal with LBP? (15)
5. What are the 'best' (i.e. most cost-effective, most satisfying, least iatrogenic) strategies for treating LBP? (14)
6. What can be done to improve the quality and value of LBP research? (13)
7. Is there a need for a new paradigm for thinking about LBP? (13)
8. How can we improve self-care strategies and stimulate self-reliance among persons with chronic or recurrent LBP? (11)
9. How do patient and provider beliefs and expectations influence outcomes of care for LBP? (9)
10. Can the development and dissemination of guidelines improve outcomes and reduce costs of care for LBP? (7)
11. What are the best strategies for diagnosis? In particular, what is the reliability, predictive value, and clinical utility of common symptoms and diagnostic tests? Can 'gold standards' be developed? (6)
12. What is the role of patient preferences in treatment outcomes? (6)
13. What are the predictors, determinants and risk factors for chronic disability in LBP patients, including physical, psychosocial, mental health and behavioral factors? Can subgroups at high risk for chronic LBP or therapeutic failure be identified? (5)
14. What are the most pertinent LBP outcome measures for researchers, clinicians and patients, and how can better measurement scales be created and validated? (5)

cont'd p. 418

15. What strategies are effective in educating physicians about various aspects of LBP and reinforcing physician effectiveness in communicating and counseling? (4)
16. What impact do benefit systems (such as workers' compensation or social security disability) have on LBP? (3)
17. How do persons who seek care for LBP differ from those who manage their problem without professional care? (3)
18. What can individuals do to prevent LBP? (3)
19. What are the appropriate relationships between manual therapists (such as chiropractors) and primary care physicians? (3)
20. Should primary care physicians treat LBP in all its presentations or would it make more sense if some segment of these patients was seen instead by back care specialists (e.g. orthopedists, chiropractors, physical therapists)? (3)

This forum felt that much traditional research on back pain has little relevance to primary health care. This list is very different. It does not include any strictly biomedical questions. It shows the very different interests and concerns of patients and providers in primary care, where most back pain is treated. It places back pain in a much broader, clinical and psychosocial context. Borkan & Cherkin (1996) summarized these areas:

- the daily challenges facing patients with back pain and their providers
- providing effective and cost-effective health care for back pain
- more effective methods of routine assessment and management
- changing knowledge and behaviors in patients, providers and society
- radical change in how we view low back pain – a new paradigm.

The forum hoped that this list would help to shift the focus of future research and encourage funding agencies to give priority to these areas.

The CSAG report into health services for back pain in the UK also listed main areas for future research and development:

- diagnostic triage and referral systems
- an integrated service for the management of nonspecific low back pain in primary care
- physical therapy and manipulative therapy
- a dedicated rehabilitation service for patients with nonspecific low back pain who do not recover with routine primary care management and who fail to return to work by about 6 weeks
- audit of health care delivery and outcomes for patients with back pain.

CONCLUSION

I am well aware that this is the bare outline of a future back service. We still have many uncertainties about the best way to provide health care for patients with nonspecific low back pain. The answer will vary with local circumstances and resources and needs. We may now have more questions than answers, but at least we can see some of the issues more clearly. The urgent need is research and development to test these and other ideas in different settings. There is wide scope for pilot schemes and experiment. What is not in any doubt is that we must provide better health care for patients with nonspecific low back pain. The starting point is to recognize the need and a willingness to try to meet that need.

BIBLIOGRAPHY

AHCPR 1994 Clinical Practice Guideline Number 14. Acute low back problems in adults. Agency for Health Care Policy and Research, US Department of Health and Human Services, Rockville, MD
Bombardier C, Esmail R, Nachemson A L 1997 The Cochrane Collaboration back review group. Spine 22: 837–840
Borkan J M, Cherkin D C 1996 An agenda for primary care research on low back pain. Spine 21: 2880–2884
Coulter A, Bradlow J, Martin-Bates C 1991 Outcome of general practitioner referrals to specialist out-patient clinics for back pain. British Journal of General Practice 41: 450–453
Croft P, Papageorgiou A, McNally R 1997 Low back pain. In: Stevens A, Rafferty J (eds) Health care needs assessment, 2nd series. Radcliffe Medical Press, Oxford, ch 3, p 129–182
CSAG 1994 Report on back pain. Clinical Standards Advisory Group. HMSO, London

Davis D A, Thomson M A, Oxman A D et al 1992 Evidence for the effectiveness of CME. A review of 50 randomized controlled trials. Journal of the American Medical Association 268: 1111–1117

Deyo R A, Phillips W R 1996 Low back pain: a primary care challenge. Spine 21: 2826–2832

Deyo R A, Cherkin D, Conrad D, Volinn E 1991 Cost, controversy, crisis; low back pain and the health of the public. Annual Review of Public Health 12: 141–156

Evans R G, Barer M L, Marmor T R (eds) 1994 Why are some people healthy and others not? The determinants of the health of populations. Aldini de Gruyter, New York

Feuerstein M, Beattie P 1995 Biobehavioral factors affecting pain and disability in low back pain. Physical Therapy 745: 267–280

Fordyce W E 1995 Back pain in the workplace: management of disability in non-specific conditions. IASP Press, Seattle

Frank J W, Kerr M S, Brooker A-S et al 1996 Disability resulting from occupational low back pain. Spine 21: 2908–2929

French S (ed) 1992 Physiotherapy: a psychosocial approach. Butterworth Heinemann, Oxford

Korr I M 1974 Andrew Taylor Still memorial lecture: Research and practice – a century later. Journal of the American Osteopathic Association 73: 362–370

Liebenson C 1996 Rehabilitation of the spine. Williams & Wilkins, Baltimore

Little P, Smith L, Cantrell T, Chapman J, Langridge J, Pickering R 1995 General practitioners' management of acute back pain: a survey of reported practice compared with clinical guidelines. British Medical Journal 312: 485–488

Nachemson A 1983 Work for all: for those with low back pain as well. Clinical Orthopaedics and Related Research 179: 77–85

RCGP 1995 The development and implementation of clinical guidelines. Report from General Practice No. 26. Royal College of General Practitioners, London

Robertson J T 1993 The rape of the spine. Surgical Neurology 39: 5–12

Rossignol M, Abenhaim L, Bonvalot Y, Gobielle D, Shrier I 1996 Should the gap be filled between guidelines and actual practice for management of low back pain in primary care? The Quebec experience. Spine 21: 2893–2899

Waddell G 1996 Low back pain: a twentieth century health care enigma. Spine 21: 2820–2825

White A A, Gordon S L (eds) 1982 American Academy of Orthopaedic Surgeons symposium on idiopathic low back pain. Mosby, St Louis

23

Epilogue

We have come a long way from where we started. Or perhaps in a sense we have come full circle. And we still have a long way to go.

Back pain is a 20th century health care disaster
• Human beings have had back pain throughout recorded history
• Back pain has not changed: it is no different, no more severe and no more common than it has always been
• What has changed is how we think about back pain and what we do about it
• We have turned a benign bodily symptom into one of the most common causes of chronic disability in Western society today
• But if we can create that epidemic, we can also reverse it

Back pain is a paradox. Our ability to prevent or treat serious spinal disease is part of the success story of 20th century medicine. Tragically, much more often, chronic disability due to simple backache illustrates the failure of 20th century Western health care. The dilemma is that back pain can be the presenting symptom of many spinal diseases, but most back pain is not due to any serious disease. We get into trouble when we confuse them. The biomedical approach has not solved that problem, and there is strong circumstantial evidence that much low back disability is iatrogenic. The fault lies not in our backs, my friends, but in ourselves and how we treat our patients.

I warned you that some of the issues discussed in this book might challenge your deeply felt professional convictions and practice. Perhaps they have disturbed your professional status quo. I hope they have, and I do not apologize, because we should all be ashamed of what health care has done to back pain. Of course, we can each claim that we have achieved a great deal for individual patients. But you are blind if you cannot see that we have also done a great deal of harm to many patients with simple backache.

If we simply continue our present biomedical approach, which has failed, or just try to do more and bigger and better of the same, this epidemic will continue. That is not acceptable. We need to face up to the real and difficult questions of back pain, and to meet our patients' and society's demands that we do better. Nor can we turn back the clock, or try to return to some mythologic state of low back innocence. But we can learn from our past mistakes.

All health professionals share a common philosophy of caring for sick people. Medicine has an ancient heritage of philosophy and ethics. It is a humanistic philosophy: treating the body and the mind; healer when possible but also comforter during life's sickness. During the past century, as the practice of orthodox medicine has become more mechanistic, osteopathic medicine and chiropractic have developed their own distinct versions of that ancient philosophy. The roots and traditions of physical and occupational therapy lie in helping patients to return to normal activities and work. All health professionals spend much of their day working with patients. Physical therapy, osteopathic medicine and chiropractic are very much hands-on, with direct human contact between therapist and patient. We all, physicians, chiropractors, physical therapists and osteopaths alike, believe that we should treat the whole person. The problem is that these ideals are abstract, and we get little guidance on how to turn them into practical reality in our daily practice. We are also limited by our human nature. As we have devoted more time, training and effort to physical disease, so we have tended to neglect these more human aspects. It is all very well to say that we use science and mechanical treatment within a holistic framework, but it is too easy for that frame-

work to dissolve in the starry mists of idealism. We all agree in principle that we should treat people and not spines, but then in daily practice we get on with the business of mechanics.

The biopsychosocial model (Fig. 23.1) is not a new philosophy. Rather, it is a method, or a set of tools, to apply that ancient philosophy to our daily practice. It allows us to combine the role of healer with the more ancient role of counselor, helping patients to cope with their problem. The patient's role must also change from passive recipient of treatment to more active sharing of responsibility for their own progress.

Some doctors and therapists seem to be uncomfortable with this whole approach. They prefer to stick to nice, simple, mechanical problems that they can understand and deal with. Some actually seem to feel threatened by these new ideas. It is no longer enough to know about anatomy and pathology. The biopsychosocial approach opens a whole new perspective on how people behave and cope with illness. It reveals the limitations of our treatment and of our professional skills. It exposes us to the difficulties and stress of dealing with emotions. We must accept that patients are not neat packages of mechanics or pathology, but suffering human beings. Professional life may be much simpler if we stick to physical treatment of

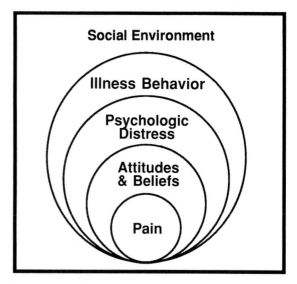

Figure 23.1 The biopsychosocial model.

mechanical problems, but health care demands that we treat human beings.

Some people may argue that I have played down the physical problem of back pain. I would deny that. I have stressed again and again that I believe that back pain starts with a physical problem in the back. Back pain is very real, it causes a great deal of human suffering and disability, and it needs health care. Basic science and biomedical research are the foundation for better understanding and treatment in the future. But they are only half the story. Back pain and disability also involve these equally important psychosocial issues that we ignore at our patients' peril. This book has focused more on these non-biologic issues to try to redress the balance.

- Back pain arises from a physical problem in the back
- The problem is how we react and what we do about it.

I do agree that over the last 10 years the balance of back pain research has perhaps swung too far towards these psychosocial issues, to the neglect of the physical. We need much more and better research into the physical basis of nonspecific low back pain, although I would argue that this should focus more on dysfunction than on anatomic and structural lesions. Of course we need better physical understanding and treatment. Hopefully, the pendulum will swing back over the next 10 years. At the same time, I hope that we will continue to treat patients as well as their backs.

We must also change the health care system

- Clear and accurate diagnostic triage, and appropriate referral
- Most medical specialist services are designed for patients who need investigation and treatment of serious spinal pathology or nerve root problems that fail to resolve. They are inappropriate and may be harmful for patients with simple backache
- Most patients with simple backache should be managed mainly in primary care. We should design that service to meet the needs of these patients
- This requires a fundamental change in professional practice and a shift of resources

We really are talking about a revolution in health care for back pain. Health professionals, patients and society must all adopt a new approach. All health professionals must face radical change in their practice. Patients and society must change their ideas and what they do about back pain. But health professionals cannot escape the final responsibility. We provide the health care. We must also give patients and society a new understanding of low back pain and disability, that alone makes real change possible.

I end this book more optimistic than I began. There are still a lot of dinosaurs and sacred cows to be shot. We still need much research and development. But I believe that we can now glimpse a better way ahead, even if much of the detail is still obscure. The back pain revolution *is* beginning. Clinical management *is* changing. We do now have the first faint hints that the epidemic may have peaked. Back pain is a challenge and an opportunity. The lessons of back pain may even serve as an example and test-bed of a new health care approach for many benign, nonspecific symptoms. That is the challenge and the excitement of back pain at the start of a new millennium.

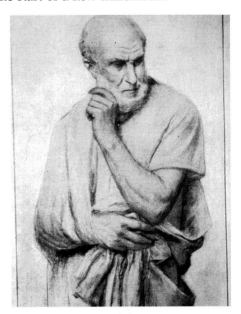

Figure 23.2 Hippocrates. Health care is about helping suffering human beings. The challenge is to combine treatment of their physical disorder with care of the whole person.

Index

Underlined page numbers refer to illustrations and tables.